HOW TO BE YOUR OWN VETERINARIAN
(sometimes)

**A Do-It-Yourself
Guide for the
Horseman**

RUTH B. JAMES, DVM

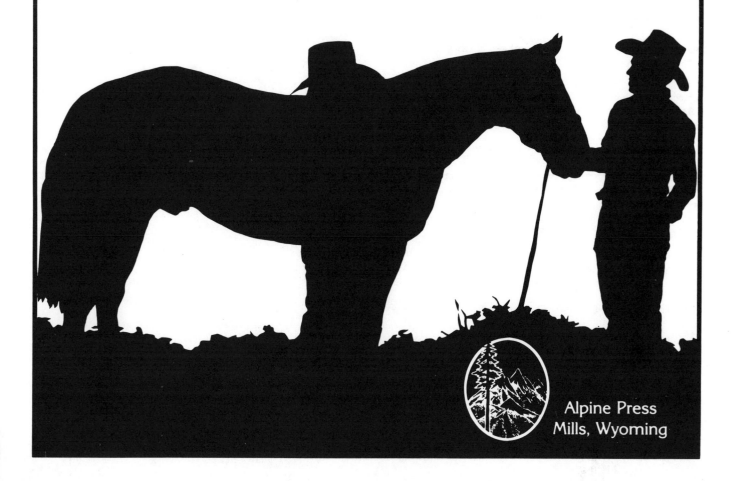

Alpine Press
Mills, Wyoming

Inquiries should be addressed to Alpine Press,
    P.O. Box 1930, Mills, Wyoming, 82644.

Published by Alpine Press
            P.O. Box 1930
            Mills, Wyoming 82644

Final Editing by Ed Barc.
Illustrations by Terry Flanagan.
Cover photo by Ruth B. James, D.V.M.
Back cover photo by Deane Stanton.
Interior photos by Ruth B. James, D.V.M.
Custom photo processing by Norm and Evelyn Grant,
    Grant's Photographic, Tempe, Arizona, 85281
Typeset by Kachina Typesetting, Inc.,
    Tempe, Arizona 85283.
Printed by Cushing-Malloy, Inc.,
    Ann Arbor, Michigan 48107
Printed in the United States of America.

Library of Congress Catalog Number 85-080557
ISBN 0-9615114-0-0

I would like to thank Western Horseman for their kind permission to
reprint portions of the following articles, written by myself, which first
appeared in their pages:

"Back Problems: Causes and Cures," November 1976.
"How to Shoot a Horse," August 1977.
"Longeing and Hot Walkers . . . Possible Dangers," October 1977.
"More Efficient Exercise for Older Horses," April 1978.
"A Horse's Color—It Can Make a Difference," May 1979.
"The Fat Horse," October 1979.
"Choosing the Broodmare," January 1980.
"Getting the Mare Ready for Breeding," February 1980.
"The Nuts and Bolts of Horse Feeding," April 1980.
"Laminitis—Causes, Symptoms, Treatment, Prevention," January 1982.
"Mallenders and Sallenders," May 1982.
"Spavin," June 1982.
"Everything You Wanted To Know About Mare's Milk," February 1984.

To
JOHN MURPHY
Who Died

To
LADY NIGHT SAN
Who Lives

and To
HOWARD
Who Puts Humpty Dumpty Back Together Again

WITH LOVE

He Was O.K. Yesterday, Then Bingo!

"Doc, I called you just as soon as I seen Ol' Buck was sick.
He's been a little poorly but he never missed a lick.

Last winter he got picky and wouldn't eat his grain
So I gave him Doctor Bell's; tied garlic in his mane.

Then several months ago when he started losin' weight
I gave him Copenhagen and a pound of Catfish bait.

He come down with the splatters and all his hair fell out!
So I fed him Larramycin and a couple of smoked trout.

Then last week after ridin' he got stiff as pine!
His navel needed "smokin" so I used some turpentine.

He went plum down on Sunday, His kidneys, so I guessed.
I doctored up his water and tied him facin' West.

Last night I got to thinkin'. You were here two years ago.
You gave him some concoction for a cough and runny
nose.

I wondered if your treatment, which then improved his luck,
Had later turned against him and poisoned my Ol' Buck?"

Anon.

Taken, with slight adaptation, from
   the Arizona Livestock Board Newsletter

DISCLAIMER

To help insure the reader's understanding of some of the medical descriptions and techniques in **How to Be Your Own Veterinarian (Sometimes)**, brand names have occasionally been used as examples of particular medications or equipment. However, the use of a particular trademark or brand name is not intended to imply an endorsement of that particular product, or to suggest that similar products offered by others under different names may in any way be inferior. The author has not received any compensation from any of the cited companies which would result in a conflict of interest or bias in the use of any particular product. Nothing contained in this book is to be construed as a suggestion to violate any trademark laws.

Although every effort has been made to present scientifically accurate and up-to-date information based on the best and most reliable sources available, it should be understood that the results of medical treatments depend upon many factors, including proper diagnosis, which are not under the control of the author or the publishers of this book. Therefore, neither Alpine Press nor the author assumes responsibility for and make no warranty with respect to results that may be obtained from the procedures herein. Neither Alpine Press nor Dr. Ruth James shall be liable to any person for damage resulting from reliance on any information contained in **How to Be Your Own Veterinarian (Sometimes)** whether with respect to diagnosis, drug dosages, treatment procedures, or by reason of any misstatement or inadvertent error contained herein.

Also, it should be noted that neither the author nor Alpine Press manufactures, packages, ships, labels, or sells any of the drugs or equipment mentioned in this book. Accordingly, neither can be held responsible for results that may be obtained with products manufactured by others.

The reader is encouraged to carefully read and follow the label directions provided by the manufacturer for any product which may be used. If there is a conflict between instructions contained in the book and those provided by the manufacturer, those provided by the manufacturer should be followed.

ACKNOWLEDGMENTS

In the long process of writing this book, many people have helped me. I would like to thank those who so generously loaned materials which I needed (and put up with their not being returned, it seemed, forever). Among these are Bob Ashcraft, Dr. Alan Miller, Dr. Jim Shelly, Dave Hathcock, Dr. Jim Morrison, and Mel Bramley. Thanks are also due Kevin Proctor, who provided the Newscript program for the TRS-80, Model III computer upon which the book was written; without the program and the machine, I'd either still be typing, or have given up long ago! Thanks also to the wonderful ladies at Arizona Veterinary Supply Company who so cheerfully checked my information on drug names and manufacturers.

Howard Walworth of Walworth Quarter Horses graciously loaned his horses, his facilities, and his assistants for endless hours of photography, for which I am extremely grateful. Thanks are also due to those who worked so long and hard on the photos with me—Sue Achenbach, Lorraine Morris, and Mary Johnson, as well as to the models, Pat Scully, Chris Breedt (a special young man from Rhodesia); also to John and Katharine Deegan who posed for the cover photo. I am grateful to Ed Connelley for his patience while working on photos, and to Al Coury, Jr., who provided the location for several photo sessions.

My thanks to those who took the time and effort to read the manuscript for me: Dr. Ray Allen, Jodi Enochs, Janice James, and Dr. Harvel Alishouse.

I am thankful for the very special friends who encouraged me when it seemed that I would never finish, and who believed in the worth of the project when I was beset by doubts. Among these are Doug and Sue Achenbach, J. Brian Freeman, Jerry Buk, Rick NeVille, Howard Walworth, Ray Deskins, John Vitela, Phill Morrison, and Deane Stanton. I also owe a debt of gratitude to all the teachers who have helped to shape my thinking, and to the clients and animals who have taught me so much. Anyone who has helped me and not been mentioned herein has been omitted because of my fallible memory, not because of any desire to do so.

CONTENTS

Introduction

1. Helping Your Veterinarian to Help You   1
2. Knowing Your Horse: The Normal Animal   4
3. Horse Management   17
4. Feeding the Horse   26
5. Reproduction and Foaling   56
6. Soundness   90
7. Lameness   110
8. Back Problems   159
9. Horse Restraint and Safety   163
10. Treatment Methods   180
11. Medications   198
12. Bandages and Bandaging   211
13. Injuries and Their Treatment   217
14. Respiratory Problems   239
15. The Digestive System   251
16. Eye Problems   271
17. Skin Problems   276
18. Internal Parasites   297
19. Hernias and Castrations   308
20. Toxins and Poisonous Plants   314
21. Miscellaneous Conditions   327
     References and Notes   343
     Recommended Reading   345

INTRODUCTION

When I was a child, the arrival of our veterinarian was greeted with mixed emotions. On one hand, there was happiness at seeing Dr. Lynn Leadbetter, a special person whose kind manner and dry sense of humor never failed to impress me; on the other hand, there was the knowledge that the charge for his visit would strain our already marginal budget. I know that he often charged my family less than his normal fees because he knew we could scarcely afford them; his kindness has never been forgotten.

About two years ago, I finally had to admit that I was a financial failure as a veterinarian. I could not bring myself to charge what my services were realistically worth. I was not charging enough to make a living wage because I felt so much sympathy for those whose animals were ill or injured. This was brought home to me after I spent a large part of one day suturing two enormous cuts on the front legs of a colt who had fallen through a cattle guard, and found myself presenting a bill for some $74! I could not bring myself to make money from my clients' and friends' misfortunes.

As a practicing veterinarian, I saw the unnecessary calls because nothing was really wrong with the horse. I saw other horses who were neglected until their injuries took months instead of weeks to heal. I saw horses who were left untreated until a minor colic became a life-threatening twisted intestine which necessitated surgery.

I decided to write this book to help the horse owner treat simple problems himself, to call the veterinarian sooner when it is necessary, and to know the difference between the two. Not incidentally, I hope to be able to save the horse owner some money with this knowledge. If I can save each person who buys this book just one veterinary call, it will have paid for itself. If I can also prevent the heartache of losing the use (or even the life) of the horse that you love, and save that animal some pain and suffering, then the two years that I have devoted to writing it will have been well spent.

When you get this book, please read it at least lightly from cover to cover. In doing this you will come to know my thinking on treatment of injuries and illnesses, and also which problems are considered minor or which need veterinary help immediately. This first reading will give you an idea of how to begin and where to look for specific information when your horse is ill or injured.

I have tried to emphasize preventive measures which may be taken to keep many problems from occurring so that you may never need to treat them. Many illnesses, such as founder, are in large part preventable, but may be nearly incurable or permanently damaging once they have occurred. Preventive medicine is the cheapest form of veterinary care—and the most effective in the long run!

Chapter 1

HELPING YOUR
VETERINARIAN TO HELP YOU

The purpose of this book is to help you to work with your veterinarian; to help you determine when you need him; and to help him to help you. If you follow some of the suggestions, you should be seeing less of him (or, of course, her). This makes it doubly important that you have a good working relationship with him when you really do need him. A little effort will result in better health for your horses and a lower veterinary bill.

Your first contact with a veterinarian can make a great difference in your future relationship with him, and can save misunderstandings and bad feelings. If at all possible, choose a veterinarian who works with horses and enjoys doing so. If a practitioner who does only equine work is available in your area, he may be your best choice. The next best selection is a veterinarian who works mainly with large animals, but enjoys working with horses. In some areas, the only veterinarians available have specialized in cattle or hogs and will work on horses only with reluctance. This is usually due either to a personal dislike of horses or to a fear of them. Working with one of these practitioners may be less than satisfactory; on the other hand, because of their disinclination toward horses, they may be more willing than others to help you do your own work.

Find out if the veterinarian will come to your premises, or whether the animal must be hauled to his clinic. This will depend on both his facilities and yours, and whether his practice is mainly based in a clinic, or mostly mobile. In some cases, you can save a substantial amount of money by taking the animal to him. On the other hand, it may be essential with some injuries or illnesses that he be able to come to your place.

If you have poor facilities which are exposed to bad weather and not even a stout post to anchor a spoiled, recalcitrant horse, don't be surprised if the veterinarian is reluctant to come when you need him and can't get the horse to his clinic. Good facilities are absolutely essential for your safety, the veterinarian's safety, and that of the horse.

If you are having routine work done, such as tube worming, try to call several days in advance to make an appointment. This will allow the veterinarian to schedule your call along with others in the same neighborhood. Some veterinarians split the mileage charges among several owners; this can result in dollars saved, especially if you live some distance from his office.

During your first conversation with the veterinarian or his staff, don't be shy about asking how much he charges for his services. What are the mileage charges, what is the call charge (the fee for his visit to your premises), how much does he charge if you bring the animal to the clinic, and how much extra is charged for night, weekend, or emergency calls? This information can help you determine whether to have the veterinarian come out or to haul the animal to him, and may help you to decide whether to call Sunday night or wait until Monday morning. Additional fees will, of course, be charged for medication or treatment, laboratory work, and other services beyond the base fees. If money is a problem, it may be well to inquire as to the cost of treatment after he has given you a diagnosis and before he begins medication. He may be able to choose the least expensive of several alternative treatments and save you some money in that way.

During this first consultation, ask how he likes to be paid. Does he prefer to be paid at the time the animal is treated, or does he provide charge accounts with later billing? Is there a discount for cash payment? None of us likes to have to chase our money, as we prefer to be veterinarians instead of collection agents. Keeping your bill paid will help to insure a rapid response when you have an emergency in the middle of the night. If you find that you are unable to pay your veterinarian's bill, don't just ignore it—call him and talk about it. Tell him how much you are able to pay and when—and then stick to the schedule you have set for yourself. Most of us try to be understanding when our clients have unexpected emergencies and are unable to pay their bills. And, most of us do a certain amount of pure charity work. None of us likes to be "beaten out of our money," and have little sympathy with people who try to do so.

Understand your veterinarian's needs. Find out if he prefers to work in the barn or out in the open (sometimes weather may leave little choice in the matter). Will he need your help or will he bring his own assistant? For some surgery, he may need several helpers to safely restrain the horse so the animal does not hurt himself or those around him. If he requests help, be sure to have it there. If the veterinarian does not have water in his vehicle, he would appreciate a clean bucket of warm water and some paper towels from your house.

The veterinarian is fitting your animal or animals into the rest of his time schedule. Words that we all hate to hear are "While you're here, doc . . .". If you need other animals treated, dogs vaccinated, etc., be sure to mention these items when you make the initial appointment so that your veterinarian can allow time for them in his schedule. Keep a list of work that you need done "when the vet comes" so that you can let him know these needs in advance.

It helps to be straightforward when talking with your veterinarian. Don't worry that you don't know the technical terms for everything—we're used to being addressed in plain English (and sometimes worse). If the vet uses terms that you don't understand, don't be embarrassed to ask for an explanation. This is more likely to be an oversight on his part than an attempt to overwhelm you. The only stupid question is the one that is left unasked.

If you need to discuss a problem which embarrasses you, speak with the receptionist or another person on the veterinarian's staff if it is easier for you. Many people are embarrassed to discuss problems involving the animal's reproductive tract. There is no need to be bothered by this, but rest assured that you are not the only client who has this problem.

Give the veterinarian as much factual information as you can when first discussing the illness. You are better acquainted with your individual animal than your veterinarian. It will be your everyday observations that determine that there is a problem. This is a vital part of the preliminary diagnosis. Don't play it down. On the other hand, don't jump to conclusions. Many veterinarians are called to treat "colics" that turn out to be completely different ailments. It is often better to tell the vet what your animal is DOING, not what you think the problem is. As he becomes more familiar with you and your animals, he will know whether or not you know what you are talking about, and how astute you are in dealing with your animals and their problems. He will then have a better basis to know what questions he needs to ask you and how to sort out the information that you give him. This preliminary information may not seem important to you, but let your vet decide whether it is or not. What may seem minor to you may become meaningful later after further examination and observation, laboratory tests, and watching the course of the disease.

Don't be afraid to give your impressions of change: the animal is acting better or worse, feeling stronger, or remaining the same. This is especially important in treating diseases which take some time to heal. If a problem is not responding to one medication, it may be necessary to change to another. As the person seeing the animal several times a day and administering his medication, you are the one who is best able to make these determinations. Don't be afraid to call the vet and ask him if the animal should be getting well faster or changing more rapidly. He can then either give you information over the phone, or decide that he needs to re-examine the animal in person.

Wait to give the animal's detailed medical history until the veterinarian arrives. Most of us would rather have it then, while we are looking at the animal, than over the phone. We may have forgotten it by the time we arrive at the farm and you will have to repeat it anyway. Give any information which is pertinent to the problem at hand. For instance, while the vet is examining a mare with reproductive problems, it helps to be able to tell him her past breeding and foaling history, heat dates, and any treatments which have been administered in past years.

Accurate health records will help you to be able to give this information. Keeping your records in order also allows you to do routine work on time, thus keeping your horse from getting diseases or health problems, all of which will help to save you money in the long run.

Cooperate with the vet in any way you can. If you know about when the vet is going to arrive, he will appreciate having the horse caught, haltered with a stout halter and good lead rope, and tied. We do not appreciate having to hold roundups for wild horses (many vets charge for same). Offer to hold the animal while he examines it; having someone familiar at hand may help to calm the horse.

Have adequate lighting. If no light is available, a drop cord, lantern, or vehicle lights would be greatly appreciated. Having a couple of extra flashlights available at night is helpful. Veterinarians appreciate clients who assign a child with a flashlight to light their way back to the truck for extra equipment or medication.

A clean place to work is also helpful. If the vet has to work on an animal in a dirty stall, provide canvas, carpet, or feed sacks for him to stand or kneel on. This is especially important when the animal is lying down or must be anesthetized (as with a severe cut or a foaling problem). This may even make the call less expensive!

Warn the veterinarian if your animal is difficult to treat. However, it's more diplomatic to say "He can sometimes be a problem to treat," than "My horse hates vets!" Some of this dislike may be due to the animal's previous experience. Some of it is also probably because many horses are sensitive to the smells of other animals or to medication odors which vets carry on their hands, clothing, and boots (even with best of sanitation procedures).

Make sure you understand the veterinarian's instructions regarding treatment and aftercare of your animal, preferably BEFORE he leaves the farm! If you are not sure, don't hesitate to ask him to repeat them, or to jot them down on paper for you. Most of us would rather go over instructions an extra time than to have to recall every word that we said when you call back two days later. If you don't know how to do the treatments or techniques that he has prescribed, ask him to give you a demonstration.

Carry out treatments as instructed, even if it means getting up in the middle of the night. Correct timing can be important, especially when certain antibiotics are given. Keep a sheet of paper in the barn and make notes if the vet has asked you to record the animal's temperature, feed consumption, bowel movements, or other information. Also jot down any questions which you would like to ask the next time you call the vet. This will help to make the call brief and more efficient. If your veterinarian has asked you to call him with more information on the animal, or with a progress report, find out what number you should use, and if it is all right to call after hours; some veterinarians actually prefer to receive these calls in the evening. I like to take them late at night when I have time to sit still and think; other vets would rather get them first thing in the morning so they can include the animal in the day's calls if a recheck is necessary. It's often worthwhile to call even if you haven't been asked, to tell him that the animal has recovered; vets like to hear good news, too.

If you call a veterinarian to treat an animal which has been examined or treated by another vet, be sure to give him the details of the first treatment. Some medications can mask symptoms or cause others to develop. If the previous veterinarian has made a diagnosis which is in error (which we can all do), it will save time for the veterinarian if you tell him as much as you can about what was said and what treatment was given. Discontinue any medication which was given to you by the first veterinarian; failure to do so may result in a conflict between the old and new medication. In some cases, this may confuse the diagnosis by complicating signs of the disease, while in others it may actually be dangerous.

Let your veterinarian know that you have books on horse health, and which ones you read and use. Some veterinary and animal care books are hopelessly outdated and should be consigned to the history shelves. Ask if he can recommend any specific books which he recommends for you to own or borrow and read.

Find out how he would like you to handle emergencies until he arrives. Even if you call late at night, he may be at another emergency and not to be able to get to you for a while. How does he like to have wire cuts or other injuries treated until he can get there? Some veterinarians have information sheets for emergencies, while others teach short courses for their clients. Almost all will take some time to discuss their preferences if they know you are interested. It is a good idea to have the veterinarian out to your place at least once a year for tube worming and tooth care. If nothing else, this will help to keep you in his mind. Also, it helps to assure that he remembers your existence favorably when you have a problem in the middle of the night; not to mention that he'll know how to find your place. It also gives you a chance to go over any health problems or questions that you might have. The object of this book is to help you to work WITH your veterinarian, not make him feel defensive about his profession.

Remember that your veterinarian may not be just one person working alone. His staff members are also available to help you with your problems, and can help you communicate with him.

Working with your veterinarian to assure your animal's health can be a very rewarding experience. It can also save you a great deal of time and money.

Chapter 2

KNOWING YOUR HORSE: THE NORMAL ANIMAL

Behavior
  Posture
  Movement
Voice
Appetite
Digestive System
Skin and Coat
Mucous Membranes
Abdomen
Feces
Urine
Vaginal Discharge
Brain and Central Nervous System
Other Indicators of Animal Health
  Temperature
  Pulse
  The Stethoscope
  Normal Heart Rate
  Respiration Rate
  Gut Sounds
Blood
  Anemia

Being your own veterinarian begins with knowing your own animal, and knowing what is normal for that individual. You must know what is normal before you can know what is abnormal. Observe the animal from day to day and note changes that occur. It is extremely valuable to know what is "normal" for horses in general.

For example, veterinarians are occasionally called out to examine a mysterious swelling on a horse's belly, about 4 inches behind the cinch area and about eight inches from the midline of the animal's belly. Owners look under the horse and see this bump—really noticing it for the first time—and call their veterinarian in a panic to find out what has happened to their horse. If they had taken a moment to look, they would have found that the animal has a lump just like that on the other side because it is a perfectly normal muscle! So, before you call your veter-inarian about a mysterious swelling, compare. Does your animal have something like that on the other side? And does your other horse or your neighbor's horse have one?

Comparison extends to judging the animal's attitude (its normal actions, reactions, and performance). Is he lying down more than normal? Is he more docile than normal—or more upset? Is he performing up to par? These criteria are important for judging the animal's physical condition, as well as his health. It is also important to know the names of various parts of the horse so that you can tell your veterinarian where a problem is and to be able to understand his explanations to you.

BEHAVIOR

Behavior is another area to observe. It is based on mental attitude (disposition or temperament). Is a normal-ly calm animal suddenly grumpy and pushy, chewing on and kicking the other animals? Mares in heat often exhibit these symptoms when there is no stallion around to show you that they are in heat. Observing these actions should make you suspicious of them. One good example of a behavioral clue is a mare who would cow-kick when she was cinched up—but only when she was in heat. Other mares, though, may not show any signs of heat unless they are tested with a stallion or a gelding who acts like a stallion. Behavior varies from animal to animal and from breed to breed. What would be outrageous behavior from most Quarter Horses might be considered normal for a Thoroughbred or Saddlebred.

Determine as much as possible what behavioral changes in your horse are caused by stress and environ-mental changes. How does the animal react to storms? Does he trailer well, or does he quit eating and drinking for three days and get gaunt until he finally settles down to a routine when you haul him? Does he do better with a companion or without?

POSTURE

Your observation of the animal's posture may be the first clue that something serious is wrong. Sick animals often assume unusual positions, stances, or attitudes. They may be restless, as contrasted with a healthy animal who often stands or lies quietly. Abnormal postures do not always indicate a disease. However, if they are accompanied by other signs, they may indicate the location and seriousness of the illness.

A horse with colic, for example, may stretch, much like a dog getting up in the morning. One client had a mare who usually stretched every morning, about the time she was fed. She would put her front feet forward, and pull her rump back until her belly nearly touched the ground. The first time he saw her do that, he carefully watched her for signs of colic. There were no other indications of abdominal problems. Continued observation showed that this unusual stretch was a normal ritual for this mare.

Variations in posture may not indicate a specific disease. A horse who shifts his weight continuously from one leg to another usually has pain somewhere in one of his legs. It may come from a muscle, joint, or tendon.

If he completely refuses to bear weight on the leg, this is a more serious posture. It tells you that something more severe is wrong with the leg, but not necessarily WHAT is wrong. The problem may be in the foot, knee or hock, or as high as the shoulder or hip. It may be an indication of anything from a severe stone bruise to a fractured bone.

Extreme changes to the animal's normal posture often occur with severe disease problems. One example of this is a horse with acute founder or grain overload. The animal will often display a peculiar stance, along with a reluctance to move, or even to allow one foot to be lifted.

Tetanus (lockjaw) is another example of another abnormal posture. The animal may become so stiff and tight with the muscle spasms which accompany the disease that his front legs stick forward and his rear legs push out backward, making the animal resemble a sawhorse. His head will be pulled up and back, his tail may be rigidly extended, and his ears will be stiffly upright.

MOVEMENT

Movement is closely related to posture. Abnormal movements are often the first sign of injury or disease

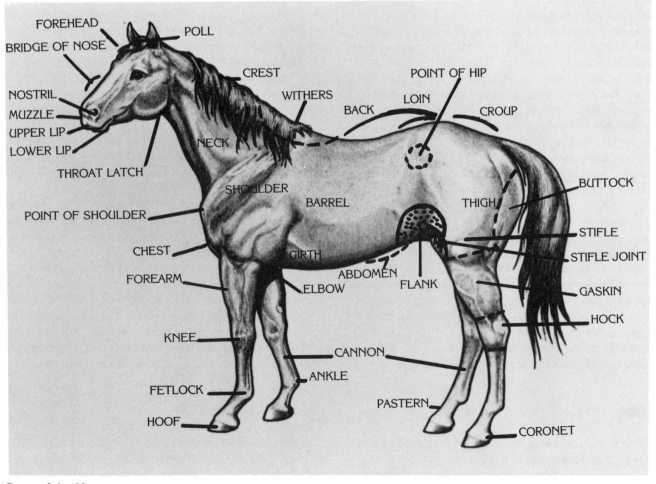

Parts of the Horse

processes. They can signify that the animal is annoyed or uncomfortable. A barrel or cutting horse who is spurred may react immediately with an angry switch or crank of his tail. A horse with his ears laid back flat against his head is signalling to his owner or another horse that something is going on that he doesn't like. This is a good time to find out what is bothering him before you become the recipient of a flying hoof or a nip from his teeth.

Movements such as pawing, shaking the head, yawning, or scratching may indicate a serious problem, or may signify only that the animal is irritated or annoyed. It is up to you to compare these movements with the animal's normal actions and decide which is which.

The sequence of movement of the legs is called the gait. These movements can be compared to previous motions of the same animal, or to similar movements of other animals. The term "way of going" is often used to express the combination of movements which make up the gait. Stumbling, clipping, interfering, and forging are just a few words used to describe abnormalities in the gait or way of going. One of the first signs of lameness may be a change in the animal's way of going.

Again, you must know what is normal for your horse. One of my clients owned a lovely 28-year old cutting horse gelding—a really great animal and superb teacher. The animal had been through much wear and tear in his lifetime, and moved very stiffly. This was his normal, everyday gait. However, just put him in front of a cow and his movement totally changed. He forgot all the pain and moved! For this horse to be stiff and sore at a walk was perfectly normal; for him to have been stiff when in front of a cow would have been abnormal.

A stiff gait may also be social in nature, as when a horse approaches another horse whom he does not know. He often struts the last few steps to the other animal on "tiptoes," snorting and sniffing, with his neck arched.

What is a normal gait or way of going for one breed is often completely abnormal for another. Quarter Horses, for example, generally have a definite walk, trot, and lope, with the legs moving almost entirely back and forth, like hinges. Easy-gaited horses (such as Missouri Foxtrotters, Tennessee Walkers, and the Paso breeds) may have an entirely different way of going. Many of these individuals look like eggbeaters coming toward you when you are used to looking at walking-trotting horses. Yet these movements are normal to these breeds. If your Quarter Horse suddenly starts paddling like a Paso, it's time to seriously question what is wrong with him.

VOICE

The horse's voice is a means of communication, both with other horses and with humans. Stallions tend to have a shrill whinny which can be heard for quite some distance, while mares and geldings neigh more softly. A soft nicker can be a way of saying "hi," while a louder nicker often means "feed me!" Snorts may be used to signal fear or alarm, or may mean excitement or pleasure depending on the circumstances. Know your horse's voice and what it means. This is especially useful if you have the animal stabled near your house. Many horse owners sleep through normal horse sounds, but learn to distinguish the noises which mean the neighbor's horses have escaped and come into the yard.

APPETITE

How well your animal is eating is one of the best indicators of his overall health. When you are feeding the same carefully measured amount of feed every day, it is easy to tell when your animal is not eating and may have a problem. Don't panic if a horse eats lightly at one meal, but look closely for a cause if a hearty eater suddenly eats less for several consecutive meals. Check to see if someone else is feeding the horse, or overfeeding him at other meals. If he leaves food, is he not eating hay, grain, or both? Are there any signs of illness?

The animal's activity also has a bearing on his appetite. Moderate exercise may make the horse ravenous, while overwork may leave him "too tired to eat." Loss of appetite is also seen with colic or other digestive problems, as well as with fever and severe pain. A depraved appetite, in which the animal may chew on bones, paint, or other peculiar feedstuffs, may be seen with some mineral deficiencies, as well as with some mental disorders. Or, it may merely be due to boredom. If the animal does not eat as well as you feel he should and does not appear to be ill, the mouth and teeth should be checked to see if there are any problems. The feed should be inspected to see that it is not moldy, soured, or contaminated by foreign materials.

An evaluation of the animal's appetite should also include monitoring his thirst. With some illnesses, the horse may stop eating, but continue drinking. Animals drink more water than normal with fever, diabetes mellitus, and some digestive system and kidney problems. If your horse is sick and you have an automatic waterer, it is a good idea to shut it off so you can monitor the intake. Give the animal water from a bucket or other container, firmly anchored so that the horse cannot dump it over or otherwise spill it. In this way, you can tell IF the animal is drinking, and how much water he is consuming.

DIGESTIVE SYSTEM

After you have evaluated the animal's appetite, go on to check the digestive system. The mouth should be examined (see teeth section for further examination of the normal mouth). Check to see that the teeth are normal and that there are no sores, ulcers, or foreign bodies present on the tongue or gums. Saliva may drip from the mouth with any of these conditions or when the animal has a hay cube or other foreign object lodged in the mouth. This may also occur with the administration of certain drugs or when the animal is unable to swallow. A dry mouth may be seen with fever and some medications (see Mucous Membranes).

SKIN AND COAT

The skin is a good indicator of the animal's health and of the level of care that he is receiving. It should be clean and healthy, free of dirt and parasites. A certain amount of scurf ("dandruff") is normal in range horses and those not groomed regularly to remove this loose material. Animals who are fed a high level of oil will have very shiny hair. Those kept in sandy pastures or bedded on sand often work enough of it into their coats to dull them, as well as drying them so that the ends of the hairs stick out slightly, giving the animal a rough appearance.

Compare your horse to others in the same pasture or kept under the same conditions. Exposure to sun often dries the animal's coat enough to make it look rough, as well as less shiny than others. For this reason, show horses are often allowed to graze outside only at night, or are kept covered with sheets to keep the sun off them. The long coats seen in the northern states and in high mountain areas in winter often make horses look like "wooly bears." A normal winter coat should look healthy, even though it is long and furry. A well-fed animal will often have a shine even on his winter coat.

Skin abnormalities may include missing patches of hair, scrapes or bites, sores, or abnormalities in the sweating pattern. Contagious diseases such as mange, ringworm, and lice are often noticed to involve more than one animal. Warts or tumors may be found, and should be examined closely to determine whether they need to be removed or just observed.

MUCOUS MEMBRANES

These are the membranes which line the body openings: the nostrils, mouth, eyelids, anus, prepuce, and vagina. The membranes of the eyelids (also called conjunctivae) and the membranes of the mouth are a good location to evaluate the animal's overall health. This is usually called "checking the animal's color."

A bright red conjunctival sac may merely mean that the horse's eyes have been irritated by dust or are infected. However, if the membranes in the animal's mouth are the same color, this may indicate a serious problem affecting the whole body. If the horse has white skin around his eyes, he may be prone to irritation of the conjunctivae by sun; he may have red eyes much of the time, especially in the summer. This is another example of needing to know what is normal for your individual horse. An animal who is short of red blood cells (suffering from anemia) or who has suffered blood loss may have very pale mucous membranes.

A dark red (purplish or dark blue) color is called cyanosis, and indicates a lack of oxygen in the blood; it is seen with some heart problems and a few poisonings. A yellow coloration is called jaundice or icterus. It usually indicates a liver problem. With some diseases, small hemorrhages, or spots of blood may be seen under the membranes. These may be as small as the head of a pin, or may be large, irregular blotches. Any of these symptoms may indicate a serious illness, and should be checked by your veterinarian.

Dry membranes may indicate a fever, or may be caused by the administration of certain drugs, such as those given to control the symptoms of heaves. Also note any peculiar odors in the mouth. An infected tooth, for example, may cause a foul, rotten odor.

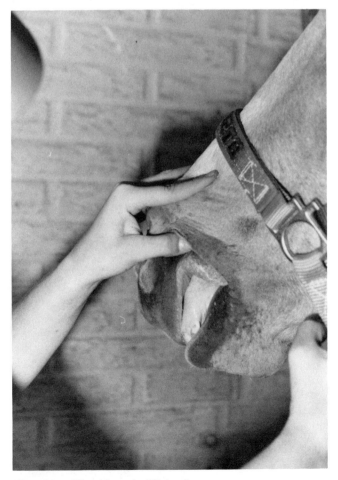

Checking The Horse's "Color."

ABDOMEN

The size and shape of the animal's abdomen depends on a number of factors, including the breed, sex, age, and conformation of the animal. It varies with what the animal has been fed and how he is used. A sagging, enlarged abdomen may be due to an abdominal tumor or an accumulation of fluid in the abdominal cavity. More commonly, however, it indicates that a mare is pregnant, or that the horse has been kept on a bulky diet, such as hay or pasture with little or no grain, for some time. It may also show that the animal has had little exercise to help keep the muscles toned up and in shape. The abdomen may suddenly increase in size with a gaseous colic.

Reducing the size of an horse's abdomen to improve its appearance is often simply a matter of feeding more grain and less hay or roughage. If you can also exercise the animal, the program will progress much more rapidly, and the animal's overall appearance will be better, because of the increased muscle tone.

A thin abdomen may be due to a disease of the digestive tract or to fever. Starvation or long-term marginal nutrition may leave the horse looking thin and hollow. A "tucked-up" abdomen may also result when diarrhea causes emptying of the digestive tract.

FECES

Feces is the technical name for the waste products of the intestinal tract, also known as manure, dung, stools, or bowel movements. The animal's manure often gives important clues to what is going on in his digestive tract. It is normally yellowish to green to brown, depending on the type of feed. A normal adult horse will pass as much as 30 to 40 lb. of manure per day, in eight or 10 separate bowel movements.

Normal horse droppings should be fairly well formed, but soft enough to flatten slightly when they hit the ground. Hard droppings may indicate a lack of water, lack of exercise, or dry or indigestible food. Overly soft droppings may result from much hard work or excessive fatigue. They may also be due to too much fresh grass or alfalfa, too much bran, or problems with the digestive tract.

Feeding too much concentrated grain and too little roughage often causes feces which are covered with slime or mucus; these may also have a very unpleasant odor. A large amount of unchewed grain may indicate that the animal has tooth problems or is eating too fast; however, a certain amount of unchewed kernels are normal in horses fed whole oats or corn.

Keeping an eye on your horse's manure can help you to adjust his feed to what is best for him, or to change to a feed which he can more efficiently utilize. Horses who are prone to colic should be given enough bran to keep the feces slightly loose—so that they form into a soft pile. They should not be so loose as to be considered diarrheic. Occasionally worms, especially ascarids and bots, may be seen in the manure.

Diarrhea is not common in horses, and can be a symptom of a severe problem when it does occur. Diarrhea should be carefully noted for color: yellow, white, or black. Is there blood or mucus present?

A diarrhea is often seen in the foal when the mare comes into her foal heat. Foals with this diarrhea are normal in all other respects; they eat and play normally and look bright and healthy. Any other signs of illness in a horse with diarrhea, such as loss of appetite, colic, or lethargy, are indications to call your veterinarian immediately. By the same token, extremely dry feces, or lack of feces, indicate that you should be observing the animal closely for other signs of illness. They may also occur if the animal does not have enough water.

URINE

Normal horse urine is clear to whitish to yellow or reddish-yellow. It may be transparent or cloudy. The cloudiness is caused by the presence of crystals in the urine and is usually normal. Horse urine may be the consistency of water, or it may be so thick and filled with mucus that it is actually stringy. Either is normal, depending on the individual. There should not be any lumps or clots in the urine. A dark red or brown color occurs when myoglobin is passed in the urine because of the breakdown of muscle tissue. Fresh red blood may occur with stones in the kidney or bladder. Either of these should alert you to call your veterinarian immediately.

VAGINAL DISCHARGE

Mares normally have a vaginal discharge during their heat (estrus) cycle. It may be straw-colored to white, and may stain the hind legs, matting the hair with the fluid. Dried mineral crystals may leave white, salty-looking crusts on the skin. The discharge may be slightly pinkish, but should not be bloody.

Mares with chronic vaginal infections may drain continuously. A thick greenish-yellow pus may run down the hind legs, causing the hair to slough and leaving large bald spots down the inside of the hind legs. Do not buy a mare with this problem if you want a sound broodmare. Even if you clear up the infection, the mare may have suffered enough damage to the lining of the uterus that she will never become pregnant or carry a foal to term.

After a mare has foaled, she will drain fragments of membranes and fluid for a week to ten days. This discharge is usually reddish or brownish in color. It should not have an unpleasant smell. If it has a fetid odor, have the animal checked by your veterinarian, as there may be an infection of the uterus which will need antibiotic treatment.

BRAIN AND CENTRAL NERVOUS SYSTEM

Since we cannot examine the brain directly, we have to rely on external signs to tell us what is going on inside the animal's head and spinal column. Brain problems may be first seen by attitude and mental changes—the animal becomes dopey or sleepy, or may instead be nervous, upset, and excited. Problems in some areas of the brain or spinal cord may be shown by a staggering or uncoordinated gait.

Nervous signs may be seen from damage caused in the brain by several poisonous plants. The "locoed" horse who has permanent brain damage from eating too much locoweed is a good example of this. Another example is the irreversible destruction of brain cells caused by yellow star thistle or Russian knapweed.

Paralysis of a single limb or one group of muscles (such as sweeny) is caused by injury to a motor center in the brain or, more commonly, to a nerve leading to the involved area. Paralysis of the rear half of the body may result from injury to the spinal cord. This may be due to pressure from blood oozing from a broken blood vessel inside the spinal column or from a tumor. It may also be due to a severed or severely compressed spinal cord, which frequently occurs with fractures of the spinal column.

Paralysis of the entire body may be caused by severe damage to the brain. Or, it may be due to physical or nutritional exhaustion, where the animal is too weak and too ill to rise. It often occurs shortly before coma and death.

Coma is the term used when the animal loses consciousness. It may be caused by exhaustion of the body's resources by various disease processes, or by certain poisonous plants or other toxins. It is frequently the last stage before the animal dies.

OTHER INDICATORS OF ANIMAL HEALTH

Your horse's temperature, pulse, and respiration are important monitors of his general health. Use them in addition to examining his overall attitude, behavior, and movement to determine whether you have a problem, and if so, how serious it is. Always check the animal's temperature, pulse, and respiration before you examine him further or exercise him. If you see any of these readings elevated from the normal, do not immediately assume that the animal is ill, but correlate it with other observations on the animal's condition and activity.

TEMPERATURE

This is one of the best indicators of animal health. Use a rectal thermometer made especially for large animals. These thermometers are large and stubby, and quite thick so that they are strong and less likely to break. If you get one with a ring in the end, it can be equipped with a small alligator clip from an automotive store and a short (10 to 12 inch (25 to 30 cm.)) length of heavy nylon thread or fishing line. This can then be clipped onto the tail to help prevent breakage if the horse swishes his tail and pulls the thermometer from the rectum. Thermometers should be stored in a cool place; leaving one on the dashboard of a vehicle in summer usually ruins it.

Begin by shaking down the thermometer. The easiest way to do this is to hold it by the ring end between two fingers and the thumb. Shake it downward with a short snapping motion of the wrist. This often has to be repeated 10 or 15 times to get the mercury toward the bulb end. It should be shaken down to about 95 degrees. How low you shake it is not critical unless the animal's temperature is well below normal (hypothermic). If this is the problem, shake it all the way to the bottom and see if it

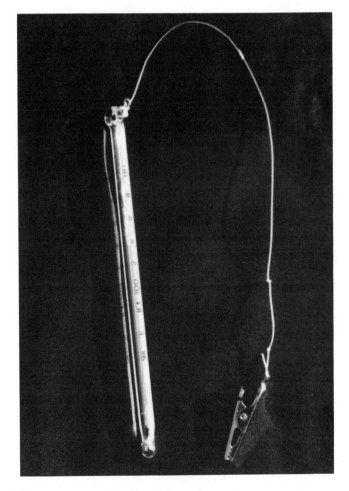

Thermometer with clip and cord.

comes back up at all. It is helpful to lubricate the thermometer with petroleum jelly or a similar product before inserting it.

Take the horse's temperature by standing at his left hind leg, facing the rear, and pushing your hip slightly into his leg so that you can move with any movement and are less likely to get kicked. Hold the tail in your left hand, grasping it six or eight inches out from the root. Hold the thermometer in your right hand. Slowly but firmly raise the tail up and to the side with the left hand, while inserting the thermometer with the right. Push it gently in until only about a half inch is sticking out. Then, clip the alligator clamp to the hair of the tail near the horse's body. Leave the thermometer in place for two to three minutes. Reverse the procedure to remove it, unclipping it from the hair and grasping the string before taking it out. When you have removed it, wrap a few strands of tail hair around the thermometer and pull it through them to clean it before you read it.

Normal temperature for the horse is approximately 99.5 to 101.4 degrees F (37.5 to 38.5 degrees C). Foals and yearlings may have normal temperatures up to 102 degrees F (39.0 C), especially if they are nervous or excited.

Normal temperatures may run slightly higher in hot, humid weather, or if the animal has been in direct sunlight. Under these conditions, temperatures of 102 degrees F (39.0 C) are not uncommon. The temperature is often elevated if the animal has just been exercised. Temperatures are usually a degree or so higher in the afternoon than they are in the morning. When you are checking the animal's temperature several days in a row, try to do it near the same time; this will give a more accurate indication of changes from day to day than will taking it at different times.

Exposure to cold weather or winds or drinking large amounts of cold water may lower the animal's temperature briefly. Body temperature is slightly higher one or two hours after a meal. Animals who are in unfamiliar surroundings or handled by strange people may also show an elevated temperature.

Fever is the term used when an animal's temperature is above normal. An elevated temperature is seen with fever due to illnesses, as well as with sunstroke (heat

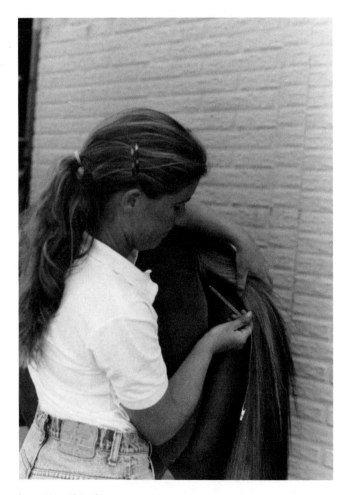

Inserting the thermometer.

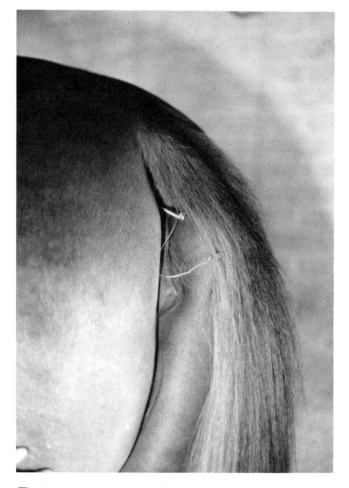

Thermometer clipped to tail.

exhaustion). It is well worth the effort to take your horse's temperature morning and evening daily for a week or so when you know the animal is healthy. This gives you a base reading to use to determine whether the animal is warmer than normal or not. Don't worry until a horse's temperature goes over 102 degrees F (39 C), especially if the day is hot or the animal is excited.

Do not be in a hurry to reduce a moderate fever. Fever is one of the body's defensive mechanisms. The rise in body temperature makes the animal a less hospitable host for many bacteria and viruses, and helps the body to kill off the organisms which are attacking it. When the temperature goes to about 103 to 104 degrees F (39.5 to 40 C) or persists more than two to three days (to the point where the animal has stopped eating and is becoming weak), then something needs to be done about reducing it. Of course, you should be treating whatever is causing the fever meanwhile, but the fever itself is not the problem in most cases—the real difficulty is the disease which is causing it.

There may be outward signs that the horse is running a fever. He may be trembling and sweaty. His skin may feel cooler than usual. The coat may seem to "stand up," and he may be hump-backed and miserable-looking. Take the animal's temperature and record it for your veterinarian.

If the horse is shivering, or it is cold or windy outside, he should be brought into shelter if at all possible. He should be blanketed and have deep bedding so that he will be warm and not lose heat to the ground or floor if he wishes to lie down. Animals who are running a fever often have little or no appetite. They may be thirsty and depressed. Again, it is important to remember that the fever is not the problem—it's part of the healing mechanism. Your horse's survival may depend on quickly finding WHY he has the fever.

PULSE

The pulse which you can feel in an artery is an intermittent wave caused by the heart forcing blood through it. The arteries alternate between expansion and contraction, and it is this "pulse" that we palpate (feel) and count. One of the easiest places to take the horse's pulse is at the edge of the jawbone. Here the facial artery crosses the jawbone from inside to outside. You can feel the pulse in it

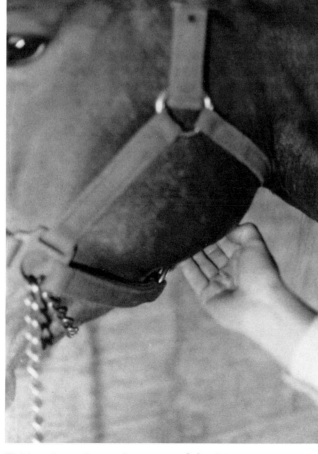

Taking the pulse at the curve of the jaw.

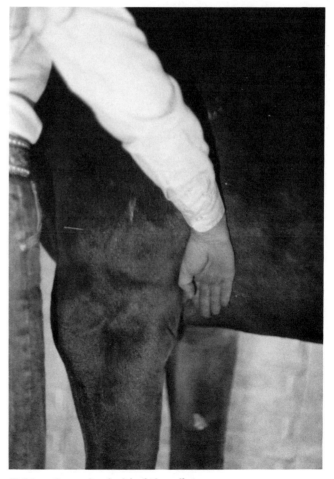

Taking the pulse behind the elbow.

by pressing it gently against the jaw bone, using the balls of the first and second or second and third fingers.

Another place to take the pulse is just behind the horse's left elbow. Do this by pushing the back of the hand, flat, firmly against the chest wall. This way, the heartbeat can be felt against the back of the hand.

Some people check the heart rate by pushing their ear against the chest wall behind the animal's elbow; try this method if you do not have a stethoscope.

The digital arteries on the legs are sometimes used to check the pulse. If you can normally feel the pulse there, this is helpful in determining whether there are foot problems or not, as you can feel changes in its character and strength.

Some animals will show a pulse in the jugular vein when they are at rest and especially if the head is level or hanging downward. This is normal for some horses. If other signs of heart disease such as fainting and fading are seen, it may mean that one of the heart valves is leaking blood backward into the jugular vein.

If your horse seems "short of breath," and his heart rate INCREASES rather than decreases while he is resting after being worked, you should have him examined by your veterinarian. These may be signs of fatigue or heart trouble, and the animal should not be worked until the cause is determined.

THE STETHOSCOPE

A stethoscope is an instrument well worth having to make it easier to hear the sounds of internal organs. Inexpensive models made for nurses are available. One of the keys to being able to hear anything with a stethoscope is to find one that fits your ears. Try before you buy! If it doesn't fit in one direction, take it out of your ears and turn it 180 degrees, then try again. Some stethoscopes fit markedly better one way than the other. The earpieces should snugly fit your ears without pressure or pain; they should not be so loose that they rattle around. Some stethoscopes offer two different sides, one flat and the other bell- or cone-shaped. For most users, a stethoscope with a flat side is sufficient.

After you have found an instrument that fits, the next step is to practice with it. The head of the stethoscope must be pushed firmly into the animal's side. Learn what the squeaking of the animal's hair sounds like against the

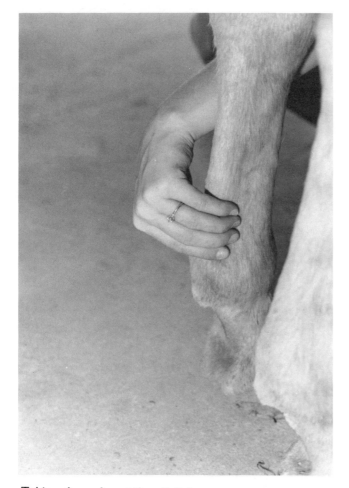

Taking the pulse at the digital artery.

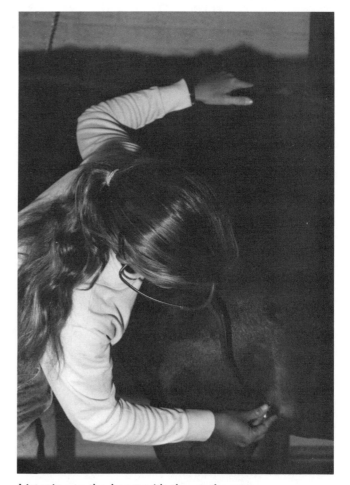

Listening to the heart with the stethoscope.

head of the stethoscope and against its tubing. Then, learn how hard you have to push to make firm contact with the animal's chest wall to avoid that noise.

Listen to a spot on the chest wall behind the left elbow for eight to ten seconds. Now, move two or three inches; compare what you hear with the sounds at the previous location. Are they more distinct or more muffled? Louder or softer? Cover a large area behind the elbow to determine where you can best hear the horse's heart. Examine the left side first; then, go to the animal's right side and repeat the procedure. On which side were the sounds clearer? If you'd like to hear lung sounds, go over the animal's whole chest in the same manner.

When using the stethoscope, the animal should be standing quietly. He should not be allowed to feed. Rattling chains and other noises should be kept to a minimum. When you are getting used to a stethoscope, have people in the area remain quiet. After you have learned to listen with the stethoscope, you will become accustomed to ignoring outside sounds, but it helps not to have them around in the beginning.

This is another place where practice makes perfect. What at first is an unintelligible bunch of thumps will sort itself out into a distinct pattern of sounds. The loudest one will be a loud "lub," followed by a slightly softer "dub." This pattern is then repeated. Sharp ears may pick up two softer sounds in addition to the major two. These are normal, but cannot be heard in most horses. Count only the "lubs," or you will get a pulse rate twice as high as it really is. Note the number of "lubs" per minute.

Horses occasionally have what is called a sinus arrythmia. This gives an irregular heartbeat. If you are listening with a stethoscope, it will sound as if the animal's heart skips an occasional beat. This is normal, as long as the animal does not show fainting or other signs of heart problems, and as long as the heartbeat becomes normal when the animal is exercised. If you have trouble making sense of the heart sounds, ask your veterinarian on his next visit to listen with you and help you to understand them.

NORMAL HEART RATE

An adult horse's normal, resting heartbeat varies between 26 and 40 beats per minute. A foal 2 to 4 weeks old will have a heart rate of 70 to 90 beats per minute; one 6 to 12 months old will be between 45 and 60 beats per minute, while 2 to 3 year old horses are usually around 40 to 50 beats per minute. The pulse is usually slightly faster in the evening than in the morning. The pulse may be raised by hot weather, exercise, excitement, or alarm. It may be slower than normal with severe exhaustion, old age, or excessive cold. (1)

A heartbeat of more than 60 beats per minute in a resting adult horse should be considered abnormal, especially if the horse is showing signs of colic. Any time one

of my clients has a horse with these symptoms, I want to hear about it immediately! A heart rate over 80 is often a very unfavorable sign. It often is seen with colics which are later fatal, and diseases such as salmonellosis.

Heart rates well over 200 beats per minutes have been recorded in horses during extreme work efforts. A well-conditioned horse that is ridden hard can top a hill with a heart rate well over 100 beats per minute. After a ten-minute rest stop, he should recover to 72 beats or less. An animal who does not recover to this limit is either not well conditioned or is ill, and is being severely stressed. Continuing to ride or work the animal can lead to collapse, thumps, and exhaustion.

RESPIRATION RATE

Respiration rate refers to the number of inhalations (or exhalations) per minute—the number of times the horse breathes in (or out). Do not count both in and out, or you will have a rate double what it really is. This is usually easy to count in the horse. Just stand back and observe the ribs moving in (or out). Do this from a distance, with the animal standing. If you have a stethoscope, place it

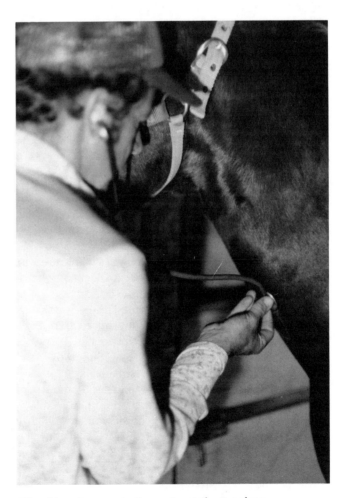

Checking the respiration rate at the trachea.

over the trachea, on the underside of the horse's neck, about eight inches down from the throatlatch. The air can be heard to move in and out. Again, count as it moves in or out, but not both.

The normal respiratory rate for the horse is between 8 and 16 breaths per minute. As with temperature and pulse, respiration is usually faster in foals. It increases with work, hot weather, overfilling of the stomach, and pregnancy. A fat animal will have a respiratory rate well above what is considered normal. Respiratory rate is also related to body size, exercise, and temperament. It is often elevated when the animal is examined by strangers, as at a trail ride, or by a veterinarian.

A measure of a horse's fitness can be made by the speed at which the respiration rate as well as the heart rate return to normal after work. In most horses, the heart rate will be around 36 and the respiration rate around 12 when he is at rest. This is a ratio of 3:1.

With hard work, a well-conditioned animal may recover to a pulse of 70 and respiration rate of 35 after 10 minutes rest, giving a ratio of 2:1. An animal who is not showing adequate recovery may have his pulse and respiration rates equal to each other after 10 minutes rest. The failure of both to drop into normal limits indicate that the animal has been severely stressed and should not be allowed to continue on the ride or to do other work.

A horse's respiratory rate is said to be "inverted" when the respiratory rate is higher than the heart rate. This is generally more serious than when they are just equal, and even more reason to pull the animal from the event and have him examined by a veterinarian as soon as possible.

GUT SOUNDS

Another area of examination is open to those with a stethoscope, that of intestinal sounds. These are the tinklings and bubblings made by gas as it percolates around and through the liquid and solid contents of the digestive tract. A fancy word for these sounds is "borborygmus." By listening to both sides of your animal's flank area for several minutes each, you can get an idea of what is normal. This can be done with the stethoscope, or by putting your ear on the animal's flank. These sounds have a flow and timing to them—not an exact rhythm, but a certain ripple and flow. We are not interested in specific numbers here, but rather in how the sounds of a sick horse compare with those of a normal horse.

When your veterinarian listens to the horse's flank and hears no sounds at all, he will, among other things, suspect an impaction or other colic problem which is causing a lack of gut motility. If he hears a rapid churning, with considerable tinkling of gas bubbles, he will suspect what is called a gaseous or spasmodic colic. These are not infallible rules, but when correlated with other findings from his physical examination, they will add to his sus-

picions in one direction or another. What you are looking for is merely whether the sounds are more or less active than is normal for your animal. And, as with any of the other tests, you have to know the normal before you can detect the abnormal.

BLOOD

Blood is a fluid tissue consisting of a liquid, called plasma, and numerous cells. It is sometimes considered to be a connective tissue because of its cleansing and communicating functions from one part of the body to another.

Red blood cells are small round discs containing hemoglobin. This chemical can combine with either oxygen or carbon dioxide, whichever is in greater concentration. Because of this characteristic, they can take up carbon dioxide in the tissues where it is in greatest supply, and move it to the lungs. There, more oxygen is available, so the cells dump the carbon dioxide (where it can be exhaled) and pick up a fresh supply of oxygen to carry

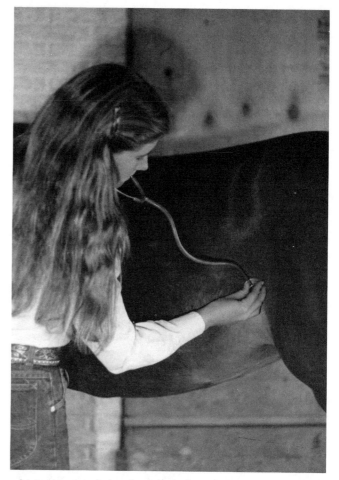

Listening to abdominal sounds.

back to the tissues. A smaller-than-normal supply of red blood cells is called anemia.

White blood cells are one of the body's first defenses against infection by viruses and bacteria. The white blood cell fraction of blood also includes the platelets which are involved with blood clotting.

Plasma is the term used for the fluid fraction of unclotted blood. It carries nutrients from one part of the body to another. For instance, it carries fats, amino acids (from the breakdown of proteins in the food), and carbohydrates, taking these to the cells of various tissues. There, the plasma picks up waste products, leaving them in the kidneys and liver for removal from the body.

Plasma also delivers hormones produced by glands within the body to other sites where they are needed. For instance, hormones are produced in a mare's pituitary gland in response to longer days in the spring. They are then carried by the blood to her ovaries to tell them to produce eggs and come into heat to get ready for the breeding season.

Serum is the fluid portion of the blood which remains after the blood has clotted. Serum contains the antibodies which prevent disease and infections.

Blood is important to temperature control in the body by moving heat from deeper tissues to the surface where it can be dissipated. It also helps maintain water balance and a constant pH (acid-base balance) in body tissues.

Approximately 8% of an animal's body weight is

TABLE 1–1

Normal Blood Values for the Horse

From R. D. Frandson, "Anatomy and Physiology of Farm Animals," Lea & Febiger, Philadelphia, 3rd Ed., 1981, reprinted with permission.

Red Blood Count:	7 million cells per cubic millimeter
White blood cells:	9 thousand cells per cubic millimeter
Hematocrit (percentage of cells):	42%
Hemoglobin:	12.5 grams per 100 ml. blood
Blood pH:	Average 7.4 (ranges from 7.35 to 7.43)
Coagulation time (minutes):	11.5
Blood volume (percent of body weight):	9.7
Differential white count (per cent):	
Neutrophils:	55
Eosinophils	4
Basophils	1
Monocytes	10
Lymphocytes	30

*Data compiled from standard references, including Benjamin, Dukes, Payne, and Spector.

blood. That would mean that a 1000-lb. horse has about 80 lb. of blood (roughly eight to ten gallons). Most horses (assuming they are normal at the time of injury) can lose from several quarts to a gallon of blood without any damage from the blood loss itself. Of course, if this is combined with a pooling of blood in the abdominal viscera due to shock or other reasons, the additional blood loss may be very serious. Horses, especially those who have gotten into a wire fence and been cut, have the talent of taking a little blood and spreading it a long ways, making it look as if they are bleeding to death. Occasionally, a horse can bleed to death due to an injury, but it is rare.

Blood transfusions may be given to animals who are in severe shock or have suffered from significant blood loss. Horses who have never previously been transfused are unlikely to have a reaction to the other animal's blood, as they do not have antigens against the other blood groups as humans do. However, if the animal has ever had a transfusion, he might possibly react when another one is necessary some time in the future (say, more than three or four weeks after the original transfusion). A record of any blood transfusions given your horse is valuable for this reason.

When giving transfusions, many veterinarians try to pick a horse for a donor who is unrelated to the recipient animal; they may prefer to use the most cold-blooded and common animal available. For instance, for a highly bred Arabian, this author has used a part-Quarter Horse mare, rather than one of the other Arabians on the farm, thus hoping to further reduce the remote chance of any reaction. If enough time and a laboratory are available, cross-matching may be done to insure that the donor is compatible with the recipient.

Blood pressure in horses cannot be measured with a human blood pressure cuff—it simply does not work. Blood pressure can be measured in the horse, but it takes special instruments and techniques. It is rarely done except in university hospitals when special monitoring is needed.

A horse's heart will pump enough blood in four minutes to fill a 55-gallon drum. If he is galloping, he will move the same amount of blood EACH minute.

ANEMIA

Hemoglobin values are important to the race horse trainer who wants to make sure that his animal is operating as efficiently as possible and is not anemic. For this reason, many trainers want the animal's hemoglobin level to reach 16 grams per 100 ml. of blood. They may feed iron and liver extracts and special mineral preparations to help achieve this level. How important this hemoglobin level is is not known for certain. If the low hemoglobin is discovered with a hemoglobinometer, it may not be significant.

Horses who have anemia will have reduced oxygen-carrying capacity of the blood; they may have less energy and ability to do work than normal, and may have pale mucous membranes. They may have significantly less red blood cells than normal animals.

If the animal is indeed anemic, it is important to find out why. Is there a deficiency of B vitamins or iron which are needed to produce red blood cells? Is the animal affected with worms who are draining blood from him? Or is his bone marrow not producing enough red blood cells? Is a disease process involved? Anemia is seen with diseases such as equine infectious anemia (swamp fever), and with equine piroplasmosis and ehrlichiosis. Has he recently suffered an injury causing severe blood loss? It is often necessary for your veterinarian to run a number of laboratory tests to determine the exact cause of anemia.

Chapter 3

HORSE MANAGEMENT

Fences
Root Cellars, Septic Tanks, and Other Traps
Shelter
Bedding
A Clean Environment
Grooming
Foot Care
Exercise
    Circular Work—Possible Dangers
    Overweight and Exercise
    Longeing
    Exercise for Mature Horses

Horse management might seem to be an inappropriate topic for this book. However, management can prevent many horse diseases and injuries. Indeed, it can be the cheapest form of preventive medicine and can save untold dollars in veterinary bills and loss of animal use. Let's discuss some points of horse management which can prevent injuries to your horse and save you money:

FENCES

In its most elemental form, horse confinement may be nothing more than a barbed wire fence around a piece of prairie, restricting the horse or horses to a given piece of real estate. And therein lies one of the greatest causes of horse injury—barbed wire. Horses get into barbed wire in many ways. Some of them tend to be handy with their front feet and paw at it, thus trying to saw off their feet. Others are run into it while being chased by larger or more aggressive horses in their group. Horses also panic at things, real or imagined, and run blindly. This might happen during a storm, or for no apparent reason at all. The horse may crash into the wire in the course of this flight. Horses also tangle with barbed wire while reaching for the proverbial "greener" grass on the other side. They look for

ways to stumble into the remains of old fences which are now down on the ground, lying in wait. They also trip and stumble same while trying to step over or leap fences which are poorly maintained.

The prevention for the barbed wire problem is simple: don't keep a horse in an enclosure fenced with it. If you are building the enclosure yourself, use barbless twisted wire, or woven wire or chain link. Concrete reinforcing mesh makes cheap fence panels for corrals or smaller enclosures. Use of these metal products avoids the biggest problem with wooden fences—that of being eaten by the horses. This brings us to wooden fences.

Wooden fences are attractive and go a long way toward beautifying a piece of land. They are not the best horse fences in the world because many animals have a tendency to eat them. A horse may go for years without having so much as a nibble on the fence. Then overnight, one or more of the animals decides to chew the place down, and it looks as though it had been attacked by a herd of beavers. When one horse starts chewing on the wood, he often starts others doing it.

Some of these wood-chewing horses will get a colic from swallowing the splinters. At the very least, they usually get large sores in their mouths, cheeks, or tongue. There may be sizeable ulcers from where the splinters have lodged. The animal may also have a decreased appetite because of the pain that occurs when he eats.

Some people claim that a mineral deficiency is involved here, and a few owners have success feeding certain mineral supplements, saying that the chewing problems immediately stopped. Another cure is to paint the fence with an anti-chew substance. These may or may not last for a period of time, depending on how wet your climate is. The other cure is to go to some type of metal fencing, such as pipe, sucker rod, or wire.

Wooden fences have several other disadvantages. They may splinter sharply if a horse runs into a board or attempts to jump a fence and crashes down on top of it. Nails or other fasteners often protrude or work out, thus offering still another hazard waiting to tear the horse's hide. Wooden fences should be inspected frequently for nails or splinters.

If you can afford them, oil field sucker rod or pipe fences avoid many of the disadvantages associated with wooden or wire fences. Pipe fences should have the bars close enough together so that the animal cannot get his head out between them. Otherwise, the animal will probably rub a large spot out of the middle of his mane. The bars should be either spaced far enough apart that an animal who gets a leg between them can get it out again, or so closely that there is no chance of this. It is often safer to only run the fence to within 16 or 18 inches of the ground, rather than going closer and leaving a small space where a horse may catch his feet while lying down.

Any corners should be squared where they meet other panels. Panels with rounded corners which were sold some years ago as being "safer" for horses have instead proven to be less safe as they allow animals to catch their feet in them while pawing over the top at their neighbors. One or both forefeet may become hung in the "V" between the panels. At that point, the animal is on top

of the pins you have to remove to take the panels apart. His whole weight is hanging on his legs and the pins. Often the only way out is to remove the bars with a cutting torch. Needless to say, by the time the animal has hung there long enough to be discovered and you have gone for a cutting torch, he is going to be battered and possibly crippled. As a final point, you can imagine the hazards of using a cutting torch around a horse.

Steel cable fencing is often used, especially where cheap supplies of used cable are available. Cable fences are often built with round steel posts, with the cable being threaded through holes cut in the pipe. When fitted with turnbuckles in each length so that the fence can be tightened when it sags, cable can make a good-looking, functional fence. It is fairly safe when kept tight. One hazard to watch for, however, is fraying cable which may cut the horse.

Fencing made of rubber belting has come into vogue lately as being safe. It definitely limits the amount of cuts and bruises that occur. However, under some circumstances, the rubber can wear and become frayed. The horse may then eat these ragged edges, resulting in a

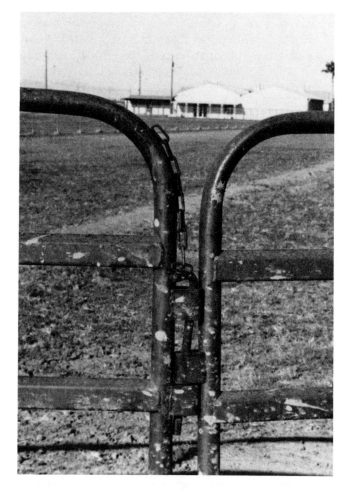

Rounded corners may be hazardous to your horse.

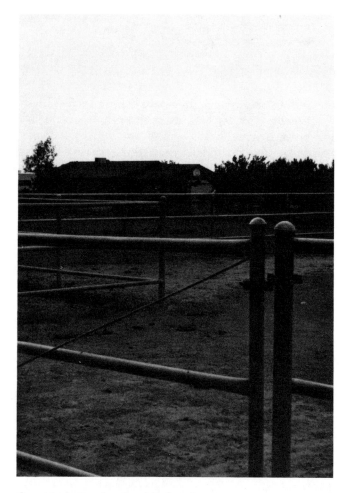

One kind of safe, durable fencing.

foreign-body impaction and/or colic. This is especially a problem with foals and yearlings who are young and bored. If carefully maintained, it can be good and safe fencing. Only time will tell if there are other problems with it.

ROOT CELLARS, SEPTIC TANKS, AND OTHER TRAPS

Root cellars and horses don't mix. Tragedies involving horses and root cellars occur in several ways. The animal may push into the root cellar, from curiosity or perhaps from hunger for something that he can smell from the past. He is unable to get out the door as it squeezes shut when he pushes on it. Or, he may stand on the roof and have the old, rotten boards collapse. One of the saddest calls this author has ever made was to examine a horse who survived one of these falls. He was not the tragedy—his starvation and dehydration would be repaired with several days of carefully spaced small feedings and waterings. The heartbreaking part were the two fine mares who had been standing beside him on top of the cellar when it fell in—who now lay dead inside it, victims of the injuries which occurred when the rotten roof boards collapsed.

If there is a root cellar or similar structure in your pasture, either fence securely around its perimeter so that horses cannot get on top of it (as they are prone to do with higher mounds of earth), or have it totally collapsed and filled so that it does not present a danger.

One client nearly lost her aged gelding when he fell into an abandoned septic tank which she did not know was in the pasture. The flexor tendons on one hind leg were totally severed, either when he went through the cover of the tank, or from debris in it. He was lucky to escape serious infection, but he required four or five months of intensive, expensive nursing before he was healed. Carefully examine your property for these hazards and eliminate them.

SHELTER

Shelter may be a luxury in mild climates, especially if the animals have access to good tree cover in their pasture. It is an absolute necessity if you are foaling mares in January in Chinook, Montana. It is also necessary if you live in Phoenix in summer and there are no trees in the pasture. In Phoenix, shelter may be no more than a sun shade up on pipe or wooden legs to cover the animals in the heat of the day. In the Montana example, it may be necessary to have a good, tight barn. For foaling; it may even need to be heated. Your needs will depend heavily on your location.

Barns should be on well-drained ground. If they are open-sided sheds, they should be backed into the prevailing wind. In most areas, this usually means that it will be open to the south or east. Stalls within a barn should be as roomy as is practical. It is good to have a run for each stall if possible so that the animals can get exercise and be inside or outside as they wish. Ventilation is important in a barn to keep it from getting damp and foul if it is shut up in cold weather; drafts should be avoided.

While shelter is nice to have, in many areas it is not an absolute necessity. For several years one of my clients brought twelve horses through the winter in Wyoming on a pasture with no trees or shelter. They were given heated water, all the hay they could eat, all the pasture they could scrounge, and grain when it was less than 20 degrees F below zero (−29 C). There was a week of 40 degrees F below zero (−40 C) weather, and a whole month where it did not get UP to freezing! The horses came through the winter fat and in fine shape, with no illness or frostbitten ears. This is certainly not ideal care, but illustrates the extent to which feed and care can make up for lack of shelter when none is available.

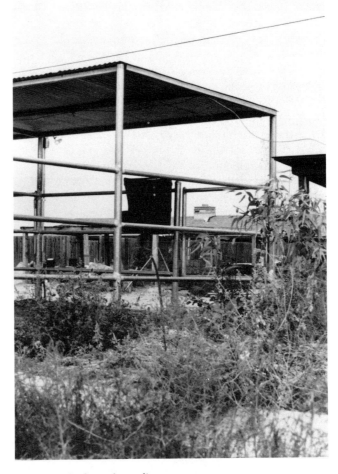

Sun shade for a hot climate.

BEDDING

The type of bedding which is available to use in your stall or barn will depend heavily on where you live. In timber areas, wood shavings or sawdust may be obtained from a local sawmill at nominal cost; sometimes, they are free for the hauling. Excessively fine shavings should not be used, as they may be dusty and cause coughing. Make sure that no black walnut shavings are present, as they can cause a severe founder in horses.

Straw is a common bedding. It is found in grain-growing areas of the country. Because it can be baled (similar to hay), it is often shipped long distances for use where other bedding is not readily available. Straw should be clean and free from dust, molds, or spoilage which may cause your horse to cough (and possibly develop heaves or to cause illness if he eats it). Some horses will eat enough straw that it cannot be used for their bedding.

Sand is used for bedding in many parts of the country where other materials are not available, especially in the southwestern states. The sand should be fine and clean, free of rocks or other foreign material. Sand has the disadvantage that it will often dull the animal's coat after he has slept on it for a period of time and worked it into his hair. For this reason, it may not be good bedding for show horses unless they are covered with blankets or a sheet. Of course, if you own a horse who never lies down, it's no problem. Sand gives good footing and helps cushion the hooves of horses who have been foundered. One disadvantage is that it is heavy to remove when it is soiled and it must by replaced periodically when it becomes soaked with urine.

Other materials such as rubber mats have been used for bedding. These are easy to clean, but may not give adequate cushioning for the horse who lies down a lot. Coarse materials, such as tree limbs which have been run through shredders, are better than nothing at all, but do not absorb urine well, and are rough enough that they may cause skin irritation on some horses. Whatever bedding you use, it should be harmless to the horse whether he lies down on it or eats it, and should be absorbent enough to allow it to soak up urine so that it can be removed easily. If it's also a material that enriches the soil when you spread it, so much the better.

A CLEAN ENVIRONMENT

A clean environment is one free of hazards. Clean up any toxic wastes such as pesticide cans and old batteries which may poison your horse. Eliminate stagnant water or marshes if at all possible. This will help to eradicate mosquitoes which carry sleeping sickness, among other diseases. If you cannot remove standing water, it may be possible to introduce top-feeding fish such as Gambusia which eat mosquito larvae. Your local health department can often tell you where to get these fish.

Smaller puddles may be treated individually. You may see mosquito larvae ("wrigglers") in low spots in your yard. Take an oil-soluble insect repellent (such as Farnam's Wipe) and sprinkle a few drops on top of each puddle. Within an hour or so, all larvae should be dead. This will not eliminate all mosquitoes in the area as they can come from many miles away, but should lessen the problem. Be sure that no pets, wild animal, or birds will be drinking from the puddle if you use this sort of treatment. Eliminating stagnant water also helps avoid the spread of disease form one animal to another through urination or defecation in the water.

GROOMING

Grooming is important to the confined horse. It is not so necessary for the range horse as he is free to roll in sand or grass as he desires to help get rid of insects and clean his coat. He can wade into a creek or river and will often splash water on his belly with his feet for cooling, or will lie down and nearly roll to slop water over his back or cover himself with mud. On the other hand, the horse who is kept in a stall has none of these options; he may not even have access to a clean spot to roll. He must rely on the goodwill and caring of his owner to clean his coat and keep him groomed.

The purpose of grooming is to help remove dirt and dead skin material ("scurf" or dandruff) and to help distribute oil from the skin surface over the hair coat. Most people begin by using a currycomb in one hand and a brush with the other, moving the currycomb ahead of the brush to loosen unattached dirt, and following with the brush to smooth the hair.

Manes and tails should be carefully combed if you wish to keep them in good condition and not remove too much hair. Burrs and weed material should be picked out or cut out, if necessary. The horse's tail acts as an important flyswatter. The longer and fuller it is, the more efficient it is. Keep the strands separated rather than allowing them to clump or wad together.

Horses may be bathed if they are extremely dirty, or if it is necessary to treat them with medicated shampoo for certain skin conditions. Do the procedure only on a warm, preferably sunny day. If it's cold or windy, wait. Having the animal clean may not be worth having him chilled and stressing him so that he becomes ill. Use lukewarm water, if at all possible, and a shampoo which is recommended for horses. Using shampoo made for humans, or products such as dish detergent, may cause excessive drying of the animal's skin.

Rinse the horse thoroughly as soap residue may result in severe skin irritation, especially under the saddle area. If the animal has been ridden or worked, cool him out carefully and thoroughly before washing him. Suddenly pouring cool water on a hot horse may result in severe shock or founder.

Horses are often covered with thin blankets called sheets, especially if they are shown. One client had a show mare who was extremely susceptible to mosquito bites, which would cause huge welts all over her body. This made it impossible to put a saddle on her. Because the owner lived in an area with a large mosquito population, he kept a light sheet on her all summer. When animals are covered in this manner, it is important to groom them frequently—daily, if possible. This helps to keep dirt from accumulating under the sheet. It also helps you to spot any oncoming skin problems before they become severe. This mare actually appreciated her sheet, and would come nickering to the owner and stick out her head for it if it were not promptly replaced after she was ridden. A sheet will also keep the sun from drying and bleaching the animal's summer coat, which is important if the horse is shown.

Many people blanket their horses in the winter. If the horse is living outside in a cold climate and is going to be used there, he should be allowed to grow a natural winter coat. A horse who is blanketed will have a thinner coat than one allowed to hair up normally. He will also be more susceptible to chilling when he is used outdoors without his covering. Horses with heavy winter coats who are ridden in the middle of winter may prove nearly impossible to cool out because of the thick hair. Walk the animal until he is cool when touched on the chest muscles. Then, blanket him and leave him overnight (or until evening if he is ridden in the early morning). At this time, remove the blanket and let him return to his normal relationship with his environment.

A horse who is blanketed and hooded in the winter needs grooming even more than an animal kept in a sheet in the summer. Hoods should be removed during the day whenever possible. An animal who is hooded all the time will itch severely, and will often rub out his mane by scratching against anything available. A show mane may be ruined in only one or two days.

Make sure that the hoods and blankets are safe and will stay in place. One of the best blanket designs is closed on the front and slips over the horse's head. It has one belly band, in the cinch area, and straps around the hind legs. The animal can run, buck, kick, or roll in this type of blanket without losing it or getting tangled and having problems. Whatever kind you use, be sure that it is safe and secure.

FOOT CARE

An old proverb says, "No hoof, no horse," and it is certainly true. Having the best-looking champion horse in the world does not get you over the next mountain if his feet are bad. Horse's hooves are made of a hard, horny material. They grow down from the coronary band much as our fingernails grow from the base. The hoof material must be kept moist enough that it does not crack or split,

but dry enough that diseases, such as thrush, do not occur.

The ground surface of the hooves should be cleaned frequently—daily if at all possible. This allows the removal of stones and manure which may cause the animal discomfort and contribute to disease. Cleaning also allows an examination of the lower part of the foot, or sole, which is so important to the horse, as well as an inspection of the shoes to see if they are loose or excessively worn, or have other problems.

A hoof pick is an inexpensive (usually less than $1) and handy tool to clean the horse's hooves. One may also be carried conveniently on a saddle (tied on to a saddle string, or in a small pocket) for use while riding. Begin at the back of the hoof and work to the front, carefully picking the hoof clean. Note any black or oozing spots (which may indicate that the animal has thrush), or areas of soreness or softness in the sole.

A hoof knife is a handy tool when you wish to pare the foot clean for further examination. Use the sharpened edge to scrape a thin layer of hoof material from the sole until you have a clean, fresh surface over the entire area. Look for reddened or blackened areas, for signs of pus, holes, or slit-like areas (where a nail may have entered).

Cultivate a relationship with your farrier (shoer). He may be as important as your veterinarian in keeping your

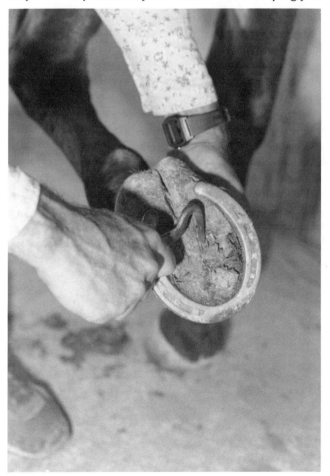

Cleaning the hoof with a hoof pick.

horse healthy. If your horse has no health problems, he may be even more important!

The horse's shoes should be reset when necessary. Reshoeing (or resetting the old shoes) too often may make it difficult for the farrier to attach the shoes, because not enough new hoof will have grown out to allow space between the old nail holes and the new ones. Thus, the new nails may tear out chunks of the hoof and may, in some cases, result in losing the shoe. This is inconvenient if you are at home; it may be a disaster if you are fifty miles up a rough canyon in a wilderness area. For most animals, about seven to nine weeks between shoeing seems to work well.

If the hoof is allowed to grow too long between shoeings, the excessive length will usually change the hoof angle, as the toe grows faster than the quarters on most horses. This extra length will put extra strain on the horse's tendons, and may lead to a bowed tendon as well as potential joint problems.

Feet which are left untrimmed for long periods of time may splay out, crack, and then break. This is especially a problem at dry times of the year. This may leave gaping holes if an attempt is made to shoe the animal, and can result in loss of his use for a month or two while he is growing enough new hoof material so that shoes can be nailed on.

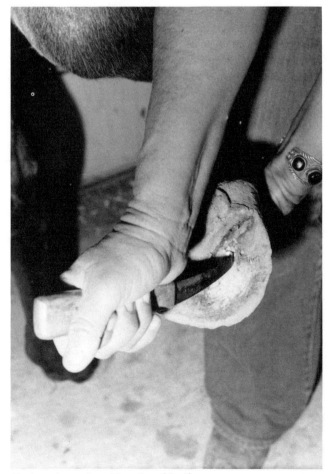

Paring the sole with a hoof knife.

It may be necessary to shoe some horses as frequently as every six weeks. This is especially true of horses with problems such as navicular disease or founder who are unusually sensitive to changes in hoof angles. These animals may experience severe pain if allowed to go too long between shoeings. So, it is a kindness as well as good maintenance to reset their shoes frequently. Allowing a foundered horse to go too long between trimmings may result in enough change of angle that the coffin bone penetrates the sole of the hoof and results in loss of the horse.

EXERCISE

Exercise is important to horses of all ages. Forcing an animal to "exercise" was not necessary when horses were used for everyday transportation or work. Then too, none of us needed to go to an exercise spa to "work out" when physical work was a part of daily life. Our horses, just like ourselves, have become soft and are victims of a leisure society. It is up to us to take the horse out of his box stall or corral and work him.

The type of exercise that we give an animal can have a great bearing on his longevity and usefulness. Perhaps the luckiest horse is one who is worked moderately and frequently, preferably on a daily basis. And the unluckiest? It's probably a tossup between the horse who is strictly confined and gets no exercise at all and the one who is left without work all week and then worked to death on weekends, whether in the mountains, on the hunt course, or in the arena. This poor fellow is the equivalent of the human weekend athlete who kills himself off with sporadic heavy bouts of tennis or other strenuous exercise, followed by a week of misery and pain from pulled tendons and strained muscles because he is not in good physical condition. Unfortunately, the horses usually doesn't have any say in the matter and can't refuse to be dragged into this sort of activity. The weekend athlete horse, like the human of the same kind, is very prone to injuries which may leave him crippled and useless. The time which the horseman devotes to conditioning the horse is an investment in the health and continued usability of that animal, just as a regular exercise program is an investment in his own health and well-being.

Training or conditioning an animal involves strengthening bones, muscles, ligaments, and tendons so that they will take the work that is demanded of them. It also involves developing the cellular systems which produce energy in the muscles of the heart and body. The type of exercise used will depend on the type of work the animal is asked to do.

CIRCULAR WORK—POSSIBLE DANGERS

Many horsemen view hot walkers and longeing as great inventions. These tools offer freedom from riding a horse every day, or are used to condition the horse who is too young to be ridden, especially when getting him toned up for halter competition. Unfortunately, we have seen numerous instances of temporary or permanent blemishes—even injury caused by these devices and methods.

One problem is the animal with the not-too-straight front legs, especially those tending toward bench knees. When these animals are worked at an early age with heavy longeing, they often develop severe splints. They would have been less likely to show splints if they were worked at a later age and not stressed by the hard, circular work. Take a moment and think about the mechanics involved when a horse is moving in a circle as compared to moving in a straight line. You will understand how injury can occur through the circular work.

Windpuffs are a blemish that are generally seen on older horses or horses who have been overworked on hard surfaces. They are also seen on young race horses. Once these blemishes on the fetlock area have occurred, they usually remain for life. Swellings of other joints can occur in the same manner, especially in the carpal and hock joints. The injury is caused by the pounding that is absorbed by the tissues in the joints. It's disappointing to see a promising young show horse with these swellings which may be counted against him in the show ring.

Longeing and hot walkers can cause these problems because the horse is always in a turn, usually a small one. Instead of the concussion hitting squarely on the whole joint surface, as it would when the animal is traveling straight, it's unevenly distributed with more weight applied to one side of the bones and joints than the other. Compounding the problem is the fact that these animals are often under two years of age. Their epiphyseal plates (the areas from which the bones grow) are not yet solidly formed and are still basically held together by cartilage. This is an ideal situation for damage to the joint surfaces and/or epiphyseal cartilages.

OVERWEIGHT AND EXERCISE

The tendency of many people who show or judge horses to see fat as beautiful contributes to leg problems. Weanlings, yearlings, and short two-year olds are often pushed to put on extra weight. They are frequently kept two to three hundred pounds heavier than they should be for their stage of development. This weight is piled on top of joints, bones, and cartilages that are not mature and are quite susceptible to injury. This causes extra concussion each time the horse takes a step. Combined with work in circles, the weight can add greatly to the stress and strain that causes blemishes and/or permanent damage. The final result is often a limited or shortened using life of the horse.

LONGEING

Colonel Alois Podhajsky, in his book "The Complete Training of Horse and Rider," discussed longeing at the Spanish Riding School at Vienna, home of the Lipizzaner. He emphasized the fact that Lipizzaners are not started into schooling (or longeing) until age four, and points out that hard work before that age can be injurious to the horse and shorten his useful working life. For confirmation of his opinions, look to the race tracks. The relatively high number of young race animals who are quickly retired or put down gives evidence that they were worked too hard, too soon. While we seem to put horses to work at a younger age in the United States as a matter of economic necessity, young horses who are longed should be so with finesse, and for very short periods of time.

The late Col. Podhajsky was considered to be one of the finest trainers of horses and riders in the world. He went on to say that longeing should be more than just making the horse go around in a circle. The horse should be taught to move on the longe line lightly and with collection and coordination, not lugging and pulling at the line with head crooked to the inside or outside of the circle.

Colonel Podhajsky also mentioned the importance of longeing the horse in as large a circle as possible. Correct longeing should be more than just a mad dash around an owner who stands like a post in the center of the circle, or a total substitute for working the horse on days when he doesn't feel like riding.

What is the solution to the problems of longeing and hot walkers? Simple—get out of the circle. Lead or pony the young horse in a straight line on soft footing. If you jog, how about taking that young equine with you and helping him learn to lead well at the same time? I do, often! But don't do as one of my clients did. After she had been told not to longe a young colt, she called me and told me that she had worked him and he was very lame. When asked what she had done with him, she replied that she had taken him behind the pickup, down to the gate and back. Well, "down to the gate and back" is about three miles on a packed-clay road that is about as hard as concrete. Instead of joint damage, the colt was road foundered! Fortunately, there was no permanent harm done, and the next time she used a softer place to work the animal. Also, it was recommended that she start him at a much shorter distance than three miles.

Ponying is a good technique for hardening and shaping up the show horse who is too young to be ridden. Pony the young one with a gentle, reliable horse who will not kick or injure him. This is also a good way to work two animals at one time, which can save valuable time in exercising them.

When working the young animal, it is very important to: 1) work the animal in a straight line; 2) start slowly and gradually work up to longer distances and harder work as the animal gets into shape; 3) keep the animal's weight within reason for his age and size—extra pounds put more stress on bones, ligaments, and joints that aren't ready for it; and 4) pick the best footing available. Work the younger animal mainly at a trot, but only after he is warmed up thoroughly. These techniques also work well for the fat, out-of-shape horse that you want to get back into working trim.

Circular work can be used with the older horse with less danger than with the younger animal, but is surely boring and can definitely be overdone. Discontinue circular work if the horse shows lameness, and re-evaluate your training program. If the problem persists after work is stopped and the animal rested for several days, consult your veterinarian. Use a walker with the longest arms that your space and pocketbook will allow.

Treadmills have been introduced which allow the animal to work in a straight line. It remains to be seen if they will replace the hot walker and reduce problems that walkers cause.

EXERCISE FOR MATURE HORSES

Suitable exercise for older horses depends on the type of animal, his training, the amount of time you have to work him, facilities available, and many other factors. Riding the animal is usually good exercise. Horses, like people, get tired of doing the same thing over and over, and often become spoiled and sour when forced to do so. This seems to be especially true of horses used for speed events, such as race horses and barrel and gymkhana horses.

Most horses, like most people, benefit greatly from a change of pace. It is a real treat for a highly trained event horse to go for a trail ride in the mountains or through a forest. It is tremendously relaxing and helpful for a barrel horse to go out and rope calves or round up cattle. This type of change helps to keep the animal's mind fresh.

When you're out riding like this, relax the pressure—both on the horse and on yourself. Often we get so hung up on asking precision of the animal that we take him out and ask him to turn "exactly three feet from that tree," thus making what is supposed to be "free time" as hard as everyday work. You don't need to let the animal get away with anything, or forget his manners or training—just try being a bit less strict with him for a change.

Any exercise program should be started gradually. If you have just brought the animal in from pasture, an hour or so of riding is plenty for the first three or four days; this should be mostly at a walk and trot. Gradually add periods of loping or cantering, extending their duration as the animal gets into shape.

You can estimate the horse's condition by watching how hard he breathes, and how long it takes him to recover after you have stopped exercising. How heavily the animal sweats is also an indication of his fitness. More precise measurement of his condition is often used with endurance and competition trail horses, where the rider takes the animal's pulse after hard work, and takes it again after the animal has been at rest 10 minutes. It should drop to 70 beats per minute or less. This drop indicates that the animal is in suitable physical condition for rides of

twenty to one hundred miles in length, depending on the animal and how long and how hard you have been working him.

Any exercise period should begin with a warmup and end with cooling out the animal. Old-time horsemen often said to walk the first and last mile, and it's not a bad idea. A proper warm-up period will help prevent injuries, and is especially important with horses who are asked to run, stop, and turn sharply, such as cutting and reining horses.

As the animal becomes older, it seems that more warmup is needed. Attention to this important detail will help to extend the useful life of the horse. When cooling the horse, walk him until the chest area (between the front legs) is cool when touched. If possible, also walk the animal until he is dry, if he has been sweating. In the winter, this is sometimes impossible. In that case, put a sheet or blanket on the animal, depending on the weather. Leave it on overnight and remove it the next morning if the animal is not regularly blanketed.

If you are short of time and yet are trying to condition your horse for strenuous working events or for endurance or competitive trail riding, the following are some more efficient exercises that you could use. They are definitely NOT recommended for use all the time because they are too strenuous, and because both horse and rider benefit greatly from the relaxation and training provided by pleasure trail riding. These techniques are not advised for young horses, either. Horses pushed hard with this type of conditioning should generally be four years old. Five would be even better.

Going up and down hills adds greatly to the stress of a given distance; a mile uphill is much more work for the horse's heart and lungs than a mile on the flat. This is valuable when getting a horse into shape for endurance and competitive riding. It makes the horse watch where he is going and makes him place his feet carefully. It helps him learn to bear the rider's weight over varying terrain with greater coordination. It also gets the animal's legs into shape for hard work.

If the hills are gentle and the footing is good, the horse can be trotted or loped when the rider feels that he is in shape and is handling the hills well at slower speeds. Be sure to maintain control; it is easy to let the horse pick his own speed to the point that he charges up hills and gets into the habit of doing what he wants rather than what the rider wants.

Galloping is especially valuable for conditioning race horses and endurance horses. The horse can gradually be worked up to a two-mile gallop daily. This should end up totaling five to seven miles per ride as follows: walk a mile or so to warm him up, and then trot at least a mile to really get the animal loosened up. After a two-mile hand gallop, walk another one to three miles as needed to calm the animal and cool him out. Galloping is good for getting the heart and lungs into shape and is also good for conditioning the legs.

When conditioning a trail or endurance horse, a

program of two-mile gallops three days a week, alternating with long flat trots or hilly work on the other days, is valuable. This gives a hard program of conditioning with enough variety in work and terrain to keep both the horse and rider from being bored.

When galloping, watch out for loss of control. Don't let the horse get into the habit of a mad dash at full speed. That can result in a runaway, out-of-control horse who is a hazard to himself and his rider. Also watch that the gallop is on good footing for the safety of both horse and rider, so that the horse is not likely to step into a hole or get stone bruises on the soles of his feet.

As mentioned previously, longeing is not recommend as a method of exercise or conditioning because of the many problems it can cause. It is best used as a training method, for the horse over four to five years old, when used with care and not to excess.

Ponying is a valuable method when conditioning two race or trail horses at the same time. Ride one and pony the other, alternating every other day. This allows the rider to condition two horses in the time it would take to work one, and is also good for general training. It is very useful when the rider gets stuck on a mountain with two horses and has to get them both home. That can be a miserable adventure when neither horse will lead from the saddle, or if the horse being ridden kicks at the other.

Work in deep sand is definitely NOT recommended for young horses, as it can easily lead to sprains, strains, and bowed tendons. For older horses, it can be especially valuable for getting the legs into shape. Work up gradually and don't overdo it, as it is very hard work. Dry irrigation canals and dry washes in the western states often have sandy bottoms that are ideal for this type of exercise. Plowed farmland can also be used.

Work in water is very good for the heart and lungs. Swimming horses who have injured legs will maintain cardiovascular fitness without concussion to the joints. Horse swimming pools are great facilities if you have access to one. Rivers or lakes can be used, and the ocean is good for those of you who live on the coasts.

Remember that NOT ALL HORSES CAN SWIM. Therefore, never swim a horse by yourself, especially the first time. Have someone standing by with a rope in case you need help. If you are going to swim in a lake or river, ease the horse into deep water gradually—so that if he can't swim, he can quickly get back to shallow water.

If the horse is saddled, loosen the cinch a couple of notches so that he can breathe more easily. A horse forced to swim with a tight saddle may be unable to breathe and may drown. On the other hand, if the saddle has a back cinch, make sure it's snug (but not tight) against his belly so he won't catch a back foot in it when he begins swimming.

A swimming horse needs total freedom of his head, so if you are using a tie-down on, remove it. If he can't get his head up, he will drown. Be sure there is no boggy mud or quicksand on the bottom in which the horse might get stuck.

Many horses learn to enjoy swimming, and willingly wade right in after a few days. If a horse is swum in a pool, he can often be worked by just one person walking alongside as he swims.

Work in snow adds much more stress than other kinds of work because of the heavy going and cold air. The horse must be well warmed up before really pushing into deep snow. Footing should be good enough so that there is no danger of injury to horse and rider due to slipping and falling.

If much work is going to be done in the snow, it may be worth putting ice calks on the horse's shoes to give him better traction. Or, you might want to remove the shoes to help eliminate the snow-balling problem. Some people feel that cleaning the animal's hooves and then coating them with butter or salad oil helps them to shed the snow more efficiently.

The cold air makes it difficult to cool the horse out, and almost impossible to get him dry if he's sweaty. It is often advisable to blanket the horse overnight and remove the blanket the next morning.

People who foxhunt often give their animals a "hunter clip." There are several variations on this basic haircut. The animal may be clipped with a coarse clipper, leaving the hair under the saddle for extra padding and protection. Or, it may be removed over the upper part of the body and left long on the legs. These horses are walked until they are cooled and then are kept blanketed.

Pulling a sled loaded with rocks, sandbags, or other weight can help with a conditioning program. Or, you can just tie onto an old tractor tire, railroad tie, or similar object. A car hood can be used as a sled and loaded with whatever weight you desire. Adjust the weight of the object or sled to coincide with the animal's condition, increasing it as the animal gets into shape. This work is especially useful for rope horses. It is good for any horse's general education, and will help teach him to pull calves, firewood, game meat, or anything else that the rider wants moved. One of my clients conditions her winning barrel horses by having them pull, daily. Do be careful that on a slick slope, the load doesn't overtake the horse and slam into his hind legs.

If either you or the horse have not pulled before, ask a horseman who is familiar with this training to help you the first time or two. Someone who trains rope horses or harness or draft animals is a likely candidate. This helps avoid the possibility of a wreck and injury to yourself or your horse until he becomes accustomed to this new (and initially frightening) activity.

Start with a light load and work up to the desired weight. Use a rope dallied around the saddle horn; do not tie hard and fast, for safety's sake. Or, you can use a harness and collar if they are available. Make sure that the collar fits properly.

Chapter 4

FEEDING THE HORSE

Roughages
  Pasture
  Grass Hay
  Alfalfa Hay
  Alfalfa/Grass Hay
  Grain Hay
  Straw
  Miscellaneous Hays
  Hay Cubes
  Chopped Hay with Molasses
  Silage
  Complete Feeds
  Miscellaneous Roughages
  Selection of Hay
  Blister Beetle Poisoning
Grains (Concentrates)
  Oats
  Corn
  Other Grains
  Grain Mixtures
Feed Supplements
Bran
Urea
Vitamins
Minerals
Salt
Water
Wood Chewing
The Digestive System
When To Feed
  Feeding Schedules
  Working After Meals
  Feeding the Tired Horse
How to Feed
  Watering the Horse
  Wolfing Feed
  Feeding When Camping With Horses
  Finding Pasture

How Much to Feed
  Measuring Feed
  Overfeeding
  Feeding the Idle Horse
  When Your Horse Doesn't Eat His Feed
Special Situations
  The Growing Horse
  The Pregnant Mare
  The Lactating Mare
  The Breeding Stallion
  The Working Horse
  The Thin Horse
  The Fat Horse
  Feeding the Sick Horse

Horse feed may be divided into two general categories: roughages and concentrates. Roughages are feeds such as pasture, hay, and silage. Their bulk is essential to proper functioning of the horse's digestive tract. The fiber in them is felt to be important in scrubbing harmful accumulations of bacteria from the intestinal walls, thus helping to prevent digestive problems. Roughage is important to help prevent colic as it stimulates good intestinal motion.

Concentrates are feeds which are low in fiber and high in usable nutrients. They include grains such as oats, barley, and corn, as well as products such as wheat bran, cottonseed meal, and linseed meal.

Roughages are the foundation of most horse rations, while grains are the icing on the nutritional cake. Many horses can (and indeed, do) thrive on hay alone, with no grain. Horses cannot remain healthy if fed only grain, no matter how much they are given.

Concentrates are the easiest way to provide the calories necessary for a hard-working horse. If the animal is not fed enough grain, he will first burn body fat for energy, and then will burn muscular tissue, resulting in a thin (and less efficient) horse. On the other hand, a horse who is an easy keeper and not being worked will thrive on a good-quality hay alone. Salt and water round out the list of necessities.

Horses have been given many unusual feedstuffs throughout the world. Desert horses in Arabia are fed dates and camel's milk. Danish horses are said to like dried swamp peat and beet molasses. Icelandic ponies are fed dried fish, which has the same nutritional value as oats but contains more vitamins. (2) Eggs and broth made from a sheep's head are said to have been used as horse feed in India. Lime leaves and the seeds of carob trees have been used in Spain and Italy. Nearly any edible roughage you can name (including such things as peas) has probably been used as horse feed somewhere in the world.

Feed must contain enough nutrients, (protein, fats, carbohydrates, fiber, vitamins, and minerals) to enable the horse to support his body in good health. It must include enough calories (energy) to allow the horse to do the work demanded of him. An excess of calories is merely turned into fat, which may be harmful to the animal's health and is certainly a waste of money. The feed must contain enough fiber (also called roughage) to keep the animal's digestive tract moving properly. Protein provides the building blocks for muscle growth and the basic ingredients for cellular maintenance. Foals and weanlings need around 16% protein, while mature horses can get by on about 8% protein. (3)

Some natural fat is found in most horse rations. Rations have been compounded with large amounts of fat added to give extra energy to animals who are being worked extremely hard, such as endurance horses. These animals literally cannot eat enough grain alone to keep them from losing weight when they are working. Fats help to provide essential fatty acids which keep the skin and coat in good condition. Fats act as solvents to help the animal take in fat-soluble vitamins such as A and D. They may increase the palatability of some feeds, and they help to keep down dust in the grain mixture. They also help the grains to go through machines which form feed pellets. Feeding a concentrate ration high in fat may decrease the complications (e.g., colic and founder) which may occur when animals are fed high levels of grain alone. Fats are most often added to grain rations by putting in corn oil or linseed or cottonseed meal.

An adequate supply of vitamins and minerals is necessary to keep all body systems healthy and functioning properly. Some conditions may increase the animal's need for a particular vitamin. For instance, toxins produced by certain molds (called mycotoxins) may be present in some feeds. These may increase the animal's need for vitamin K to allow his blood to clot normally.

Minerals become necessary additions to the animal's ration when soils are depleted of nutrients. For instance, selenium has been shown to be deficient in many areas,

and this mineral is being added to animal rations. This mineral also shows how too much of a good thing can be toxic: in large amounts it can cause severe problems, including sloughing of the mane, tail, and hooves. A little is a necessity, and too much is a poison, demonstrating the need for moderation in feeding. It is a good idea to find out where the hay you feed your horse is grown and check if that growing area has any mineral deficiencies. Hay is often shipped and fed long distances from its growing area.

Nutritional deficiencies may be seen in animals who are fed inadequate amounts of nutrients. Stress may bring on deficiency problems in animals who receive marginal nutrition. Sudden changes in weather (temperature and moisture) can severely stress animals, as can irregular feeding and poor management. Muddy corrals and inadequate housing in bad weather can severely stress your horse. When deficiencies occur, they are rarely seen as single disease problems. For this reason, the symptoms which occur with each deficiency will not be discussed. Most commonly seen are multiple deficiencies which involve several nutrients; for instance, a calcium deficiency may also involve phosphorus, vitamin D, and vitamin A imbalances.

Most nutritional deficiencies may be cured if they are discovered and corrected soon enough. If permanent changes (such as rickets) have occurred in the body, the damage may not be repairable. When large amounts of a missing nutrient are added to the diet, it is important not to create an imbalance with this addition. The best cure for nutritional deficiency is to not let it happen by keeping the animal on an adequate plane of nutrition throughout his life, avoiding periods when the feed is inadequate (either in quantity or quality).

The type of feed used for your animal depends in large part on what is available in your area, and may also depend on economic factors. Since the average horse will eat about 5½ tons of feed (including hay or pasture and grain) per year, small differences in feed costs may result in large savings over a period of time. (4) For instance, there may be a two- or three-fold difference in price between a premium native (mountain meadow) hay, and a locally-grown alfalfa hay. While the "native" hay is probably the ideal feed, the price differential makes alfalfa the logical choice for most horse owners.

Convenience must also be considered when choosing horse feed. The best hay in the area may only be available in five-ton stacks, which may make it totally impractical for feeding. Grain which is available only in hundred-pound sacks may be a poor choice if fed by a teenage girl. Convenience also includes a consideration of waste: if so large a quantity must be purchased at one time that there is much waste, cheap feed may end up being the most expensive in the long run.

Cost is a major consideration with horse feed; high-priced feed may be the least expensive if it is high in nutrients and palatability so that it is well utilized with little or no waste. The best ration in the world is worthless if it is unpalatable and the animal won't eat it. Feeding it to your own animal and seeing how well he does on a ration is the final test of how well it works. In addition, modern horses are bred for a faster rate of growth than were horses at the turn of the century. Some deficiencies will only show up with a higher growth rate. Thus, nutrient requirements which were determined sixty or eighty years ago are not adequate for today's highly bred animal. With some of these criteria in mind, let's take a look at some of the more common feedstuffs used in the United States.

ROUGHAGES

PASTURE

Pasture is the ideal feed for the horse. It most nearly resembles what a horse would eat if left entirely to himself in the wild. Free grazing allows the horse to choose which plants he wants to eat (assuming that it is not so over-grazed that he must eat all available plant material, good or not). It allows him to graze a bit at a time, when he is hungry. Left totally to himself, a horse will alternate periods of grazing and rest around the clock. It is not uncommon to be out in a pasture at night and hear the soft munch, munch of horses eating a midnight snack.

A good pasture is also labor-saving; the horse mows and packages the feed. All the owner must do is make sure the animal has adequate water and salt and is in good health. It relieves the owner of the need to be present twice a day to feed the animal.

Many types of grasses and legumes are used for pasture. They range from dry buffalo grass prairie to lush irrigated Kentucky bluegrass, and from alfalfa fields to coastal Bermuda pastures. Small grains such as wheat, oats, rye, and barley are often planted for temporary pastures in winter or spring when regular pastures are short or dormant. While these plants are in their active growth stages, they supply plenty of vitamins, and are high in protein, especially early in the season. As they reach maturity, their palatability decreases. They may become tough and woody. Lowland or marshy pastures may contain deep, beautiful green grasses. Unfortunately, these grasses are often both unpalatable and low in nutritional value. They may deceive the horse owner into thinking that he has plenty of pasture, when in reality the horse will not eat these grasses unless forced to do so.

Sorghum and sudangrass hybrids may cause several disease problems when used as pastures and should be used with extreme caution. Valuable animals should not be grazed on these pastures. The problems which may be seen include permanent paralysis of the urinary bladder and cyanide poisoning.

Some horses will need supplementation while on pasture. At the very least, loose minerals should be provided in boxes. Many people put out two boxes, one with loose salt, and the other with a complete mineral mixture. This allows the horse to eat more salt if he is sweating heavily or the weather is hot. Hay may be needed if the pasture does not supply enough forage, or in special conditions as mentioned below.

If pasture is used for winter feed, it shares many of the same problems as hay late in the spring. The plants have bleached out to a light tan, meaning that the Vitamin A content is extremely low. Mature forages (especially grasses) are also low in protein and phosphorus. It is often necessary to supplement pastured horses with grain and a vitamin/mineral supplement late in the winter. Some grasses hold their nutrients against the leaching effects of rain and snow better than do others. The tough, wiry grasses and sedges of the western prairies, for example, furnish more nutritious winter feed than do many common pasture grasses. Clover and other legumes make good feed even when mature, if all the leaves have not fallen or been blown from the stems.

Pasture also may present a problem early in the spring, when the grass is growing extremely fast, and is what farmers call "washy." It has an unusually high water content, and the animal literally cannot eat enough of it to get the nutrients he needs. A horse may be standing in grass up to his belly and starving because of this. This problem is very common in the Pacific Northwest and in other parts of the country where there is a lot of precipitation. It can happen anywhere in a wet spring. The fact that this early grass is very laxative does not help the situation any. The problem is easily remedied by feeding the horse some grain, and a vitamin supplement if recommended for your area. Often, grain by itself will do the trick. Or, the animal can be given supplemental hay. He can also be allowed to graze only a few hours and then brought in and fed hay.

When starting a horse who normally eats hay onto pasture, do it gradually, especially if the pasture is green and growing. This gradual introduction is extremely important when putting the horse on legume (alfalfa or clover) pasture, to avoid colic, founder, or other digestive problems. Feed the animal his normal morning ration of hay, and grain, if you are feeding grain. When he is finished and full, turn him out to graze for one to two hours the first day, and then shut him back into his pen or stall. Watch carefully for signs of laminitis, colic, or diarrhea. If the first day's grazing is successful and the animal does not show any ill effects, do the same each day for two or three more days. Then, leave the animal out for three to four hours a day for another two or three days. By this time, he should be adjusted to the pasture and can be turned out to graze full-time.

If the horse has a history of founder (laminitis) or colic, it may be worth taking as much as two to three weeks to accustom him to fresh green pasture. Remove the animal from pasture at the first sign of digestive or foot problems.

There is a good reason for allowing the animal to become accustomed to the pasture gradually. The forage is digested by bacteria in the horse's intestine. It takes different kinds of bacteria to digest fresh green grass than it does dried grass hay. Allowing the horse to become used to the pasture gives his bacteria time to adjust their numbers in order to efficiently digest the new ration. Some of the unneeded ones will die off, and the critters needed to break down the new feed will have a chance to multiply for their task. Letting the bacteria get into tune with the feed goes a long way toward preventing digestive upsets. This gradual changing routine should be used with any new feed, whether roughage or grain.

It is best to turn a horse out onto a new pasture early in the day, especially if he has never been in it before. This gives him a chance to become familiar with the fence boundaries and hazards, such as banks and streams, before it becomes dark. This avoids many wire cuts caused by animals running through a fence that they did not realize was there. It also gives the horse time to get acquainted with his pasture-mates, if there are any.

Pasture should not be allowed to get too tall, as the grass becomes less nutritious and less palatable. It should also not be allowed to be grazed too short, as this can harm the grass roots, causing damage to the pasture which will take months or years to heal. Because they prefer immature pasture plants, horses may graze some areas to the ground, while allowing others to grow quite tall. This can be countered by dividing pastures into small fields, and putting enough horses into an area to graze it quickly and heavily, and then rotating the animals to another pasture. It can also be fixed by mowing (clipping) the tall grass so that it will grow again from the roots.

Pasture which has been flooded should not be used for horses. The horse eats the forage, along with sand that has been left on it, and may soon develop a case of sand colic.

Horses may be grazed on lawns, but should not be allowed to do so if the grass has been treated with weed killers, insecticides, or fungicides, or materials to kill earthworms or gophers. If the lawn is hedged with oleanders, care must be taken that the animals do not graze this extremely toxic bush. Several common garden flowers, such as foxglove and iris, are toxic. Grazing animals should not be allowed access to them. Check the plants in the area you plan to use for grazing to see if any might be harmful.

Mares who are hard to breed may benefit by being placed on lush green pasture. This seems to aid conception in some animals. In pigs and sheep, feeding fresh green material before breeding is called "flushing," and is a common springtime prebreeding practice.

GRASS HAY

This is one of the best dry roughages available for horses. The type of grass hay which is available varies from one part of the country to another. Bluegrass makes a fine-stemmed, high-quality hay, as do the native meadow hays of the high valleys of Colorado, Wyoming, and Montana. Bermuda grass hay is common in Florida and Texas. There are also a great number of cultivated grass hays, such as brome grass, orchard grass, fescue, etc. Timothy, or other good quality grass hay, has long been the standard against which other hays are judged.

One of the greatest advantages of grass hay is that it is much less likely to be dusty or moldy than legume hay. While it is comparatively low in protein, the amount it contains is still adequate for horses who are not working hard and are not pregnant or lactating. Horses who are growing or lactating will need supplemental grain when fed most grass hays.

Grass for hay should be cut in prebloom or early bloom stage, when it is highest in protein. At this stage, it is also lower in fiber and high in palatability and digestibility.

Please note that grass clippings ARE NOT a form of grass hay! Grass clippings should not be fed to horses for a multitude of reasons. If they contain weed killers, fertilizers, or fungicides, they may actually be toxic to the horse. They are prone to cause choke because they are in small pieces and the horse does not have to chew them in order to swallow them. Thus, he does not mix adequate saliva with them, and because they are dry, they may get stuck partway down the esophagus. Or, they may get all the way to the stomach and down into the intestine, resulting in an impaction and colic (which is sometimes fatal). All in all, the small amount of feed that can be gotten from most lawns is not worth the risk of feeding grass clippings. Let the animal graze the lawn and mow it himself if you wish to feed this material!

ALFALFA HAY

Alfalfa is a legume which is very rich in nutrients. It is high in protein, often as high as good grain. It is rich in calcium and vitamins A and D. It is very palatable, and is relished by most horses.

This hay is available in most parts of the country. In many areas, more than one crop of it is grown per year. The hay is then referred to as "first cutting, second cutting," etc. The first cutting of the season starts growing in the spring as the weather begins to warm. It takes longer to grow than the other cuttings, and thus often has very coarse stems and fewer leaves than later cuttings. Unless it is of very good quality, first cutting alfalfa hay generally makes much better cattle feed than horse feed. Many horse owners will buy only a few bales of first cutting, to tide them over until the second cutting is taken. Then they stock up on second or third cutting, and store some in a dry place for winter use.

In some parts of the country, there may be up to eight or nine cuttings per year. In these areas, first cutting still may be the winter hay, which is too coarse and stemmy. The other cuttings are not too different from each other, unless they've been rained on or otherwise damaged. Areas which have blister beetle will usually have less of this pest in the first cutting, or in cuttings very late in the season. If you are in one of these areas, this is a major consideration (see Beetles).

Alfalfa hay is cut by most hay producers when about 10% of the plants are in bloom. Letting it mature until all of it is in bloom results in a coarser hay, with much lower protein and vitamin content. Also, when it is harvested too late, many leaves are lost, leaving it with less nutritional value. Try to get hay which is cut and baled at the proper time for the best nutritional value for your hay dollar.

Good quality alfalfa hay may actually contain more protein and digestible energy than is needed by mature, non-working horses, especially if these animals are "easy keepers." This type of animal can easily become overweight if fed a good legume hay on a free-choice basis. For these animals, the amount given should be limited to what is needed to maintain a normal weight.

Dehydrated alfalfa may be made into pellets and used as a large part of the ration. This product is often called "dehy." It is well accepted by horses (see Pellets).

ALFALFA/GRASS HAY

This is a mixture of alfalfa and grass and is a very good hay to feed horses. Many horsemen prefer it over straight grass or straight alfalfa hay because it has more nutritional value than grass hay, but with less of the complications (such as occasional colic) which some people feel they get from alfalfa hay.

This combination is better than straight grass hay because of its greater amount of protein and vitamins for use in pregnant or lactating mares, growing young horses, and hard-working animals. It is a good hay to use when having your horses fed by children or inexperienced persons who may cause them problems by overfeeding them on alfalfa.

GRAIN HAY

Hays made from small grains are fed in some parts of the country. Oat hay is made from the same plant from which we get oats for grain, but is cut slightly green with the stalk attached, allowed to dry, and baled. Oat hay should have good, plump oats on it. It should not be so dried or so late-cut that all the hulls have opened and the oats have fallen out. If this has occurred, the feed value is severely reduced, nearly to the level of oat straw. Good oat hay is cut while the grain is at the milk or early dough stage; at this period, most of the nutrients are in the leaves instead of all being in the grain as they are later.

The same sort of hay is often made from other grains, such as wheat or barley. Barley hay often has rough beards on it which may irritate the horse's mouth.

STRAW

In some areas, the oats or other grains are combined off the stalks, and the stalks (called straw) are cut and baled and used for horse feed. The same type of feedstuff may be produced from wheat, rye, or other grain. It can be used to add bulk when animals are fed a completely pelleted ration. Straw may be dusty, and sometimes contains dirt or other contaminants, which may be harmful to the horse.

Straws are very poor horse feed, as they are usually completely yellow; all the carotene (vitamin A) is gone, and the feed value is low. If you are going to feed the horse both the oat straw and the oats, why not cut it while still green and a lot higher in feed value and feed the whole thing as oat hay?

In an emergency, horses can survive on straw, but, for the long haul, it is not nutritionally adequate, even for the non-working animal. It is said that in Europe, oat straw is coarsely chopped and fed with the horse's grain ration. In this case, the grain would supply many of the nutrients otherwise missing from the ration.

IMPORTANT NOTE: Chaff from wheat and rye should never be used as horse feed. The sharp beards from the grain heads can become lodged in the mouth or throat and may cause serious problems. They are said to be the basis of intestinal concretions ("stones") which may later form intestinal obstructions. (5)

Oat chaff is said to be safe if fed in very small quantities and mixed with corn fodder or coarsely chopped hay, but may cause serious problems if fed in large amounts. It can be used to add bulk to the ration of horses who are given only pelleted feed, but again in small quantities.

Rice hulls are a poor quality feed which are very high in fiber. They may be used with a pelleted ration as mentioned above for oat chaff. Some feel that their sharp edges may be irritating to the mouth and digestive tract.

Any hulls or chaff which are fed should be as dust-free as possible. They should be clean and free from mold, or they should not be used for horse feed.

MISCELLANEOUS HAYS

Many grasses and grains which have not been specifically mentioned above are grown and made into hay. Millet is occasionally grown for hay. It should be cut early. Millet should not be fed as more than half of the roughage ration as there is some evidence that when fed in large quantities, it may cause serious lameness and swelling of the joints.

Sweet clover may be grown and cut for hay. If it becomes spoiled and is fed over a period of time to horses (or other animals), it will cause the animal to have a very prolonged blood clotting time. This can be fatal if the horse is subjected to surgery (such as castration) or injures himself as with a wire cut. Bear in mind that the hay need not appear moldy or damaged for the toxic principle to be present.

Horses should be removed from clover hay and given another feed for a couple of weeks before any surgery is performed, for safety. If your horse is eating sweet clover hay and requires emergency surgery, be sure to tell your veterinarian that he is on this feed. Your veterinarian may wish to check the animal's clotting time before starting surgery. It may be necessary to give the horse a blood transfusion during or after the operation if excessive bleeding occurs.

Other legumes may be cut for hay in various parts of the country; for instance, peas are occasionally cut and stacked for horse roughage.

HAY CUBES

Hay cubes are like miniature bales of hay, approximately $2 \times 2 \times 4$ inches. They are generally made from alfalfa. The hay is cut in the field and partially dried in windrows. When it reaches the appropriate moisture content, a large machine is run into the field and the is hay processed into cubes on the spot. Then it is put into large trucks and hauled to storage or delivered in bulk. It may also be bagged and sold in that form.

Hay cubes have several advantages. They are easy and clean to handle and store. They may be stacked in any dry spot: an empty, clean stall, or in a shed, building, or bin. Many people stack hay cubes on the ground outside and throw a tarp over them. This may result in mold on the bottom layer just as it would with hay stored the same way. Watch when you are buying cubes that you do not get any which have been stored on the ground somewhere before they reached you. As with any other hay, they should be bright and green.

Hay cubes are easy to measure precisely. It is much easier to dip up half a bucket of hay cubes than it is to estimate a constant amount of hay, especially if the bales vary in size and weight. Hay cubes are clean. If stored in a clean area, inside out of the weather, they have much less dust and mold than most hay. This makes them good for horses with severe heaves. They are light in weight and convenient to feed.

Any feed which has that many advantages must have some disadvantages, and hay cubes certainly have their problems. They may be made from poor quality hay—hay that is too weedy or tough or diseased to put into bales and sell. The best defense against this problem is knowing the dealer or farmer who sells the cubes to you.

The confined horse who is fed hay cubes is often bored because he eats his meal in 10–15 minutes and then stands around the rest of the day rather than taking one to two hours to munch his dinner when fed hay. Since it takes only a small quantity of the cubes to feed the horse, the horse does not get the amount of chewing to which he is accustomed. It's similar to people on liquid diets: they may get all the nutrition they need, but they always feel hungry because they do not get enough chewing to feel that they have eaten anything. This often causes the horses to eat any wood in sight.

Because the horse is always hungry, he may wolf down the cubes. They go down quickly because the hay is already chopped into small pieces. Since he is eating quickly, he does not chew the cubes as finely as he should before he swallows them. By the same token, the shorter eating time and faster eating keeps the animal from mixing in as much saliva as he should. All of this leaves the hay going into his digestive tract both inadequately chewed and inadequately mixed with saliva, which leads to impactions and colics. These are much more common in horses who are fed hay cubes.

Several large stables have fed nothing but cubes and sing the praises of their cleanliness and convenience. When questioned closely, they almost routinely seem to lose a horse to colic every year or two—more deaths than are seen in stables feeding hay. For this reason, I do not recommend that owners feed hay cubes to a normal horse, but only use them for horses with heaves or other special health problems. A stable with a hundred horses may accept the loss of a horse every year or so ($\frac{1}{2}$ to 1% loss per year) as normal, and even as a fair trade for the ease of feeding hay cubes. But if you have one horse and he dies from the problem, that is 100% of your herd!

Some horses do not relish cubes when first started on them, but usually will begin eating them within a day or two.

CHOPPED HAY WITH MOLASSES

A mixture of chopped hay with molasses is a common feed in California and other parts of the country. It is generally a good mix, as it has no dust and horses find it very palatable. One or two flakes of clean, high-quality hay should be fed with it, once or twice a day. This helps to give the horse the amount of chewing that he needs, making him feel fuller, and helps to prevent wood-chewing problems. Large amounts of this feed (in sacks) can be stored in a relatively small amount of space, and probably with much less fire hazard than is present with baled hay. This is especially important in stables where many people are around. This hay product can also help avoid many of the problems with hay quality that occur in California because of the frequent seasonal rains. Problems are similar to those noted for hay cubes. In addition, the molasses is a very high energy feed and may cause your horse to become fat if fed to excess.

SILAGE

This is made from corn or other feed grain which is chopped while quite green and compacted into an airtight silo or pit. The end result is a sort of "pickled corn." Good silage has a distinctly fermented smell, but should not smell sour or moldy. Moldy silage may cause horses to become severely ill or even to die. This toxicity may be due to the molds themselves, or to other poisons, such as botulism toxin, which may form in the process of spoilage. Frozen silage is reported to cause colic. (6)

Make sure that no urea has been added to the silage; encountering an area in the silo where this feed additive is excessively concentrated may cause toxicity when the silage is fed. For these reasons, some authorities recommend that silage not be fed to valuable horses, or those used for racing or hard work.

A type of bacteria causing a disease called listeriosis may grow in silage and cause abortion. Thus, silage is not a suitable feed for pregnant mares. Because silage is high in moisture and may distend the animal's abdomen when fed in large quantities, some horsemen feel it unsuitable for performance or working horses.

Silage is generally an acquired taste for horses; once accustomed to it, the animals usually maintain good flesh and good health. When starting a horse on silage, put a bit of it on top of the animal's hay, gradually increasing the amount of silage and decreasing the amount of hay. It is better, if possible, to feed some hay along with the silage. In most cases, silage is fed as no more than half of the roughage, with hay being used for the other half.

This feed is usually found around feedlots or dairies. Often the horses are fed silage right along with the cows, and they seem to do quite well on it.

COMPLETE FEEDS

These are commonly known as "pellets." Hay is ground very finely, and to it is added a grain mixture, vitamins, minerals, and salt. This feed contains everything that the horse should need. Pellets do have a number of advantages. Like hay cubes, they are very convenient to transport, store, and feed. There is less waste than with hay or grain feeding. Horses may look more attractive because they do not have "hay bellies." Pellets take minimal labor to feed, there is less dust, and the horse is not able to pick through the feed and only eat what he wants. Feedstuffs which a horse would not normally eat can be combined in a pelleted feed and thus utilized.

For the normal horse, pellets are unnecessary. The normal horse needs both his chewing action to feel full and roughage to keep his digestive tract moving normally. Throughout the eons of evolution, his intestines have evolved to digest large amounts of rather coarse feeds. The horse critter does not cope well with finely cut, small quantity feedstuffs.

Some people use pellets in addition to grain. They would be much better off, economically, to feed a bit more hay and a compensating amount of grain mix instead of paying to have the feed so highly processed because this processing is not needed by the healthy horse. Feeding pellets to horses may also result in fence or tail chewing as the animal seeks to satisfy his urge to chew. Some authors suggest stopping this by feeding a small amount of hay. That negates most of the advantages of feeding pellets in the first place (no dust, ease of storage, etc). If you are going to feed any hay at all, feed a normal amount and forget about the pellets.

Pellets may be used instead of hay cubes and grain for the horse with heaves. There seem to be fewer problems with horses who are fed pellets than with those fed hay cubes. It would seem logical that since the hay cubes are more coarse, they would be better feed for the horse than pellets. Observation, so far, has not proven this to be true. Given the choice, feed a horse with heaves pelleted feed instead of hay cubes.

Pelleted feed may also be required of people going into certain wilderness areas. If you know that you must feed your horse pellets on an upcoming trip, begin about three weeks ahead to accustom him to them. Start by giving one to two pounds per feeding. As you increase the amount of pellets, decrease the amount of hay and grain proportionately. Watch the animal for signs of colic and stop the pellets if any signs are observed.

Pellets are a good choice for feed for the old horse who has few teeth left and cannot graze enough, or eat enough hay or grain to stay in reasonable condition. Because they require little or no chewing, they can often keep one of these animals in much better condition than if he is forced to eat grain and hay.

Pellets are often used to partially or completely replace hay for horses who are prone to impaction colics. They lessen the intestinal filling and distension that may occur when the animal is given hay alone. Pellets may also flow through the digestive tract more easily than hay, again reducing the problems in these animals. Pellets also usually result in softer manure, which should help to lessen the chance that impaction will recur.

Pellets should not be fed to horses who are prone to choke. Softer foods, such as grass or moist mashes, are preferable.

MISCELLANEOUS ROUGHAGES

Feather meal and dried poultry wastes have been successfully used in small amounts in horse rations. Experiments have been conducted feeding corrugated paper boxes and computer paper to horses (and you thought the computer age didn't go with the horse!). The paper is ground and added to pellets, making up as much as 50% of the animals' ration. Supplemental protein, vitamins, and minerals are needed to balance the ration. The paper must be free of heavy metals, such as lead. Currently, it is recommended that these unusual feedstuffs be used only for mature, idle, non-valuable animals.

SELECTION OF HAY

Hay is perhaps the most common horse roughage in the United States because so many horses are confined or stabled. Many kinds of hay are used, depending on the area of the country. Regardless of the type, good hays have several characteristics in common.

Quality hay should have good color, ranging from a deep, dark green for alfalfa hay to a bright, light green for oat hay. This indicates that the hay was cut and processed at the proper time and that there are plenty of vitamins in it. Poor quality hay may be responsible for vitamin A and thiamine deficiencies, among others.

The stems should be fine; some hays are so coarse and tough that a horse would scarcely eat them unless starving, and then would not eat enough to stay in good condition. There should be plenty of leaves on the hay, whether grass or legume. Much of the nutritional value is in the leaves. If they are gone, all that is left is a bundle of stems, with a much lower food value.

Some grasses and feed grains such as barley have awns or beards on the seed. These are rough, sharp spikes which stick in the horse's lips and gums. Feeding hay with these present may cause raw, bleeding ulcers, or sores with bunches of these awns embedded in them. While the animal may be treated by removing the awns from the sore and applying an antiseptic to the spot, the only permanent cure is to take him off the offending feed.

Good hay should smell fresh and clean and be free of moldy, musty, or dusty odors. It should also be free of visual signs of mold or mildew: these show up as white patches or black spots. Molds may stimulate allergic reactions and subsequent cough which will eventually lead to heaves. Some molds are toxic and will produce outright poisoning.

Reject any bales which are exceptionally heavier than the rest, especially if the hay is freshly baled. This often means that they were baled too wet and will spoil or mold. The moisture in bales which are too wet may cause spontaneous combustion, causing the stack or barn to burn. If in doubt, open a bale—it should be cool and dry, not hot and damp.

Good quality hay should be free from weeds. At best, weeds cost you money: you are paying for them instead of for usable hay. They may be plants that the horse will eat, but are often not as high in nutritional value as the grass or legume. They may have sharp awns; foxtail and cheat grass (downey chess) are two of the most common of these. Both can cause severe damage to the horse's mouth. At worst, the contaminating weeds can be poisonous plants which may make your horse ill or even kill him. They also bring weed seeds to your premises—and who needs more weeds? Buy hay that is as weed-free as possible.

Hay should also be free from trash. In some areas, it is common practice to bale hay from roadsides. This may contain anything from beer cans to crushed bottles to heaven-only-knows. A horse will usually pick through this type of feed to get the hay without eating anything that he shouldn't. But what if he licked an insecticide container that someone discarded by the highway? Or got some of the soil sterilant that some highway departments use to keep weeds from growing into the edge of the pavement? Hay from roadsides may also contain abnormally high levels of lead from auto exhaust fumes which may cause problems in the long run.

If you feed "highway hay," don't just throw a flake to the horse. Pull it apart and sort out any junk which may be inside. As an elderly neighbor used to say, "It's better than licking at a snowbank." But, given the choice, quality feed usually doesn't cost—it pays. It is often worth paying a premium to a grower for his guarantee that any spoiled bales, or ones with more than just a few weeds, are returnable for exchange or credit.

BLISTER BEETLE POISONING

This problem will be discussed here because toxicity occurs when alfalfa hay containing blister beetles is fed to horses. These beetles are a group of insects including over 200 species. They are found from the eastern coastal states to Utah, Texas, and New Mexico, and from southern Canada to Mexico. They are small beetles, usually less than a half inch long. Some species have black stripes alternating with orange or yellow ones, while others are black, gray, or gray with tiny black spots. These beetles vary in their size, shape, and color, and feed on various plants in different areas. Those with stripes are most commonly implicated in cases of toxicity to horses. They all contain a substance called cantharidin. They belong to the same family as the "Spanish fly."

SIGNS

The first sign of blister beetle poisoning may be colic or abdominal pain. It may be so severe that the animal throws himself to the ground and thrashes violently. This pain is due to the irritating action of cantharidin on the membranes lining the stomach, digestive tract, and urinary tract. Colic usually occurs within one to two hours after the horse has been fed. Since the symptoms depend on the amount of cantharidin the horse has ingested, a horse who has gotten only a small amount may show mild colic, with pawing, stretching, looking to his side, and general nervousness. He may show shock and be lethargic. He may be depressed and weak, with rapid respiration, and may sweat profusely.

The horse may splash in his water, playing in it with

his lips and tongue, without drinking. He is trying to relieve the burning in his mouth caused by the cantharidin. Some animals may show ulcers in the mouth. Irritation to the animal's mouth and throat may have occurred when he ate the beetles. Several hours to a few days after the horse has eaten the beetle-infested hay, he may show frequent urination, passing only a small amount each time. This is because of irritation to the lining of the bladder and urethra. The urine may be tinged with blood. Severe poisoning is reported to cause low blood calcium and magnesium. These lowered electrolyte levels may cause stiffness or an exaggerated "goose-stepping" gait. Some horses may show a contraction of the diaphragm with every heartbeat, leading to a peculiar fluttering-type breathing ("thumps").

Death may occur as little as three to four hours after feeding or may be as much as five days later. Some horses, if they have not taken in too many beetles and have minimal internal damage, have survived the disease. Most horses who survive three days will recover. (7) In some cases, horses may die suddenly with no clinical signs, but most animals are sick for several days before death occurs.

A test is available at some laboratories to test for cantharidin. The only problem is that it takes a gallon or more of urine and requires a week's time. The horse will be either dead or recovered by the time the test is back. At that point, it is more of academic than practical value. Identification of beetles found in the hay can also confirm the diagnosis.

TREATMENT

No antidote is known for cantharidin. As with many other subjects in this book, prevention is the best course of action. Examine the hay for blister beetles before feeding it and if you find any—don't feed it! Because the toxin is so rapidly absorbed, immediate treatment is usually recommended if blister beetle poisoning is even suspected. Horses being fed alfalfa hay who are suffering acute colic or undefined illness should be treated as if affected by blister beetles, when the problem is known to be present in the area where the hay was grown.

This is definitely an occasion to call your veterinarian immediately! Be sure to tell him if you have noticed beetles in the hay, or suspect blister beetle poisoning. The treatment is similar to that used for many colics, so there is no conflict if the problem turns out to be colic from something else. One of the treatments that is commonly used is to pass a stomach tube and give the animal activated charcoal. This is then followed by a quantity of mineral oil, as is used in many colics. Drugs may be given to treat the shock which occurs, and fluids may be given intravenously for the same reason.

If one horse on a farm or stable is affected, the suspected hay should be removed from all the horses and a clean supply which is known to be safe should be substituted. The rest of the animals should be carefully observed for signs resembling colic which may signal the onset of beetle poisoning.

HOW TO GET HAY WITHOUT BEETLES

Blister beetles complete one generation per year. The adult beetles mate in the summer. The females lay eggs in shallow holes in the soil. The eggs hatch in the fall. The larvae immediately begin searching for the grasshopper eggs on which they feed. Grasshopper eggs are laid in clusters of up to 30 or more within an inch or two of the soil surface during the late summer and fall. Blister beetle larvae eat the egg clusters, and then winter in the soil and emerge as adults in late spring or early summer. This suggests that years with heavy grasshopper infestations will be followed by heavy blister beetle years.

The adult beetles generally emerge the first of June or later. In many areas, this allows the first cutting of hay to be harvested before the adult (and toxic) beetles become active. Beetle activity ceases in early fall; this should allow late cuttings to be free of beetles in many areas. If you are in a beetle area, this may be a major consideration in hay purchase.

Beetles feeding on alfalfa prefer the blossoms if they are available; if not, they will eat leaves. They also eat many other plants; among them are peanuts, puncture vine, soybeans, goldenrod, and goathead. Since the beetles are attracted to alfalfa flowers, cutting a field before it reaches 10% bloom will help reduce the chances of beetle infestation.

Modern haying equipment contributes to the blister beetle problem. Swathers cut the hay and crush the stems to promote faster drying. In the process, the rollers crush any beetles which are on the alfalfa at the time. The beetles are gregarious and tend to locate in large swarms in one place in a field. This may allow thousands of beetles to end up in one bale of hay. With old-fashioned mowers, the hay is cut, and raked into windrows for drying, which takes several days. This gives the beetles time to leave the hay and fly elsewhere.

If the hay producer can allow the extra drying time, it is worth cutting the hay without crimping to avoid killing the beetles and to give them time to leave the cut hay. Don't cut areas that are obviously infested with beetles. It is also possible to spray entire fields with short residual insecticide just before harvesting. Spray fence rows and field borders as well. Or, you can inspect fields shortly before cutting and spray any infested areas that are found. Malathion at 1.0 to 1.25 lb. active ingredient per acre may be used, or Sevin at 0.8 to 1.0 lb. active ingredient per acre. (8) When using these or any other pesticides, read and follow the label directions. To use them any other way may be dangerous and is definitely illegal. There is no waiting period between spraying and cutting with either of these products. Storage of contaminated hay does not decrease the risk of toxicity, because the cantharidin is a very stable toxin.

The number of beetles needed to cause symptoms in the horse is variable. As few as five to ten beetles may be all that are required in some cases, while in others, the animal may need to eat 200 or more. Contrary to popular opinion, one beetle is not enough to kill a horse. However, enough beetles have been found in one 5–½ lb. flake of hay to kill 29 horses. This makes it possible for the animal to get a lethal dose in only one or two bites of hay. For this reason, hay should be examined carefully in a blister beetle area. One flake may be perfectly clean, while the next may have enough beetles to kill several animals.

As a hay buyer, you need to know your alfalfa supplier. Don't be afraid to ask what precautions he has taken to avoid beetles in his hay. If at all possible, examine each flake of hay for the presence of beetles. You must look closely for them, as they may be finely crushed after being through the conditioner on the swather. (You can usually tell hay that has been crushed in the field to aid in drying—the stems are crimped.) The color of the beetles is usually dulled by the drying so that they are easily missed. Another solution is to stop feeding alfalfa hay. However, it may be difficult to get any other kind of hay in some areas. And, alfalfa is a more nutritious feed than many other kinds of hay. If you wish to continue feeding alfalfa hay in a blister beetle area, the price of safety is, as they say, "eternal vigilance."

GRAINS (CONCENTRATES)

Before specific kinds of grain are discussed, a few comments will be made on grain in general. Whatever kind of grain you are buying should be clean and free from dirt, dust, weed seeds, and extraneous materials. If many weed seeds are present, at best, you are paying good money for poor quality feed; at worst, you may be getting large enough quantities of toxic seeds to cause your horse to become ill. Grains should be plump and characteristic of their species, showing that they have prospered in their growth and have been harvested at the proper time.

Grain should be free from signs of mold; mold indicates that it was either harvested too green, or that it had been allowed to become damp or was improperly stored after harvesting. Grains such as rye are especially susceptible to infestation by a fungus called ergot. Ergot shows up as hard, black kernels that look like misshapen seeds. Small amounts of ergot in grain can cause abortion, or more dangerous problems, such as loss of circulation to the feet. If you are buying grain locally, buy from someone upon whom you can rely and who knows what he is doing, and then keep an eye on the grain for any suspicious material. When buying products made from processed grain, such as pellets, about all that you can do is to rely on the reputation and quality control of the feed company.

Quality grain should also be free from large amounts of grain dust and small particles of broken grain, often called "fines." It is important to distinguish this material from vitamin and mineral additives that have merely fallen off the kernels in a grain mix. Grain for foals and older horses with poor teeth should be crimped, cracked, or rolled to make it more easily digestible. It may even be steam-treated to partially cook it as a part of the rolling process.

OATS

Oats are the most popular grain given to horses. Their bulk helps to prevent founder or impaction. They are fed in several ways. Some people feed whole oats (generally the cheapest form of oats). Others prefer oats which are rolled or crimped. These oats are run through a mill and flattened so that the hard outer shell of the grain is broken. There is considerable debate and difference of opinion among horsemen as to which is the most efficient, and in the end, most economical form. One author states that crimping oats may improve their utilization by 7 to 10 per cent. (9) Many whole oats are passed in the animal's manure, quite as whole and undamaged as when they were eaten. Horses often do not chew their food as much as they should, and this contributes to the passage of whole oats through the digestive tract. Animals get more benefit with less waste from rolled or crimped oats. Young foals or horses with poor teeth will definitely need rolled or crimped oats.

Oats are often dusty and may contain large amounts of weed seeds and other foreign material unless they are carefully cleaned. Oats often vary considerably in the number of pounds per bushel—the heavier the weight, the better the oats. In general, unless there is no other way, grain, including oats, should be bought by weight rather than by measure. This assures that you will get full value for the money spent. Buy from a reputable seller, and watch what you buy.

CORN

Corn is a good feed for horses who need to gain weight; conversely, it is easy to make a horse fat on this grain. While it is usually rather low in protein, it is high in carbohydrates (calories or energy), making it a good choice for the hard-working animal who is not staying in condition on oats or a grain mix. It contains twice as much energy as the same volume of oats; therefore, you can get by with feeding about half as much corn as you do oats. It is this high energy content that gives corn the reputation of "making an animal high," which it will do if you feed him the same quantity as you were feeding of oats! So, adjust the amount fed accordingly. Corn is also high in fat, which puts a healthy, shining coat on a horse.

Corn's high calorie content makes it ideal when horses need additional energy, such as with hard work, or in cold weather. It lowers the amount of bulk that the animal has to carry in the digestive tract, while still giving the energy necessary for work.

Corn is often the least expensive grain available, and should be considered when providing energy is the main reason for feeding grain. Several forms of corn are available:

Whole corn is not a suitable feed for most horses, especially those who are young or have poor teeth. It has the same problem of not being adequately chewed, and passing through the animal undigested as mentioned above for whole oats.

Corn on the cob is a good feed for the horse who wolfs his grain as fast as he can, causing digestive problems. Having to bite the grain off the cobs forces the animal to slow down. This is the only good reason for feeding whole corn (other than having an abundant supply of it and needing to use it for horse feed). Ear corn has the advantage of storing well without spoiling as easily as shelled corn. It is also less prone to mold.

Corn may be fed after being coarsely ground, cobs and all. The cobs help to provide bulk and fiber in the animal's diet. This, like other highly concentrated, rich feeds, should be given after the animal has had his fill of hay. Corn which is finely ground (especially without the cobs) may cause founder or colic. In fact, this is true of all grains which are finely ground.

Corn that has been steam flaked is a superb feed for horses who need extra calories (see Thin Horse). Corn is such a hard grain that it must be steamed before it can be flattened by the flaking machine. The grain comes out of the flaking machine damp and it must be dried before bagging, or it may mold. Check the grain carefully for signs of mold: bluish, grayish, or greenish streaks, or a musty odor. Do not feed the corn if you see any of these signs.

Occasionally, a feed store will try to sell you cracked corn for your horse. Cracked corn is broken into small, hard pieces which resemble tiny chunks of gravel. This grain is so fine that most horses have trouble picking it up and getting it back into their mouths so as to be able to chew it. The horse finds this frustrating, and will usually dribble a large amount all over the ground, resulting in considerable waste. For this reason, cracked corn is not suitable horse feed.

OTHER GRAINS

Barley is sometimes used for horse feed. It is higher in protein than oats, and supplies more total digestible nutrients (TDN). It is much heavier than the same volume of oats. When feeding barley, it is especially important to start the animal on it gradually and to feed the entire hay ration before giving the animal his grain to help prevent colic. As with oats, barley should be rolled or crimped. It is helpful to feed barley mixed with other grains, or along with wheat bran to help avoid colic. Some people have cooked barley prior to feeding it to horses, but studies have not shown that cooked barley has any benefits over that which has been crimped or rolled. Make sure that the barley has been adequately cleaned to remove the beards.

Many other grains are used as horse feed according to their availability and price, including wheat and rye. Rye should be carefully checked or bought from a reliable source to avoid contamination with ergot. Rye containing ergot should NOT be used for feed. Rye is best mixed with molasses or other feed to increase its palatability. Horses do not seem to like rye, and may not eat it if fed by itself. This problem can be avoided by feeding grain mixtures which do not contain more than one-fourth to one third rye by weight. Both rye and wheat should be rolled or crimped for most efficient use.

Milo and sorghum are especially popular in the southwestern states. These grains are also best crimped or rolled before feeding. Some experts feel that these grains should not make up more than one-fourth of the total grain amount. When fed in large quantities, they seem more prone to cause digestive problems and founder than do oats. In this manner, they are somewhat like corn. If you are going to feed one of these grains and have no experience with it, ask your veterinarian or county agricultural agent about it.

GRAIN MIXTURES

Grain mixtures vary in content from one part of the country to another, and from one season to another, but the overall nutritional content is fairly consistent. These mixtures go by names such as Omolene, Show Flake, Trophy, etc. Most feed manufacturers have their own brand of horse grain mix. These contain oats and corn as a basis, with wheat, barley, and other grains added according to price and availability. Most of these mixtures have vitamins, minerals, and salt added. Many horsemen prefer to feed them rather than feeding separate grains, such as oats or corn. My own horses are fed one of these mixes as a general feed, and given rolled corn when they mainly need calories.

Feed companies pay nutritionists to balance these mixtures, and thus the horseman gets the benefit of far more expertise than most of us have in every sack of grain that he buys. Grain mixtures should have plump, distinct grains, and a minimum of "fines" or dust-like material. Some small particles will be present when vitamins, minerals, and bran are added to the mix. They are usually bound together with molasses, which also adds palatability and calories. The mix should smell fresh and clean. Some of these mixtures smell good enough, in fact, to eat for breakfast! These mixtures can draw flies because of their high molasses content and should be kept in covered containers to avoid this problem.

If the grain is steam flaked or rolled and is bagged too wet, it may mold. It will be grayish and caked together, with a foul, moldy odor. Do not feed ANY grain which has molded—return it to the feed store. It can contain enough mold toxins to poison a horse or cause severe colic.

Most grain mixes are in the 10 to 12% protein range, which is adequate for most horses. Horsemen feeding foals in a creep feeder may wish to use a 16 to 20% protein mixture if it is available. This high protein mix may also be used for pregnant or lactating mares who are not doing well on a 12% mix.

Grain cubes (also known as "cake") are a convenient treat for horses—much better than sugar or other sweets. They can be bought from your feedstore, often in small quantities (by the pound). They are a good reward for use when training, and handy to carry in your pocket when catching horses. Buy the largest cubes that you can get, usually about ¾ × 1¼ inches, chopped in pieces from an inch to four or so inches long.

Under most circumstances, grain cubes should not be fed as the entire grain ration. The grain in them is finely ground and so concentrated that the animal can eat them very rapidly. This could prevent him from mixing the grain with enough saliva, possibly leading to colic.

FEED SUPPLEMENTS

Calf Manna (The Carnation Company, Milling Division, Los Angeles, California) is an example of a commonly used feed supplement. It is a mixture of vitamins and minerals in a milk-product base which gives more fats and more B vitamins than are found in most feeds. This product was designed as a feed for small calves who are taken off milk, or in addition to milk. However, it has come to be used for young horses who are in need of extra nutrition. It is also a good supplement for older horses who are thin or ill and need extra-good quality feed. Give 1 cup once or twice a day to a thin adult horse (see Thin Horse). Feeding an excess of Calf Manna or similar products to young horses may cause epiphysitis (inflammation of the growth centers of the long bones) if it results in a vitamin or mineral imbalance when added to the rest of the animal's ration.

Molasses is a common feed component and is used in nearly every commercial grain mixture available. It may be made from either sugar cane or sugar beets; both have the same feeding value. It is tasty and is often used to help make feed palatable. Some horses, however, seem to prefer feed without molasses. Molasses reduces the dust and helps bind the vitamin and mineral additives to the grain so that they do not all end up in the bottom of the feed bin. Unfortunately, molasses may occasionally be used to make poor-quality grain attractive to the animal. It is slightly laxative. As a source of energy, molasses should not generally exceed 10% of the concentrate ration. In hot, humid climates, large quantities of molasses may cause the feed to become wet and mold easily; less of it should be used in the grain mixture in these areas.

Soybean meal is one of the best sources of protein. It is especially well digested by foals and young horses. It is added to grain mixtures to raise their protein content.

Cottonseed meal and linseed (flaxseed) meal are often used in horse feeds as protein supplements. The oils (fats) which they contain are helpful to the animal's coat. In large amounts, they may cause digestive disturbances. Linseed meal is well accepted by horses. It is often used in a pelleted form to avoid dustiness. Excessive quantities of linseed meal may be laxative, limiting the amount which can be fed. If too much linseed meal is given to a pregnant mare, she may produce so much milk that her udder becomes tight and she will not allow the foal to nurse. Why? Her udder hurts.

An old-time method for feeding linseed was to buy flaxseed at the drugstore and put a handful in a teacup. Cover it with water and let it set overnight. Then, pour the mixture over the morning grain. This was given two or three times a week to improve the horse's coat. (10)

Cottonseed meal is not very palatable and must be mixed with grain which the animal likes. Otherwise, its value and use is similar to linseed meal.

Peanut meal is occasionally used in the United States for protein supplementation in horse rations. It is commonly used in some foreign countries. It is high in fat and becomes rancid easily; for this reason, it should only be fed fresh and should be carefully stored in a cool, well-ventilated area. Because of this problem, it is not a good feed for young growing horses. It is very palatable. Peanut hulls are sometimes used as a component of pelleted feed, to provide roughage.

Sunflower meal may be fed as a protein supplement. It is low in lysine (an essential amino acid) and for this reason should be fed as only a limited part of the ration. It should only be fed to older animals until experimental results confirm its usefulness for foals and young growing horses.

Fish meal is a good quality protein supplement. If it contains too much bone and fish heads, it will be lower in protein value, although still a valuable source of minerals. Meat meal is sometimes used in horse rations and may be a good quality source of protein, as is meat and bone meal.

Dried skim milk is both palatable and digestible. It contains lactose, which is the best source of carbohydrates for young horses. The protein which it contains is of very high quality and it is rich in vitamins and minerals. High price usually limits skim milk as a protein supplement for horses. It is often used in milk replacers and in foal rations to supplement mare's milk. It is also used as a base for some vitamin and coat supplements.

Protein blocks are often valuable as pasture supplements when the pasture is turned brown by drought or freezing. Brown pasture has a lower protein content and many of the vitamins are no longer present in adequate amounts. These blocks supplement protein and vitamin A, in a grain base. They come in 50-lb. units, the size of a salt block. They can be fed free-choice, in a sheltered place so that rain or snow do not damage them. It is best to keep them up off the ground as they absorb moisture from the soil and you'll lose part of the block.

Root crops such as carrots and turnips make good variety feed for horses. In general, a pound or two per day are the maximum that should be fed. Excessive quantities may cause colic and other digestive problems. Potatoes make good horse feed, but may cause indigestion if fed raw and in large quantities. They are best steamed or boiled if you are feeding large amounts. Horses often enjoy apples as a treat, and animals who are pastured in orchards may eat large numbers of apples. Some horses like cucumbers or watermelon, as well as many other vegetables and fruits. As with any unusual feedstuff, moderation is the key word to feeding these materials. Also, be sure your horse chews his food because swallowing chunks of these items can cause choke.

Citrus pulp is a common feed in some parts of the country, and is a good addition to horse rations. This is the pulp and seeds which are left after oranges and grapefruit are pressed for juice. It is a bulky feed containing much fiber, and a good energy source. It may be fed up to one-quarter of the ration of mature animals, but should be used in lesser amounts for young, growing horses. Molasses may be added to rations containing large amounts of citrus pulp to improve their palatability. Beet pulp may be fed in the same manner as citrus pulp.

Gelatin has been recommended by some owners and trainers as stimulating hoof growth. Two experiments have been conducted which found no benefit from feeding it. These were fed up to ¼ lb. per day experimentally, which should be enough to show results if it were going to work. (11)

Materials such as sunflower and almond hulls and apple skins may be used as feeds, especially if they are incorporated into a pelleted feed. Ground corrugated paper boxes and corn cobs have also been used in the same way.

Corn oil can be a valuable supplement to add calories to the diet while allowing a decrease in the amount of grain fed. This reduces the chance of founder and digestive upsets that can occur when feeding a large amount of grain. Feeds high in oil content are being given to endurance horses who cannot eat enough grain to supply their bodily needs. High-oil feeds would probably also be valuable for the older horse or animal with bad teeth who cannot eat enough grain to stay in good condition. It is

also very helpful for putting a gleaming, shiny coat on a horse, especially for show purposes. (12)

BRAN

Bran is the name given to the coarse outer coatings of grains. Wheat bran (sometimes called red bran) is most common in the United States, although other types of bran, such as rice bran, may occasionally be fed. Wheat bran is most popular among horsemen. It is highly palatable, although horses not accustomed to it may need to be started on it gradually to acquire a taste for it. It has a mild laxative effect and helps to stimulate the digestive tract by adding bulk and holding water. It is high in protein, averaging 16%.

Owners should add approximately one to four cups of bran to a horse's diet daily, mixing it with the grain. One well-known horseman and writer, Louis Taylor, wrote that he fed his horses a two-pound coffee can of bran twice a day. (13) The amount needed will vary with the individual animal, the type of feed, and other factors. Add enough so that the manure is just softly formed into lumps. This use of bran helps to prevent many of the colic problems that go along with confining a horse and feeding what are, to him, largely artificial feedstuffs. This, along with a religiously regular worming program, helps many horses who are prone to chronic colic. Some horse owners who keep horses in sandy corrals or pastures feed bran regularly to help prevent sand colic.

Small amounts of bran may be fed dry, mixed with the grain ration. It often helps the animal to eat more slowly and chew more thoroughly. This is good for horses who tend to colic because they do not chew their food thoroughly. Larger amounts of bran should be dampened to prevent it from balling up in the esophagus and causing a choke.

Bran may also be fed as a mash; this is good to give to a mare who has just foaled. Many horsemen use it for hard-working horses who are normally fed large amounts of grain daily. They give it on days when the animal is not worked, to help prevent colic and "Monday morning sickness." This is most usually seen with draft horses who are worked hard, and race or endurance horses in hard training. A bran mash is sometimes helpful in mild cases of colic, if you cannot get veterinary help. It is good for animals with mild constipation. It can also be given to horses who are going to be shipped long distances, to help prevent digestive problems.

Make the mash by measuring two to two and a half gallons of bran into a large bucket or pan. Add enough boiling water to make it moist, stirring as you add it. Place a cloth or cover over the container, allowing it to steam. Feed when the mash is lukewarm or cool. Or, you can just mix in enough cold water to make a mixture the consistency of moist sawdust. Years ago, it was thought that the steaming released nutrients; this has been disproven.

Bran, in any form, has a large amount of readily available nutrients, and the steaming is not necessary to make them usable. It does, however, make large quantities of bran palatable. If you've seen bran, you know that it strongly resembles dry feathers. It would be difficult for a horse to feel like eating a gallon or two of it, dry! Bran mash should always be prepared fresh and fed as soon as it has cooled. If allowed to stand for a period of time and become sour, it may produce a serious colic.

An excess of bran may be harmful, causing a problem known as "bran disease," "miller's disease," and "big-head." These are common names for a problem called nutritional hyperparathyroidism. Because there is too little calcium in the blood when the animal is fed large quantities of bran, the parathyroid glands secrete excess hormone. This, in turn, causes removal of calcium from the animal's bones to supply the needs of his blood. This removal of bone calcium leads to an enlarged head, thus the name "big-head." In addition to the gross signs seen on the animal's head, there may be degeneration of joint cartilage and tearing of ligaments from their attachment to the bone. These can result in obscure lamenesses. Beware of feeding too much bran without other compensating, calcium-rich feeds, such as alfalfa hay.

UREA

Urea is a nitrogen-rich compound which is often used in cattle feed and occasionally for horse feed. One pound of urea is equivalent to nearly three pounds of protein. Bacteria in the caecum of the horse use the urea to manufacture protein which is then used by the horse.

Research at Colorado State University has shown that urea is utilized by older horses for maintenance. It is less well utilized by foals and young growing horses. Mature horses have been tested with up to a half pound of urea in their daily ration. Urea was once thought to be toxic to horses, but now appears to be tolerated by grown animals in moderate amounts. Colorado State University's research has also indicated that feeding range protein blocks (normally used for cattle) to broodmares caused no ill effects on mares or their foals. This should decrease the concern of owners who run horses and cattle together and use feeds containing urea for the cattle.

Urea can be toxic to the horse if fed in abnormally large amounts. If you are feeding grain with urea mixed into it, make sure that the urea is well distributed throughout the mixture and that no lumps are present. Silage which has been treated with urea should probably not be fed to horses because of the chance that the animal may get an excessive concentration of the substance at any one feeding.

Young foals may be susceptible to urea toxicity; for this reason, it is best not to use feedstuffs containing urea for anything but mature horses. It should not be fed to young animals or valuable horses until further research is done on its utilization and safety. (14)

VITAMINS

Additional vitamins are generally unnecessary if the horse is getting an otherwise adequate diet. They are also not needed if the animal is getting a good-quality complete grain mixture. Additional vitamin A is needed in many northern states in the spring by horses who are fed only hay or pasture. By late winter to early spring, the alfalfa or grass is bleached to a very light color, indicating that most of the vitamin A has leached out. This can lead to skin problems (especially decreased resistance to ringworm), reproductive problems (subfertile stallions, mares who refuse to come into heat), and foals born with inadequate stores of this essential vitamin. These animals need a vitamin A supplement, which is best fed with a bit of grain. Vitamin supplementation should also be used if recommended by your veterinarian for some special problem. Other than these applications, much of the money spent for vitamin supplements is spent unnecessarily.

Just because a little of a vitamin is good does not necessarily mean that a lot is better. Excess doses of vitamin D, for instance, can lead to mineralization of the heart and blood vessels, as well as ossification of other soft tissues. If the problem is not immediately fatal, some animals may recover; recovery is likely to be prolonged, taking six months or more. (15) Large excesses of vitamin A may cause poor growth, hair loss, signs of nervous system problems, anemia, and liver dysfunction. Bone problems may also develop. Excess vitamin A is often incriminated in problems such as epiphysitis. (16)

Conversely, one study found that National Research Council (NRC) recommendations, which are used by many people as standards, may actually recommend too little vitamin A for growing horses. The NRC recommends approximately 20 International Units of vitamin A per lb. of body weight per day. This study recommended between 2 and 5 times that amount, but NO more than 100 I.U. per lb. body weight. (17)

MINERALS

Additional phosphorus is needed in certain parts of the United States. The mountain states east of the Rockies, extending in a belt from Mexico to the Canadian border, and the Basin States of Idaho, Nevada, and Utah, are generally short on phosphorus. Lack of this mineral often results in foals who are born with extremely weak and crooked legs, and in mares who fail to come into heat and breed properly. Phosphorus supplementation may also be needed when animals are fed large amounts of alfalfa hay, which can be very high in calcium. Dietary calcium and phosphorus interact in that an excess of one can lead to a functional deficiency of the other.

Selenium is a mineral which may cause problems in either excess or deficiency. If too much is present (as with certain poisonous plants), selenium toxicity may occur. If there is not enough, a selenium deficiency may cause a problem called "white muscle disease." This is a muscular dystrophy seen in young foals, especially in the eastern United States. Foals with white muscle disease are weak and reluctant to move. When they do move, their gait is often stiff and stilted. They may have muscle tremors while standing. The muscles may appear swollen and feel hard or rubbery when palpated. The inability to move and suckle the mare may literally lead to starvation. The temperature may be elevated, as well as the pulse and respiratory rate. Muscle damage may cause the urine to appear brownish, much like a horse with azoturia. The foal may die because of damage to the muscle of the heart.

If a dead foal is examined, the muscles may be gray or white, and will look more like fish than horseflesh. Treatment is to inject a vitamin E and selenium mixture. This is given intramuscularly. Or, a similar compound can be given to the foal as a drench, mixed with a little water. Supplementing the mare prior to foaling may not be enough to prevent the problem in severely deficient areas. Selenium supplementation is also used for horses who exhibit azoturia or tying-up (see Azoturia).

Iodine is another mineral which may cause problems in areas where it is deficient, such as the northern United States. Lack of it may cause goiter, especially in foals. In some cases, goiter can occur because certain plants being fed to the horse tie up the available iodine. Cabbage-family plants, including brussel sprouts, kale, etc., can cause this problem. Animals who are fed these should have extra iodine supplementation. Young animals are most susceptible to iodine deficiency, although reproductive problems may be seen in mares who are short of it. Iodine is also considered necessary for disease resistance. Feeding iodized salt is enough to take care of most animal's needs in iodine-deficient areas.

For some reason, an excess of iodine can also cause goiter. This problem is said to be most commonly seen when animals are fed kelp, especially if it is used in addition to other sources of iodine.

Some people like to set out trace mineralized salt blocks. These are made for cattle, and are so hard and rough that many (perhaps most) horses will not voluntarily eat them. Indeed, some animals will not lick them even when they are starving for minerals or salt. The only good way to put out minerals for horses seems to be loose, in a small box.

For large pastures, feeders are available with a hood over them. These have a weathervane-sort of top so that they swivel away from storms to keep the contents dry. They mount conveniently on top of a piece of pipe. If the animal is in a stall, a small box can be placed in one corner. The animal can then be offered one or more trace mineral/salt mixtures, allowing him to make a choice.

SALT

Salt is a mineral (containing sodium and chlorine), but is discussed separately because of its extreme importance to the horse. Horses doing hard work may lose several ounces of salt per day in their sweat. In hot weather, the animal may lose the same amount while doing nothing. This can lead to fatigue and exhaustion. Mares who are lactating heavily also have a great need for salt. Lack of salt will eventually lead to decreased milk production. Salt helps to increase feed palatability and utilization. Inadequate salt may result in a decreased growth rate.

Many horses won't eat anything but plain iodized salt, and will ignore other "flavors" completely. If your horse will not lick a salt block, put a small box or bin in one corner of the stall, and offer loose, granular salt. Some animals will readily eat salt with trace minerals when it is offered loose, but they may continue to refuse it if it is offered in blocks. This is a good way to get trace minerals into your horse. Horses should have salt available, free choice, at all times, in a form they will eat.

Salt poisoning may occur if horses are starved for salt, and then allowed free access to it, especially if they do not have adequate water at the same time. Signs may include colic, frequent urination, diarrhea, staggering, and weakness. Paralysis of the hind legs may be seen. If your horse has been without salt for a long time, start him back on limited salt intake for a few days and gradually get back to free choice. (18)

WATER

It may seem odd to list water as a nutrient, but it is of the utmost importance to good food utilization and good health. Horses need a constant supply of reasonably pure water at all times, not just once or twice a day. While animals can often drink water that humans would not consider suitable, there are some kinds that are harmful.

Much alkali water in the western United States contains selenium. If this mineral is taken in excessive amounts, it will cause the mane and tail to fall out and the hooves to fall off. Water which leaches through mine tailings may have a very high content of some toxic minerals such as arsenic. Nitrate is not usually a problem in horse water. Nitrites in large quantity, however, may tie up hemoglobin in the blood, resulting in rapid death. Low levels of nitrite may be associated with infertility and late-term abortions in mares, and poor growth rate in young animals. (19)

In some areas, highly mineralized water will cause a

chronic colic and diarrhea in horses. These problems will stop as soon as pure water is hauled to them. This has been seen in a well that was surrounded by wells which were not causing horses any harm. So, do not assume that because your neighbor's horses have no problems with water, it will not cause trouble for your animals. If in doubt about your water, call your city, county, or state health department. They will tell you where you can get the water tested. Be sure when you send in the sample to let them know that it is being used to water horses.

An adult horse may drink as little as five gallons a day, especially if the weather is cold. Ten gallons a day is about average, and in hot weather, he may consume much more. The amount consumed in cold weather may not be sufficient to prevent colic and other digestive problems. The water should be heated by a tank heater if at all possible (see Winter Care). It need not be hot; 40 to 55 degrees is warm enough. Horses will drink more of the warmed water, resulting in better feed efficiency and fewer colics and digestive problems.

If a thirsty horse is watered right after he has eaten, this may wash much of the stomach contents into the small intestine before they have had time to become properly mixed with digestive juices. This causes a loss of nutrients; it may also result in indigestion, colic, or founder. Water a thirsty horse, then allow a half hour to an hour before giving him his feed. Of course, the horse should be thoroughly cooled before he is watered to avoid these problems. Give him a few sips of water at a time until he is completely cooled.

WOOD CHEWING

Some horses chew on any wood around their corral or stall. This must be differentiated from cribbing. Cribbing involves a whole ritual of movements, including sucking in air as the animal cribs. Wood-chewing does not involve this sequence of actions; it merely tears up barns and corrals. Begin prevention by feeding the animal a good salt and trace mineral mix, free choice. This cures the problem with animals who are chewing because they are deficient in salt or minerals. Changing the ration to include more hay may sometimes stop the wood chewing because the horse chews all he wants to while eating.

Next, consider boredom as a cause of the problem. A companion (such as another horse or goat) may stop the chewing. More exercise or riding may give the horse some variety in his world. In some animals, this is probably a bad habit (much like humans chewing their fingernails). It may be almost impossible to cure. In addition, one wood chewer in the stable may teach it to the others. At this point, investigate painting a repellent substance on all wood surfaces or replacing wooden fencing with woven wire or metal fencing. In some cases, these are the only possible cures, short of selling the horse.

THE DIGESTIVE SYSTEM

The structure of the horse's digestive system determines how he digests feed, so it will be discussed here, before we go into more details about methods of horse feeding.

The digestive system begins with the horse's large, sensitive lips, which gather food and help bring it into the mouth. If the food is grass or other pasture, it is mowed with a combination of shearing action of the incisor teeth and pulling action of the lips. The tongue helps move the food back into the mouth, between the molar teeth which will grind it. Saliva from salivary glands (the largest of which is behind the jaw, below the ear) is added to the food and mixed with it. This helps to provide lubrication when the food is swallowed into the esophagus, as well as adding enzymes which begin to digest the food.

The muscular action of the pharynx forces the ball (or bolus) of food into the esophagus. The pharynx has a trapdoor action so that the food cannot return through the mouth. This is why a horse who vomits will have food coming out his nose. An animal who is choked by a blockage of the esophagus will have food, saliva, or water running from his nostrils for the same reason. The palate also effectively prevents the horse from breathing through his mouth. The swallowed food is forced down the esophagus to the stomach by progressive waves of muscle contraction around the esophagus.

Large pills (also called boluses) should not be given to horses because of the danger they may become lodged in the esophagus and destroy the lining of this tube before they can be noticed or removed, thus leading to scarring after the animal heals. This scarring leaves a constricted spot when the scar shrinks, and the animal may choke more easily in the future.

The horse has a very small stomach, with only a one- to four-gallon capacity in the mature animal. Contrast that with the cow: a cow's rumen (only one of its FOUR stomachs) may hold as much as 50 to 60 gallons of feed at a time! Overall, the horse's digestive system is more nearly like that of a pig than like that of the ruminants.

Food passes through the horse's stomach quickly, and not much digestion takes place there. The site where the esophagus enters the stomach and the place where the small intestine leaves it are fairly close together. For this reason, water passes quickly through the stomach and small intestine to the large intestine and caecum. By comparison, not only does the cow store food in her 55-gallon drum-sized stomach, but she later regurgitates it at her leisure and rechews it before sending it on to the second stomach—we call this "chewing her cud." With such a small stomach, the horse is frequently hungry. Given a choice, he will eat small amounts nearly 24 hours a day.

As the horse eats, the partially digested food passes into the small intestine in a continuous stream. During a large meal, the stomach may be serially filled and emptied as much as three times. This rapid passage means that the feed will have limited contact with the enzymes and acids secreted by the stomach lining, resulting in inefficient digestion. The emptying process is slower when the animal stops eating.

Hydrochloric acid is added in the stomach to help digest food. A digestive enzyme called pepsin is also added here; it acts on the protein in the food, starting to break it down. A small amount of the nutrients in the feed are absorbed in the stomach, but for the most part, digestion in the stomach is limited and is preparatory to more complete digestion in the intestines.

If the horse does not have water available all the time, he should be watered before eating. If he is watered on a full stomach, much of the material in it may be washed into the small intestine without being adequately digested. For this reason, it is also advisable to feed some hay before giving the animal his grain, so that it will remain in the stomach longer to allow more complete digestion.

The small intestine is 60 to 100 feet long, and only holds 10 to 12 gallons. It is about two inches in diameter. The food material here is very fluid and passes through quickly. Here, bile, which is secreted by the liver, is added, as well as enzymes from the pancreas.

The fermentation which breaks down the cellulose in the roughage the horse has eaten takes place in the large intestine. Most of the absorption of nutrients from the food mass also takes place here. The large intestine is divided into the caecum, large colon, small colon, rectum, and anus. The caecum is a long pouch that holds 4 to 8 gallons. It is about four feet long. The large colon is about 12 feet long and holds 12 to 20 gallons.

In these two compartments of the digestive tract, bacteria digest cellulose. The horse cannot utilize the food value of the cellulose directly. The numerous bacteria in these areas of the digestive tract break down the cellulose. The horse then absorbs the smaller chemical components produced by the bacteria, as well as breaking down and digesting large numbers of the bacteria themselves.

Keeping these bacteria happy is a key component of good horse nutrition. In fact, it might be useful to think in terms of "feeding the bacteria" rather than "feeding the horse." The balance of particular types of bacteria in the digestive tract varies with the kinds and amounts of feed

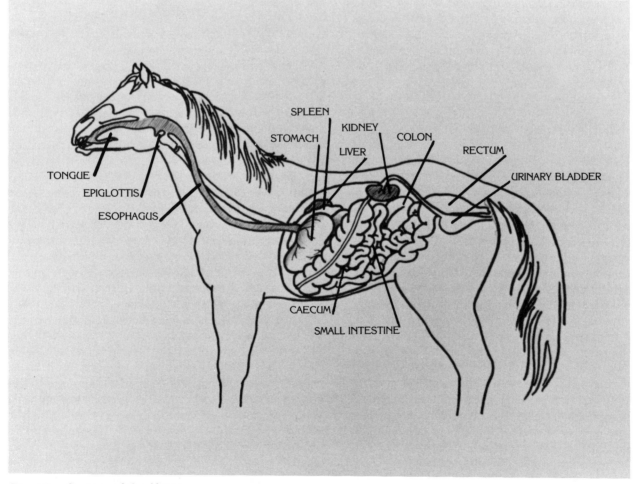

Digestive System of the Horse.

being given the animal. When the type of feed or the relative percentage of a given feed component is changed, the numbers of each type must be adjusted to digest the new ration. This is why gradual changes are so important in the horse's diet.

The small colon is 10 to 12 feet long and about four inches in diameter. This is where water is removed from the waste material and the balls of manure are formed. The rectum is the last part of the digestive tract, about 12 inches long. It extends from the colon to the anus, which is the end opening of the digestive tract.

WHEN TO FEED

We have just discussed the fact that the horse has a very small stomach for his size, and that digestion is more efficient when the stomach is not completely full. Overloading the horse's stomach not only makes digestion less productive, but may put pressure on the diaphragm, making breathing difficult. Because of their small stomachs and normal eating habits, horses get hungry frequently, just as we do. Horses in nature, when left to themselves, graze day and night, continuously putting small amounts of food into their systems. The closer you can come to what fits the horse in the wild, the fewer digestive problems your horse will have.

Horses who are fed once a day tend to get too hungry. When finally fed, they eat too rapidly and may also overeat, resulting in colic and other digestive problems. Excessively irregular feeding schedules may give the same difficulties. Twice a day is the absolute minimum for feeding the confined horse. Three times a day is even better—this procedure is followed in many show and racing stables. Trainers who are trying to maximize the animal's efficiency and yet avoid problems with colic or founder may even feed four times a day. This technique is also used by owners of young show horses who are trying to avoid digestive problems. A horse will gain more weight on less feed when he is fed more frequently because of the greater digestive efficiency.

The horse should be fed a portion of hay at each feeding. His grain ration is divided among the feedings so that it will not overload the animal's stomach with a large amount of rich food at any one time. Feed hay first, then give the grain an hour or so later.

FEEDING SCHEDULES

Some horsemen and nutritionists recommend that two daily feedings be spaced exactly twelve hours apart. While this may be ideal, feeding on so rigid a schedule can lead to riot and sedition in the horse barn if you are not there on time. Some horses who are always fed at the same time become so accustomed to the routine that they kick the barn door or paw the corral panels if they are not fed precisely on time. This can lead to costly repairs, both to the facilities and to the animal who cuts his foot or otherwise injures himself while carrying on in this manner.

Your schedule may not allow you to always be at home at a certain time. Therefore, feed within a range approximately 12 hours apart—say, between 6:00 and 7:30 in the morning and again between 6 and 8 in the evening. Keeping the animals on a slightly less regimented schedule will not normally cause colic or other digestive problems, and will result in a quieter, less impatient bunch of horses.

And what if you are going to be late for feeding time? If you know in advance, it's easy to premeasure the animal's grain and set it in a safe place (where the horses cannot get it before feeding time). Also, break off the amount of hay that you want the animal to have. This makes it easy to call a friend or neighbor—even one who knows absolutely nothing about horses—and have them dump the animal's feed into the feeder. If you end up getting home on time anyway, that feeding is ready to be fed.

Some horses who have problems with chronic colic benefit by being kept on a very rigid time schedule. One client has a stallion who invariably colics if she is late in feeding him. If you have an animal with chronic colic, a strict schedule might be worth a try.

What about the horse on pasture? It is usually best if he is left free to graze day and night, as is natural for the beast in the wild. The exception to this is when the heat during the day is extreme, or insects are annoying the horse. In this case, you may wish to bring the horse into a confined paddock or barn during the day.

WORKING AFTER MEALS

Do not work the animal hard immediately after a meal. His stomach and intestines are filled with food and water, requiring more space than before feeding. This extra space is gained by slightly filling out the abdomen, and by the stomach bulging forward against the diaphragm. This reduces the size of the thoracic cavity, and may prevent the lungs from expanding as fully as they normally would. This may cause labored breathing and considerable discomfort.

Working the animal hard shortly after feeding may also interfere with digestion. Blood which would have normally have gone to the digestive tract is shunted to the muscles, slowing the intestinal motions and reducing the amount of digestive secretions which are produced. This can result in colic or impaction, and will also result in loss of nutrients.

FEEDING THE TIRED HORSE

Do not feed a horse right after he has been worked, especially if he is tired. His muscles have been working hard, and much of the body's blood is in them. This leaves less blood to produce digestive enzymes. In addition, hard exercise causes an actual shutdown of part of the blood flow to the digestive tract, making it much less efficient and more prone to colic, founder, and other upsets.

Give the exhausted horse small amounts of water (eight to ten sips) every five minutes or so, until the animal is thoroughly cooled out and no longer thirsty. Then, give him a small quantity of hay and let him eat it. An hour or so later, feed the rest of his hay. After he has finished that hay (and only then), feed his grain ration.

This delay gives the animal time to relax and rest a bit before he has to cope with digesting feed as rich as grain. It gets his saliva flowing so that by the time the grain is fed, it will be well mixed with it. This helps avoid impactions caused by eating large amounts of grain and NOT mixing them well with saliva. It also puts the grain on top of a good feeding of hay, thus diluting it so that it does not arrive in the intestines all in one concentrated mass as it would if the animal ate it before eating the hay. All of these things help to avoid digestive problems.

If a horse has been off feed for more than a day, whether due to lack of communication between those who are feeding him or because of illness, put him back on full feed gradually. As usual in problem cases, give good-quality hay first, and worry about grain later, after the animal's digestive tract is working normally.

If the animal has also been short of water, by all means do not allow him to drink all that he wants. Allow eight to ten swallows, and then give the same amount every five to ten minutes. When the animal's thirst is quenched and he is no longer desperate, you can allow him water, free choice.

HOW TO FEED

There are as many schools of thought on methods of feeding horses as there are horsemen doing the feeding. Feeding the roughage portion of the diet on the ground is considered by many to be the most natural way. However, this allows the animal to re-infest himself with worms from the manure that is invariably dropped in the area. In sandy areas, the animal may eat small amounts of sand with the feed. Over a period of time, this can lead to a severe or possibly fatal sand colic.

It is generally best to feed hay from some sort of feeder to avoid waste, and to keep the horse from soiling the hay, either by dropping manure on it, or by trampling it into the dirt of the corral. Wall-mounted hay racks are good. They should not be so high that the animal has to reach far above his normal head position to eat. This results in hay leaves falling into the horse's eyes, with subsequent ulcers or eye infection. It's also uncomfortable. It is good to have a pan under this type of feeder so that hay leaves fall into it, and can be eaten from there.

Otherwise, the animal pulls out what hay he can and drops the rest, including many of the leaves, on the ground. He then picks the rest of his meal from the ground, which is what you were trying to avoid in the first place.

Large tires, fitted with plywood bottoms (bolted on for safety), make good horse feeders. They enable the animal to take his food from ground level, as the horse eats in the wild. Hay racks with a bottom tray may be used for feeding several animals. All feeders should be checked for safety. They should have rounded corners, with no protruding edges or bolts to catch and tear the horse's hide. Any openings should be small enough that the animal cannot get his head through. Hay may be fed from a large wooden box.

Do not make a hay-feeding enclosure too tight. One horse owner had a horse who tore his hay from the rack, tossing his head violently, and spread hay all over the place. He built a large, hooded manger that came around the horse's head. It prevented the animal from wasting hay. However, it held all the dust and mold in around the animal's nose (and there is a little, even in the cleanest of hay), and caused the animal to acquire a severe case of heaves.

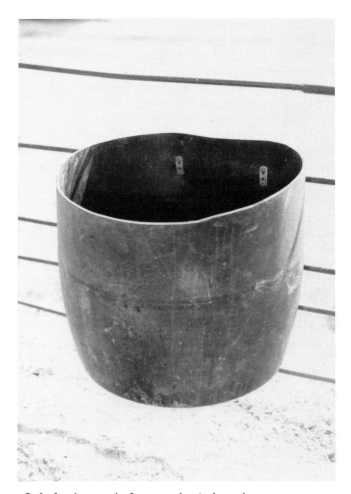

Safe feeder made from a plastic barrel.

Make sure there is adequate feeder space or enough feeders if horses are fed in a group. You may find that one horse bullies the others, or that one horse is consistently driven out of the group, thus not getting enough food. If this happens, simple stalls (or dividers) with a manger in the front and shields to keep the horses from stealing each other's food may solve the problem easily and inexpensively. Put a chain or butt bar behind each one, and shut the animals in while they eat so that none can steal the other's food. After a few weeks, if the animals eat quietly and finish about the same time, they may be fed without shutting them in, allowing them to leave when they are finished. The animals will become accustomed to their own stalls and will automatically go to them if you use the same one for the same horse every time.

If you are feeding hay to pastured horses, and cannot set up a feeding stall arrangement, feed the hay in flakes thrown AT LEAST 20 to 30 feet from each other. The farther apart you can space them, the less likely the bully is to run another horse off and take his hay. The hay may be scattered in separate flakes, throwing out twice as many portions as there are horses. Again, this helps to allow the shy horses to get their share by having a flake left somewhere when a bully runs them off.

Clean snow is ideal for sanitation, whether you are feeding hay or grain. Move the feeding area to another part of the pasture when it becomes soiled with manure. This also helps to spread wear and tear from the horse's weight on the vegetation beneath the snow.

When traveling, hay nets are a convenient way to feed horses. This way, there is a clean place to put their hay even if you are stuck stabling them in dirty quarters. Hay nets are also useful for feeding horses who are tied to a trailer. Be sure to tie the hay net HIGH—even perhaps higher than you would put a normal hay feeder—because the net will sag as it empties. Many horses habitually paw at them with their front feet. A combination of a low hay net and a pawing horse frequently spells disaster. Because of this danger, it is not a good idea to use hay nets to feed horses in a normal stable situation. There are fewer hazards and fewer problems with good quality, carefully planned, hay feeders.

Grain should also be fed from a feeder or container. This may be anything from the tire feeder or bottom pan of a hay feeder to a bucket or pan. As with any other feeder, it should have rounded edges and be safe. The horse should not be able to get his head or halter caught on it. Grain may be fed to numbers of horses by hanging buckets on a chain link or wooden fence. As with hay feeding, these must be spaced as far apart as possible to avoid fighting.

WATERING THE HORSE

Horses need a constant supply of clean, fresh water. A stream or river source should be checked to see that there are no minerals or contaminants which may be harmful to the horse. Ask your county health department where you can send a sample for analysis. Automatic waterers are good if they are checked daily to see that they are working. It is easy to forget them because they are supposed to be automatic. With them, it is impossible to tell how much water a horse is drinking. For the sick horse, it is often best to shut off the waterer and water the horse with a bucket so you can tell if he is drinking and exactly how much. Water buckets should be securely fastened to a wall or fence so that they cannot be tipped. They collect less dirt if fastened about chest level to the animal. Also, the animal cannot paw the bucket or put his foot into it at this height.

Galvanized tanks or old bathtubs are commonly used for water containers. They grow algae badly and should be dumped and scrubbed frequently, especially in summer. A new toilet brush or broom makes a handy cleaning tool which can be used with household cleaner or disinfectant to get out the dirt. Be sure to rinse well after scrubbing to get out all traces of cleaner.

In summer, tanks may be filled according to their size and the number of animals using them. For instance, a large tank used by two horses may be filled only half full. This way, the animals have drunk it nearly down by the time it has become dirty with algae and the dirt which has blown in. The next time you fill it, dump it and clean it well. When done at every filling, this is usually enough to keep the tank clean and water fresh. Extremely large tanks which cannot be dumped for cleaning should have drains. In some cases, a couple of goldfish or carp may help keep the tank clean by eating some of the algae which grows. Besides, if you have a little time in an otherwise busy schedule of caring for your horse, goldfish are pleasing to watch.

WOLFING FEED

If the horse bolts his grain rapidly, one cure is to put large (5 or 6 inches and bigger) smooth rocks or chunks of block salt in the bottom on a large feeder. The animal must nose around the stones to get his feed, thus slowing eating down to a more reasonable rate. The grain may be fed spread over a large area in the feeder (not on the ground) so that the horse cannot get large mouthfuls. Coarsely chopped hay may be added to the grain to slow his eating. Feeding ear corn so that the animal has to chew it off the cob can also be helpful. It is especially important to feed the entire hay or roughage ration first to one of these animals. Only after he has finished should he be fed his grain. This may mean two trips to the barn, but it may save the animal from a colic or worse.

FEEDING WHEN CAMPING WITH HORSES

If you are feeding grain without a feeder, put it on top of a flake of hay to help keep the horse from having to eat it off the ground. When camping with horses, nosebags are ideal grain feeders. Some horsemen recommend using them to help get shy horses to come to you. Begin with the horse in a corral and put a nosebag on him with some grain in it. Wait for him to eat it, and then approach him to remove it. The theory is that in learning to come to you to get the nosebag off, the horse associates you with feed and learns to come under all circumstances.

If you are camping with horses and find yourself without a nosebag, you can feed grain off the top of a saddle blanket, holding the horse by the lead rope until he has finished the meal. Be sure that you put the grain on the TOP of the blanket, leaving the horse-side down. Otherwise, grains may catch in the fibers and irritate the animal's back when the blanket is used the next day. The blanket must be brushed clean of sticks, twigs, and grain the next morning before use. Flat rocks also make good grain feeders. The point is, keep the grain off the ground.

FINDING PASTURE

Locating good pasture for your horse may be quite a project, especially if you live close to a large city. Begin by finding people whom you trust. The pasture may be nothing more than a vacant lot but the owner should be someone in whom you have confidence. Limited access by other people to the pasture is a plus. While it may be inconvenient to go through someone's yard to get in to feed or ride your horse, by the same token, it gives your animal extra security. Someone trying to steal the animal would have to go through the same efforts to get him out. In addition, having someone who will keep an eye on the animal, even if they do not know much about horses, is preferable to having the animal unwatched. It's even better if you can find someone who knows horses and is more likely to call you if they think the animal is ill or injured.

Fences should be horse-tight and safe. It is, of course, ideal if they are made of something besides barbed wire. Chain link, woven wire, wood, or some other material is much less likely to inflict damage upon your animal. The pasture should be free from trash, such as old cars or loose wire, on which your horse may get injured. Other hazards may go along with trash. The horse may become poisoned by chewing on an old car battery or getting into a pesticide can that has been discarded. It is well worth spending time to clean up the pasture yourself if it is satisfactory otherwise.

If you are boarding the horse in a common pasture with many other people's horses, look at the other animals in the field; are they mares or geldings or a mix of everything? Has someone left a two-year stud colt in there, uncut and ready to breed your prized mare? Any time you put a new animal in a pasture, there will be some kicking and biting and fighting while the animals determine the new pecking order. In a pasture with little turnover (no new animals being introduced), the animals get their differ-

ences worked out, and all know where they fit in the ranks with a minimum of problems.

In a pasture where new animals are constantly being added, the horses never seem to completely settle down. In one of these pastures, your horse may always be a mass of kicks and bites. Horses in these pastures are more prone to other injuries, too. It is not uncommon for a nasty horse to drive a more timid one into a fence or even through it, resulting in a severe wire cut. It is often worth paying a premium to keep your horse in a pasture with a smaller number of animals and less turnover.

Be sure that there are not so many animals on the pasture that all the good feed is eaten and the animals are left with weeds or, worse yet, poisonous plants. One client had a horse boarded in a pasture that had been eaten down to the bare dirt. A careful search found one dandelion that the horses had missed—in approximately 40 acres! What was left was a poisonous plant called Russian knapweed. It, like most poisonous plants, is something that most normal, well-fed horses will not eat. When there was nothing left, the animals began to eat it. Two of the horses suffered severe brain damage before their owners discovered what was happening. These horses had to be euthanized; the damage was permanent and there was no chance of recovery.

Check on the other horse owners. Are they conscientious about worming and other care? If they are not, you would be advised to look elsewhere for pasture.

The cheapest pasture may cost the most in the long run. If you are not familiar with what good pasture should look like, ask a horseman friend to check it with you. You may be able to get someone from the county agricultural agent's office to look it over. They will usually do this at no charge. Or, how about getting a high school or college botany, range management, or agriculture teacher to take a look at it? It is much better to be safe than sorry.

Shade is needed to protect pastured horses in hot climates. Shelter can make a big difference in how your horse comes through the winter and how much feed he needs to do it in colder areas. Good water is an absolute necessity. Be aware that in some areas, running streams dry up in the summer and may leave your horse without any water at all. In some areas, horse owners commonly haul water to dry pastures with tanks on small trailers or in the back of a pickup. Decide whether this extra bother will make up for the lesser price that you will pay for such a pasture.

If the pasture is green and lush, accustom the horse to the fresh new feed over a period of days. If it is dry and cured out, as it will be in the northern areas in the fall, you may be safe in just turning the horse out after a morning feeding of hay.

HOW MUCH TO FEED

Veterinarians are often asked how much a horse should be fed. The answer usually is, "It all depends. . . ."

Horses have the same problems with being fat and thin that humans have. Some are called "easy keepers" and can get by on a very small amount of feed. Others can be fed all they can eat and still remain thin. As with people, it depends on the individual's own metabolism, the amount of activity, how efficiently the animal chews his food, how well he digests it, and a host of other factors.

The best answer to the question is "Enough, but not too much." Seriously, when someone wants to know how much feed to give his animal, he must first consider what his animal is doing. Is he an endurance horse expected to undergo rigorous training and then travel 100 miles in 24 hours? Or is she an old, overweight broodmare who is never ridden? Look at your animal. What are you asking of him? Is the animal calm and sedate or one who is nervous and paces the fence continuously? Is the animal hot-blooded or cold-blooded? An animal with a large amount of Thoroughbred or Saddlebred breeding will generally require more calories per pound of body weight than will one of Quarter Horse or pony parentage.

Is the animal a mare or stallion? During the breeding season, the stallion may be so excited by the mares around him that he will walk the fence continuously and nearly forget to eat, resulting in his becoming extremely thin. One client had a Saddlebred stallion who paced so much and ate so little that he looked like a skeleton during breeding season. Later in the year, when he was no longer used for breeding, and the mares were all out of heat and gone home, he returned to a normal weight.

What sort of body build does the animal have? A tall thin horse usually requires more groceries to maintain the same body condition than does a short, chunky one.

How often do you use the animal? And how hard? There is a world of difference in feed requirements between a race horse in hard training and a backyard animal that is used for a four or five-mile walk a couple of times a week. What feeds are available in your area? Is the weather cold or hot? A horse in the middle of a windy winter in Montana will need significantly more feed than will one who spends his winter in Hawaii. It takes a lot of calories of feed to replace the heat lost to a driving wind or winter rain. How the horse looks to you is another consideration in determining how much to feed. What is fat to one person is thin to another. Even the horse's disposition enters into this: a horse in a group who pushes the others away from feed may become overweight, while at the same time contributing to the other animals' being thin.

Many tables and charts have been published which tell you how much to feed a horse. They are still only guidelines, much as calorie charts and counters are to humans; you still have to adjust the feed to the animal.

Begin by feeding approximately 20 lb. of good quality hay per day, divided between a morning and night feeding. The hay, by itself, may be quite enough for a nonworking horse or an easy keeper. If this does not provide enough calories to keep the animal in the desired body condition, or does not provide enough energy to do the necessary work, grain may be added to the ration.

In general, hardworking horses are fed proportionately less hay and more grain. This is because they have trouble eating enough hay to provide enough calories (energy) for their needs. A hardworking animal, such as an endurance horse, may be so tired that he does not eat his full ration of hay. The grain therefore puts in easily digested energy and concentrated calories. The same sort of regimen is used for race horses. They are fed just a few pounds of hay and may receive as much as 20 to 25 lb. of grain per day.

More hay and less grain tends to put a large belly on a horse (called a "hay belly" or "grass belly"). To reduce one of these equine "beer bellies," feed proportionately less hay and more grain. Hardworking horses who are overfed on hay will be uncomfortable when they are exercised—another reason for giving more grain and less hay to the performance or using horse.

The rule for feeding horses is: FEED ONLY ENOUGH OF A NUTRITIONALLY BALANCED RATION TO KEEP A HORSE IN CONDITION FOR THE AMOUNT OF EXERCISE HE GETS. How do you tell how much that is? Easy—just LOOK at your horse! Don't overfeed! A fat horse is not a fit horse. If he's too fat, he's getting too much to eat for the amount of exercise that he is getting. Cut back on his grain accordingly. If you get down to no grain and he's still too fat, feed less hay. Make cutbacks or additions gradually so the animal has time to get used to them (remember the bacteria?).

Whatever amount you use initially, feed it for approximately three weeks. Then, look at the horse!! Is he fatter or thinner than when you started? If there is a scale handy, weighing the animal can give an accurate indication of his weight changes. Make sure that the scale is accurate. Many scales made to weigh large trucks are not reliable when used for something that is considerably lighter, like a horse. And like a bathroom scale, one that is inaccurate is worse than none at all.

A weight tape is a handy tool to keep track of the animal's weight changes. These may be purchased from feed stores, tack shops, or through saddlery catalogs. Lacking this, any tape measure may be used. You could even use a string or cord and tie knots in it as the horse grows or shrinks in girth—a lot like punching another hole in your belt when you've eaten too much spaghetti! Measure around the animal's heart girth area, just behind the front leg. Is the animal getting larger or smaller than when you started?

Other clues to changes in the horse's weight may be used. How much fat is on the rump area? Is there a hollow groove down the middle of the back? If there is a hollow groove, the animal is much too fat! How much fat is over the ribs? Can you see the ribs? Are they more or less prominent than they were before? In winter in areas where the animal has a heavy coat, don't rely on your eyes. Feel the animal's ribs with a bare hand every couple of weeks.

Otherwise, the animal may become thin under his winter woolies before you realize what is happening.

Another good measure of weight change is how the saddle fits. This is especially true with a western saddle. Notice how much distance there is between the end of the cinch ring and the dee ring on the saddle. Is it increasing or decreasing? The rear cinch gives you an extra idea of the animal's condition. In which hole does it buckle? Is it tighter or looser than the last time you rode the animal? This will give you both an idea of the animal's weight change, and an idea of how good the animal's physical condition is. As the animal goes from unconditioned to conditioned, the belly muscles tighten and become more firm. You can take the back cinch up farther as these abdominal muscles strengthen with exercise. Hard work does the same thing for the horse's abdominal muscles as sit-ups do for ours.

MEASURING FEED

Now, how do you measure the feed? If you've never fed a horse before, it may be worthwhile to weigh the hay for the first couple of days. You can use any handy scale to find out how much 20 pounds is and to adjust the feeding from there.

Another good way to begin is by knowing how much each hay bale weighs. For instance, if your bales are averaging 70 lb., a 1000 lb. horse will eat about ⅓ of a bale per day. Divide the bale into three pieces. Feed half of each one of these pieces per feeding (morning and night). Feed this amount for about three weeks, noting changes in the animal's weight as mentioned above.

If the animal is still thin, there are two choices; either increase the amount of hay, or add grain to the ration. You will probably already be feeding enough hay, so start by adding a one-pound coffee can of grain per feeding (morning and night). Many horse nutritionists will be critical of these methods, saying that the only way to feed is to measure the feed with great accuracy (i.e., weigh each feeding). However, if you feed the same amount per feeding, it doesn't matter whether you measure it in pints, portguzebies, quarts, or quadroons. What does matter is that you feed the same amount at each meal. After several weeks, you can see the effects of feeding this amount. It will take the same amount of feed to keep the animal in the same condition no matter how you measure (or weigh) it.

When feeding grain by volume (such as a coffee can), you must remember that different grains have different weights per volume. Oats may weigh as little as 0.7 lb. per quart, while corn may weigh 1.8 pounds per quart. Take these relative weights into account when deciding how much grain to feed your animal.

After testing a given amount of feed on a given animal, you can then adjust upward or downward, as needed. Adjusting the amount of feed for a group of horses is done on the same principles; you just have to look at the condition of individual members of the group and decide whether they need more or less feed overall. Watch for the bully and the really timid animal.

Now for a few hints on keeping your animal in the shape you want; it helps to have the same person feed the animal all the time. Then you don't have one person feeding a large amount of extra feed or a great difference in the amount fed from meal to meal. If children are feeding, make sure they understand that the animal could become ill or die from overfeeding. This helps overcome their urge to "be kind to the horsie" and dump in an extra measure or two of grain because the animal likes it.

If the animal is being fed a large amount of grain, it is especially important to reduce the amount of feed on days when the animal is not being worked. This avoids the problems of azoturia or Monday morning sickness.

If the hay tends to be dusty, dampening it with a garden hose and nozzle that makes a fine spray or with a watering can will help to keep down the amount of dust that your horse inhales and will help to prevent the animal getting heaves from the hay. It will also help to avoid aggravating the problem if the horse already has the heaves and you find it necessary to feed hay.

OVERFEEDING

One of the most serious consequences of overfeeding is obesity and the whole host of complications that go along with it. Colic and founder are often caused by too much feed. (For further discussion, see Fat Horse).

FEEDING THE IDLE HORSE

Feeding too much grain to a horse who is not working can cause azoturia and lead to serious, permanent damage to the horse. The grain ration should be cut in half on days when the animal is not worked. The harder the animal is being worked and the more grain he is being fed, the more important this rule is. Horses who are unused for longer periods of time should have their rations adjusted so they do not become fat.

Horses whose legs tend to stock up (swell up with fluid overnight or when they are rested) should have the amount of feed they receive carefully correlated with the work they are doing. Reducing the grain ration will help to avoid this swelling. In addition, an animal who tends to stock up should never be left for long periods without exercise to help move the fluid out of the legs. These animals badly need enough exercise or activity to help keep the circulation in their legs active.

WHEN YOUR HORSE DOESN'T EAT HIS FEED

Let's say your horse normally eats all his groceries and licks the feed pan clean. But this evening, he didn't want his grain. Check him carefully for symptoms of illness. Then, check the feed. Have you just opened a new sack? There may be something wrong with it. It may be moldy and thus unattractive to (and unhealthy for) the horse. Or, a large amount of vitamins or minerals or other substances may occur in a small amount of feed because of improper mixing or improper measuring of feed ingredients. A sample of feed could be taken to a laboratory for analysis. Your country agricultural agent can usually tell you where to send it. An excess of vitamin D, for example, may lead to calcification of the heart, rapidly leading to the animal's death.

A horse who doesn't eat either hay or grain should be carefully watched and checked by a veterinarian if he does not eat at his next meal, or if signs of illness develop. Also, check with others who may have fed him: children, neighbors, or friends. He may not be hungry simply because he has already eaten.

If your horse does not eat all his grain at every feeding, chances are good that you are either feeding him too much, or that he does not like the particular type of grain you are feeding. It could also mean thata he needs some dental attention. No more grain should be given than the horse will clean up within an hour or two after it is fed. This, of course, does not apply to creep feeders for young horses, where grain can be left in front of them at all times.

SPECIAL SITUATIONS

THE GROWING HORSE

Foals should be started on supplemental creep feed at two to three weeks of age (see Foal Feeding). Animals who are accustomed to eating hay and grain will come through the shock of being taken from their mothers much better than those who have to learn to eat as well as leaving mother at the same time. The latter, instead of growing, may actually go backward in size and development for a period of time. Avoid setbacks at weaning time if at all possible.

Young foals may gain two to three pounds per day; this gain slows to around ¼ to ½ lb. per day for the two-year old animal. The young animal will make 55 to 60% of his growth during his first year. It is good economics to feed the growing horse well during his first year. This is especially true for the first winter for animals in cold climates, where they must both eat to keep warm and to grow. Pounds put on the horse during his first year can be put on for a fraction of the cost of pounds put on in later years. Some animals may never recover from a poor start in that first year and never reach their full potential. These horses are said to be "stunted."

For the animal to reach this rate of growth, the feed must be adequate in both quantity and nutritional content. Weanlings who are being raised for race or show will be fed more concentrates and less hay than those who are pushed less intensely. Their ration must include all neces-

sary nutrients for the rapid growth which is expected of them. Animals who are too fat should have their rations reduced so as to avoid epiphysitis and other leg problems caused by excess weight. Good quality forage should make up the bulk of the diet. Legume hays such as alfalfa contain far more nutrients than do grass hays or pastures. If you are raising the animal on grass, it may be necessary to supplement phosphorus and protein; this can be given in the form of a grain or concentrate supplement.

Yearlings who are not being fed for race or show can be allowed to develop a bit more slowly and naturally. They can be fed mainly on roughage, whether a high quality hay or good pasture. The roughage should contain a minimum of 11% protein (12% is better) if concentrates are not fed. If the forage falls below this level, protein supplementation will be needed. Horses raised on grass pasture alone may not get adequate amounts of protein, calcium, and other nutrients. These horses may have a slow growth rate, and may never reach their full size potential.

THE PREGNANT MARE

The pregnant mare should have good quality feed in order to grow a good quality foal. Some mares will develop a stout foal when fed only pasture or hay. Indeed, some western range mares never see grain except when caught. If the mare's diet is lacking in any essential nutrient, it will be taken from her system by the foal, depleting her own body supply. The weight of the foal, fluids, and membranes range from 10 to 12% of the mare's body weight. A full, rich diet results in a healthy mare, a healthy foal, and nourishing milk.

During the last three months of pregnancy, the foal will take up a great deal of space in the mare's abdomen. If at all possible, her ration should include more grain and less roughage (pasture or hay) during this period. Protein content of the ration should be around 12% during this period, but depending on the individual mare, may have to be as high as 14%.

A confined mare will need good quality hay or other roughage. It must have enough calories to provide for both the mare's own body and for the fetus developing inside her. If she begins to get thin, supplement her as needed with a grain mixture, adjusting the amount to keep the mare from becoming too fat.

A mare who is too fat may have trouble at foaling time because the opening in the pelvis through which the foal must come is partially filled with fat.

Excessive fat and lack of exercise may also contribute to preparturient edema, in which the mare gets a shelf of swelling along her legs and down her belly. This swelling may hang down 4 to 6 inches or more. The fluid adds an incredible amount of weight; when added to the weight of the foal and the normal abdominal contents, it may lead to rupture of the prepubic tendon. This allows the foal to drop down a foot or so, along with the intestines. The tendon is usually so stretched and shredded as to be unrepairable. While this condition is very rare, it almost certainly results in death of the mare (or the necessity to put her out of her misery) and loss of the foal besides. Better, instead, not to let the animal get fat.

In areas which are deficient in phosphorus, a supplement high in this mineral is needed for the pregnant mare. If you are feeding several pounds of grain daily, it will probably provide enough phosphorus to be adequate for the foal. Lack of phosphorus may cause the foal to be born with crooked legs. These may bend in several directions, or the foal may be so coon-footed that the heels touch the ground. The problem is much more readily prevented than corrected. It is much easier to feed the correct minerals to the mare and let her put them into the foal than it is to try to add them in after the animal is born (see Phosphorus).

Feeding the mare additional vitamin A shortly before foaling (say, for the last month) will help to increase the vitamin A content of her milk. Excessively rich feed before foaling may contribute to a tight udder and result in the mare not allowing the newborn foal to nurse. If this happens with a confined animal, the mare may be milked out (she may need to be tranquilized in order to be able to do so if she is really uncomfortable). If it occurs in a mare who is not closely watched or is a pastured animal, the foal will probably die because the mare does not allow it to nurse.

THE LACTATING MARE

After the mare has foaled, do not give her any grain for the first 48 hours. For the first 24 hours, give her a little hay. Feed a bran mash after she has foaled to help clean out her digestive system and get it circulating normally again. Overfeeding the mare right after birth and during her foal heat may result in a diarrhea (called scours) in the foal.

During the last few weeks of pregnancy and the first week or two after foaling, she needs a normal amount of good quality feed. This should be increased as the foal gets larger and her milk production increases. Feed the mare enough so that she can produce milk and keep up her own body weight as well as possible.

Some mares habitually become thin enough when they are nursing a foal that they look like milk cows. A mare with this type of metabolism may need to have the foal weaned earlier than usual in order to avoid too great a drain on her body, and to allow her to put energy into getting her body ready for rebreeding, if that is desired.

Make sure the mare has plenty of water. It takes water to make milk. Salt is also important to milk production— be sure the lactating mare has free access to plenty of it in a form she will eat.

If the milking mare is lacking in nutrients, she will have decreased milk production, and will be unlikely to breed back while she is nursing the foal. Mares on less

than adequate nutrition often foal every other year, failing either to come into heat or to conceive, or both, while they are nursing a foal. Feeding all the necessary nutrients will allow the mare to raise a good foal and to get her body ready to breed back.

When the foal is weaned, the mare's grain ration should be cut by at least half for a week or two. For some mares, it may be desirable to entirely remove grain from her diet until she has dried up. Some mares may have to be put on limited amounts of roughage for several days. This will help to decrease her milk production and allow her to dry up with less pain. Do NOT milk out the mare, as this will stimulate her to keep producing milk, which is the opposite of what you want. If you wish to put her back to her regular amount of grain after she has dried up, do it gradually. But, remember that half may be quite sufficient now that the milk is not being taken from her body.

THE BREEDING STALLION

Breeding stallions require nutrition similar to that listed for the pregnant mare. Every attempt must be made to have the animal in good flesh (but not fat!) going into the breeding season. If his appetite drops as his interest increases, feed more grain as needed to maintain him as close to normal body weight as possible. If he shows a severe loss of weight, it may be necessary to change from oats to a more palatable grain mix, or from a grain mix to rolled corn. Good quality roughage is especially important in keeping a breeding stallion in good flesh and condition.

Several years ago a client stood two stallions for the breeding season. The 14-year old stallion was a veteran breeder and knew what happened at that time of the year. He was a tall, rangy horse, weighing about 1100 lb. He was fed on the side of the corral opposite to where mares were teased. He would take a mouthful of hay from the feeder and walk over to the teasing bar, chewing as he went. When he reached the bar, he would look over to see if any mares were being brought to him (optimist!). By the time he walked back to the feeder, he had finished the mouthful of hay and was ready for another. At the height of breeding season, he was being fed 20 to 25 lb. of hay per day. In addition to this, he received a gallon can of grain mix and a gallon can of cracked corn morning and night. By the end of the breeding season, he had lost about 75 lb. All the exercise walking back and forth had made him very trim and fit-looking (he was also being ridden lightly for approximately an hour a day). The second stallion was young and inexperienced and not nearly so excited. He required less than half the feed of the older horse, while weighing nearly the same.

During the nonbreeding time of the year, a high-quality pasture will supply most or all of the nutrients required to keep most stallions in good condition. As with other pastured horses, he should have access to loose salt and mineral mixtures, as well as plenty of clean, fresh water. If the pasture is inadequate, high-quality hay should be used for supplemental nutrition. Small amounts of grain may be necessary to keep some animals in good flesh.

THE WORKING HORSE

Race horses are asked to make a maximum effort at a very young age. Their arbitrary birthday of January 1st assures that many "two-year olds" will run before they are actually 24 months old. Since training begins some time before their first race, it is not uncommon to see animals in the neighborhood of 16 months being worked. These factors contribute to the large number of early breakdowns that occur. For this reason, optimal nutrition in the young working horse is of the utmost importance. It is imperative that all necessary nutrients are present in the ration, preferably in slight excess so that the animal is assured an adequate quantity of each.

It is important to remember, however, that many vitamins and minerals MUST be balanced in relation to each other, and that excesses of some may cause deficiencies of others. Use a reliable purchased grain ration, or consult a book such as Cunha's "Horse Feeding and Nutrition" for the concentrate part of the animal's ration. Feed the best quality hay available. The working horse is an athlete. As such, he must not be overweight. A trim, thrifty, well-muscled animal is lean and ready to work, whether for performance or racing. Be sure not to allow the animal to become too thin; if this occurs, the animal will have lower reserves for his efforts, and less muscle mass with which to make the effort.

Special diets have been compounded for endurance and hardworking horses which contained fat to help provide energy. Some endurance riders swear by these special concoctions. A trial conducted by the New York State College of Veterinary Medicine tested diets with 8% fat added; no difference in performance was found between animals fed this diet and those fed a standard ration. Diets containing 12 or 24% protein were also tested. They were not shown to have any beneficial effects. On the other hand, they also did not have any harmful effects, as had been hinted by other studies. (20)

The working horse's disposition can, to a large extent, be regulated by the amount of feed that is given. Some horses "cannot stand prosperity." They will get too "high," and be hard to handle or impossible to ride. Some will buck or otherwise act like broncs if they are getting too much in the way of carbohydrates. The horse's mood can be balanced in large part by the amount of feed (especially grain) that he is given. If he is too "hot," give him less feed.

On the other hand, attempting to adjust an animal's disposition can be carried to extremes. In many cases, it is better to exercise or work the animal more if he is really feeling frisky than to try to starve the playfulness out of him. Lack of proper nutrition can result in undeveloped

muscles, poor feet, slow recovery from work, and susceptibility to disease. An animal subjected to this type of deprivation to get his mind into line may never recover from it physically, and may always be below normal. He may never attain his full growth or performance potential. This is a place where a common sense balance is very important!

THE THIN HORSE

Sooner or later, we all seem to be confronted with a thin horse or horses. When the problem is a whole pasture full of thin horses, it's generally easy to find the cause, which is usually some sort of management problem. Thin animals are most commonly due to too little feed, or to a pasture that is eaten down to where the greens that are left are either unpalatable or poisonous to the animals and which they will not eat voluntarily. Check for this by walking the pasture to see exactly what kind of plants are present, and in what quantities (see Pasture).

If the horses are being fed hay, they either need a better quality of hay, or more of what they are already being fed. It may be necessary to supplement their diet with grain. If you feed grain, put it in separate feeders, if at all possible.

Let's look at some of the causes of the individual thin horse. Obviously, if he's by himself, check the pasture for overgrazing and poor quality feed as outlined above. Worms often come to mind as the cause of the thin horse, and with considerable justification, as they commonly are the cause! Is your horse on a routine worming program? He may need worming more often than other horses, especially if he is under two years of age. A thin horse should be wormed once a month for three months, using a different wormer each time.

The horse should be tube wormed the first time using wormers for both roundworms and bots (this is a job for your veterinarian). Then, paste worm the horse the next month with a wormer for roundworms. Whether tube or paste wormer is used for the third treatment depends on how much progress is being made. If the animal is still having severe problems with worms, he should be tube wormed again. Otherwise, paste worming can be used (see Worming).

If the thin horse is in with others, it may be necessary to remove him from the group, confine him, and feed him separately. You may be able to get him back into condition by feeding extra feed apart from the bunch every time that you see him. If you can give this animal the extra feed twice daily (or even three times), it will probably not take long to plump him back to normal. If you are only seeing the horse a couple or three times a week (as in a large boarding pasture), it will likely take longer to get the animal back into condition. Be careful when supplementing the animal on an irregular schedule not to feed so much grain each time that the animal founders or gets a case of colic. Do not feed a horse on an irregular schedule more than about two pounds of grain per feeding. It is much better to get the animal in where he can be fed small amounts of extra feed on a regular basis rather than to try to pour it all into him in a few feedings a week.

Dental problems cause at least as many thin horses as do worms. This is especially true of the older horse—say, past the age of ten. Check your horse's teeth as described in the chapter on dental problems. If his grinders are in good shape, then look for management problems.

The new or inexperienced horse owner often does not know exactly what he needs to feed to keep his horse in good flesh. On the other hand, the experienced horse owner may not be feeding quite the quantity or quality of feed needed for an individual animal. With a thin horse, change or upgrade feeds as follows:

1) Hay. If feeding grass hay, switch to a good quality grass/alfalfa hay or straight alfalfa hay. This is a lot like changing from lettuce to ice cream if you want to gain weight.

2) Grain. Change from whole oats to rolled oats, or from rolled oats to a grain mix. Or, go from a grain mix to steam-rolled corn. This has the most calories per pound of any of the commonly available feeds.

3) Supplements. One of my clients will buy a 50 lb. sack of Calf Manna for a thin horse. This feed supplement is made for calves. When combined with the rest of a "better nutrition program," it often works wonders. Feed 1 to 1–½ cups twice a day with the animal's grain. This client comments that he has never had to buy a second sack for a horse whose only problems were nutritional.

4) Vitamins. Add these if necessary. They are usually needed only in areas where the feed is deficient in nutrients or if your veterinarian feels that they are required.

Start with better and increased feed gradually! Do not founder your horse (see Founder). Work the animal up to full feed over a period of 2 to 3 weeks. Reduce the amount and richness of feed immediately if the animal shows soreness in the feet or any signs of colic.

SOCIAL PROBLEMS ASSOCIATED WITH THINNESS

One of the first questions with a thin animal is whether he is the only animal who is thin in the group or herd. Is he a very young or very old animal? Let me point out several social problems by telling you about a starvation case that I was called to treat. There were two horses in the pasture. One was hog-fat and the other was a true starvation case. This was very puzzling initially because there usually is not that great a difference between two animals who are fed together. Closer examination revealed several problems: First, the "pasture" which looked so good to the owners was in reality eaten bare of all edible grass and had only sagebrush left standing. This plant is of low palatability and minimal nutritional value to the horse. They will eat it only if starving. Secondly, the hay that was

being fed was more than a year old and of exceptionally poor quality, with very little nutritional value. Thirdly, upon questioning, it became obvious that the husband was throwing out what little hay that was fed all in one pile. The older, stronger, dominant gelding ate it all, pushing the thin, weak three-year old filly completely away from the food. She was literally starving while he was rolling in blubber. This is typical of social problems which may cause one horse in a bunch to be thin while the others are fat.

There was another social problem involved here: the owners. Further questioning revealed that the husband didn't like the filly and loved the gelding, which was his horse. These people barely had money to feed one horse, let alone two. The filly belonged to his wife, and he didn't care that the animal was starving. Another strike against the animal was the worm load that she was carrying. When I examined her, she was weak enough that she was staggering. Upon rectal examination, the damage caused by worms in the arteries to her hind legs could be felt. This was part of the cause of the staggering.

How was this problem treated? The people were talked into worming the filly in order to remove the worms that were causing so much damage in her arteries and that were also competing with her for food. They wanted her vaccinated at the same time. This was not done, because to attempt to immunize her in her run-down state would probably not work, and the vaccine (and expense thereof) would be wasted. A proper feeding program was outlined to help bring her out of the starvation. Then they were convinced to attempt to sell her to someone who would be able to care for her properly. The next week I was cheered to receive a call from her new owner. We spent considerable time on the phone outlining a feeding and health care program for the filly. When called to her new home to worm her two months later, I found a plump, shining black filly running gaily around the pasture.

When a horse is the lone thin animal in a larger group, he should be observed carefully at feeding time. Is he getting any feed at all, or are the other animals driving him away from it? Often, a submissive animal is obvious because he will have bite marks all over his body; he may also show evidence of being kicked, such as large bruises or sizeable spots where the hair has been scraped off. Some of these animals truly look as if they had been to a war and lost.

Feeding a thin animal more frequently than usual will often help it to gain weight. The practice is definitely worth trying. The same treatment is recommended for humans who wish to gain weight—eat lots of high-calorie snacks and meals spaced throughout the day to provide a steady flow of nutrients into the body. Plenty of fresh water is also important in plumping up the thin horse.

OTHER CAUSES OF THE THIN HORSE

After you've ruled out or corrected the feeding, worming, tooth, and any social problems (both horse and human) as outlined above, where do you go from there if the animal is still thin? If you've changed feeding programs, give the new regimen at least a three-week try before giving up and deciding that it is not working. Measure the horse at the heart girth before you start the program and again at the end of three weeks, to see if there has been any gain. Otherwise, the animal may be gaining weight, but because you are seeing him every day, you cannot see the change and think that you are getting nowhere. If you really are getting nowhere, it's time to call your veterinarian and have him thoroughly examine the horse. Thinness may be caused by diseases, such as equine infectious anemia (swamp fever), chronic liver or kidney disease, or internal tumors which affect digestion; however, these are very rare. Don't look for exotic problems until you've ruled out all the common ones.

THE FAT HORSE

Some horsemen feel that "fat is the most beautiful color." The Arabs, who are masters with horses, disagree, saying, "The enemies of a good saddle horse are idleness and fat." Fat is neither attractive nor healthy, and that goes for all animals—humans as well as horses. Fat covers a multitude of sins. Most horsemen have seen horses with exceptionally poor conformation—peaked croups, slab sides, and absolutely no muscle condition—plumped out by excess feed to the point where a judge placed them, for heaven only knows what reason, over horses in good, normal condition and possessing far superior conformation.

The situation has gone so far in some breeds that the halter animals exhibited for conformation are a completely different group of animals from those shown in performance classes for their working ability. The Quarter Horse and Appaloosa are examples that come immediately to mind, with some Arabians not far behind. In these breeds, the halter horses are too fat and out of shape to compete in performance events. Instead of placing fat, judges should give preference to animals in normal condition. It is much healthier for the individual animal, and it's much easier to judge the basic body and bone structure that is so important for breeding stock, if it is not obscured by blubber. Saddlebreds, for example, are usually shown in normal working trim and no premium is placed on overweight.

Excessive fat on young horses can cause permanent damage, especially when combined with work. The extra poundage stresses bones, muscles, ligaments, and tendons which are immature and not strong enough to carry the load. Damage to the epiphyseal plates from which the long bones grow can be caused by excess weight. If this cartilage is examined under a microscope, it appears crushed and thinned. It looks exactly the same as the damage resulting from experimental crushing of the same cartilage. The resulting damage, called epiphysitis, can lead to abnormal bone growth with possible permanent bone damage and crippling.

Strain to the ligaments around the joints can give rise to windpuffs, bog spavins, and related injuries. These rarely cause permanent lameness, especially if the cause is corrected promptly. However, they almost invariably result in permanent blemishes and disfiguration.

Young horses suddenly pushed with too much grain may develop a swelling of the pastern area. This is a type of ringbone related to rickets and is called rachitic ringbone. If the horse's rations are quickly returned to normal, permanent bone damage can sometimes be avoided. This type of problem may also be seen in horses who are fed extremely large amounts of various vitamins and supplements. In an attempt to be kind to the animal and to get maximum growth out of it, the owner pushes so many different minerals into it that he throws the animal into an imbalance, usually in the calcium/phosphorus ratio, resulting in the same problem.

Excess fat in older horses results in stress with a capital "S." The heart has to work harder in order to pump blood through the added bulk. Lungs also function overtime to move oxygen through the extra body mass. Feet are called on to carry the extra weight. Those who think that weight doesn't create problems should look at the massive draft horses. Some lamenesses which are very common in that type of horse, such as ringbone, are directly related to their weight. Too much weight on too-small feet leads to lameness problems and can be a predisposition to navicular disease. This is especially seen in some Quarter Horses (especially members of certain lines) that weigh 1200 pounds or more and stand on extremely small feet.

Founder is often seen in a particular type of overweight horse. These animals commonly have a very large crest on the neck, especially if the animal is a gelding. They tend to be overweight and chunky. There may be a hereditary predisposition to the problem, especially as seen in Shetland ponies and some Morgans. Hormones produced by some plants might be involved in causing the laminitis or founder. The owner of one of these founder-type animals must make a real effort to hold down its weight. This can be a project as these horses are often exceptionally easy keepers. Limiting the weight to a normal level helps minimize complications in the feet and makes the animal more comfortable.

Obesity causes a general lack of well-being in the horse just as it does in humans. The animal doesn't feel as well as he should. He is less agile and maneuverable. These animals clearly have less endurance and stamina, as shown time and time again in North American Trail Ride Conference (NATRC) and endurance-ride competition. An overweight horse rarely finishes a ride and if he does, clearly shows himself at a disadvantage compared to the animal in normal body condition. This is demonstrated by poor recovery on pulse and respiration checks and also by the general distress shown by the animal.

Overweight animals have problems with anesthesia and surgery if they are ever sick or injured (this goes for humans, too). The animal stands less chance of surviving his problems due to general lack of body tone and cardiovascular fitness. Fat holds anesthetic agents; thus it takes a greater quantity of the drug to anesthetize an overweight animal. This leaves a greater quantity of anesthetic in the body to be detoxified. The animal is down longer and has less chance for recovery. There is a greater probability of complications. Surgery itself is more complicated due to fat in the surgical area. The surgery takes longer, leading again to a longer down time. Fat can also lessen the strength of the surgical incision if the surgeon accidentally incorporates any into the closure (and it's extremely tough to avoid it in a fat animal).

Breeding problems are frequently seen in overweight stallions and mares. Mares who are too fat often do not come into heat properly. They cycle late or not at all. They must often be given hormone injections in an attempt to bring them into heat—shots they would never need if they were in normal condition. A mare should be on a rising plane of nutrition and preferably gaining weight when bred. It is better to start a mare a bit thin and have her gaining than to have her too fat. This is called "flushing" in other species and is well known to contribute to fertility and increased conception rates. The result is a higher conception rate in fewer heats and with fewer services.

Stallions who are overweight may show lessened interest in breeding, due to being overweight and in poor physical condition. Extra fat in the scrotum insulates the testicles and raises their temperature, often leading to lessened fertility and viability of the sperm. Being overweight puts extra weight on the stallion's hind feet when he mounts the mare. This is especially important in a stallion with any hind-leg problems. One of my clients had a stallion with a fractured hind coffin bone. The owners were able to breed him through the summer with special shoeing to support the broken bone and careful attention to his weight to keep him slim and trim.

Overfeeding can affect a horse's disposition. The overfed horse is often hard to handle due to an excess of energy. This is especially true if he's been receiving too much grain in relation to the amount of work he's doing. Although he may not have the stamina to last very long, he can be pretty hard to control until he "runs out of gas." A comment was made in the past about one of the top cutting horses; it was said that he "could not stand prosperity." This animal was one of the best cutting horses in the world when kept on reasonable-to-slightly-short rations. If fed too much, the horse turned into an uncontrollable, man-eating bronc who was a hazard to himself and to all around him.

Reducing an animal's rations back to normal often results in a dramatic improvement in disposition and manageability. A memorable example is a team of draft horses which belonged to one of my friends. When overfed, the horses were dangerously uncontrollable and ran away. When their rations were cut back, they again be-

came the gentle giants my friend had originally purchased. My own cutting mare furnishes another example of using rations to fine-tune the using horse. If she is a bit short on calories, she will not be as sharp and snappy as usual. When her roll backs are sloppy and slow and her spins are less-than-great, I know that she needs a bit more grain than she has been getting. On the other hand, if she is so high and silly that it's hard to do anything with her, it's time to cut back a bit. Never underestimate the power of feed control in fine-tuning the working horse. Balancing the amount of work and exercise with the amount of feed being given can make the difference between winning and losing, especially with horses in classes like western pleasure. They need to be fed and conditioned so that they will look good, but yet not be so high that they will not display the sterling manners that make a winning western pleasure horse.

When a saddle is placed on a fat horse, there is a tendency for it to roll due to a combination of factors. The excess fat tends to make the overall shape of the horse more round and allows it to turn more easily. The loose rolls of fat tend to turn with the skin. The saddle must be cinched excessively tight to try to keep it from turning. The combination of the saddle rolling and a too-tight cinch often results in saddle or cinch sores.

Considerate people who wouldn't dream of asking a horse to carry a 500-lb. rider think nothing of asking the same horse to carry a 250-pound rider and 250 pounds of extra weight on his body. The animal would be healthier, happier, and more comfortable with the 500-pound rider—at least he could get rid of the whole thing at the end of the day and not have to carry around half of it all the time.

Several years ago, a leading trainer was asked by a horse magazine how he got rid of horses that were too poor to fit his breeding program—the real dogs. His answer was that he poured the grain to them and fattened them up. The he put them in the front paddock as visitors came into his farm. His comment was that he couldn't get them fattened up fast enough—people bought them as soon as he put them out!

Why does a horse get fat? Just like a person who becomes overweight, he is getting more calories than he needs. Disposition enters into the amount of feed that a horse requires. Some breeds and lines tend to be easy keepers. These individuals often have a "don't care" attitude toward life—nothing much bothers them. They are often passionately devoted to their vittles—the time they are most likely to trample you is on the way to the feed trough.

After you've taken the horse's breed and disposition into account and see that he's overweight, what do you do? Look over his total feeding program and see where you can cut down. Some horses, just like some of us (including myself), have to be on a perpetual diet in order to maintain a reasonable weight. You might as well accept the fact right now that if your horse is fat and you would like to have him down to a reasonable weight, he will have to eat less than he would like to have. In fact, he will probably be partly hungry much of the time. And, he will probably beg for more. Turn, please, a deaf ear, and have a healthier horse. And, not just incidentally, fewer medical problems and veterinary bills, which is what this book is all about.

Start by cutting grain down sharply or out altogether. Grazing may be limited or cut out, especially with a foundered horse. With a stabled horse, the next step is to reduce the amount of hay. Also consider changing to a low-calorie hay: grass instead of alfalfa, for example. Give the overweight animal more exercise, but be especially careful to start him gradually and work up to longer distances and harder work.

Several years ago, this author was called to look at a stable full of horses that had recovered from influenza some months previously, but were still hacking and coughing. The most prominent thing noted on examination was that all were grossly overweight. Each horse had a trough down the middle of its back formed by a ridge of blubber on each side of the backbone. Conservatively, these horses were 300 pounds heavier than they should have been. The horses' lungs could have handled a normal amount of weight, but were severely stressed carrying the extra fat, with the result that they were still coughing two months after a fairly minor ailment. When the owner was questioned, he said, "I couldn't bear to see them hungry." This man wasn't doing his horses any favors by giving them excess food. He was killing them with kindness! Love your horse and feed him well, but please don't kill him with kindness.

FEEDING THE SICK HORSE

Sick horses should have free access to plenty of good quality, clean, easily digested feed. Ideally, the feed should be high in protein. Good alfalfa hay is one of the best feeds for a sick horse. If the animal is not accustomed to alfalfa hay, the change should be made gradually, over five to seven days. Reduce the amount of grass hay until you are feeding only alfalfa. If you suddenly switch to alfalfa hay, the horse may end up with diarrhea or colic on top of his other problems.

Offer the animal one or two types of grain. Sweet feeds with molasses are especially palatable to some sick horses. Give small amounts of feed frequently, and change them if the animal does not eat them. Feed which has been contaminated with saliva can become sour or mold, and will be refused by the animal. Offer a variety of foods so that the animal can take his choice, and keep trying different ones in an attempt to come up with something that will please the horse.

Horses who have been off feed for several days may require injections of amino acids and other medications to correct the negative nitrogen balance that occurs and to get the animal eating again. Consult your veterinarian on this. Additional B vitamins may be helpful for horses who have been eating little or no feed for several days. They are also helpful for horses who have had diarrhea and may not be absorbing adequate amounts of these vitamins from their digestive tracts.

Occasionally, supplementation or force feeding is necessary for the animal who does not eat. Your veterinarian may pass a stomach tube and give the animal nutrients, vitamins, and minerals. Dehydrated cottage cheese is often made into a slurry and given several times a day with a dose syringe. This product is very nutritious and can make a big difference with a sick horse. Dehydrated alfalfa meal is also used in supplemental mixtures. Some animals with long-term disease problems may have to have a stomach tube passed and sutured into place so that you can feed them regularly through it during convalescence. Horses can be kept going for long periods of time with a liquid diet if necessary.

Animals who have not eaten for five or more days may require intensive treatment, including intravenous therapy in addition to feeding nutrients via stomach tube. Again, this is a job for your veterinarian. Intravenous feeding is especially used with foals who have diarrhea and can or have become quickly weakened or prostrate because of their limited reserves.

The horse's immune system is rapidly weakened when he stops eating. The problems caused by this lack of food should alert the owner to take extra care to see that animals have feed available when they are hauled long distances. Animals who are not eating will have an increased susceptibility to disease and should be isolated as well as possible, while receiving extra nursing care to bolster their poor defenses.

Chapter 5

REPRODUCTION AND FOALING

Choosing The Broodmare
Getting the Mare Ready for Breeding
  Artificial Lighting for Mares and Stallions
  Breeding History
  Heat Cycles
  Breeding Exam, Mares
  Caslick's Operation
  Opening the Mare
  Cervical Cultures
  Endometrial Biopsy
  Laparoscopic Examination
  Timetable for Breeding the Mare
  Pasture Breeding vs Hand Breeding
  Teasing
Breeding
Contagious Equine Metritis
Pyometra and Metritis
Embryo Transfers
Artificial Insemination
Prostaglandins
Other Hormones
Pregnancy Diagnosis
  Rectal Palpation
  Blood Test
  Ultrasonic Examination
Care of the Pregnant Mare
Abortions
Foaling
  The Membranes
Early Foal Care
  Immature and Premature Foals
  Barker and Dummy Foals
  Neonatal Isoerythrolysis
Foaling Complications
  Uterine Torsion
  Caesarean Section
  Induction of Labor
  Tears in the Vagina, Cervix, or Uterus
  Prolapse of the Uterus

Rupture of the Uterine Blood Vessels
Navel Ill and Joint Ill
Foal Septicemia
Foal Feeding and Care
  Mare's Milk
  Colostrum
  Mastitis
  Mare's Milk as Human Food
  Feeding the Orphan Foal
  Feeding the Older Foal
  Weaning

CHOOSING THE BROODMARE

No matter how many horses you have, the broodmare is the foundation of any breeding program. She must be selected with care in order for a breeding program to be successful. Before the breeder can select a broodmare, he must first define his goals. What is he expecting to produce? Does the mare have the genetic background to produce it? The chances of producing a winning cutting horse are much greater when both parents are proven cutting horses. A foal with stakes winners on both sides of his pedigree has a far greater probability of winning races than one from a casual, guesswork mating.

If you are breeding for type, start with a broodmare who is as close as possible to your desired goal. If you want stretchy, tall Quarter Horses, start with that type. Don't buy a bulldog mare and breed from there. It takes a lifetime of work to hit breeding goals and it is difficult under the best of circumstances. Don't handicap yourself by starting with the wrong animals.

A good example of dedication to goals is Hank Wiescamp, who is well-known for his single-minded pursuit of a particular type of Quarter Horse. Whether or not you like his type of animal, you must admire the work and commitment that he used to reach his ideal.

Most of us need to take a good look at the mare we already have to see if she is, or is not, what we need to breed. Appraise her objectively. Too many people decide to breed their mare to the neighbor's stallion solely because they think it will be fun to raise a foal—"a good experience for the kids." A haphazard breeding like this often results in a poor quality foal that is neither usable nor saleable when he matures.

In the current depressed economy and poor horse market, perhaps another question to ask is whether you should breed the mare at all. Recently, one of my clients sold a nicer-than-average Quarter Horse filly for $20 more than the stud fee. That's not much return for a year of the mare's time and two years of feed, training, vet bills, shoeing, and care!

On the other hand, the good, sound working mare who is winning trail rides, working cattle, or winning races or performance classes might be exactly the one to breed. She has proven that she has the conformation, intelligence, and disposition to do something. She has the soundness to work and to keep on working.

Too many people, however, breed the failures and keep the good mares working. Thus, the "losers" contribute a disproportionate number of offspring to the genetic pool. Too often a cutting mare, for example, is shown for five or six years while the ones that didn't make it are at home having foals. As a friend once said about a pair of Catahoula cow dogs that she had bought, "If they can't work, we can always breed them." For what? To produce more little dogs who can't work cattle? Unfortunately, we too often fall into the trap of "those who can, work; those who can't, breed!"

Most horsemen who have been around racehorses have seen large pastures full of Thoroughbred mares that broke down in race training—the popped knees, splints, bone chips, and other problems. These mares were home having foals while the ones who could run and STAY SOUND were out winning money, not reproducing. The winners are the very horses that should have been kept and cherished as broodmares. In many breeds, too, mares are used for breeding without ever being ridden. No one knows whether they have the disposition, soundness, or intelligence to do anything. It is far better to choose a mare for breeding who has proven her usefulness.

The broodmare should be free from hereditary faults and unsoundness. Splints, ringbone and sidebone, bog spavin, bone spavin, thoroughpin, navicular disease, and stringhalt are among the unsoundnesses that often have a hereditary basis due to poor conformation that either causes the problem or predisposes the animal to it. Curb, when accompanied by curby conformation, is a similar problem. Cataracts are occasionally seen as a hereditary problem. These unsoundnesses must be distinguished from blemishes, such as windpuffs and scars, which do not affect the mare's function or soundness. Cosmetic blemishes are generally unimportant in the broodmare if she is not being shown.

Parrot mouth is a hereditary problem that can cause the breeder considerable grief. The parrot-mouthed mare whose front teeth don't mesh enough for her to graze may not be a problem to the owner who loves her and doesn't mind giving her the special feed and attention she will need all her life. However, her foals may be unsaleable. One client had a parrot-mouth race horse who started running and broke down. The owners would have been willing to turn him out to pasture and keep him because they were fond of him or train him and use him as a riding horse—he would have made a good one. However, he could never graze normally and thus could not be pastured. He could never be used as a stallion because of this hereditary defect. As a result, he was put down—a waste which could have been avoided had his dam (or sire) been chosen with greater care. A word of caution: careful selection of breeding stock greatly increases the chance of success, but even then an occasional throwback will show up to disappoint you.

Breeding soundness and conformation are important to the broodmare. In a breeding mare, the anus should be directly above the vulva so the manure and its juices fall away from the vulva. A mare with the flat croup favored in some breeds, such as the Arabian, often has an anus 2 to 4 inches ahead of the vulva. Manure drips into the vulva and provides a continuing source of bacterial contamination. This produces a chronic vaginal infection that often keeps the mare from conceiving.

This type of mare can be helped by suturing the vulva partially closed from the top to keep it clean. This is done before breeding. She has to be bred very carefully to avoid tearing. She must be cut open before foaling and resutured afterwards. She will frequently need treatment for the uterine infection that follows the vaginal contamination. All this runs into a lot of trouble, more difficult conception, and extra costs.

Mares of this type would not conceive in nature and the problem would eventually be eliminated from the horse population. We have propagated it by breeding for certain unnatural conformational traits, such as the flat croup, and by continuing to suture and breed mares with a tipped vulva. Mares with normal conformation but who are excessively thin can also have the anus several inches ahead of the vulva. Their anus will return to its normal position when fed so that the mare's weight is back to normal.

Your veterinarian should be able to do a rectal exam of the mare's reproductive tract to see if it is in good order. The ovaries should be normal and functional, the cervix not scarred, and there should be good tone and no abnormalities in the uterus.

A word here about auctions—watch out! Breeders sometimes dump their problem mares. One of my clients bought three mares at an auction. One mare turned out to have a chronic infection in the uterus that no amount of treatment would clear up. The horse was not rideable, so she was sent to the canners.

The second one did not come into heat, but acted like a stallion. Examination showed a tumor on one ovary the size of a small watermelon which was producing male hormones. Surgery to remove the tumor was successful, but the other ovary had been so suppressed by the male hormones that it never did come back into production. Then, there was the skull fracture to repair when this mare, in her role as a "stallion," smashed headlong into a board fence and caved in the bone over her sinuses. She also had a laminitis from being previously foundered and could not be ridden. She was put down.

The third mare did turn out to be normal, but the profit from her did not make up for the vet bills, feed, time, and complete waste of the other two horses.

When possible, get a good reproductive history with any mare that you buy. Knowing what worked before if she had any problems helps assure getting a foal the next time the mare is bred. Also, knowing what didn't work can give your vet ideas as to what to do without wasting time trying the same treatment over again.

Other chronic conditions might cause the mare (and her owner) difficulty. Heaves is a good illustration of this, as is laminitis. These problems are neither contagious nor hereditary, but can interfere with usefulness and mobility, as well as requiring extra care and maintenance. For example, some good broodmares will have varying degrees of laminitis, acquired by being foundered somewhere along the way. Care needed by one of these can vary from just oftener-than-usual hoof trimming to frequent new sets of special shoes. These animals are definitely not sound as riding horses, but might produce another few foals for the owner who will cater to their problems. Leg injuries that make locomotion difficult, such as popped knees on turned-out race mares, can cause similar problems.

Tumors may shorten the life of the broodmare. Especially check gray mares that are being considered as broodmares for the presence of melanomas, which may show up as black nodules anywhere on the body, but especially on the face, under the tail, and between the hind legs.

While an animal with one of these problems might still be a candidate for a broodmare, the owner should evaluate whether he is willing to expend the time, effort, and money that would be needed to keep her in condition, or whether he would be better off with another animal without these problems.

A broodmare should be free from disease. A Coggins test will help to assure that she does not have, or is not carrying, swamp fever (equine infectious anemia). Imported horses are normally tested to be sure that they do not have piroplasmosis, a tick-borne disease. The mare should be examined for venereal diseases, such as the contagious equine metritis which swept Kentucky in 1978.

Vices are definitely undesirable in the broodmare. Several that come to mind are biting, striking, cribbing, weaving, and stall walking. A point to remember is that the mare will often teach these vices to her foal.

Good conformation is a must for the broodmare. Straight legs contribute to the utility and saleability of her foals. They also lessen the likelihood of injury to the using horse. The most beautiful horse in the world, with a crooked leg or two, should hold no appeal for the breeder. Breeders often explain a crooked leg as being due to an early injury. This author tends to consider them hereditary in the absence of scars, or until proven otherwise. There are certain lines of horses in almost all breeds that are noted for bad legs, so the problem is definitely heritable. Some people will buy a crooked-legged broodmare and say that they are going to breed her to a straight-legged stallion and get straight-legged foals. In my experience, this rarely works.

Good looks in the mare are a must for the breeder of halter horses. They enhance the saleability of the foal—everyone likes to own a good-looking horse. For the show animal, a working horse with good conformation and attractive features will place above the animal with equal working ability, but common looks. Beauty in the aged broodmare must be looked for with an experienced horseman's eye. When these old gals are turned out without exercise, grooming, and other upkeep, they can look pretty saggy and shabby, especially if they have several foals in a row. Remember to look for the basic bone structure—straight legs, etc., rather than judging cosmetic appearance.

Breed conformation or type is noteworthy. The mare should produce offspring that are normal for the breed she is supposed to represent, both for saleability and showability. The Arabian breed, for instance, points out that breed type is more important than conformation in judging their halter (breeding) classes. They point out that without breed type, one may have an outstanding and excellent horse, but not necessarily an Arabian.

Needless to say, registration papers usually enhance the economic value of both the mare and her offspring. Unregistered or unusual crossbred animals are often difficult to sell unless well-trained, and often will not sell for enough to begin to pay the costs of raising them.

Some people forget that it is very important that the broodmare be a good mother. "Mothering ability" includes caring for the foal when it is born—licking the membranes off its head so it can breathe, staying with it and allowing it to nurse, and keeping aggressive adult horses away. It also involves having a high level of antibodies against disease in the colostrum to give the foal protection against common horse diseases until it is old enough to be vaccinated. She should also produce enough milk to raise a good, sturdy foal.

Mares who do not lick the membranes off the foal at birth, or who desert it, are a common cause of foal loss in range mares (and in stabled mares if the owner is not present at exactly the right time).

One of my clients had a mare who wouldn't let her foal nurse unless he held her halter in one hand and held a chunk of 2×4 against her forehead with his other hand. He never had to use the club—just the threat was enough. But he had to be there every time the foal needed to nurse for the first three or four days of the foal's life. After that, the dingbat would finally accept her foal and care for it.

It can easily be seen how impractical this animal would be for a range breeding operation. Mothering ability is hereditary, too; this mare's daughters were as incompetent as she was at mothering. After a few years of coping with them, this man finally sold the mare and all her daughters.

The serious breeder should discriminate against the "accident-prone" horse as a broodmare. Another client had a broodmare who lost foals two years in a row. The first year, she foaled in the range herd and the foal was kicked to death, apparently by some of the geldings in the bunch. The second year, she foaled on the bank of a stream and the foal fell into the water and drowned. The third year she had another live foal—this time in the confines of a fenced hay yard so that the two previous losses would not be repeated. She somehow managed to step on the foal and break its leg. After considerable time and sizable vet bills, the leg healed, but the foal never became sound enough for use.

All accidents, you say? Yes, but the other mares did not have these disasters and came in each fall with a usable foal at their sides. In this, we should agree with Tom Lasater who developed his Beefmaster breed of cattle by rigid selection. One of his criteria was that if the cow did not bring in a calf in the fall for whatever reason, he eliminated her from his herd. While we may not remove a mare from the herd on the basis of one lost foal, after the second loss, she should be taken off the free lunch program and replaced with a mare that will bring home a saleable offspring.

Disposition is paramount for a broodmare. Whether bad character traits in the horse are inherited or learned may perhaps be debated, but it is frequently seen that a mare (or stallion) with a bad disposition has foals the same. Since this is often seen when the foal is weaned early or orphaned, at least some case must be made for heredity.

As mentioned previously, the using mare should be given preference, because she has already proven that she can get along with people; the fact that she can be ridden and worked proves the presence of intelligence and the ability to do something. Mares should at the very least be halterbroken, especially if they are going somewhere else to be bred. It also helps to have them stand tied, to be able to work with ropes around them, to trailer them, and to work with their feet, hind end, and tail.

A broodmare should ideally be a horse of sterling soundness. I realize that many are not. The broodmare owner must evaluate whether he likes the individual and her bloodlines enough to live with her problems. Can you AFFORD to maintain a problem horse? One mare that comes to mind was a foundered mare with the heaves. She could not be turned out to pasture because the grass made the laminitis so bad that she could not walk. When kept in and fed hay, she coughed continuously due to the heaves. Definitely a no-win situation. Worth it? The owner thought so. I'm not sure—I know she wouldn't have been worth it to me!

Choose YOUR broodmare in light of the total horse: conformation, soundness, ability, and genetic background. Don't lose sight of your breeding goals. Pick the broodmare most likely to produce the type of foal you want. Decide before adding her to your herd whether or not you want to live with any problem that she has.

GETTING THE MARE READY FOR BREEDING

With high hopes for an outstanding foal who will grow up to become a national champion, you hauled your best mare all the way from Minnesota to California to breed to Mr. Super Stud. But, she didn't come into heat because she was exhausted from the trip. Then she came down with influenza and they nearly lost her. After they got her back into condition to breed, they discovered she had a uterine infection and wouldn't settle. By the time the breeding farm got all the problems fixed, it was August and too late to breed her to get an early racehorse foal.

Far-fetched? Not at all. Most breeding farms can tell you stories like this, and some that are worse. What makes these stories even sadder? They usually could have been prevented! PLANNING is the key to getting a healthy foal, and it must start months before the mare even gets near the stallion.

Planning should start five to six months before the breeding season with the decision as to which mares are going to be bred so they can be properly prepared. Choose the stallion(s) early, selecting on the basis of conformation, disposition, bloodlines, availability, and your budget. Book early to be assured of a spot on his breeding schedule. With many stallion owners, early bookings often assure a lower stud fee than later in the season.

Choosing a stallion who is a proven breeder gives more assurance of getting a foal than with a doubtful or unknown horse. A live foal guarantee is sometimes more costly, but may be worthwhile to the mare owner by insuring that he will either get a foal or be able to breed back to the stallion again the next year at no extra charge other than mare care. There should be a clear understanding as to whether a cash refund of the stud fee will be made if the stallion owner is not able to honor the rebreeding. Read over the breeding agreement and make sure that you understand it and that its terms are acceptable.

Mares to be bred should be on a nutritionally adequate feeding program. They should be gaining weight, but not overweight. It is better to start with a mare who is too thin and start feeding her up (thus having her gaining), than to start with a mare who is too fat and must be slimmed down by the stallion owner before she can be bred. Fat mares often do not come into heat until they are brought down to a normal weight. It is ridiculous to pay mare care fees to have the stallion owner put your horse on a diet! Fat mares may have a significantly lower conception rate than mares in normal condition when they finally do come into heat.

Adequate vitamin levels should be provided in the feed or in a vitamin-mineral supplement. Vitamin A is especially important in bringing mares into heat and having the reproductive tract ready for breeding. Mares in the northern states who are fed hay or pasture may be especially lacking in vitamin A in the spring if the roughage is bleached out. Vitamin A can be fed as a supplement or given in the form of an injection.

Phosphorus is important for reproductive health. There is some evidence that adequate phosphorus levels also help prevent crooked-legged foals. Phosphorus is deficient in the soils (and thus in the feeds) in the Great Plains and intermountain areas of the West. It may be given as a feed supplement. Feeding grain will often supply part of a horse's phosphorus needs. One of my clients had a ranch where every foal was born with crooked legs. The mares had been kept on pasture year-round. When they were brought in and fed phosphorus supplements for several months before foaling, the leg problems were completely eliminated.

Tractability is a desirable trait for the broodmare and is imperative if she is sent to someone else's stallion to be handbred. One especially important part of her general training is halter-breaking. It would seem obvious to most people that mares in this situation should be halter-broke, but one breeding farm had a customer deliver three mares to be bred. We found that none of the three could be caught, haltered, or led—they were broncs right off the range. Mares like this present a real danger to themselves, to the handlers, and to the stallion.

Several other facets of training are important for the broodmare. She should be trained to load in a trailer if she is being hauled to the stallion. This saves upsetting and/or injuring her when she is hauled. She should allow all her feet to be picked up. She should be accustomed to ropes on and around her, as many stallion owners put breeding hobbles on every mare to reduce the chances of her kicking and crippling the stallion. She should calmly stand tied wherever she is left. She should allow people to handle her hindquarters and tail—for washing, tail wrapping, and reproductive examination.

ARTIFICIAL LIGHTING FOR MARES AND STALLIONS

Artificial lighting is now used to bring difficult or late-cycling mares into heat early in the season. It is also widely used to get mares into heat during the winter. The majority of mares are out of heat and have no interest in the stallion from about December until March. In nature, this schedule is determined by the length of night and allows foals to be born in the spring and summer, when they will have a better chance to survive. However, man has decreed that the horses of many breeds will share January 1 as a birth date. This means that if your foal is born in August, he is an official "year" old the following January 1, when, in reality, he is only five months old. There is an obvious advantage to having foals born as soon after the official "birthday" as possible. This advantage is especially important if the resulting animal is being shown or raced.

For this reason, artificial lighting is used to stimulate mares into heat during the period when they are normally out. This technique, for example, was used on a 27-year old Quarter Horse mare. This mare had bloodlines such that if the owners could get one foal, it would be worth a great deal of money. However, in Colorado where she lived, she did not come into heat until June. Her cycles were very irregular, and by the time they had settled down enough for the veterinarian to figure out what the mare was doing, it was September and she was out of heat for the season. Starting her on a lighting program resulted in her cycling regularly and early enough in the season so that she could be bred and settled.

Lighting of this type is generally started the first of December, but can be started in January and February. You don't need to start it gradually—just begin "16-hour days" right away. This simulates the long days of summer for the mare, stimulating the pituitary gland to push the ovaries into action and start the mare coming into heat. Only light is necessary for this, not heat, so the barn doesn't need to be heated. Put the lights on timers so they come on a little before sunset and go off at 8:30 pm, and then come on again at 4:30 am and go off after sunrise. You might have to adjust the time schedule according to the number of daylight hours in your region; your goal is 16 hours of light. Either incandescent or fluorescent lights can be used. A 200-watt bulb over every stall or every other stall is enough. After the lighting program is started, it takes approximately 40 to 60 days for the mare to begin coming into heat, so plan the lighting period accordingly. (21)

The theory that "if a little bit is good, a whole lot is better," works as badly with lighting as it does in many other areas. Dr. E. Palmer, speaking at the Equine

Reproduction Symposium in Australia showed that 20 hours of light gave less stimulation than 14–½ to 16 hours. He found that the length of the night was more important than the length of day because the mare's body seems to measure the length of the night period from sunset onward.

Some farms put their breeding stallions on the same lighting program as their mares, to get them tuned up and ready to go for the earlier-than-natural breeding season. This does seem to help bring some stallions into greater sperm production earlier in the season.

Incidentally, the same lighting schedule can be used to help animals shed their hairy coats so that they are slick and fancy looking for the winter show season. This method is healthier than using heavy blankets or heated barns, which may increase the danger of respiratory diseases due to chilling when the animal is used without his "clothes." It also gives a finer appearance than body clipping. Heavy hair coats may cause problems with cooling out wet horses after working in cold weather. The disadvantage of this technique is that some animals will begin to hair the next August as soon as the days become shorter!

BREEDING HISTORY

The mare's records should be in order. Perhaps the most important are her breeding records. Records of all previous breeding problems and treatments should accompany the mare to the stud farm. One of my clients who was standing a stallion worked all summer trying to settle a mare whose owner swore up and down that she didn't have any breeding problems. After trying for three months to get her settled, we called the farm where she had been bred the previous season. Yes, they said, she was a real problem. The only way they were able to get her bred was by using saline infusions into the uterus.

When treated this way, the mare responded by settling the next time she was bred. When the mare owner was confronted with this information, he admitted that he had deliberately not told us about it! And what good did it do him? It cost him an extra three months of boarding and veterinary bills. Don't keep a mare's problems secret! This can result in getting a late foal or no foal at all, not to mention a lot of unnecessary expense.

Health and immunization records should also go with the mare, including her present vaccination status and any previous health problems she has had. They might not mean much when the mare is in good health, but may make the difference between life and death if she has an emergency and the veterinarian is unable to contact the owner.

Last but not least, have all registration records in order. If you just bought the mare, get her papers transferred to your name immediately. Sometimes it can take months to get all the correspondence ironed out. The stallion owner will often want a copy of the mare's pedigree for his records. A photocopy of her registration papers is often the most convenient way to do this.

HEAT CYCLES

The mare's heat cycle is also called the estrus (also spelled estrous or oestrous) cycle. This is the period during which she will produce a fertile egg (ovulate) from the ovary, and will accept the stallion. Mares only come into heat during the longer days of the year. In the northern states, this may mean only between May and September, while in the southern states, a breeder may have mares in heat nearly all year long.

Most mares come into heat every 21 days; that is, 21 days from the time the mare comes into heat, she will start into heat again. Mares vary from about 18 to 31 days in their heat cycles. Older mares or those who are on poor nutrition may have longer than average cycles. Heat periods are also longer early in the season before they have been established in a regular rhythm.

Ovulation, or the fertile period generally occurs 24 to 48 hours before the mare goes OUT of heat. Thus, no matter how long she is in heat, if it is a fertile heat, ovulation will occur shortly before the end. Since the sperm only live about 24 hours in her genital tract, it is necessary to breed her shortly before she goes out of heat.

Most breeders begin breeding the mare on the second day of her heat cycle, and then breed her every other day until she goes out of heat. This helps to assure that viable sperm will be in the mare's genital tract when the egg is released from the ovary. If you have a problem mare, your veterinarian may palpate her ovaries through the rectal wall to determine when she is ready to ovulate so that you can breed her at that time.

A mare who has just foaled will come into heat about nine days later, although this may range from about 4 to 18 days. This is called the "foal heat." She can be rebred at this time if she foaled cleanly and without complications (no retained membranes, tearing, or bruising, or infection). If you are taking the mare to a stallion, haul her when the foal is six or seven days old so that she will be there if she should come into heat a day or two early. It will also give her time to settle down to the new premises before breeding.

If she has had problems or injury to the reproductive tract during foaling, you can wait until the next heat period (18 to 21 days after the foal heat). This will give her time to heal and get ready to rebreed. Alternatively, prostaglandins can be given about a week after she is out of foal heat. This will bring her into heat about 15 days after she has foaled, giving her additional time to rest, but not so long as waiting until the second natural heat after foaling.

A mare is never too old to breed if she is in good health and if she is bred to a stallion who is expected to produce a foal of reasonable size. Foaling is easier on mares who are younger because their pelvis is held together with more cartilage than bone. But, there is no good reason to avoid breeding an older mare if you want a foal from her. You may wish to keep a closer eye on her than you would on a younger animal when she does foal.

BREEDING EXAM, MARES

Ideally, all mares should be examined by a veterinarian prior to breeding. This is especially important the first time a filly is bred to determine that she is reproductively normal. Recently, a client brought me a three-year old filly who had been bred several times during an earlier heat period. Each time, there was a bit of fresh blood from her vulva. At the last breeding, the stallion punctured the vagina, necessitating extensive and lengthy treatment by another veterinarian. The owner wanted me to examine the animal and determine why he could not get her bred. Incidentally, she had not come into heat until she was given an injection of a hormone.

Examination showed that the animal's vagina was only about six inches deep (it should have been about 12 to 14 inches if normal), and ended in a cul-de-sac rather than a normal cervix. No sign of a cervix was seen, nor was it observable with rectal palpation. It was also not possible to find a normal uterus. Apparently the animal had been born with just part of a reproductive tract. Examination before breeding would not make her reproduce any better, but it surely would have saved the owner's time and expense in attempting to breed her, as well as the time and money invested in healing the vaginal perforation. In the long run, as with many other preventive procedures, a prebreeding examination would have saved the owner some money, to say nothing of the pain it would have prevented for the horse!

Your veterinarian will begin by evaluating the mare's reproductive history and noting any problems that she has, such as failure to conceive, irregular cycles, foaling problems with her last pregnancy, failure to carry pregnancies to term, etc. He will correlate this with her overall condition and state of health.

His next step will probably be a rectal examination; here, he reaches a gloved hand into the mare's rectum. Feeling gently through the rectal wall, he can determine much about her reproductive tract. He will check to see that the uterus has good tone with no obvious defects. The cervix is examined to see that it is normal. The ovaries are palpated to see that they are normal in size and shape and that there are no cysts or other defects. Many veterinarians can tell whether the animal is ready to ovulate or not. At the same time, he will examine the mare's external genitalia to see that she has no scars or tears.

He may examine her vagina and cervix with a speculum (a device which holds it open and allows him to look in). He may take a bacterial culture from the cervix with a long swab at the same time.

Animals with apparent hormone abnormalities may need a series of laboratory tests to determine what is wrong and what treatment is necessary. One of my clients had a mare who rarely came into heat; when she did, she would not conceive. When we finally did bring her into heat with prostaglandins and breed her, she aborted early in the pregnancy. Other symptoms, such as a poor hair coat and the tendency to stay thin on good feed, suggested hormonal problems. We ran some special blood tests, and found that the animal was severely hypothyroid, and would need supplementation of thyroid hormones in order to breed normally.

CASLICK'S OPERATION

A normal mare's anus should be directly above her vulva, so that manure falls clear of the vagina. Some mares have poor reproductive conformation and have the anus placed two to six inches ahead of the vagina. This is especially common in mares with flat croups, such as Arabians. These mares are said to be "tipped." This arrangement allows the bit of liquid that often follows a bowel movement to run into the vagina, giving the mare a

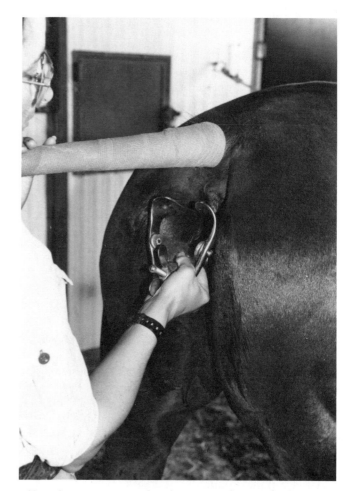

Mare being examined with a vaginal speculum.

chronic vaginal infection. A mare with this infection will usually fail to conceive until she is treated. Older mares, or those who are very thin, may appear "tipped." If the only problem is loss of weight, returning the animal to normal condition often corrects it.

If the lips of the vulva are loose and slack instead of being pulled tightly together, the mare may take in air as she moves. On the racetrack, these mares are called "windsuckers," because they often pull air into the vagina as they run. As with the mare who has poor conformation in this area, this defect will cause a continuous vaginitis (irritation or infection in the vagina). Some trainers feel that this affects the animal's performance, causing her to run less well than she otherwise would. Most mares on the racetrack are routinely stitched shut. Some mares do not have vaginal lips that hang loosely, but may show "windsucking" conformation by having numerous horizontal rows of wrinkles across the lips of the vulva, rather than having them pressed tightly together in a straight line as is normal.

If she is "tipped," the vet may recommend that the mare be sutured. This is often called just "suturing." It is also called "Caslick's surgery," or just plain "Caslick's."

The vet will twitch the mare and deaden her genital area with a local anesthetic. He will then remove a small strip of tissue from each side, usually with a pair of scissors. Then he will suture the two cut areas to each other. The areas are trimmed so that they will grow together. Without trimming them and making fresh new edges, it would be just like stitching two of your fingers to each other: they would not knit together.

The suturing must be carefully done, with no gaps in the suture line. A pinhole is enough to continue the animal's infertility. Most veterinarians suture the animal closed to just below the level of the pelvic brim. This should leave sufficient room for her to urinate. If she is sutured too tightly, the urine will not flow out, but will pool on the floor of the vagina and may go clear into the uterus, causing the very problem you are trying to prevent. Sutured correctly, the mare can still be bred (while sutured), using care and a breeding roll (described below).

Depending on the type of suture material that is used, it may be necessary to remove the stitches in 10 to 14 days. It is important that some types of suture material not be left in place. If not removed, the stitches can collect manure and filth and help to continue infection in the

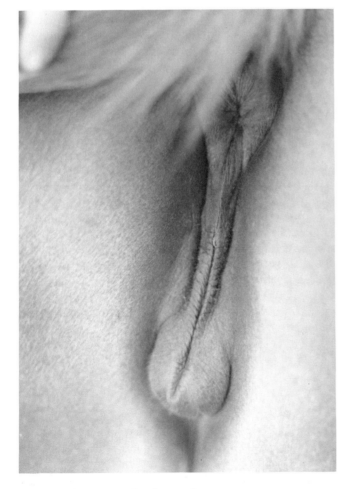

Mare with a normal vulva and anus.

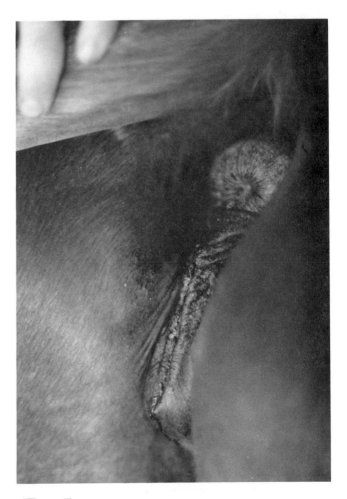

"Tipped" mare.

mare. Often, when a mare is tipped, surgery to remedy the problem is all that is necessary to fix her breeding problem and make her fertile again.

My practice is to go through a mare band in the fall and suture any mares that are open (nonpregnant) whose breeding conformation indicates that they need it. At the time of surgery, the animal's vaginal walls are often severely reddened and may be streaked with pus, indicating a definite infection. If nothing else is done but suturing them shut, most mares will be found to be free of infection in the spring when they are cultured before breeding. It's amazing how easily the body can clear up the infection on its own if we just fix it so that manure isn't dripping into the vagina several times every day!

A surgical technique has recently been described in which the surgery is done just inside the lips of the vulva, and is thus invisible from the outside. This makes it even more important that a mare be examined before breeding. Otherwise, tearing may occur when she is bred if the owner does not realize that she has been sutured. Pregnant mares who are purchased should be examined for the same surgery, to make sure they will not tear out when they foal.

WARNING: A mare who has been sutured needs to be opened before she foals. Since we have reduced the size of the opening through which the foal must come, it may tear out horribly if she is NOT cut open. They never seem to tear out in a nice straight line; the result is usually a jagged-edged wound that is often damaging to the mare as well as painful. They nearly always cost more to repair than merely resuturing the Caslick's after the foal is born.

When it is evident that the mare is about ready to foal (within two or three days of it, as nearly as you can tell), get her in and restrain her in a set of stocks if you have them. Put a twitch on her. Wash her genital area with a mild soap such as pHisohex, then rinse her with a tamed iodine solution (such as Betadine). Wash and rinse your hands in the same manner, as well as a sharp pair of scissors (preferably surgical scissors). Or, you can use a disposable scalpel. If worst comes to worst, a sharp pocket or hunting knife, cleaned as above, can be used. Insert your index and second fingers into her vagina, spreading them widely apart. Pull them outward so that the skin stretches tightly over them. Then, cut up the midline, to approximately the top of the suture line. The mare will bleed a small amount, but this is no problem. No medication is needed on the cut. A twitch is usually sufficient to do this bit of work, especially if you cut quickly and cleanly. No anesthetic is necessary.

If you arrive at the foaling of a sutured mare who is not opened, you can quickly open her in the same manner. If she is lying down trying to have the foal, a twitch may not even be necessary. Nature somewhat deadens the pain sensation around the mare's perineal area just prior to foaling. Again, by quickly cutting her open, you can save much trouble and pain which could be caused by tearing.

The mare can usually be resutured without anesthesia within a half hour after the foal is born, as this area is naturally made less sensitive during the birth process. Or, she may be resutured several days after foaling. Many mares are opened and closed in this manner every year for their entire lives. It's definitely not ideal to breed this sort of conformation into our animals. Unfortunately, as long as their offspring are worth large amounts of money, people will continue to put up with this sort of nuisance in order to get foals from these mares.

When you deliver the mare to the stallion to be bred, be sure to tell the stallion owner if your veterinarian has advised the use of a breeder's stitch or the use of a breeding roll with the sutured mare. A breeder's stitch is used to support the sutured area of the vulva after a Caslick's operation. It is usually made with heavy, carbolized umbilical (cotton) tape, and helps prevent the sutured area from tearing out when the mare is bred. It is generally left in place until she is checked in foal and then removed, as the cotton tape can act as a wick to pull bacteria into the vagina. If the mare has been sutured very tightly, it may be necessary to open her before she is bred. This keeps her from tearing open, and prevents bruising or hematoma on the stallion's penis. She is then resutured after breeding.

A breeding roll is a piece of wood about three inches in diameter and three or four feet long, covered with a soft padding such as carpeting. It is held between the mare and stallion during breeding (above his penis) to keep him from going too deeply into the mare. Again, the object is to avoid opening up the sutures. Needless to say, sutured mares should not be pasture bred, as they may tear easily, even if the sutured area is completely healed.

OPENING THE MARE

Old-time breeders "opened" mares before breeding. This meant that the fellow inserted a washed hand and arm into the mare's vagina, and thrust one or more fingers into the cervix to open it. Apparently the theory was that it would allow the semen to better enter the uterus. This is NOT a good practice for two reasons. It can introduce infection into the vagina and/or uterus, and it breaks the vacuum which is normally present. This vacuum helps to literally suck the semen into the uterus and helps to increase the conception rate. So, "opening" the mare may actually decrease rather than increase conception rates.

CERVICAL CULTURES

Another procedure that your veterinarian will perform in the course of a breeding soundness exam is a cervical culture. Using a long swab, he will reach into the mare's cervix and take a sample of the material there. This gives an indication of the state of health of the uterus, telling him what kind of bacteria, if any, are present.

He will take this sample to his clinic or to a commercial laboratory where the swab will be rubbed onto a special sterile medium made of blood, gelatin, and other special nutrients. The medium designed to nurture any bacteria that are present. These cultures are incubated at body temperature. They are usually examined 24, 48, and perhaps 72 hours after they are placed onto the medium. If any bacteria are present, the laboratory will usually put them onto different types of media to see what kind they are. They may also run what is called a "sensitivity test," or just a "sensitivity." This tells your veterinarian which kind of antibiotic will kill the bacteria that are present, and saves a lot of time, trouble, expense, and effort in treating the animal with something that doesn't work. It allows your veterinarian to go directly to a drug that will specifically attack the infection. Streptococcus and E. coli are the bacteria most commonly found in uterine cultures.

Your veterinarian will treat the mare's infection with the proper antibiotic, usually diluted in a quantity of sterile water or saline solution. He may treat for as many as three to four days in a row. The solution is placed directly into the uterus, usually with a long piece of tubing. We often wait for a period of time—as much as a week or two, and then culture the cervix again to see that we have gotten the infection killed in the uterus.

If the infection is gone, and there is no other problem, the mare is ready to breed. If it has not been cleared up, the lab will run another sensitivity test. Frequently, a whole new pattern of sensitivity is seen on the second culture. This means that we have killed out all the bacteria which were sensitive to the first antibiotic. This has allowed some others who were not sensitive to it to grow and to flourish without competition. At this point, your veterinarian will treat with the antibiotic that is now recommended for the situation. This procedure may have to be done several times before the uterus becomes sterile and ready for breeding. Breeding is useless as long as the mare remains infected, because even if the sperm and egg do unite, the infection will keep the embryo from implanting itself on the uterine wall. It will just be flushed from the uterus and the mare will come into heat again.

Every mare owner who is sending a horse out for breeding should have her cultured before she leaves his premises. If you do not, and she is infected, she will not get pregnant anyway and your mare-care money will be wasted. If the stallion owner requires that all mares be cultured and you have not had it done, he will have it done for you. If she is infected, he will have her treated, and again she is standing there costing you a whole lot more than if you had treated her at home.

Some mares with uterine infections will have so bad a problem that they continually drain pus from the reproductive tract. This may run down the hind legs and cause the hair to fall out. The chances of curing mares with severe pyometra (pus in the uterus) is small. Even if the infection is cleared up, it may have caused permanent, irreversible damage to the uterus.

ENDOMETRIAL BIOPSY

If a mare has had a chronic infection, there may be so much damage to the lining of the uterus that she will never conceive. After the infection is cleared up and a reasonable attempt has been made to breed the mare to a stallion of known fertility under good management, she should be further examined. About half of the mares with chronic infertility will show endometritis (an inflammation of the lining of the uterus). About 85% of them will show fibrosis of the uterine lining. (22)

Diagnosis of endometrial fibrosis, as this problem is called, usually entails a uterine biopsy. For this examination, the veterinarian takes an instrument called a biopsy punch and removes a few small pieces of the uterine lining. These are sent to a laboratory which preserves the material in a special solution, slices it into extremely thin sections, and stains the sections with a dye. This allows the cells to be easily seen when examined under the microscope. The slices are scrutinized to see whether or not a viable uterine lining exists, or if it is damaged. If damaged, the extent of the damage can be approximated.

If there is not enough uterine lining present, the embryo cannot adequately attach and will not get enough nutrients to survive. The mare will carry the foal for a short length of time, abort, and come back into heat. This may show up as a horse with longer-than-normal heat cycles. These are caused by her getting pregnant and then losing the foal at a very early stage of development. The uterine biopsy can be a valuable diagnostic tool in determining whether or not a mare can ever carry a foal to full term.

LAPAROSCOPIC EXAMINATION

Laparoscopic examination may be used with mares who are problem breeders. This involves making a small incision in the horse's flank. Then, a long thin instrument called a laparoscope is introduced through this opening. This is somewhat like a thin telescope, with fiber optics to carry light to the end of it within the animal. The veterinarian then looks through an eyepiece, and can see the uterus, ovaries, Fallopian tubes, and other internal organs. The mare should be kept off food for 24 hours before examination to allow her intestinal tract to partially empty and become less active, making it easier to see what things look like inside the abdomen. This examination will often discover the reason for a mare's infertility and may help to predict whether she can be cured or not.

TIMETABLE FOR BREEDING THE MARE

4 TO 6 MONTHS PRIOR TO BREEDING

Select the stallion who will mesh well with your mare and make the necessary arrangements to breed her to him. This may include paying a booking fee to reserve a breeding.

6 TO 8 WEEKS PRIOR TO BREEDING

Call your veterinarian and arrange for a general health check and reproductive examination of the broodmare. Try to schedule this exam for the first or second day of a heat period, if at all possible. Her teeth should be checked to be sure that she is eating efficiently and floated if needed. Wolf teeth should be removed if they are bothering the mare, as should any caps that are hanging on. A fecal examination should be done and the mare wormed, if worming is due or indicated at this time.

The reproductive examination will usually include a rectal exam to check the condition of the ovaries, cervix, and uterus. A sterile swab for culture of the cervix should be taken. If there is any bacterial growth, the vet will return and administer antibiotics based on the sensitivity pattern found in the culture. A mare with a tipped vulva will need to be sutured at this time and treated for infection already present in the uterus.

Routine immunizations should be administered during this visit, depending on the time of the year. The mare should have a tetanus booster if she is on a regular tetanus toxoid program. Otherwise, she will have the first of a pair of initial tetanus shots. She should be vaccinated for influenza. Rhinopneumonitis vaccine is vitally important to the broodmare and should be administered if she is not pregnant. "Rhino" shows little or no respiratory symptoms in the broodmare, but results in abortions and foals born weak that often die within a few days. The vaccination is a simple, inexpensive, and safe way of preventing this loss. If this is the proper time of the year, encephalitis (sleeping sickness) vaccine should also be administered.

3 TO 4 WEEKS BEFORE BREEDING

This veterinarian visit should also be scheduled to catch the mare in heat, if at all possible. If she showed any infection on the first culture and was treated, she should be recultured to be sure that the infection has cleared. The second course of vaccinations (if necessary) should be given at this time. Blood should be taken for a Coggins test, required by most stallion owners, and generally mandatory for interstate transportation of horses.

The vet should make his final visit three or four days before your departure, to clear up any problems the mare might still have. He should bring her health records up to date and have them ready to accompany the mare. He will write the health certificate to allow the horse to be transported across state lines. Get information from the vet regarding any medication or treatment that the mare needs. Also, obtain a supply of any needed medicine and get complete information on any treatment that is to be continued.

The farrier should visit and pull the mare's shoes and trim her feet. Most stallion owners require this to help prevent injury to their stallion. Doing it at home before the mare leaves allows the mare owner to have his own shoer do the job.

DELIVERING THE MARE

Plan to deliver the mare to the stallion four to seven days before she is scheduled to come into heat, if at all possible. Hauling the mare and taking her to a new place will often result in her not coming into heat or not showing heat enough to be bred. If this occurs, the stallion owner will have to wait 21 days before she is in again. Delivering her a few days ahead of time allows her to rest, to get used to her new lodging and neighbors, and to be ready to show heat when she comes in.

Be sure to give the stallion owner any special feeding instructions that are necessary for her health. A good example is a mare who requires extra bran in her grain to keep her from getting colic. If she requires special feed, take some along or make arrangements for the stallion owner to buy some for her. If the mare is sutured, be sure to tell the stallion owner.

PASTURE BREEDING VS HAND BREEDING

Perhaps the ideal way to breed mares is by turning them loose in a large pasture with a stallion. This is used to some extent in the western states, where a ranch owner will turn a stallion in with his mares. A good range stallion has the experience and sense to breed the mare when she is in the right stage of her heat period. Using this method, many mares can be bred who cannot be settled by hand breeding. Occasionally, the owner of a valuable mare who cannot be gotten in foal will turn her out in a bunch like this. If the stallion is able to get her bred, the resulting pregnancy will often stabilize her hormonal situation enough that she can be hand-bred to the stallion of choice the next year. It's definitely a method to try when all else fails.

Unfortunately, this natural situation is often impossible in city areas and in the east. And, owners of very valuable stallions cannot risk getting them kicked or injured and losing the use of them as breeding animals. As a result, most of our mares are "hand-bred." This involves keeping the mare and stallion in separate stalls or corrals. They are brought together only for teasing or breeding. In nature, a stallion may breed a single mare eight or ten times a day. If we are trying to breed the same stallion to a number of mares, we cannot permit this. A mature stallion may be hand-bred to two or three mares per day. Often, he is only bred morning and evening. Extra mares may be brought back into heat with prostaglandins after they have gone out in order to spread the stallion around. A mature stallion may handle 40 to 50 mares in a short breeding season (say, February to May). He can handle more if the season is extended into August as it may be in the northern states.

Often, a mare who has not been around a stallion will come into heat within 24 to 48 hours after being moved to premises with a stallion. It is often hard for the owner who does not have a stallion to tell when the mare is in heat, as some of them do not show any signs at all unless there is a stallion around. For this reason, it is often desirable to take the mare to the premises where she will be bred, rather than trying to determine when she is in heat and then hauling her to the stallion. Also, hauling will upset some mares enough that they will go out of heat. Young fillies, by the way, will usually come into heat some time around a year of age. They often seem to do so when it is most inconvenient, such as when you are going to trailer them with a stallion. It is important to remember that they are becoming mature, especially if you don't want them bred!

TEASING

The mare is exposed to a teaser to determine when she is in heat. This allows her to show sexual behavior so that only mares who are in heat are exposed to the stallion. This saves him from possible injury. In a small breeding operation, she may be tried with the stallion who will eventually be used to breed her. In larger operations, the teaser may be a stallion (sometimes a pony stallion) or a studdy-acting gelding who is kept just for that purpose.

The mare is led up to the teaser stallion, usually across the fence from him. In large operations, the mares are often run in large bunches into a long alleyway and the stallion is led down the line of mares. He is allowed to sniff each one and will show interest in those in heat. Many breeders check mares every other day during the time they are out of heat, so as to not miss the next heat cycle. They will then check them every day as they are coming into heat and during the heat.

If you are teasing just one mare at a time, it is usually best to do so on opposite sides of a solid fence. This is so the stallion cannot get a foot into the fence in his excitement. Also, the mare cannot kick through the fence and hurt either herself or him. Horses are large, fast, and have tremendous strength. When they are in the grip of sexual excitement, both horses and handlers are in great danger of being hurt if extreme caution is not exercised.

Most handlers lead the mare up to the stallion head-first, and allow them to sniff noses. Some mares, when not in heat, will object so violently to him at this time that they may snort and scream, often lashing out with their hind legs or trying to whirl and get away from him. The mare may flatten her ears and bite at the stallion. She may resent being handled. She may swish her tail angrily. The stallion may scream sharply. If you know him well, you can often pick out this short, sharp noise as an indication that he's saying she's not in heat. Until you know a given mare better, you should at this point assume that she is not in heat. Some mares will urinate from nervousness when they are not in heat. Only repeated teasing will tell when

these mares are "in." Often the stallion's actions are a better clue than those of this type of mare.

Mares who are nursing foals may not show heat, especially if the foal is not near. Many breeding facilities have a small pen for the foal near the teasing area so that the mare can see him. Then, she will be more likely to show normal estrus signs. Mares who are teased just before feeding or before they are turned out, may be excited and not show signs of heat. Try to tease at the same time each day, so that both mares and stallions may become used to a routine. Some mares will show signs of heat only when twitched.

As the mare comes into heat, she will be more inclined to stay near the stallion and to nuzzle him. Often she will push her neck toward him, allowing him to nibble and sniff her. As she comes further into heat (say, the next day), she will turn sideways to him and allow him to push and smell her flanks. She may totally turn her hind end to him. In turn, he gets more and more interested and nuzzles and nibbles. He may nicker and snort rather than scream.

The stallion may show a "fleering" or "Flehmen" response to the mare's odor. This is a sharp curling of the upper lip. It has also been called a "horse laugh." It is common to many domestic and wild animals and usually indicates the animal's interest in an odor. It does not necessarily indicate that the mare is in or out of heat—only that the stallion is interested and is checking her.

If there is any danger of transfer of venereal disease, the teaser should not be allowed to touch the mare, only to get close. Teasers have been known to spread venereal problems on their nose from one mare to another.

The mare in heat will usually lift her tail and hold it more or less erect over her back (or she may hold it to the side). She may open and close the lower end of the vulva, an action known as "winking." She will often spread her hind legs and drop her rear end, squatting slightly. This stance looks as though she is trying to urinate, but is held for long periods of time. Indeed, the mare may urinate; her urine will contain odors which further stimulate the stallion. When these signs are seen, she is ready to take the stallion.

Some mares will come into heat and not show any signs of it. This is a behavioral problem. As mentioned above, it may occur in mares who are worrying about their foals. It is also seen in nervous and maiden mares. These horses should be carefully introduced to the teasing system. Gentle teasing and close observation will allow the owner to determine when some of these animals are in heat. Trial and error may help to find a method of teasing which works for a particular horse. Shy mares are best checked individually rather than in groups.

If the mare's heat pattern cannot be determined at all, it may be necessary for your veterinarian to palpate her every day or every other day for a period of time until he can tell when a follicle is sufficiently developed on the ovary that the mare is ready. She can then be bred using tranquilizers and hobbles, if necessary. Or, if facilities permit, she can be artificially inseminated. Mares who stay out of heat for prolonged periods of time can, if necessary, be treated to bring them into heat. Again, your veterinarian should be consulted for the latest treatment of these problems.

BREEDING

When the mare is clearly showing signs of heat, she should be moved away from the teasing horse to the breeding area. Breeding should usually be done away from both the stallion's pen and the mare's pen. Even if it is only a different corner of the driveway, having a special breeding area fixes in the stallion's mind what he is supposed to do there. Also, it helps to keep him from acting in a manner appropriate only to breeding when he is in other places.

Wrap the mare's tail to get her ready for breeding. There are rubber tail wraps with Velcro closures that can be used or you can use Vetrap or Elastikon tape. This helps to keep hairs from being carried into the vulva as the stallion enters her, thus keeping her cleaner and helping to prevent infection. Begin at the root of the tail and wrap outward for 10 to 12 inches. Then, wash the mare with a mild soap, such as pHisohex.

Rinse her well with a solution of Betadine or other mild disinfectant. It is important to watch what you use in a mare's perineal area, as it is very delicate. It is easy to scald her in this area by using too-strong products, irritating soaps, or not rinsing her adequately. An easy way to wash her is by using large chunks of cotton from a roll. This is easy on the mare and sanitary. Finally, she should be rinsed with clean water. If any disinfectant is left on her perineum, it may be carried in as the stallion enters her and may kill the sperm. The stallion should be led to the breeding area. When he has an erection, his penis should be washed in the same manner, again rinsing well.

Breeding procedure from this point is pretty much a matter of personal preference and depends a lot on the handler, the facilities available, and how the stallion has been trained. One person can usually handle a well-trained stallion and properly restrained mare, or a mare who is known to be gentle and easy to breed. Several

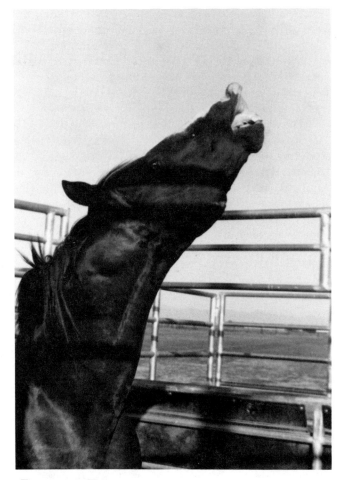

Fleering or Flehmen response.

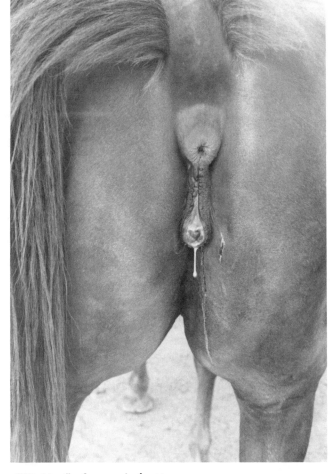

"Winking" of mare in heat.

handlers may be needed with inadequate facilities and fractious animals.

One of my clients had a number of mares and several stallions. She was often left to breed unknown mares by herself. She had a safe place to tie the mares—a stout post in the middle of a stretch of fence. The mare could swing no more than 180 degrees against the fence. She would tie the mare to the post and wash and prepare her. She would then put a sideline on the mare's left hind leg, not really tying it up, but just restraining it lightly so that it could not kick backward at the stallion. You can use a set of breeding hobbles instead; they are convenient and help to restrain both hind legs instead of just one. They are good protection for a stallion who has been trained to mount from the rear.

After preparing the mare, the woman would get the stallion. She used a halter with a chain under his chin. The chain was never needed with this stallion, but gave her an extra measure of security. A stout lead rope about 15 feet long was used. It gave her enough rope to hang onto the stallion while he was on the mare and yet be well out of the way in case he would come off roughly or swing his front feet. He never did, but it pays to be safe rather than sorry. She always wore a hard hat when breeding. Again, she never needed it, but. . . . At the reproductive facility at Colorado State University, all handlers wear motorcycle helmets while handling stallions or mares in a breeding situation. They report that this practice has saved them several possible injuries or deaths.

It is important to keep the stallion under control as he approaches the mare. A stallion who rears or waves his front legs is a hazard to his handlers. Even if you feel safe most of the time, it only takes one small blow with a front hoof to kill you. My great-grandfather died that way. Most handlers let the stallion talk and snort and become interested—as long as he walks beside them like a gentleman. The horse should lead on a slack shank, rather than dragging his handler. Whatever you do, stay at the animal's shoulder rather than out in front of his feet.

My client would now lead the stallion out, tie him to a hitching rail, and wash his penis as she had washed the mare. She would then bring the stallion to the mare's left side (the one with the sideline) to prevent him from being kicked. She would let him sniff the mare's flanks and nuzzle and talk until he was fully erect. At this point, she would give him slack and say, "Up!" He would mount the mare from the left side, then swing himself around and enter the mare.

Ejaculation is often signaled by a sharp jerk or two of the stallion's tail, called "flagging." If you can see the underside of his penis, you may notice the urethra pulsing as he ejaculates. If the stallion will tolerate being touched while he is in the mare, you can gently place a hand on the underside of the penis and feel the urethra pulsing. This is the surest way of knowing that he has ejaculated. Some stallions may flag and become limp without ejaculating. If

there is any doubt, the horse should be checked as above. Most stallions show sharply decreased sex drive and interest after they have ejaculated. As he comes out of the mare, you may see a few drops of fluid on the end of his penis.

The stallion usually relaxes at this point and slides off the mare. It is important to back the stallion away from the mare to avoid his being kicked. Mares do not often kick, but it's better to be safe and train the stallion in safe habits that will help him to keep working a long and useful life for you. It is good at this point to again wash the stallion's penis and sheath. He can be rinsed with clean warm water or a mild antiseptic solution. This helps to remove mucus which has come from the mare's genital tract. It is important not to over-disinfect the stallion's penis. A certain amount of bacteria are normal to good genital health, both in the mare and the stallion. If these are removed, harmful ones generally take over, often causing infertility problems which were not present initially.

My client would then put the stallion back in his pen. She would then return immediately and take the sideline off the mare. She then would lead the mare around for five minutes or so, at a walk. The five-minute walk helps to prevent the habit that some mares have of squatting and getting rid of some of the semen. By the time you have led them for five minutes, they have generally lost the urge to squat.

It is important to train a young stallion properly for breeding. He needs to learn that breeding occurs in a certain place in a certain halter, and that he is to act like any other horse the rest of the time. It is worth taking the time to establish good breeding habits and manners. A young stallion needs gentle guidance, firm discipline, and a clear definition of what he may do where. During the learning process, he may try to mount the mare's side or neck, often before he is fully erect. He should gently be pulled off the mare and repositioned as you want him to learn.

Guide him from front to rear on the mare with the lead rope, pulling him back down when he tries to mount the wrong way or before he is ready. He may become confused if you try to help him too much. Allow him to take his time and get interested at his own pace. It may be necessary to try him both morning and night for several days before you will get a mare bred. Needless to say, it's good to start a young horse on a gentle mare who will stand quietly for him. That way, you can give him your full attention rather than dividing it between him and the mare. It is best if one person consistently handles the young horse so that the same signals can be used from one breeding to the next.

Masturbation is common in breeding stallions. Since the horse does not ejaculate, it should not affect his semen quality. However, some people feel that it affects his sexual drive so that he may be less interested when presented to a mare. Adequate work and a large corral for exercise may help to reduce the problem. If it continues, the horse may be fitted with a plastic ring to prevent his getting an erection. Called a stud ring, it is slipped just behind the head of the penis and must be removed before a mare is bred. It must be kept carefully cleaned by daily washing, or it may cause irritation and infection. Masturbation is thought to be more common in stallions whose penis and sheath are dirty. Cleansing as described previously may help these animals.

CONTAGIOUS EQUINE METRITIS

Contagious equine metritis (CEM) is a highly contagious genital infection of mares. It is a venereal disease, spread by sexual contact. It was first described in 1977 in Europe, Australia, and the United States. Mares may have endometritis (an infection of the lining of the uterus) and infertility. Affected animals do not have any sign of disease anywhere else in the body. Both mares and stallions can be carriers, without any visible signs, yet be able to transmit the disease to other horses through sexual contact. Mares may be treated with antibiotics, but some still remain carriers. Some mares will recover and conceive without antibiotic treatment and still remain carriers. In addition to its spread by sexual contact, the disease may be spread by people who are washing or handling mares or stallions. It may also be carried on the nose of a teaser stallion from one mare to another.

A large percentage of infected mares come back into heat shortly after being bred to a stallion. Some will have a thick, mucus discharge from the genital tract; this may be mixed with pus. The discharge occurs 1 to 6 days after service and may persist for up to three months. Not all mares have a visible uterine discharge. Foals nursing the mares remain healthy.

CEM is treated with antibiotics after a culture and sensitivity are run to determine which antibiotic will kill the bacteria which are involved. Most animals who are treated and who recover seem to have normal fertility during the next breeding season.

Sanitation between animals in breeding situations is very important. Disposable gloves and disposable towels, as well as quality disinfectants, should be used by those handling horses for breeding in order to avoid spreading the infection between animals. Artificial insemination is often used to prevent reinfection of the stallion once he has been treated and pronounced clean.

A strict screening program is used to screen imported stallions so that infected animals are not brought into the country. Outbreaks in the United States are promptly quarantined, and all affected mares and stallions are treated. (23)

Kentucky, in particular, has put into effect strict import requirements for mares coming into the state to be bred. A series of cultures are required. In addition, blood tests may be necessary to confirm that the mare has not been exposed to the disease. These may take a month or more. You should plan for the time and expense necessary for this testing when shipping mares into Kentucky to be bred. In addition to the state regulations, some breeding sheds may have even more strict requirements. Check before shipping your animal to them. These strict measures were put into effect to save the Thoroughbred breeding industry which is so important to Kentucky. At this point, CEM appears to have been eliminated from the state. They are, however, taking no chances that it will reappear and devastate the industry as it did when it first appeared.

PYOMETRA AND METRITIS

Pyometra means "pus in the uterus," while "metritis" refers to an inflammation of the uterine lining. They commonly refer to an infection in the uterus which may be caused by bacteria, fungi, yeasts, or other organisms. With pyometra, the mare may not cycle at all. She may have a sticky, yellowish, or greenish drainage from the vulva. There may be enough of it to drain down the animal's hindlegs. This material will cause the hair to slip (fall out) if it is left on the skin for a prolonged period of time.

Mares who have a uterine infection which is less serious are said to have a "metritis." These animals may come into heat and cycle normally, but will not become pregnant. They may have pus in the uterus, but not so much that it drains visibly from the mare's genital tract.

Call your veterinarian if your mare has either of these problems. He will examine her genital tract and take a culture swab from the cervix or uterus. This will be sent to a laboratory for culture and sensitivity tests. Repeated treatments may be necessary to clear the animal of infection. In some cases, enough damage may have been done to the uterine lining that the mare will never conceive or carry a foal to term.

EMBRYO TRANSFERS

Embryo transfers are done between a mare who is unable to conceive or carry a foal and a recipient mare who will carry the fetus. This practice is used with an old mare who has enough damage or fibrous tissue in the uterus that she can no longer carry a foal to term. It is also used with very valuable mares. The mare may be bred naturally to the stallion or artificially inseminated. The tiny embryo is then taken from her body about eight days after she ovulates. This is done either by flushing it from her uterus with a saline solution or surgically removing it through an abdominal laparotomy incision.

The embryo is then placed into the uterus of a recipient mare who has been treated with hormones so that she is in the same stage of her heat cycle as the donor mare. The donor mare may be given a fertility drug to help her produce several eggs rather than just one. This gives even more chances of getting one of them successfully mated with the stallion's semen and getting it to take in a recipient mare. Several breed associations have placed restrictions on the circumstances under which offspring from embryo transplants can be registered.

ARTIFICIAL INSEMINATION

Also called "AI," this technique allows semen to be collected from the stallion and placed in the mare. It is used with stallions who are so valuable that the owner cannot risk having them injured by being kicked by a mare. It is also used for horses who cannot physically mount a mare (say, a stallion with an injured hind leg). It can be used when a large number of mares are booked to the same stallion in the same period of time so that he cannot naturally cover them all. It can also help prevent spread of venereal diseases (such as contagious equine metritis) from one mare to the stallion and then on to other mares. AI can prevent the spread of nonvenereal diseases as well; examples of these are various viral and bacterial respiratory diseases.

The technique can also be used with stallions with behavioral problems, such as shyness with mares, viciousness when breeding, or delayed ejaculation. It can be used on mares with behavioral problems or those with physical problems, such as leg injuries which would not allow the mare to hold the stallion's weight at breeding. Mares who are tightly sutured can be inseminated without repeated re-opening and closing.

Mature stallions can be bred about twice a day; if more mares than this need to be bred, it is often necessary to go to AI. With good facilities and trained personnel, live foaling rates of 75 to 80% may be achieved with AI. (24)

The stallion is trained to mount a teaser mare who has been given hormones to make her appear in heat. Sometimes a dummy mare is used. He then ejaculates into an artificial vagina. This is a large tube with a soft rubber liner. The space between the outer tubing and the inner liner is filled with warm water.

After the semen is collected, it is examined with a microscope to determine how concentrated it is. It is then diluted accordingly. Good quality semen from a potent stallion can be diluted enough to cover up to 25 mares. The semen is usually used within 15 to 45 minutes. Many stud farms inseminate mares every other day while they are in heat, much as with natural cover. (25)

The mare has her tail wrapped and is cleansed as for natural breeding. The semen is deposited in the uterus, using sterile equipment to prevent the introduction of infection. Of course, she must be in the proper stage of her heat cycle. A good set of stocks to restrain the mare is important. If at all possible, stocks should be located indoors or at least in a shed out of the weather.

The legality of artificial insemination varies from one breed association to another. Some associations require that the mare be covered naturally at the same time. Some have also required that stallions used for artificial insemination have their blood type on file. This is then compared with the mare's blood type and the foal's blood type in cases where parentage is questioned. This testing is extremely reliable and lessens the possibility of owners attempting to register foals to the wrong mare or stallion.

At the present time, it is not possible to consistently store frozen stallion semen and have enough sperm survive to give satisfactory conception rates. Because breed associations have discouraged storage, little research has been done and little is likely to be done in the future.

PROSTAGLANDINS

These are the new wonder drugs of the last few years in equine reproduction. Prostaglandin F2 alpha is used for treating dysfunctions of the reproductive cycle in mares. The drug is given to mares who do not come into visible heat and are not pregnant or who come into heat erratically. It can be used to bring a mare in shortly after she has gone out of foal heat so that instead of waiting 21 to 25 days for the second heat, she may be bred about 15 days after she foals. This allows her reproductive tract a bit more time to rest and get ready for pregnancy, but still brings her in earlier than she would come in by herself. It can be used to shorten the time between heat cycles when a mare is missed or too many mares are booked to the stallion at the same time.

Prostaglandins are used in mares who have too long a time between heat cycles. They bring the mare back into heat and allow her to be bred sooner than her own hormones allow. They may be given for diagnostic purposes to problem mares to see if they can be stimulated to come into a normal heat at all. These drugs can also be used to synchronize heat cycles among a number of mares so that they will foal within a short period (for management reasons), or so they can be used as recipients for embryo transplants. This can greatly reduce the number of recipient mares who must be maintained at a transfer facility.

These drugs may also be used to abort early pregnancies, such as for a mare who is bred who should not have been covered or her pregnancy has been diagnosed as being twins. One dose may not do the job; it may be necessary to give it two or three days in a row. When abortion is produced in this way, the mare may not come into a normal heat for several months.

Prostin (Upjohn, Kalamazoo, MI 49001) is one of the drugs most commonly used. The usual dosage is 5 mg.

and it should be used in accordance with the label directions. In general, prostaglandins are ineffective if given less than five days after the mare goes out of heat.

Prostaglandins only work on about ¾ of the mares to whom they are given. The others often have hormone imbalances or an ovarian dysfunction so that they cannot respond. Most mares show signs of heat within 6 to 8 days after treatment. This is generally a fertile heat and the mare can be bred at this time. Mild, transient side effects may occur with the drug. These are generally not severe enough to be treated. Most mares show signs of heat with one treatment. A few will require two to three treatments. (26)

While these drugs do work wonders in some cases, they are by no means a cure-all. If the mare does not have the ability to ovulate or has other abnormalities, they will not work at all. Mares who will not come into heat should be checked by your veterinarian to determine if they are doing so silently (a behavioral problem) or if their ovaries are simply not functioning so that they cannot respond to the prostaglandin. Prostaglandins are potent hormones. They should not be spilled on your skin while giving injections. Some labeling also advises against their being handled by pregnant women or people with asthma. They are not terribly dangerous drugs, but should be handled with respect.

OTHER HORMONES

A hormone called progesterone is sometimes used to keep mares pregnant who are prone to abortion because of hormone imbalances or deficiencies. The same drug is used to keep mares and fillies who are being trained, raced, or shown from showing signs of heat. The drug is also occasionally used to help some mares toward normal ovarian cycling. Consult your veterinarian for product and dosage if you think you have need for one of these products as the products and availability change rather frequently.

Several other hormones are used to correct reproductive abnormalities in mares. Their usage is specialized and complicated so they will not be discussed here. For information on hormone problems, contact your veterinarian.

PREGNANCY DIAGNOSIS

How do you tell if your mare is pregnant? THE most common reason for a mare who has been bred to stop coming into heat is that she is pregnant. The mare who has become pregnant after breeding will often go out of heat quite rapidly. She should be teased with a stallion beginning about 16 days after the START of her last heat period. Tease her every day or every other day for eight to ten days. If she does not show any signs of heat, this is

usually because she has become pregnant. To be sure, recheck the mare 40 to 42 days after the start of the last heat period during which she was bred. If you have a stallion on your premises, it is not a bad idea to check the mare every other day throughout her cycle. If she aborts, she may come back into heat. You do not want to miss an opportunity to detect this problem, find out why it happened, and to rebreed her.

Some owners will observe certain physical changes in the mare who has become pregnant. A previously grumpy mare may suddenly become calm and docile. She may become fatter and more flabby, losing muscle tone. She may be reluctant to work. Many mares will show enlargement of the abdomen, especially in its lower third, along with a hollowing of the back. Some mares may not appear pregnant at all, even when due to deliver.

A large belly alone does not mean that a mare is pregnant. If you are thinking that she is pregnant, feeding the animal "extra well," and not exercising her at the same time, she may have a "hay belly" making the animal look as if she is in foal. This is especially true with older mares who are not worked much or are kept strictly as broodmares. They tend to have flabby abdominal muscles and, often, a saggy backbone (swayback) at the same time. All of these tend to make the animal look pregnant whether she is or not. Moderate exercise will help a pregnant mare's large belly from becoming a huge burden of preparturient edema, possibly leading to complications.

RECTAL PALPATION

Mares may be checked for pregnancy by rectal palpation. This should be done by a veterinarian because of the possibility of puncturing the rectum (which often results in the mare's death) and because it takes sensitive fingers and lots of practice. It is not something that can be done by an owner with a book in one hand and an obstetrical glove on the other. Your veterinarian will be able to palpate the mare as early as 20 to 45 days of pregnancy, depending on his talent and practice. Of course, he can check her later, but the test is often easiest earlier in the pregnancy. Overall, the test is about 90% accurate with variation between individual veterinarians.

Sometimes it is not possible to determine rectally whether the animal is pregnant or not. In these cases, some veterinarians will reserve judgment and recheck the mare the next time they are out. This practice differs between veterinarians.

Many horse owners question the safety of rectal pregnancy exams. It seems to be the concensus of most authorities that when it is done by a competent veterinarian, there is little or no danger. Groups of mares have been palpated daily for several months of pregnancy without apparent ill effects. No increase in the number of aborted fetuses has been observed. In fact, some veterinarians have attempted to abort one of a pair of diagnosed twin fetuses by manipulation through the rectum—with little or no success! Some mares do indeed abort after rectal palpation. Most veterinarians feel that these were going to abort anyway and would have done so with or without rectal manipulation.

BLOOD TEST

A blood test is available for pregnancy testing mares. It checks for hormone levels in the bloodstream. According to its manufacturer (Diamond Laboratories, Des Moines, IA 50317), it is over 97% accurate at 41 to 45 days of pregnancy and gives results in two hours. It can be used from 35 to 40 days of pregnancy to about 100 days, but is most accurate between 45 and 90 days. After somewhere between 100 and 150 days, the hormone levels in the blood which indicate pregnancy can no longer be detected by the test. Your veterinarian will draw blood from the mare and then probably take it back to his clinic to run the test.

ULTRASONIC EXAMINATION

Ultrasound methods have been used to determine pregnancy in the mare. Its accuracy is variable. At this stage of development, it is not a replacement for rectal palpation, but may be used in addition to it. It is definitely not a magic test which will work in all situations. Ultrasound is said to be quite accurate in determining that a mare is carrying a twin pregnancy. At this point, many breeders will abort the mare, bring her back into heat, and try again. For this purpose, it is best used between days 15 to 55 after the mare is in heat. The most accurate period is said to be between days 20 to 25. A study at Colorado State University determined that, at best, ultrasound was only 65% accurate for pregnancy diagnosis. (27)

CARE OF THE PREGNANT MARE

Pregnant mares should have adequate exercise to help keep them in condition and ready for parturition (the birth process). Mares may be worked hard early in pregnancy if they are accustomed to hard work all along. If a nonworking pregnant mare is to be worked hard, she must be started to it gradually with perhaps more care than would be used with a nonpregnant mare. Later in pregnancy, the frequency and duration of exercise should be lessened—say, in the last two months. Exercise should NOT be stopped. During the last month or two, long walks are generally preferable to more strenuous work, especially if the mare's belly is very large. Violent exercise, being physically battered around, or being kicked hard by another horse may occasionally induce abortion. This is,

however, uncommon. It is amazing just how durable a fetus is.

One of my clients had taken a six-months pregnant mare elk hunting. After getting an elk, he had tied it to the saddle horn and was dragging it across a narrow trail on a very steep dirt and rock slope. The mare balked and then backed up. The third time she backed up, she miscalculated and stepped off the edge. She rolled over sideways once and caught herself on the steep slope. The elk (still tied to the saddle horn) rolled past her and jerked her off her feet. This time she rolled end over end. It is really something to watch a pregnant horse roll end over end in the fetal position. She and the elk finally came to a stop about ten feet from a lake. The horse was severely bruised and shaken. She later had some problems in one leg because of damage to the underlying tissues even though the skin was undamaged. The leg required several months treatment. She carried the foal to term (in fact, a rather long term—she went 11 months and 25 days), delivering a huge, healthy filly. With all the cushion of membranes and fluid, the foal is pretty well protected. Still, the more of these problems you can avoid, the more likely you are to have a live foal.

Good nutrition is important to grow a stout, healthy foal within the mare. The mare should have a booster of tetanus toxoid four to eight weeks before she foals to make sure that she has good immunity and that she passes that immunity on to the foal.

ABORTIONS

Mares are much more susceptible to abortion than most other domestic animals. In the cow, for example, the membranes surrounding the calf actually grow deeply into receptor sites (called cotyledons or "buttons") in the uterine lining. This helps to make the pregnancy secure. By contrast, the membranes (placenta) surrounding the foal only grow slightly into the mare's uterine lining. This makes physical disruption of the attachment much more likely. Likewise, infections in this delicate area are much more likely to break the attachment between the membranes and the uterus than they are in the cow. This physical reason for the mare aborting easily is why extra care is needed for the pregnant mare.

In addition, hormones must be produced by the mare's body in the right sequence and amounts in order to get and keep her pregnant. First, one set of hormones gets the uterus ready for implantation of the fertilized egg. Then a structure (called a corpus luteum) grows on the ovary after the egg is expelled; it secretes different hormones which keep the mare pregnant. If anything goes wrong with this series of hormonal changes, the fetus will be aborted. Some hormones are also produced by the foal and the membranes around him which help to maintain pregnancy, especially during the second half of gestation. Disturbances in hormone production and distribution anywhere in this process may result in abortion.

Certain virus diseases may cause abortion. One of the most common of these is rhinopneumonitis. This disease is seen in young horses on a farm as a respiratory disease. It then appears in the mares, often some months later, as a number of abortions late in pregnancy. Occasionally, foals are born weak and die within two to three days. Viral arteritis is another virus which can cause abortion.

Bacterial infections may cause the mare to abort early in the pregnancy. These mares usually show up as ones who pass their first heat following breeding without showing signs of heat. The owner assumes, rightfully, that the mare is pregnant. Then, when teased on the second heat (at 42 days), she is found to be in heat. The mare had actually become pregnant on the first breeding and then aborted very early in the pregnancy. Often, no signs are noticed in connection with one of these early abortions. Bacteria such as Staph, Strep, and E. coli are among those causing this type of problem. Contagious equine metritis may do the same.

Some feedstuffs, such as grain with ergot contamination, may cause abortion. Several other plants have been shown to cause abortion, as well as certain molds on feed. Fungal infections within the uterus itself account for a certain number of equine abortions.

Mares may (and often do) abort because they are carrying twins. These usually occur between seven and ten months of gestation. Abortions due to twinning account for 20 to 30 percent of all abortions which are diagnosed. (28) Apparently, at seven to ten months, the twins reach the limits of uterine stretch or capacity and abort for that reason. Any mare who aborts at seven to ten months should be checked for the presence of another foal, especially if the membranes have not cleaned.

Mares who are pregnant may still show signs of heat. If they are bred, it may cause abortion. Nutritional deficiencies may cause abortion. If the fetus dies or is abnormal for any reason, it will be aborted.

Administration of large doses of corticosteroids, as well as some other medications, (especially certain hormones such as prostaglandin or oxytocin) may cause abortion or premature labor. Certain horse wormers—carbon tetrachloride, phenothiazines, and organophosphates—have been considered to cause abortion and should not be used in late pregnancy. Be sure to tell your veterinarian that a mare is pregnant when you have her wormed so that he can choose an appropriate medication. Do not administer drugs to pregnant mares without first consulting your veterinarian about their safety.

Fillies who are bred before they are mature will often abort. On the other end of the age scale, old mares who have foaled many times may have a severe degree of scarring in the uterus. Their uterus may be adequate to carry a foal early in pregnancy, but unable to respond to increased nutrient demands later resulting in an abortion.

Signs of abortion may be minimal, especially in the first month or two. You may happen to find a small, slippery sac and see a slight bleeding or dark brown discharge from the vulva. If you are not in the right place at the right time, you might not see anything at all. The mare is noticed to come back into heat after passing one or more cycles after apparently being bred.

For abortions later in pregnancy, the animal may be upset; she may neigh and strain. She may have little or no appetite. A bloody or mucus discharge may be present. The vulva may be swollen. The mare may switch her tail and look at her flanks, much the same as if she had colic. The udder may fill with milk. If the abortion is due to a bacterial infection, it may have a foul odor.

An aborted fetus is expelled wrapped in its membranes. If you wish to have it examined to try to determine the cause of the abortion, be SURE to save the membranes as well because they are often more informative than the fetus as to what caused the problem. Be aware that with the best of laboratory facilities and a freshly aborted fetus, we can only determine an exact cause in perhaps 50% of specimens submitted. If the foal has been dead in the uterus for some time and is not fresh, the number of positive diagnoses is even less.

It is important to recognize the occurrence of an abortion as soon as possible so that the mare may be watched carefully and assisted if necessary. The mare should be checked for swelling of and discharge from the vulva with any sign of colic or other unexplained illness or discomfort during pregnancy. A bloody or pus-filled discharge is especially ominous. If the mare does not abort the fetus within twelve hours or so, a veterinarian should be consulted to determine what is happening with the pregnancy.

If the mare has aborted a fetus and the membranes have not followed, call a veterinarian as you would for a retained placenta with a normal foaling. In fact, it is often advisable to have the animal examined after any abortion. This is especially true if there is a foul odor or if the mare is not feeling well. In any event, the animal should be treated with a systemic antibiotic, such as penicillin/streptomycin, for three to five days. She should have rest and good feed. A mare who has aborted should not be rebred for a month or longer, especially if she was not treated with intrauterine antibiotics at the time of the abortion. Many veterinarians routinely give one to three days treatment with intrauterine antibiotics to any aborted mare. This is a good investment in rapid return to reproductive health.

Normal isolation and sanitation should follow an abortion which is diagnosed as being caused by an infectious problem. If it is due to one of the viral diseases, a large amount of virus will be present in the membranes and fetus. The mare should be kept in the stall in which she has aborted. If she has aborted outdoors, she should be isolated and other mares kept out of the corral. Persons handling the mare should wear protective clothing and boots, and should disinfect their hands and footwear before handling other pregnant mares in order to avoid spreading the infection to them. The bedding for the next week to ten days should be disposed by burning. No pregnant animals should be put in the area for a month. Halters, bridles, and other tack should not be used on the aborted mare and then on other mares. The mare should be considered contagious for about a month following the abortion.

Mares who abort foals more than once may require treatment to keep them from doing so in later pregnancies. Some mares do not have sufficient levels of one of the hormones necessary to keep them pregnant. Consult your veterinarian if you have a mare who becomes pregnant but aborts at each pregnancy.

FOALING

While the foal is in the uterus, it is nourished by the blood vessels of the umbilical cord (at the navel). Oxygenated blood is brought via these vessels from the mother; the foal does not breathe until after he is born. Urine from the foal is dumped into the space between the membranes around him.

Also called parturition, "foaling" refers to the act of giving birth. The foal appears to have considerable influence on when the mare gives birth. When horses and donkeys are crossed, the length of gestation is different from a foal from two horses or two donkeys. Most mares have a gestation period around 11 months. However, they can give birth to a normal, full-term foal anytime between 10 and 12 months. Most mares go somewhere between 320 and 345 days. Using 11 months for a gestation period will give a very close estimate of due date for most mares. The length of gestation has little to do with size of the foal. Many foals who are carried 12 months are normal or small in size and are delivered normally. The fact that the mare carries the foal a long time does not necessarily mean that she will have problems foaling.

During gestation, the pregnant mare will usually become progressively larger. The size of the animal varies with the individual. Some mares become so large that the owner swears that they will have twins. All fat mares with bellies hanging down are not pregnant—a "hay belly," caused by lack of muscle tone and large quantities of hay or other roughage, will make many mares look pregnant who are not.

Other mares will not appear pregnant at all. One ranch owner described one of his mares to me, saying that they had gathered her with their range herd one summer day to use on roundup. The mare was lethargic, and the rider (who was quite inexperienced) brought this to the rancher's attention. The rancher carefully inspected the mare and finding nothing wrong with her, concluded that the problem was the rider's lack of skill. He handed the rider a switch and instructed him to "make her work and don't let her get away with anything." The next morning when the crew returned to the corral, they found a healthy foal standing next to the mare! The mare had shown none of the typical enlargement that is associated with pregnancy, carrying the foal well up inside her belly instead.

As foaling time approaches, the mare's udder often enlarges. Mares who are foaling for the first time will frequently have the udder fill, then become small again. This may occur at intervals throughout the pregnancy. Some horses do not show any udder development at all, only to have it suddenly enlarge and fill with milk after the foal is born. Older mares usually show more udder development and become quite tightly filled with milk as parturition approaches.

How do you know when the mare is about to foal? Often you don't! Mares are very much individuals and signs vary considerably from one to the next. However, a given mare will often do exactly the same thing year after year, so be sure to jot down when her udder starts to fill, how long she carries the foal, and when she begins to wax.

Waxing is the term applied to the accumulation of waxy, dried colostrum on the end of the teats. Wax is only noticed on about half of the mares. When it is seen, the mare will usually foal in 24 to 48 hours. This is not infallible; one of my clients had a mare who waxed for 30 days before she foaled (and carried the foal a full 12 months). At the end of this time, she delivered a healthy, average-sized foal.

Within 24 hours prior to foaling, the vulva relaxes and begins to lengthen and look sloppy. The mare may "drop." This refers to a sunken appearance in the muscles on each side slightly above the root of the tail. If you keep an eye on the mare, you may see this area change from its previously rounded shape. "Dropping" is due to a relaxation of the ligaments of the pelvis. The flank area may appear sunken in. The mare may wander off by herself and be irritable with other horses in the pasture.

If the horse is stabled, she should be moved to accommodations suitable for foaling at least two weeks before her expected due date. A foaling stall should be big enough for the mare to lie down comfortably and stretch her legs out to full length—preferably not less than 14 to 16 feet square. It should be bedded deeply with clean, dust-free bedding. The area need not necessarily be heated, but should be free from drafts.

The mare should be prepared for foaling by wrapping her tail from the base outward for 12 or 14 inches. Vetrap can be used, but will often slide off if the mare does not foal within a day or two. My favorite is elastic tape wrapped gently around so it holds but doesn't constrict. Wrapping it too tightly will cause loss of circulation and may cause severe skin problems on the tail. The object is not to strangle the animal's tail, but to keep stray hairs out of the birth process.

She should have the genital area washed with a gentle soap (such as pHisohex), then rinsed with a mild disinfectant (such as tamed iodine, Betadine) in water. The udder area should be washed in the same manner, being especially careful to remove any waxy, dirty material between the halves of the udder. This prevents the foal from eating this material when he is nursing. All washed areas should be well rinsed with clear water to keep the foal from ingesting any of the disinfectants.

If you are foaling on pasture, this is a good time to remove geldings from the field. They are an occasional cause of foal loss. Whether they kill the foals maliciously or whether they are just curious and injure them in that way is not known.

The pasture should contain as few hazards as possible. One rancher client lost an extremely valuable registered foal because the mare foaled near a creek with a drop of about 12 feet down into it. The foal, probably in its struggles to stand, floundered over the bank into the creek and drowned.

Mares may have false labor much as humans do. The mare will go into apparent hard contractions, strain a few times, then quit. This is not unusual and often occurs within the month preceding foaling. These pains may be brought on by severe exertion, or by blows, kicks, or falls. They may also be caused by the ingestion of ergot-infested grains or moldy feed. Early labor pains are more common in aged mares who have had more than one foal. Observe the animal carefully after such an attack to see that she does not have a case of colic.

Mares who are foaling do not like to be watched. A mare often appears to stop in the middle of the birth process when the owner walks in, just relaxing and waiting. Mares seem to have some degree of conscious control over when they foal with the result that a majority of foals are born at night. This surely dates back to prehistoric times when night was safe from the prying eyes of predators. It is usually much more satisfactory if you can watch from hiding where the mare cannot easily see you. Many large stud farms use closed-circuit TV cameras or video monitors for this purpose.

The mare's entry into serious labor is usually preceded by restlessness. Some mares show these signs for several hours, while others may show almost no signs prior to labor. The mare may sweat, either in patches or all over. She may paw the ground and look at her flank much like an animal with colic. She may be uneasy and anxious, pacing her stall. Curling of her lip (fleering) is often noticed. The mare may get up and down. She may make a bed. She may walk around with her tail raised and urinate small amounts.

Some mares may go through this series of actions several times without going into strong labor. This often occurs if the mare is closely watched. She may then act normally for several hours or even days before going through the process again.

As the mare goes into the second stage of labor, her "water" will break. This occurs when the membranes around the foal tear and the fluid which has surrounded him in the uterus floods out of the mare's reproductive tract. This fluid may be clear to slightly yellowish or brownish and is often thickened and mucoid. When this fluid escapes all at once, it is quite dramatic, sort of an equine Niagara Falls. Some mares will only have a small hole in the placenta with the fluid escaping so gradually that it goes unnoticed. An alert owner may notice the mare passing a cervical plug. This is a whitish or yellowish plug of thickened, rubbery mucus which has sealed the opening of the cervix during the pregnancy. When the cervical plug is passed, foaling usually occurs within a few hours.

When the mare has begun strong, steady labor contractions, she should foal within an hour. If she has not, call a veterinarian IMMEDIATELY. A normal foaling may take place in as little as 15 minutes, and usually does not take more than 45 minutes. Most mares finish the last stages of labor (when the foal is finally pushed out) while lying down. However, a few mares will go through the last part of the birth process while standing, especially if people are around. A mare who foals while standing will probably do the same in succeeding pregnancies. If the mare completes the foaling process while standing and you are present, help support the foal so that he is not injured by being dropped on the ground. Talk about being dropped on your head when you are born! Some mares get up and down repeatedly during labor; these actions may help to reposition a malpositioned foal. The mare may lick or eat the amniotic fluid which has come from her uterus. It is thought that this may help her to define the location for birth to take place.

If the mare is lying down when the foal's head has passed through the vulva, she will usually continue lying down until the birth is completed. If standing, she may lie down at this point. After the major portion of the foal has passed out of her vulva, she will usually stop straining and lie quietly for a period of time—often more than 30 minutes. This is normal.

When she does finally rise, she will generally lick the foal. Some mares, however, will bite or paw the foal and may need to be restrained. It has been traditional to drag the foal around to the mare's head, but this is not necessary. The mare will not usually step on her foal unless she is excited and upset because humans are around. Get out of the way and allow her to mother the new foal as she will for the first two to three hours. This time period is critical for the mare and foal to bond to each other.

When a mare gets into trouble foaling, she does so quite rapidly and quite severely because of the strength of her abdominal muscles. Foaling problems are a TRUE EMERGENCY! For this reason, many owners of extremely valuable mares either have a veterinarian in attendance when the mares are expected to foal or send them to a facility that specializes in foaling. Mares shipped to this sort of place should be sent there at least a month to six weeks before they are expected to give birth in order to give them time to recover from the trip and settle into their new surroundings. You may want to advise your veterinarian that you have a mare coming due just so you don't catch him by surprise.

Not all mares have trouble foaling; complications occur in only about 10% of equine births. The problem is that when they DO occur, they occur so rapidly and severely that the mare must have help quickly or either she or the foal may be injured or die in the birth process.

The mare's strong labor contractions will force the foal rapidly into the pelvic canal and then to the outside. Foals are normally born front feet first with the head lying between the front feet, much like a diver getting ready to go off the board. One front leg is usually slightly ahead of the other (only by six or eight inches).

If the mare has strained and there is part of the foal showing, but the foal is not completely pushed outside with the next three or four contractions, she should be examined. Wash your hands carefully with soap and water and rinse them with a disinfectant solution, such as the tamed iodine mentioned above. If you examine the mare and find ANYTHING other than the "diver" position mentioned above, send someone to call a veterinarian IMMEDIATELY. You MAY be able to correct a foal who is positioned another way. If you cannot, valuable time may be lost in locating a veterinarian and getting him on his way to you. Let him be on the way to you while you continue to examine the foal. Better to pay for an unneeded call than to lose both the mare and the foal by waiting too long.

IMPORTANT NOTE: If you have occasion to examine a mare deeper than wrist depth, be extremely careful NOT to get your arm caught between the foal and the mare's pelvis. If it is there when she strains and there is not adequate room for it, there is a good chance of getting a broken arm! The added pressure from your arm in the birth canal can stimulate just such a contraction.

Work your hands gently into the vulva, feeling the foal's legs. If there are only legs present in the canal, you must determine whether they are front or hind feet. Imagine in your mind the difference between a small, knobby knee and a small, angular hock. Feel your way up each leg in turn to determine whether it is a front or hind leg. If the feet are showing, hind feet usually have their soles upward while front feet usually have the soles downward.

If you think you feel two hind feet, feel upward to see if you can identify the tail. A foal being born hind-end first MUST come out into the air within about five minutes of the time he is that far into the pelvis. When he is about halfway into the pelvis, the umbilical cord pinches off as it is squeezed between his mother's pelvis and his belly. He will die from lack of oxygen if he cannot get out to breathe. If you have determined that this is the problem, you will have to try to help the mare. Even if you call a veterinarian immediately, he will not get there in time to help, unless he is almost next door.

To help deliver the foal that is coming backwards, grasp the foal by both hind feet. They will be very slippery. Have a quantity of freshly laundered rags or towels handy to use to help grasp them. Pieces of clean bedsheet work well. Paper towels will work if nothing else is available.

Whatever you do, DO NOT pull straight outward! This may result in the foal wedging its hips in the birth canal and causing serious problems. Pull as if you are going to take the foal's feet to the mare's heels. This is true whether she is standing or lying down. If she is standing, you MUST pull downward. You can pull fairly hard, but work with the mare's labor contractions. Pull when she strains, allowing her to help you.

If you feel two front feet and no head, or three feet, call for veterinary help immediately. Often, the foal must be pushed partly or all the way back into the mare, turned around, or straightened out and then helped out.

Whatever you do, do not waste much time examining the mare and determining what feet are which, especially if you do not immediately feel the nose in the canal. Call a veterinarian right away. He will have a better chance of saving your foal if he can get to the problem early.

Occasionally, you will see a foal being born where the front feet are pushing up toward the mare's rectum, causing that area to bulge out. If she continues to push in that manner, she may tear out the whole divider between the rectum and vagina. Even if you do not have time to clean up, immediately grasp the feet and pull them downward and out into the open. Then, go ahead and get cleaned up.

Many times, the mare will now go ahead and push the foal while you are getting ready to help her. You have saved her the pain and misery of tearing out this delicate area, as well as saving yourself the time (as much as a year or more) and expense (often considerable) of repairing it.

When the foal's head is out of the mare, immediately remove the membranes from its muzzle. Reach into the mouth with your hand and scoop out any mucus or fluid that you can get. If the foal starts breathing, you are in business. If not, you must determine whether it is alive or not. Often the foal will be obviously dead—grayish, discolored, or deformed from having been dead within the mare for a period of time. There is, of course, no use trying to get it to breathe. Other foals may be alive, but sometimes it's awfully hard to tell. Stick your hand as far back into the foal's throat as you can. If the foal is alive, there will usually be a gagging reflex and you can feel the strong muscular push on your hand. If the foal is dead, there will be no movement.

You can also open the eyelid and observe the eyeball. A live foal usually has a glossy, full eyeball; a dead one will frequently have a dull, slightly limp globe. Touch the cornea (the clear front surface of the eyeball) with your fingertip. A live foal will show some reaction or movement when touched here; a dead one will show no reaction. If you have a stethoscope, check for a heartbeat. If there is no heartbeat, it is usually not worth trying heart massage and artificial respiration unless you know for sure that the animal was alive earlier in the birth process.

If the foal is alive (has a heartbeat) but is not breathing, you must take steps to get it breathing immediately. Sometimes when a straw is tickled deeply into the nostril, the foal will sneeze to get rid of it and thus start breathing. In other cases, a glassful of very cold water dashed over the foal's head may shock it into breathing. If you have several people, suspend the foal by its hindlegs, with the head hanging down. Reach into its mouth and clean mucus and fluid from it again. Then slap the foal alternately on the right and left sides of the chest. This both helps to move out mucus and to stimulate the animal to breathe. Keep this up for at least ten minutes, pausing every couple of minutes to attempt to stimulate the animal's breathing with a straw.

If oxygen is available, a mask can be used to flow it into the foal's nose. Either hold the animal's mouth closed or cover the entire muzzle with the mask. This action will force oxygen into the lungs. Be sure the mouth and nose are free of most mucus and fluid or it may be forced into the lungs. If you have tried unsuccessfully for 10 to 15 minutes to get the foal to breathe, suspend your efforts and check to see if the animal's heart is still beating. If not, there is little likelihood that you will be able to do anything for it. If your veterinarian is present at the foaling, there are drugs that he can give which directly stimulate the respiratory centers in the brain and will sometimes start a foal which will not otherwise breathe.

If the foal is outside the mare and is breathing normally, he may be connected to the membranes which are still inside her. As long as the mare is lying quietly and the foal is not in danger of being stepped on, leave it attached behind her. This allows the pulsing of the blood vessels in the placenta (membranes) to push a last bit of blood into the foal. This can give the foal a pint or so of extra blood, and will be helpful in giving it a good start in life.

If the foal is still attached to the membranes and they have come out of the mare, it is still a good idea to leave them attached for a few minutes. There is a natural breaking point located about three or four inches from the foal's belly. The cord usually separates here as soon as the foal struggles, or when the mare stands. If the cord does not come loose from the foal, tie a heavy string around it six or seven inches from the foal. Something like baling twine is fine. Do not use nylon thread or fine string, as that will cut through the tissue. Tie it as tightly as you can. Then, sever the cord beyond that point on the mare side of the tie with a sharp knife.

Putting iodine on the foal's navel is important to help prevent infection from going up this opening and into his body causing navel ill, joint ill, or other infection. Use either strong (7%) tincture of iodine or strong iodine and glycerine, mixed half-and-half. Put about an inch of it into a paper or plastic cup. If you have cut off the umbilical cord as described above, dip the whole length of it into the cup, soaking it thoroughly. If the cord has broken naturally, you will do the same with the stump that is left. If it has been cut and then dipped, redip it as soon as the stump breaks off at the natural breaking point. The object is to get the cord thoroughly saturated with the iodine so as to prevent any infection. If you find the foal in the pasture or corral, already born and running around, it is still worthwhile to catch it and treat it in this manner. Retreating it in the same way about 12 hours later gives additional insurance against bacteria entering the umbilical cord. Some breeding farms treat the umbilical stump this way daily for five to seven days. They report that this reduces the number of joint and navel ill infections which occur.

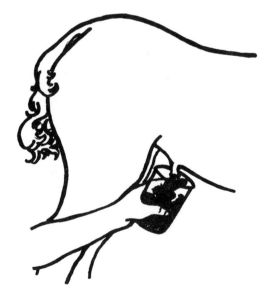

Putting iodine on a foal's navel.

The foal should be allowed to struggle and rise on his own in order to nurse. These struggles help to strengthen him. If the mare does not allow him to nurse, it may be necessary to restrain or even sedate her. Foals are stimulated to nurse by touching soft surfaces such as the mare's skin. If there are too many people around and too much handling, the foal may become confused and suck at the wall or make sucking movements into the air. Get out of the way and give the foal a couple of hours before you decide that he is having problems nursing. If he is unable to rise and nurse by about three hours, milk some milk from the mare and feed it in a bottle. Prop him up on his chest, sandwiching him between bales of hay if necessary to help his breathing and circulation. If he is weak or otherwise appears abnormal, you should have him checked by a veterinarian to see what his problem is and whether anything can be done about it.

If the foal regurgitates milk when he tries to nurse or dribbles it out his nose, he probably has a cleft palate. Open his mouth and look at the roof of it. A gap or slit may be seen where there should be a solid surface. If you see this, prevent the foal from nursing. This keeps him from inhaling milk into his lungs and getting pneumonia. Contact your veterinarian to have him examine the foal as soon as possible or take the foal to the nearest university hospital or surgically-equipped clinic. Surgical repair is difficult. It is, however, the only way to save the foal and allow it to grow up normally.

If the mare has lost her colostrum, it is necessary to give the foal an injection of tetanus antitoxin. He should also be given frozen colostrum or colostrum from a donor mare to give him the antibodies that are so important. Up to 500 ml. (a little more than a pint) may be given. (29)

Some horsemen routinely give injections of vitamins A, D, and E. An enema is a good routine practice. You can use a commercial enema (such as a Fleet enema) from the drugstore. Or you can also use a gentle soap such as Ivory (the soap, not the detergent!), mixed in six to eight ounces of lukewarm water and given with an infant syringe. This helps to remove the feces which are present in the gut. These are dark brown or blackish and are called meconium. Watch the foal carefully for the first few days to see that he is passing feces normally.

Foals who have not passed the meconium may have it become hard enough to cause an impaction; they will usually fail to nurse. This is perhaps the most common single cause of foals failing to nurse by 8 to 12 hours of age. Some foals may strain to defecate without producing anything. They may lift and swish their tails.

Straining due to meconium impaction must be differentiated from that caused by diarrhea. Usually diarrhea can be observed as the foal strains or by feces smeared on his buttocks and tail. Foals with severe impactions may show considerable signs of colic which may include depression and rolling. They may get up and down and arch their backs. If this occurs, call your veterinarian, as painkil-

lers and medication to relax the intestinal muscles may be needed. He may need to pass a stomach tube to give the foal laxatives to help him pass this material. In some foals, surgery is necessary to remove the impaction, especially if it occurs higher in the digestive tract than can be reached by an enema.

If the foal becomes raw under the tail, the area should be carefully cleansed with warm water and then coated with petroleum jelly several times a day until healed.

Occasionally a foal will get a severe diarrhea from the colostrum. If this occurs, consult your veterinarian for the proper medication and management (see Foal Diarrhea).

The stump of the umbilical cord should harden and shrivel and fall away from the body within a few days. If it does not, watch to see whether urine is dripping through it. If it is, consult your veterinarian at once. This problem is called a patent (open) urachus. This means that the tube which drained urine from the foal while he was in the uterus has not closed. Surgical treatment may be necessary to close it and prevent infection from going up it and into the foal's bladder.

THE MEMBRANES

Often the membranes are passed with the foal. The placenta may be red, brown, or purplish in color. Spread it out and examine it. The overall shape of a normal set of membranes has been described as being like a pair of "Dutchman's breeches," a heavy pair of men's pants that are cut off at the knees. There may be tears, but it should not have any holes that look like pieces are missing. It is well worth saving the membranes until you are absolutely sure that everything is O.K. If you have to call your veterinarian for any reason, one of the first things he will usually ask to examine when he arrives is the placenta. It's hard to show it to him if the dog has eaten it. Also, if the membranes are left lying around, it is not uncommon (indeed, in nature, it is normal) for the mare to eat them. The vet will want to determine if they are all there or if there are pieces missing. Their condition will tell him much about the condition of the mare's uterus.

The mare should pass the membranes within one to two hours if everything is proceeding normally. They are considered retained if they stay in her beyond this time. If portions are hanging out of her vulva, do not cut them off; their weight helps to pull the rest of the placenta loose. Merely tie them to the mare's tail and leave them for now. My preference is to have clients call if the membranes have not passed within about four hours. I'll remove them some time shortly after that. In general, they should be out of the mare by eight hours after foaling—or earlier.

After the retained membranes are removed, the mare is given penicillin/streptomycin treatment—often for three days, especially if there is any sign of infection. Your veterinarian may give her an injection to help avoid any laminitis in the feet. He may also put an antibiotic bolus, powder, or solution into the uterus to help flush it out and kill any infection which is present.

If the placenta is abnormal, or if the membranes are retained in the mare, she should not be bred on the foal heat. Retained placenta is more common when labor has been induced in the mare, or when the foal is delivered by caesarean section. It may also occur after prolonged delivery, especially if much obstetrical assistance has been given.

After the foal is cared for and things have settled down, rinse both the mare's genital area and your hands and arms with tamed iodine solution. Spread the vagina apart and look inside for tears or bruising. The vaginal walls will generally be redder than normal because of all they have been through. Bruises show up as bluish or blackish spots under the membrane. If the foal has been pulled or the mare has otherwise had difficulty foaling, reach inside to about elbow length and feel gently around the vaginal wall for cuts or tears. It goes without saying that you are in the target zone for some heavy artillery when you do this—the mare's hind feet. Be careful and take precautions in case she objects to this procedure. The membrane should be smooth all around. Tears will feel like jagged slits into which you may be able to run your finger.

If you find any tears or injuries, consult your veterinarian immediately so that he may further examine it and decide whether the tears should be sutured, or whether they should be treated otherwise. Examining this deeply is not necessary with a mare that has foaled quickly and normally and been cleaned of the membranes. If the membranes are retained, you will need to call the vet anyway and you might as well let him examine her. The less you work in this area, the less are your chances of introducing infection.

Care of the mare immediately after foaling, such as removing the membranes and suturing any tears, is extremely important to her future breeding health. If the membranes are left in place for more than about eight hours after foaling, the mare may develop a laminitis giving her the same problems in her feet as if she had been foundered on grain. Retained membranes can also start an infection which may result in pneumonia or septicemia.

EARLY FOAL CARE

The first 30 days of the foal's life are critical. Joint problems, such as joint ill or contracted tendons, can easily do enough damage to tender, young cartilage to be permanently crippling. At the first sign of these problems, your veterinarian should be consulted.

The normal foal will begin to eat with his mother, often at just two or three days of age. He will nibble hay, often lying down in it to do so because his neck at this age is too short for the length of his legs. To reach the ground, most foals must either spread their legs widely, or lie down. The mare's grain should be fed in a pan or feeder large enough so that the foal can reach in and eat, too. Fresh air and plenty of exercise are necessary. If it is possible to have the mare out on a good clean pasture, this helps to decrease the chances of scours. A creep feeder should be available to foals more than two or three weeks old to allow them to eat as much grain as they want. As long as the grain is available at all times and the feeder is not allowed to run empty, they will not overeat. If the weather is damp or rainy, the feeder should either be sheltered or fresh feed put in frequently in order that it not get moldy.

If the foal is orphaned, steps must be taken to care for it (see Foal Feeding).

IMMATURE AND PREMATURE FOALS

Premature foals have been described by Rossdale as those who have had a gestation period of 300 to 325 days. They are often undersized and have soft, silky coats. Some (but not all) of them may be slow to nurse. Immature foals were defined as those who were born after a gestation period of 325 days or more, but appear physically premature. They are of normal size but may be emaciated and often have a long, scruffy hair coat. They are also weak and slow to nurse.

Some of both types of these foals will be depressed and weak and will die in two to three days, no matter what you do or how well you nurse them. Others will need a minimal amount of supportive care and will stand to nurse by themselves within 24 hours. Still another group may require intensive care for as much as a week before being able to survive on their own. Unfortunately, it is often difficult to tell which one of these types your foal is. All you can do is to do the best that you can, but expect the worst. Then, if everything goes right and you save the foal, all is O.K. If it dies, you have expected it and are prepared for it.

Begin caring for the immature or premature foal by making sure that it gets enough colostrum, whether from its mother or from another mare. This is extremely important, as you have less than 24 hours to get antibodies from the colostrum into the animal to protect it from disease. Give as much as the foal will take—up to a quart (one liter) or more. Do NOT feed any milk replacer or other milk product until the foal has consumed the colostrum. If you absolutely cannot get horse colostrum, give cow colostrum if available before giving other products. Dairy farmers often save and freeze excess colostrum from their cows. You might be able to obtain some and keep it on hand for this eventuality.

If the foal will suck, give the colostrum with a nursing bottle. Otherwise, your veterinarian may have to pass a stomach tube down the foal's nose to feed it. As soon as the foal can be coaxed to stand while eating, always feed it standing. This will help it to seek milk from the mare. Encourage the foal to stand as long as possible. This will help to strengthen its muscles. If necessary, help to support it by the tail at first. The longer it lies down and nurses, the more it will adopt a helpless, passive attitude. Be sure to keep the mare milked out until the foal is able to nurse her empty on a regular basis.

BARKER AND DUMMY FOALS

Also called wanderers and convulsives, another name for this problem is neonatal maladjustment syndrome. The foal is born rapidly and is apparently normal. The delivery is quick and there are no problems. The foal may attempt to suck normally, walk, and follow the mare. The onset of signs is abrupt. The foal completely loses his sucking reflex and shows jerky head and body movements. He may grind his teeth, make unusual sounds (barking), and wander aimlessly. Most affected foals eventually go down and paddle or become convulsive.

Call your veterinarian if you suspect that you have one of these foals. Fluid therapy is often needed to help stabilize the foal and provide nutrition. Drugs are often given to stabilize the convulsions. Intensive nursing care is needed. It is often easiest to take the foal into a warm house rather than to attempt to provide for it in a barn or stable. With the best of nursing care and very good luck, about half of the affected foals will recover. Recovery may occur in a few hours in some animals, while others may need intensive care for several weeks. If they do recover, they usually do so completely.

NEONATAL ISOERYTHROLYSIS

This problem is comparable to the Rh syndrome in humans. It can occur when the foal inherits a blood type which is incompatible with that of the mare. For some reason (such as bleeding while in the uterus), some of the foal's blood cells enter the mare. This stimulates her to make antibodies against them. These are passed to the foal in her colostrum and act to kill his red blood cells. The sudden load of dead red blood cells in turn causes damage to the liver. This problem is rare with a mare's first foal, but may occur after that. Actually, the condition is rare, but serious enough to watch for.

Some foals are so hard-hit when they drink the mother's milk that they die within a few hours. This may be due to an anaphylactic shock (a type of acute allergic reaction). These foals will show brownish or dark-red mucous membranes.

More commonly, however, the foal will develop signs over several days. His membranes may be yellowish (icteric), and they may be pale as well. He may appear weak, tired, yawning, and may fail to nurse. His heart and respiratory rates may be elevated. He may lie down and appear unable to rise. Other foals who are less affected

may merely be less vigorous than usual and have less tolerance for stress. They are more susceptible to infections.

Contact your veterinarian if you think you may have one of these foals. Laboratory tests may help to confirm the presence of this disease, but they often cannot be run in time to save the foal. Treatment is usually started on the basis of clinical signs. It is often necessary to muzzle the foal until the antibodies in the mare's milk are gone, and to milk her out to keep her from going dry. The foal should receive colostrum from a donor mare. If possible, this milk should be checked to make sure it is compatible with the foal. When the antibodies have left the milk, the foal can be allowed to nurse his mother safely. This may take several days. In most cases, it is well worth milking the mare to keep her producing for the foal. Care should be taken to keep the foal quiet and avoid exerting him until his blood count is back to normal.

Do not breed the mare to the same stallion again when this problem occurs. In the case of valuable mares, it may be necessary to blood-type both mare and stallion to see that they are compatible in order keep from having another foal become ill or die with this problem.

FOALING COMPLICATIONS

UTERINE TORSION

Uterine torsion may occur weeks or months before the mare is ready to foal, or it may occur close to foaling time. The uterus twists around its lengthwise axis resulting in a colic. In some cases, this may be mild and recurrent while in others it is extremely violent and acute. Under some circumstances (and with a lot of luck), these may be corrected by rolling the animal. This should be done by your veterinarian after he has determined in which direction the uterus has twisted. In others, the foal may be repositioned through a flank incision and delivered normally, or a caesarean section may be performed. This is often a life-or-death situation for the mare; your veterinarian should be contacted immediately if you suspect that you have one of these.

CAESAREAN SECTION

This is the delivery of the foal through incisions in the mare's abdominal wall and uterus, rather than allowing it to be born through the vagina as it normally would. As mentioned above, it is often used to correct a uterine torsion; other indications include a pregnancy which spans both horns of the uterus, or foals who are so malpositioned that they cannot be delivered through the vagina. Monsters or deformed foals may also have to be delivered in this manner.

Like many other pieces of surgery, how a caesarean

is done depends on your veterinarian and his skills, preferences, and facilities. Some prefer to operate through the left flank, while others go in through the animal's midline. The animal is, of course, under general anesthesia while this is done. The easy part is making the incision and delivering the foal. The hard part is what seems like a mile of stitching to suture the openings. Colostrum should be milked from the mare and given to the foal as soon as possible. The foal can be introduced to the mare when she is standing solidly enough that she is not a danger to him. About half the mares upon whom caesarean sections are performed will conceive normally afterward; about a quarter of these may abort in midpregnancy. (30)

INDUCTION OF LABOR

Labor may be deliberately induced in the mare, but should generally be avoided if the pregnancy is proceeding normally and you want the best possible chance for both a live foal and a mare who will breed back normally. Generally, if induction is to be considered, the mare should have passed a minimum of 330 days since the last breeding; she must have adequate milk in the udder (not just a few drops); and her cervix must be soft and dilatable.

Induction must be done under a veterinarian's care because of the possibility of complications. Malpresentations are common with induced births. With induced labor, there is more danger to the foal than to the mare. If the membranes separate from the uterus before the delivery is complete, the foal may die before he can be delivered. If any mistake is made in judging the stage of pregnancy, the foal may be born before it is able to cope with life outside the uterus.

An owner may cause accidental induction of parturition by administering corticosteroids to a mare in late pregnancy. Other drugs may induce abortion (or early labor), including prostaglandins and oxytocin. Be very careful what medication you give to a mare in late pregnancy (or for that matter, any time in pregnancy!) Check with your veterinarian if you are in doubt.

Mares who have had labor induced may end up with foals with significantly less immunity than those who foal naturally at term resulting in weakness and greater foal loss. Some of this deficiency may be due not to lesser concentrations of antibodies in the mare, but to less vigorous sucking by the foal, who is often weaker than normal. These foals often suck less frequently and for a shorter period of time than do normal foals. A mare who is not totally ready when birth is induced may not have adequate milk in the udder until a day or so afterward.

TEARS IN THE VAGINA, CERVIX, OR UTERUS

A mare who shows any bright red blood from the vulva during or after foaling should be immediately checked by a veterinarian for tears in the uterus or vagina. A tear should also be suspected if the mare shows signs of peritonitis, such as an elevated temperature, reluctance to move, severe depression, and signs of abdominal pain. These signs may occur just a few hours after delivery, or they may be seen several days later. Tears may occur because one of the foal's feet has punched through the wall of the vagina or cervix. They may also occur if the foal is abnormally large, or the cervix is not allowed to dilate as much as possible before assistance is given with delivery.

Depending on the location of the tear, your veterinarian may or may not want to (or be able to) suture the area. He may put the horse on systemic antibiotics and may also treat with antibiotics into the uterus. He may make specific recommendations as to future breeding practices, such as when the animal may be bred, or, indeed, whether she should be bred at all.

PROLAPSE OF THE UTERUS

Prolapse of the uterus occurs when the uterus literally follows the foal out through the wide-open cervix. The old-timers called it "casting the withers" or "eversion of the womb." It may also occur following a late-term abortion. It often occurs when the mare is trying to clean (get rid of the membranes) after foaling rather than at foaling itself.

A uterine prolapse will appear as a very large bag protruding from the vulvar area with a red, often bloody coloration if the prolapse is fresh. If the prolapse is older, it may appear blackened and crusty. This is a life-threatening problem, as the mare often goes into shock after it occurs. Call for veterinary help IMMEDIATELY. The mare will often need treatment with special drugs for the shock, as well as fluids to help replace blood volume and/or blood loss. After dealing with the shock, it will be necessary for the veterinarian to administer a spinal anesthetic to help relax her, to stop her straining, and to allow him to replace the prolapsed organ. This is one of the problems in a horse that is a real emergency—get help immediately!

While you are waiting for the veterinarian, try to keep the mare standing if possible. This may require one or more persons on each side of her to steady her and help hold her up. Moisten a large towel or sheet in lukewarm water and wrap it around the uterus to keep it from drying.

If the uterus can be replaced before it has become dried or injured, the mare will usually rebreed and carry a normal foal to term during her next pregnancy. The mare may need antibiotics and other medication for several days after the prolapse has been repaired to prevent infection in it. The prolapse usually does not recur the next time she foals.

RUPTURE OF THE UTERINE BLOOD VESSELS

A ruptured uterine artery may be seen in the older mare who has delivered a number of foals normally. The foal is normal, but the mare appears to colic three or four hours after delivery. The mare goes into severe shock, sweating profusely. Her mucous membranes are extremely pale and the pulse is thin and weak. The mare may appear anxious and not wish to move. When moved, she may be weak and have a swaying gait. She may be depressed. Some animals may show acute pain and rolling, much like a severe colic. The signs usually occur after the placenta has been expelled following a normal delivery.

The foal should be removed and a ruptured artery suspected. Get veterinary help immediately, but be aware that it may not be possible to save her, no matter what treatment is given. In some cases, transfusion may be attempted; as much as 4 to 5 gallons of blood may be needed. Your veterinarian may ask you to locate one or more blood donor horses. The mare should be kept quiet, in a darkened stall. She usually improves within the next four or five hours, appearing nearly normal. The signs then reappear suddenly and severely, and the mare often dies within the hour.

Necropsy will reveal that there has been a rupture of an aneurysm (weak, thin spot) in the artery going to the uterus. The weakening in the artery is thought to be due to senile degenerative changes rather than due to worm migration in the blood vessel. In some cases, the mare may bleed into the wall of the uterus.

If the mare does manage to survive the episode, she will probably rupture the weakened artery the next time she foals, and may die at that time. This problem is a small but significant cause of mare death after foaling. Some veterinarians feel that minimizing stress in the older mare may reduce the incidence of this problem. Delay routine care, such as worming, foot care, and Caslick's operations, until several days after foaling. Older mares should not be shipped just before or just after foaling if it is at all avoidable. (31) (32)

NAVEL ILL AND JOINT ILL

These are two disease problems seen in young foals, both of which result from infection entering through the umbilical cord (navel). In some instances, the bacteria causing the problem may enter through the digestive tract. They occur in foals from a few days to three or four months old.

An abscess at the stump of the umbilicus may be the first sign. The area becomes hot and swollen and may be discolored to bluish or purple. Sometimes, there may be no signs at the navel and the foal will be noticed to be severely lame. This may be bad enough that he is walking on three legs, and the owner immediately assumes that he has been kicked. Do NOT assume that he has been injured by the mare! Call your veterinarian immediately!

The lameness is generally accompanied by a fever (up to 101.5 degrees F or more (38.5 degrees C)). The foal may be depressed. The pulse may be weak and rapid and the mucous membranes injected (reddened). Several joints may be swollen, showing that the bacterial infection has localized there. The fetlock, hip, stifle, and elbow joints are most commonly affected. The joints may feel hot to the touch and the foal may show severe pain if they are forcibly moved. The white blood count (WBC) is elevated. X-rays may be necessary to determine the extent of the damage to the joint. If left untreated, severe damage to the joint surface may occur and the animal may be permanently crippled.

Treatment includes antibiotics recommended by your veterinarian. These are usually administered for a MINIMUM of five to seven days. If treatment is started before damage to the joint cartilage has occurred, the foal may be much improved within 24 hours and will be nursing. The temperature will return to normal. Do NOT stop treatment at this time or the infection will come back. This time you will have pure pus in the joints. When the antibiotics are used for only three days, they will clear the bacteria from the blood stream (this is why the foal feels so much better). This length of time is inadequate to remove them from the joints.

Consult a veterinarian for a foal with joint or navel ill. Owner treatment, especially if inadequate in quantity or duration, may complicate the problem and lead to a joint ill that cannot be cured. Some foals may require surgery to help remove damaged tissue from the joint surface and bone. In some severe cases, the joint cartilage is damaged beyond repair and the foal will never be normal. In these cases, euthanasia is recommended for humane reasons. (33)

In some cases, a procedure called joint lavage is used. This involves anesthetizing the foal and putting two large needles into opposite sides of an affected joint. Tubes are attached to the needles and a pump is used to flush antibiotic or other cleansing solutions through the joint cavity. Incidentally, the same procedure is sometimes used in older horses to remove cartilage debris and other material which is causing destruction within a joint.

If an abscess at the navel is the only problem, it may be necessary to open and drain it. Leave this to your veterinarian and follow his instructions for aftercare religiously.

FOAL SEPTICEMIA

This is an infection which becomes spread throughout the foal's bloodstream. It may be due to bacteria, viruses, or a fungus. It may originate within the uterus before birth, or may enter the foal through the digestive tract, lungs, or umbilical cord. It is most common in foals with poor immune systems, premature foals, or those less than two weeks old. A mare who drips milk prior to foaling may lose all her colostrum by the time the foal is born resulting in a lack of antibodies. It is also seen in foals who do not receive any colostrum. Management problems, such as damp, drafty quarters, overcrowding, and filth, may make the foal more susceptible. However, it can occasionally occur under the best of conditions. A septicemia may result in an animal's death or leave it with a chronic infection, stunted, or a poor-doer.

The foal may be lethargic or depressed, even comatose. He may not be nursing, leaving the mare's udder bulging and painful. His mucous membranes may be bright red to purple as in colitis-X. The foal may be in shock. He may be jaundiced (yellow). There may be small hemorrhages inside the mouth and ears. Nervous system signs may be seen, especially coma or convulsions. The foal may show dehydration. When the skin in pinched and released, it will stand up where it has been pinched together. Check the foal's umbilical cord for swelling or drainage of urine. He may or may not have diarrhea. Joint ill—with its hot, painful, swollen joints—may accompany the septicemia.

Foal septicemia is VERY serious and often fatal. Call your veterinarian immediately if you suspect this problem. Prompt, intensive treatment is the only thing that will save the foal. Even with the best of care, the problem is so intense that many foals are lost. Your veterinarian will treat for shock and for the organisms causing the disease.

Prevention involves management to reduce stress to the foal. Foaling quarters should be clean, warm, and dry. Make sure that the foal gets colostrum. If you have reason to suspect that the mare has none, try to get some from another mare or use some that you have frozen from a normal mare. Foals from mares who have previously had problems may need preventive antibiotics for a few days. The mare should be kept up on her immunizations to keep up the degree of immunity that she passes on to her foal. The umbilical cord should be disinfected with iodine more than once. Do it right after the foal is born, and at least once or twice more, 12 to 24 hours later. On some premises, the umbilical stump is iodined daily for five to seven days. (34)

FOAL FEEDING AND CARE

MARE'S MILK

How to feed the foal depends on whether he is an orphan or is still on his mother. Let's begin with the animal who is still nursing. By all means, let the mare raise the foal if at all possible. It's a whole lot easier to help her raise the foal than to raise it yourself. Making the foal an orphan if his mother is alive should be a last resort.

Mare's milk is the natural starting food for a young foal. It is very nutritious and easily digested. It is rich in calcium and phosphorus. The fat and lactose provide plenty of energy early in the lactation. This is especially important during the first few months of the foal's life when the most rapid physical growth occurs. If the mare is on a good ration, the milk will be high in vitamin A and it is a good source of B vitamins, especially riboflavin, niacin, and B-12. The lactose (milk sugar) helps increase the absorption of calcium and phosphorus and prevents digestive upsets.

Milk is not a perfect food for feeding by itself for long periods of time. It is low in vitamin D, very low in iron, and short of ascorbic acid (vitamin C). It is also low in copper, which is essential for bone development and blood formation. Older foals kept only on milk will soon become anemic. It is a natural food for the foal, but is lacking in nutrition when used as a sole feed for the older horse. This makes it extra important that the foal be started on supplemental (creep) feeding as soon as he will eat—usually by two to three weeks of age.

A good mare has been described as "a pearl without price," referring to the good start that she gives the foal, first by growing a strong foal in utero, and secondly, by giving it a good start in life through her milk and mothering.

A mare who produces an adequate quantity of good quality milk will make the difference between having a healthy, growthy foal and a thin, poor one. In the eastern Soviet Union, Novokirghiz mares produce 3.3 to 4.2 gallons (13 to 17 l.) of milk per day, including that taken by their foals, while on pasture. Peak lactation in light horse mares has been reported as high as 53 pounds (24 kg.) of milk per day (approximately 6-½ gallons). (35) Bashkir mares will produce 330 to 550 gallons (1500 to 2700 l.) of milk in a seven to eight month lactation period. (36)

Mare's milk is usually white or slightly bluish. Colostrum may be slightly yellowish. Milk a bit out onto your hand or into a cup and take a look at it. It should be free from off-colors or blood. There should be no strings, clumps, or other abnormalities. Every mare's milk should be checked at foaling to make sure there is no infection (mastitis) present. It is imperative to examine the milk if the foal appears hungry or ill. If the mare has an infection in the udder, it may cause scouring (diarrhea) or other illness in the foal.

A mare's udder, in case you haven't noticed, only has two teats, as opposed to four in the cow. Each teat may have two to four milk ducts in the lower end. The mare's udder should be soft and pliable without heat or excessive swelling. Occasionally, a mare swells so much before foaling that she is uncomfortable and will not allow the foal to nurse. The nipples may be swollen so tightly that the foal cannot get his mouth around them. If this occurs, apply warm, wet towels to the udder to help soften it and make the mare more comfortable. Milk the mare out by hand. Then apply a soothing ointment such as petroleum jelly to help keep the udder soft. Keep in mind that anything you put on will probably be licked off by the foal, so make sure that it is edible.

In the northern states, sunburned udders (from reflection of sunlight off of snow) are sometimes a problem with mares in the winter and early spring. This occurs primarily in horses without any pigmentation on the udder, such as Appaloosas.

Incidentally, when milking a mare, get close into her flank. Some mares, especially at first, are very grumpy about being milked by a human. Milk a mare from her left side, as most animals are more accustomed to being handled from that side. Put your right shoulder into her left hind leg so that you can feel if she is going to kick and so that you are close to that leg if she does. If you are close, she won't have room enough to take a good swing and can't do much, if any, damage.

Start slowly and gently (but use a soft, firm touch—don't touch so lightly that you tickle). Massage her udder a bit, and then gently take a nipple between the thumb and forefinger. Pull from the top downward, squeezing your fingers together as you do so. The object of the game is to push the milk out of the openings at the end of the teat. A convenient container for the job is a two-quart plastic pitcher held in the opposite hand from the one you are using to milk. For those of you who might be comparing it to milking a cow, it is almost always a two-finger exercise instead of a whole-hand procedure. Remove all the milk that you can at every milking. Otherwise, the mare will try to "dry up" and stop producing milk. Some mares need to be twitched before they can be milked. If the mare's udder is tight and hard, be sure to soften it with a warm, damp towel before you start milking her as described earlier.

COLOSTRUM

Colostrum is the name given to the milk produced by the mare for the first few days after foaling. It is produced during the last month of pregnancy and stored in the udder until birth. It is very rich and differs greatly in composition from milk produced during the rest of the lactation. Colostrum has a laxative effect that helps to get the newborn foal's bowels moving normally to prevent impaction or colic. Colostrum is much richer in vitamins, especially vitamin A, and in minerals than later milk. Foals are born with only a very small amount of vitamin A in their bodies; they may receive as much vitamin A in the first day in the colostrum as they would in several days drinking normal milk. Colostrum is high in zinc, containing two to three times the amount found in regular milk. (37)

This first milk also supplies antibodies to protect the newborn animal against diseases. At birth, the blood of a foal contains almost no antibodies. For the first 24 to 48 hours, the intestinal wall allows the absorption of large, complex protein molecules, called globulins, which carry antibodies to protect the foal until he is able to produce his own antibodies. These globulins are part of the very large quantity of protein in colostrum. Milk may contain as much as 19% protein shortly after birth, dropping to about 4% 12 hours later. This shows how much a foal may be shortchanged by a mare who leaks enough milk so that her colostrum is gone by the time she foals. Mare's milk five days after parturition contains about 3% protein; after two months, this declines to just over 2%. (38)

MASTITIS

Mastitis refers to an inflammation of the mare's udder, usually due to infection by bacteria or other pathogenic organisms. This can occur at any time during her lactation, and is occasionally seen in dry mares or those who are being "dried up" after lactation. These infections are not common in the mare. Signs include a hot, painful, swollen udder. Swelling may extend down the mare's legs and forward under her belly, causing discomfort when she walks. She may have little or no appetite.

To check for mastitis, milk a bit of the milk onto a clean white paper or pan or into the palm of your hand. It may be off-colored (excessively bluish or bloody), and may contain lumps, clots, or stringy material.

Your veterinarian should be consulted for appropriate treatment. He will probably prescribe antibiotics which are to be placed in the affected side(s) of the udder through each of the teat openings for two or three consecutive days. These are the same products which are used for cattle with mastitis. This treatment is done after milking as much milk as possible out of the udder. In addition, he may have her given antibiotic injections for the same period of time. Some mares may be in so much pain that they will violently object to being handled for treatment. These mares may have to be treated with injections alone, although this is not ideal. It should be routine practice for the mare owner to milk a bit of milk from the mare's udder after the foal is born to check to see that no mastitis is present.

MARE'S MILK AS HUMAN FOOD

Mare's milk is a light, tasty, extremely sweet milk (yes, I've tried it!). In desert areas from Arabia to Mongolia, it provides both fluid and nutrition, safely carried against loss or spoilage in the mare's udder, ready for use whenever needed.

Mare's milk is made into a mildly fermented milk drink, containing 0.5 to 1.5 percent alcohol. This beverage is called kumiss (also spelled koumiss, or kumys). It is native to southern Russia and southwest China. Kumiss is produced by putting mare's milk into a container, commonly a coltskin, and adding yeast, flour, and honey. It is said to taste like sour wine.

FEEDING THE ORPHAN FOAL

Foals may be orphaned for a number of reasons. The mare may die or be ill enough so that she is not producing milk or cannot take care of the foal. She may be such a poor milker that she cannot support the foal (Why are you keeping her?). Some mares may attack their foal, making it necessary to remove the foal to save his life. Other mares may not breed while they are nursing foals; it is then necessary to "bum" the foal in order to rebreed a valuable mare. The mare's udder may be injured so that she cannot nurse the foal. Some foals may be weaned early in order that the mare may be worked or shown.

Finding food for an orphan foal can be quite a project. How difficult it is and how to replace its mother's milk depends on the age of the foal when orphaned. If he has not had any colostrum, finding some is the first order of business. Sometimes if the mare is freshly dead, enough colostrum can be milked out of her udder to give the foal a good start in life. It's a rather gruesome thought, but it might save the foal's life. If the mare appears to have little or no milk, try milking a bit out onto your hand to make sure that what is there is normal.

A maiden mare may have little or no udder development until several days after foaling, but may still be producing enough milk to feed the foal. If there appears to be no milk at all, call your veterinarian. He may be able to give her an injection to bring her into milk production; this will work on many mares. If the mare attacks the foal, you may be able to get by with tranquilizing her and holding her by the halter every two hours to allow the foal to nurse. Or, you can milk her by hand and give the milk to the foal with a bottle.

Do anything you can to try to avoid having to raise the foal yourself. One of my clients had an ill-tempered mare who would not allow her foals to nurse for the first few days unless he put a halter on her and stood with a large stick, threatening her. He never had to use it, but without it in his hand, she would not allow the foal to nurse. After three to five days of this treatment, she would finally accept the foal and raise it. So, do not give up right away if the mare will not take the foal. Shut it away from her except at feeding times so that she will not injure or kill it. Poor mothering is often hereditary. This particular mare's female offspring were as poor mothers as she was. The breeder finally sold off all the animals he had of that lineage rather than bother with them every time one foaled.

If you cannot get colostrum from the dead mother, or if the mare has no milk, try to get some from another horse owner who has a mare who is within two or three days after foaling. Breeders who have many mares often freeze colostrum from a fresh mare and save it for this type of emergency. Frozen colostrum should be thawed slowly and carefully. Attempting to thaw it in a microwave oven or otherwise heating it may lead to loss of the very antibodies that the foal so badly needs.

If no horse colostrum is available, colostrum from a cow is better than none. It has the same properties in preventing constipation and has been experimentally shown to have some antibodies that help to give the foal protection against disease. (39)

With the colostrum out of the way, the next problem is to decide how to keep the foal fed until it is old enough to eat an adult diet. There are several choices.

A SUBSTITUTE MARE

If a mare can be found who will take the foal, this is the ideal solution to the problem. Or, another mare can be milked and the milk bottle-fed to the orphan. Muzzle her foal for a couple of hours or separate it from her to allow milk to build up in the udder before milking. If you are grafting the foal onto the mare, there are several techniques that may help you.

Many factors enter into whether or not a mare will take a foal that is not her own. If her own foal was born dead or was too weak to nurse, she may be unwilling to accept a "foreign" foal. The longer the time that has elapsed between the death of a mare's foal and the introduction of a new one, the less chance there is of success. If the mare's foal and the orphan are about the same size, there is a greater chance that she will take the new baby. How strong a maternal instinct the mare has also enters into the success of the fostering. Some mares will accept a foal while humans are present, and reject it as soon as she and the foal are left alone. Other mares may be extremely hostile toward the foal, but once they accept it, go on to make very good mothers.

If the foal has been fed artificially (on a bucket) for several weeks, or if it has never sucked from a mare, it will gradually lose the sucking reflex which is necessary for it to nurse. It may also be frightened by the mare; this can occur if the mare attempts to harm the foal. Methods to help the foster mother accept the orphan foal rely on confusing the signs by which she determines which foal is hers. You may try any (or all) of the following:

1) Put a strong-smelling medicine or perfume in the mare's nostrils and on the foal's back. Mentholatum (The Mentholatum Co., Buffalo, NY. 14213) is an example of a substance to try. Feed stores or veterinarians occasionally sell a compound used for mothering calves to cows. This compound is worth a try if you can get some. Perfume is said to work at times (How about Corral #5?).

2) Milking a pint or two of the mare's milk and sprinkling it all over the foal and rubbing it into the mare's nostrils may help.

3) Cover the orphan foal with the membranes or skin from the mare's dead foal. The mare recognizes her foal by smell, taste, and sight (thus the effect of differences in foal size).

4) Put the mare in a different pen or stall than the one where she had her foal. This is a good idea to try in conjunction with other techniques.

5) Put the mare in a chute or alleyway with an opening near the udder area so that the foal can suck. Blindfold her at the same time. Also use a strong-smelling substance in her nose and on the foal. After several days of this regimen, the mare will often accept the foal.

6) Tranquilize the mare until she becomes accustomed to the foal and accepts it as her own.

7) It may help to have the mare a bit hungry. Feed her when the foal nurses to help take her mind off the foal and to help associate the foal with pleasant experiences.

It often helps to have the foal hungry before introducing him to his new mother. Do not feed him for two to three hours before putting them together. The mare should at the very least be haltered and held in hand for the initial introduction. Otherwise, she may kill the foal before you have a chance to restrain her. Make sure that her intentions are benign before turning her loose with the foal.

It is usually worth taking up to 12 hours for the get-acquainted sessions between the mare and the orphan. Favorable signs of acceptance by the mare include nickering to the baby at feeding time and readily letting down her milk. Nuzzling and licking the foal are other good signs.

If she does not show signs of accepting the foal by 12 hours, the process will usually not be successful. Try keeping the mare and foal apart for several hours and re-introducing him to the mare. She may take him on the second or third attempt. If you feel that the mare has accepted the foal, it is worth staying close by for two to three hours to make sure that everything is really working. Leave the skin or membranes on the foal for 12 to 24 hours after the mare has taken the foal. If you are using an ointment or other fragrance, refresh it periodically for the first couple of days.

COMMERCIAL MILK REPLACER

This is the next best choice to a real live mother. Use a milk replacer meant for foals, not for calves! These replacers have the fat and sugars specifically balanced to match as closely as possible the composition of mare's milk. It is false economy to try to get by with makeshift formulas if this type of product (such as Borden's Foal-Lac, Borden, Inc., Pet-Ag Div., Hampshire, IL 60140) is available. Other formulas usually result in the foal getting scours and becoming so ill that he requires veterinary treatment. This can negate any savings that may have occurred and often results in a stunted or dead foal.

Mix the milk replacer according to instructions on the can. If constipation occurs, dilute the formula with more water than is recommended for the first two or three weeks. Use an antibiotic solution in one feeding per day to help prevent scours. Neomycin sulfate solution is the drug most commonly used. Use one teaspoon (5 cc.) in one feeding each day. Do not give it with every feeding, as the foal needs a bit of time without it to be able to collect some of the bacteria which will begin to help him digest the food that he eats. The antibiotic may be given for several weeks until the foal is strong and eating other foods along with the milk replacer. Feed milk replacer or formula lukewarm in temperature rather than cold or hot.

My only disagreement with Borden's label directions is that I feel the foal needs to be fed more frequently (for the first three weeks) than they advise. Four times a day is inadequate for an animal who would normally nurse as often as 120 times per day. Feed the foal every two hours, if possible, for the first week. After the first week, feed every three hours, around the clock. This schedule goes for whatever formula you are using. This schedule is in keeping with the horse's small stomach and constant appetite. It allows giving smaller feedings each time, and lessens the possibility of upsetting the foal's digestive system by overloading it.

GOAT'S MILK

If you have a good milking goat available, it is worth trying her to save an orphan foal. She may be milked out and the milk bottle-fed. If a high stand is built, the nanny can be restrained there to allow the foal to nurse. Occasionally, a cooperative goat will voluntarily climb the stand to allow a foal to nurse. A good nanny can be a very valuable addition to a broodmare operation. Goat's milk is closer to mare's milk in composition than is cow's milk.

COW'S MILK FORMULAS

These are best used only as emergency rations until milk replacer or a goat can be found, as there is a vast difference between mare's milk and cow's milk. Some people have successfully raised foals on cow's milk, but many others have lost foals on the same diet. Use them only until you can get something better.

One formula is as follows: 2 pints low-fat (skim) milk, 1 pint limewater (have your pharmacist mix it), and 1 tsp. lactose (often found at health food stores). Add 5 cc. (one teaspoon) neomycin sulfate solution to one feeding a day only. Another emergency formula uses a teaspoonful of white corn syrup per pint of 2% (skim) milk.

FEEDING TECHNIQUES

When bottle feeding a foal, use a lamb nipple rather than a calf nipple. Calf nipples are both too large and too hard and many foals will not suck on them. You can get the foal started nursing by dipping a finger in the milk or formula and letting the foal suck it. When he is sucking on your finger, switch the nipple for the finger. A strong, healthy foal can usually be bottle fed with little or no problem.

If you prefer, you can teach the foal to drink from a bucket. Put your finger into the milk and get it wet as above. Start the foal sucking on it and then slowly lower his head into the bucket so that the foal, still sucking your finger, will begin to drink the milk. This method is more convenient for later feeding, as you can build a box to hold the bucket so that the foal doesn't tip it over. Just set the bucket in the box and leave it. You do not have to stand there and hold the bottle or change through several bottles when the foal is drinking larger quantities.

Do not teach the foal to drink from a bucket if you have any thought of grafting him onto a goat or another mare. After he drinks from of a bucket for a few days, he will lose the sucking reflex. Once he has lost this reflex, it is nearly impossible to get him to nurse. Wait to bucket train him until you are sure that you will not be putting him onto a goat or a mare.

To determine the amount to feed, follow the instructions on the milk replacer which you are using. If you are giving a formula, milk replacer directions will still give a rough estimate as to how much to feed. When in doubt, err on the side of conservatism. Feeding too much can cause scours; then the foal can dehydrate and die before you can do anything about it. Foals are small and have few bodily reserves. It is better to have a foal too thin than to have him dead. If he begins to scour (have diarrhea), consult your veterinarian immediately.

Foals who are fed milk replacer (or other liquid feed from a bucket) may lose all the hair around the muzzle after being in contact with the liquid for a week or two. This is not a problem, as it will all come back when the liquid diet is stopped.

Mare milk replacers may be used to supplement a foal whose mother is taking care of him, but not producing enough milk. Even if the mare is not producing any milk, do not underestimate the value of her mothering and care if she is able to do so. She will help to keep the foal clean by licking him. This also helps to stimulate his bowel movements. The social contact will help the animal to be better adjusted to the world of horses than orphan foals sometimes are when raised only by humans.

A companion is valuable for an orphan foal, both to keep it company and to keep it from becoming a nuisance by demanding constant attention. Another foal is ideal; if not available, an old quiet pony which will not harm the foal, an old ewe, a lamb or two, goat, or a 2 to 3 month old, healthy calf will be helpful. The companion will help teach the foal to eat, sooner than he would learn by himself. The orphan foal should be kept away from adult horses until he is 3 months old or so, unless he is grafted onto a mare who will take care of him and protect him.

Under certain circumstances, your veterinarian may wish to feed the foal with a stomach tube. If he wishes you to continue the practice, he will show you how, as well as what kind of tube to use. Do not attempt to do this without instruction and a demonstration from your veterinarian. In the horse, it is easy to run the stomach tube down the trachea instead of the esophagus. This mistake results in milk in the lungs instead of the stomach. A pneumonia will almost certainly result with the animal generally dying as there is no way to get the milk out of the lungs.

FEEDING THE OLDER FOAL

The foal will begin to nibble on roughage as he nibbles on everything else around him. This is one way of exploring his world and seeing what tastes good and what does not. If he is with his mother on pasture, this nibbling becomes grazing quite easily. Many foals will lie down in their mother's hay if it is on the ground and eat from this position.

The foal will begin to eat grain with his mother at two days to three weeks of age. Feed the mare in a pan or feeder big enough so that the foal can get his nose in and share a bit of the feed. He will soon learn to eat by himself. At this point, supplemental feed is important to help the foal get nutrients which are not present in his mother's milk, but which are necessary for his growth. Peak milk production occurs two to three months after the mare foals, and gradually tapers off after that time.

When the foal is eating well, you can build a creep feeder which will allow the foal to eat without the mother, and offer grain mixture all the time (free choice). You can also feed a fine, high quality alfalfa hay in the creep so that the foal may eat hay whenever he wishes. Young foals fed in this way will not overeat, especially when they are still getting part of their nutrition from mother's milk. This supplemental feed is valuable in reducing the load on the mare and getting good early growth on the foal.

Most people feed a grain mix with a minimum of 16% protein in these feeders; 20% mix is even better if you can get it. Don't risk mixing your own and leaving out nutrients essential for the foal's growth. Buy a good commercial creep feed. Having the foal accustomed to eating both hay and grain from the creep feeder results in a better, growthier foal. It also lessens the upset at weaning time when the foal is made to do without his mother, helping to avoid setbacks at this critical time.

Make sure if you have grain in the creep all the time, that there is some sort of protection against rain so that the feed will not get soaked and then mold and cause illness in the foal. In the beginning, especially, feed should be changed every two days at the longest. This will help to keep the feed fresh and attractive, and will allow you to keep track of how much the foal (or foals) are eating.

If the foal has crooked legs from a phosphorus deficiency, he may be fed a phosphorus supplement. The supplement can be mixed with something sticky and sweet, like peanut butter or jelly, and fed to the foal daily, rather like a paste wormer. Or, you can mix it with a bit of water to make a thin gruel, and pour it into the corner of the foal's mouth from a pop bottle. Do not hold his head too high or he might inhale some of the mixture. Most of these mixtures are not so tasty that the animal will take them by itself.

WEANING

In nature, foals usually stay with the mare for a considerable period of time. The mare may not wean the foal until shortly before she gives birth to another foal, when the foal is nearly a year old. If the mare does not become pregnant, she may not wean the foal until around two years of age. Stabled horses are usually weaned around five to six months of age.

The foal may be weaned anytime after about two months if the mare is thin and poor; early weaning is also used with mares who will not rebreed while nursing a foal. They may also be removed if the mare has a poor disposition, hopefully avoiding having the mare teach her foal bad habits.

In some cases, the foal may be left on the mare as long as seven months if she is milking well and staying in good shape. The longer the foal can be left on the mare, the more certain it is that he will develop to the best of his potential, especially if he has high quality creep feed available at the same time.

A foal makes the majority of his lifetime growth in the first 18 months, making his early nutrition extremely important. If a foal is not given adequate feed during this critical period, he may become stunted and may not develop to his full genetic potential. Some horses never make up for this early lack of feed quantity or quality.

Standard weaning practice has been to remove the foal from the mare and place him in a safe stall or corral—one with a high, tight fence so that he cannot get a leg through it, jump over it, or otherwise injure himself. Some foals are still injured when they hit the wall or fence because they are upset and excited. Putting foals together in pairs temporarily lessens the upset, but the foals later go through the same sort of excitement when separated from each other. These practices are probably unavoidable when only one or two foals are to be weaned.

The impact of this traumatic time can be lessened if a dry mare or a gelding is placed in the pasture with the mare and foal for several weeks before weaning. The mare is then removed and the foal left with the other horse for company. The mare should be taken far enough away so that she cannot hear the foal and he cannot hear her, or both of them may be upset for quite some time.

Another method of weaning works well with larger groups of mares and foals. They are all placed together in a large pasture for at least a week before weaning is to occur. In the morning, one or two mares are removed from the bunch. As above, they are taken beyond earshot of the foals. In two or three days, another mare or two may be taken out. This is continued until all the mares are removed. Some people feel that it is helpful to leave one old, barren mare or gelding with the foals, feeling that this helps to soothe them.

Chapter 6

SOUNDNESS

Age and Teeth
Head and Neck
Eyes
Ears
Withers
Back and Torso
Front Legs
    Conformational Defects, Front Legs
Hind Legs
    Conformational Defects, Hind Legs
Unsoundness
    Unsoundnesses
    Unsoundnesses or Blemishes
    Breeding Unsoundnesses
Vices

Describing in detail every factor relating to soundness in horses would necessitate a volume many times the size of this one, and would be so detailed as to require a medical degree to interpret it. What I will do instead is to give you an approach to examine a horse for soundness before you purchase him, and to help you to spot problems which you can then have examined by a veterinarian. Some blemishes and vices which can limit the usability of an animal or make him completely useless, will also be listed.

To know what you are looking for in a horse, you must first determine how the horse is to be used. A reining or race horse with a severe lameness due to an injury may be unsound for these purposes. The same animal may be perfectly suitable for light use as a child's mount. An animal who is blind (due to injury, not hereditarily) may not be a good trail horse, but may make an excellent broodmare when confined in a small corral. A stallion with parrot mouth is worthless because of the problem's hereditary aspects, while a gelding with the same problem who is kept in and fed complete feed pellets or good hay may make a good performance animal—as long as he is not made to graze for a living.

There are very few absolutely perfect horses when we consider feet, legs, conformation, disposition, pedigree, training, and ability. Those few that do exist are worth huge amounts of money—often more than we are willing or able to spend. Therefore, most of us end up with a horse which is a compromise in one way or another. Determine what you want and what features you are willing to give up to keep the price of the animal within your budget. A lightly-used child's mount, for example, can be less than totally sound if he has the sterling disposition needed to protect and take care of the child. If money is no object, step right out and buy the perfect horse.

Begin your examination by standing back a distance and looking at the whole horse. Look at the side view first. What is your overall impression of the animal? How is he put together? Are there any conformational problems that are obvious at a distance, such as swayback, over at the knees, curbs in the hind legs, etc? Move to the front and look for crooked front legs, splints, and other obvious leg problems. Go around and get a rear view to look for cow hocks, crooked hind legs, and other obvious abnormalities.

Find out a bit about the animal's background if you can. Where did the present owner get him? Knowing who raised the animal or what part of the country he came from can often give insight into how he was handled and what diseases he might possibly have. For example, horses raised in the Sandhills of Nebraska often have teeth worn far beyond the animal's actual age because he has been eating sand with his forage all his life. Some of these animals from the Sandhills are also total klutzes in the mountains because there are no rocks where they are raised and they have never learned to watch where they are going.

Always ask the owner if the animal has ever been sick, lame, injured, or had surgery. Most people will honestly tell you what they know—but they are unlikely to volunteer it unless you ask. Also ask if the animal has any bad habits or vices. You may not get an honest answer, but at least you have tried. Most people will tell you if the animal has a problem, such as rearing or running away, because they are afraid of legal liability if they do not tell you, and to keep you from getting hurt if you purchase the animal.

Ask about the availability of health records. If these are available from the owner's veterinarian, ask that they be sent to your veterinarian if you buy the animal. You can also determine from these records if the animal has been on a regular worming and vaccination program. If you are looking at a mare, complete breeding records telling when she has been in heat, when she has been bred, foaling history, and a listing of any medications that have been necessary to get her into foal are extremely helpful. They may save you a barren year or two and a lot of money in treatment.

AGE AND TEETH

Open the animal's mouth (see Mouth) and examine the front teeth. Note how they mesh and if any are damaged. Broken incisors are often found in jumpers and steeplechase horses. Unless these are causing the horse pain, they may not constitute an unsoundness. Again, how are you going to use the animal? A horse with a broken incisor may not graze well and would keep poorly if turned out to pasture. If you are going to keep him in a stall and feed him quality feed, there should be no problem.

If the horse has been on sandy pasture and his teeth are worn beyond the age that his owner said he is, the owner is probably not lying. But, you have to consider him to be the age that his teeth are and not what the registration papers say, because when his teeth wear out, that's the end of his usefulness. One of these horses may be, for example, eight years old, and have the teeth of a twelve-year old. He must, for using purposes, be considered to be twelve years old.

Now check the condition of the rear, chewing teeth. Make sure that none are missing and that a wave mouth (see Wave Mouth) or other defect is not present. Check for points which will need to be removed by floating.

Look over the gums and cheeks for any injuries or sores. Be sure the color of the horse's membranes is normal. By the time you have opened a horse's mouth and looked at his teeth, you will also have an idea how cooperative he is about being handled.

Look over the animal's teeth for age (see Ageing). Check the teeth to see whether they are baby teeth or permanent teeth. This will keep you from confusing a two-year old with a five-year old. Look for cups in permanent teeth. Check the front of the upper rear teeth for a hook if the animal is of an appropriate age. Look over the general angle of the incisors from the side. You need not age the animal to the exact year, but I hate to see 15-year old horses sold as 7-year olds.

HEAD AND NECK

The horse's head may be a very beautiful part of his body, or be totally ugly. There is an old saying that "one doesn't ride the head." This is true, but on the other hand, most owners don't like one that hurts their eyes too badly, either. If you're showing the horse, the head may make or break him.

The head and neck act to balance the movement of the rest of the body, and for this reason should not be badly attached or disproportionate. The head is an especially important balancing mechanism for the jumper or the hunter, for animals who are eventing or steeplechasing, as well as for animals doing fast, turning work, such as cutting.

Ideally, the horse's head should be proportional to the rest of his body and well attached. It should be wide across the eye area, with the eyes set well to the sides of the head. Animals whose eyes are too far to the front of their heads do not seem to see as well as those whose eyes are placed normally.

Look over the face for any bony lumps that may suggest old fractures or problems with roots of the teeth. Look along the lower jaw bone for bumps due to tooth problems. These are especially seen in animals around three years old. Check the muzzle to make sure that both nostrils flare normally. If they do not, there may be a paralysis of the facial nerve. Look behind the jaw bone for swellings or lumps which may be due to distemper or to problems affecting the parotid salivary gland. Some horses will have a swollen, scarred salivary gland due to an old infection. These do not cause any problems, but may remain enlarged for the rest of the animal's life.

Look at the poll for drainage which may indicate the presence of poll evil. See how the neck is attached to the body. It should flow well into the shoulders and not have an abrupt union at this area, nor should it look as though it had been stuck on as an afterthought.

EYES

Look at the animal's eyes, checking for any discoloration on the corneal surface and for any gray, blue, or white spots in the center deep inside (the lens area) which may indicate the presence of a cataract. Blue or white coloration is normally present in the iris in some breeds. These are called glass or watch eyes.

Blindness is often difficult to detect, even for a veterinarian. An animal who is adjusted to his surroundings will often react as if he could see. A horse who is blind on one side may shy when ridden. He may turn his head at an odd angle when approached from that side. It is always worth asking the owner if the animal can see normally. Blindness due to an injury may not be a hindrance in a breeding animal, but blind animals are usually unsafe to ride.

EARS

Observe the animal as you are handling him. A horse who can hear will generally follow you with his ears. Handle his ears gently and carefully. This will tell you that the horse is not headshy. A horse who willingly lets a stranger handle his ears does not usually have ticks or any uncomfortable ear problem. If the animal reacts violently when you attempt to touch his ears, you have to determine whether the animal is dispositionally headshy or whether he has an ear problem. Of the two, disposition is the more common.

WITHERS

The withers should be high and well-defined. Young horses may have withers lower than their rump while they are growing—until they are as much as two years old. Beyond that age, this conformation is a fault. It makes it difficult for the animal to get his hind feet under him and the animal will be much less athletic than one whose withers are higher than his rump as they should be.

Some breeds, notably the Arabian, have many individuals who have fat, rounded shoulders and almost no withers. This is especially a problem if you are trying to pack the animal or ride him in back country—it is nearly impossible to keep a saddle upright on one of these horses.

Check the withers for saddle sores, and for drainage which may indicate a fistula of the withers. Unhealed saddle sores may effectively cripple the animal until they are healed. This may take a long time, especially if the problem has become chronic; you may not be able to use the horse for several months.

BACK AND TORSO

Look at how the horse's back attaches to his rump. Note closely the top line. Abnormalities of the spinal column can often be seen or felt. Upward bulges of the spinal column, often called roach back, are occasionally found. This problem may not rule out an animal for light use, such as a child's horse. It is not a conformation compatible with hard use, such as for roping or reining, which require that the animal get his hind feet under him.

Swaybacks are also seen, especially in older animals and broodmares. They are usually sound, but are not as sturdy as a horse with a normal, nearly level back. Horses with extremely long backs often have a swing or roll to their gait which can make them very comfortable to ride. For long-term usage, a long back is weaker than a short back, and the animal may not carry weight well. Long-backed horses may experience an alteration in their gait

which makes them prone to cross-firing. Short-backed horses with long legs may overreach or forge.

Finally, check the back for saddle sores, scars, or hardened spots under the skin which may cause problems when the horse is saddled.

The ribs should be wide and well sprung and the barrel should be deep. This allows for good lung capacity. Move back to the croup. Its shape should be typical of the breed of horse you are buying. An Arabian, for instance, is, by breed standards, supposed to have a flat croup. This changes the angle of the pelvis and makes the animal less able to get his hind legs under him. An animal with an extremely flat croup, for instance, would not be good for cutting or other use where hard stopping is needed. The same flat croup would be a severe fault in a working Quarter Horse.

Don't forget to check the animal's tail. Some people have cut the muscles on western pleasure horses to make their tails limp and keep them from wringing them. Or, special nerve blocks may have been used to keep the animal from switching his tail. However, the American Quarter Horse Association has ruled against this procedure, and having a horse with a limp tail may disqualify you from the show ring. In addition, the horse may not be able to swat flies which will cause him considerable discomfort. Saddlebreds may have a set tail. Set tails should not pull to one side or the other.

FRONT LEGS

Because the horse's front legs carry between 60 and 65% of his weight, they are vitally important to the animal's overall soundness. (40) They also account for at least 75% of lameness problems. Faulty conformation makes it much easier for the animal to injure himself as he moves. Or, the stresses involved in an improper angulation of the limb may result in stress problems by themselves. Animals who are used in events which require rapid turning, such as cutting and barrel racing, have enough trouble keeping from getting tangled up in their own feet without being handicapped by crooked legs which make injuries more likely.

Look at the animal from a distance before you approach him closely. The animal should be standing quietly, with his weight well distributed among the four legs. He should be first checked while still, and later when he is moving. These examinations should be done on a hard surface, whether well-packed dirt or solid pavement. They are unreliable if you try them on uneven or sloping ground, on soft ground, or on grass.

The front legs should be straight. If you drop a line from the point of the shoulder to the ground, it should fall straight down, dividing the leg into exactly equal halves when viewed from the front. The toes should be straight forward (not turned inward or outward). A line dropped from the point of the shoulder should divide the leg equally into front and back halves when viewed from the side, as far as the fetlock joint. It will then fall just behind the heel. The knee should not deviate either frontward or backward. The angle of the hoof wall should be the same as that of the pastern. The pastern angle varies with the breed of horse. Quarter Horses, for example, often have less sloping pasterns and shoulders than do Arabians or Saddlebreds.

Check the shoulders for normal muscle covering. Lack of musculature may indicate sweeny or muscle damage. The shoulder joint should not show any abnormal swellings or lumps; moving down the leg, the elbow should also be free of these problems. The horse's chest should be well muscled and of a normal width for the given breed of horse (Saddlebreds, for example, are often narrower in the chest than are Quarter Horses). Run your hands over the knee feeling for any abnormal swellings, whether bony or soft and puffy. Bend the knee and pull the hoof gently in and out, putting a sideways pressure on the knee joint. Feel if the horse flinches at any time during this procedure.

Move down the cannon bone, looking and feeling for bony or soft tissue swellings and so on, down the foot. Examine the hoof from both the front and side, noting both the hoof itself and the shoeing job and type of shoes used if the animal is shod. Pick up the foot and examine the hoof. Clean it out thoroughly so that you can see it well. Look for contracted heels, abnormal frog, or other obvious problems.

Now check the other front leg in the same manner. When you are finished, go back and make sure that both legs match completely, from the hooves, feet, and shoeing job up past the knees to the shoulders. Both legs should be bearing weight equally. If there is any lack of similarity, try to determine where the problem is and what it is before you go any further in your examination.

CONFORMATIONAL DEFECTS, FRONT LEGS

Many abnormalities are seen in the front legs, most of which cause some sort of problems later in the animal's life, especially if he is used for hard, fast work. Some horses have such a combination of abnormalities that it's hard to isolate them all and consider them individually. Let's discuss some of the most common.

BASE NARROW

In our previous examination, it was noted that an animal with straight front legs would have a line dropped through the middle of the upper leg passing through the exact middle of his toes when viewed from the front. If his hooves instead of being on the line are standing inside it, the animal is said to be "base-narrow." It means that he is narrower at the base (his feet) than he is at the chest. This defect is commonly found in Quarter Horses with their large chests and heavy, well-developed muscles.

The animal ends up putting more weight on the outside of his foot than he does on the inside. More strain is placed on the tendons on the outside of the leg. These animals tend to have ringbone and sidebone on the outside of the foot, as well as windpuffs. The foot must be trimmed on the inside to level it. As with any conformational abnormality, observe the animal while he is moving as well as at rest before making the decision as to where he needs to be trimmed. See how he is landing on the foot. Also, see where the wear is occurring and trim the foot so it is level before shoeing.

BASE WIDE

This animal will be found to have his feet outside the vertical line down the middle of the front leg. It is usually seen in narrow-chested horses such as Tennessee Walkers and American Saddlebreds. The horse will be carrying most of his weight on the inside of his feet, putting most of the strain on the inside of the leg. Ringbone and sidebone may occur on the inside of the foot, and windpuffs may be seen here, also. The outside of the hoof usually needs to be trimmed to level it.

PIGEON TOES (TOE IN)

Pigeon-toed horses often look quite ridiculous because their toes are turned in toward each other. When these animals travel, they tend to paddle their feet outward with each step. The animal is usually also base-narrow (has his legs closer together at the feet than at the chest). Toeing in is uncommon in the base-wide horse (one who has his feet farther apart than where the legs come out of the chest). If a pigeon-toed horse also has his feet bent inward from the fetlock down, he may have severe interference problems. These are occasionally bad enough to cause fractures or other damage to the inside sesamoid bone behind the fetlock.

SPLAY-FOOTED (TOE OUT)

These horses have their feet turned outward if you look at them from the front. Often the legs on a splay-footed animal are not merely crooked at the feet, but turn outward from where the legs attach to the chest. These animals "wing" to the inside as they travel, often hitting themselves on the opposite front leg. This is worse when the animal is base-narrow than when he is base-wide.

Like the pigeon-toed animal, splay-footed horses may severely injure their sesamoid bones, as well as hav-

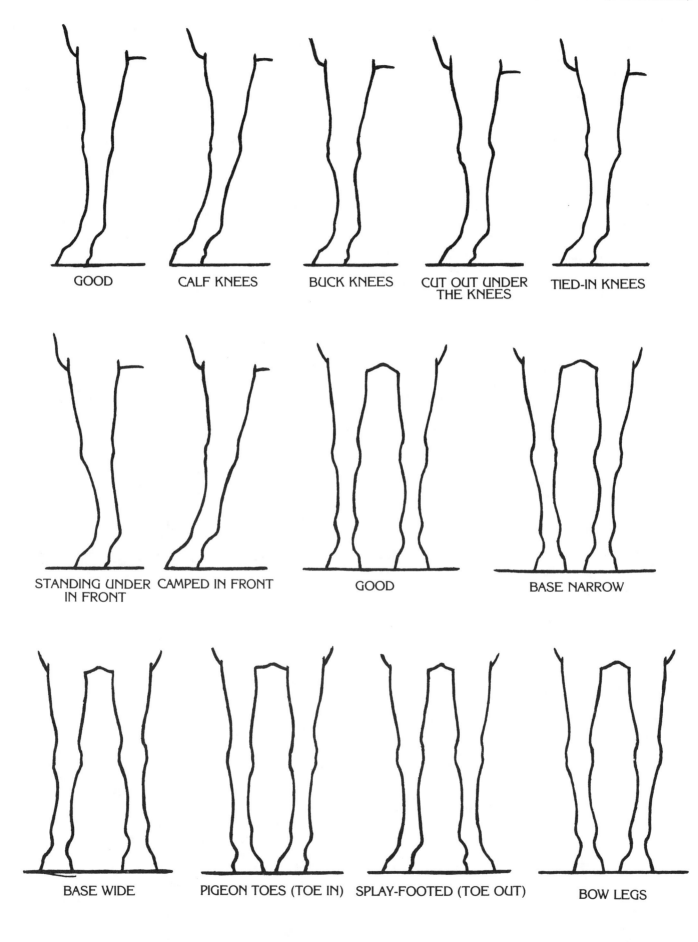

GOOD   CALF KNEES   BUCK KNEES   CUT OUT UNDER THE KNEES   TIED-IN KNEES

STANDING UNDER IN FRONT   CAMPED IN FRONT   GOOD   BASE NARROW

BASE WIDE   PIGEON TOES (TOE IN)   SPLAY-FOOTED (TOE OUT)   BOW LEGS

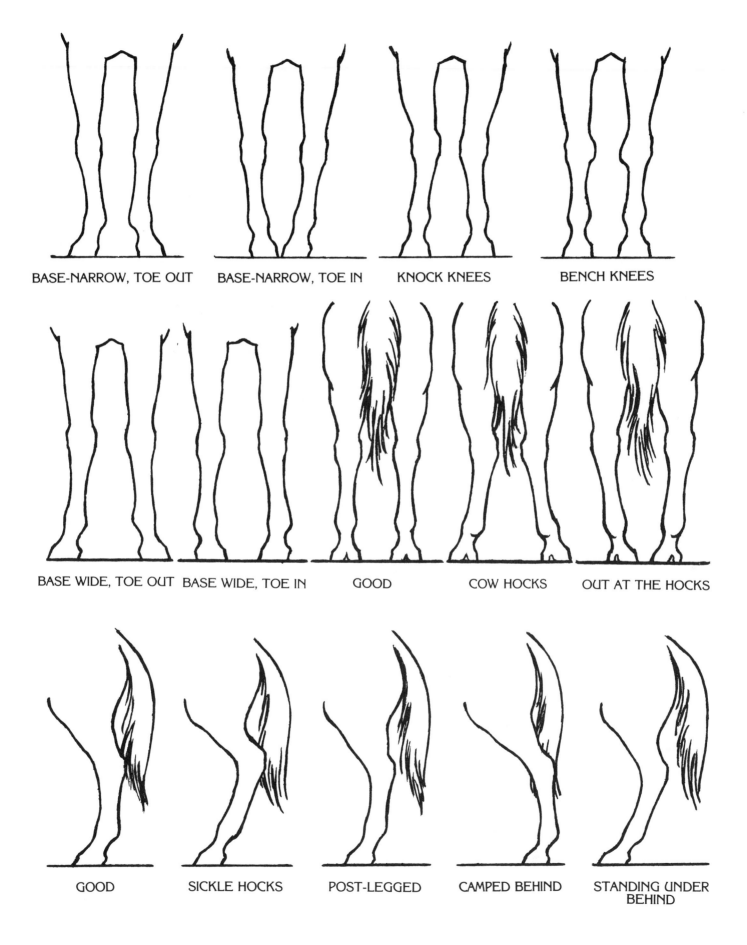

BASE-NARROW, TOE OUT   BASE-NARROW, TOE IN   KNOCK KNEES   BENCH KNEES

BASE WIDE, TOE OUT   BASE WIDE, TOE IN   GOOD   COW HOCKS   OUT AT THE HOCKS

GOOD   SICKLE HOCKS   POST-LEGGED   CAMPED BEHIND   STANDING UNDER BEHIND

ing a constant string of sores and cuts up and down the leg. Depending on how the animal moves, these injuries may extend from just above the hoof wall to mid-cannon bone. Occasional animals with high action may even clip the inside of the knee.

If you have to choose between a horse with pigeon-toes and one with splay feet, take the one with pigeon toes. He won't be as pretty, but he will usually have fewer scrapes and injuries than one with splay feet.

BASE-NARROW, TOE IN

Animals who are narrower at the feet than they are at the chest AND have their toes turned in tend to put extra strain on the ligaments on the outside of the pastern and fetlock joints. Sidebone and ringbone may form on the outside of the foot and windpuffs may be seen. These conditions result from the mechanical strains placed on the ligaments, as well as from the greater portion of the body's weight being placed on the outer wall of the hoof. The outer hoof wall will be worn shorter than the inner one. The inside wall must be trimmed a bit to help level the foot.

BASE-NARROW, TOE OUT

This is one of the worst types of conformation possible in the horse. The poor animal often looks like an eggbeater when he moves, and may hit his feet causing severe interference damage. The weight is placed on the outer wall of the hoof, while strain is placed on ligaments on the inside the leg. Fractures of the splint bones and sesamoids are common with these animals.

Observe the animal carefully while he is in motion to make sure of the corrections needed when shoeing him. These usually include lowering the inside wall and toe to make the foot level. Horses who are base-narrow and toed-in may have a way of going called "plaiting." This occurs when the horse puts one front foot almost in front of the other. The animal may step on himself, with resulting injury. Some of these horses can actually be dangerous to ride at anything faster than a walk—they trip over their own feet.

BASE-WIDE, TOE OUT

Like the animal described above, this conformation puts strain on ligaments on the inside of the leg. Ringbone and sidebone may be seen; they will also occur on the inside of the foot. The foot lands on the inner hoof wall, putting more wear on this area. The outside wall must be lowered to bring the foot back to level. These animals also tend to hit one front foot with the opposite resulting in fractures of the inner splint bone and sesamoid. Often these animals, like the animal who is splay-footed, will have a chain of small bony growths and scars inside the cannon bone from previously having hit themselves.

BASE-WIDE, TOE IN

This conformation is very uncommon. Most of the animal's weight will be borne on the inside of the leg. The injuries which occur are the same as for the base-wide, toe out animal discussed above.

CALF KNEES

Also called "sheep knees," this conformation occurs when the knees appear to be pushed backward in relation to the front line of the leg. It is a poor, weak conformation. Chip fractures commonly occur on the fronts of the carpal bones as they are crunched together when the animal moves. This injury is especially seen when he is worked hard, as with racing, roping, reining, or other work which requires hard stops. This defect also places considerable strain on the lower check ligament and the ligaments and joint capsule at the rear of the knee joint as they are stretched by the deviation of the bones.

BUCKED KNEES

Also called "knee sprung," "over at the knees," or "goat knees," this occurs when the knee joint is bent forward instead of backward as above. This is a common defect and causes fewer problems than calf knees. It is caused by excessive tension in the muscles which flex the knee. This defect places extra stress on the suspensory ligament, the sesamoid bones at the rear of the fetlock, and the superficial flexor tendon.

Bucked knees may be seen as a congenital problem, where they may be part of a case of contracted tendons. Bucked knees may also be seen in animals with rickets. If only one knee is bucked, this usually indicates severe pathologic changes somewhere in that leg.

KNOCK KNEES

Horses who are narrower at the knees than the rest of the leg put strain on the inner side of the joint capsule at the knee. They also put stress on the outer side of the carpal bones themselves as they are crunched together. The lower check ligament and suspensory apparatus may also be damaged.

BOW LEGS

Bow legs are curved outward at the knee area when viewed from the front. This is often seen when the animal is base-narrow and toes in. The strain is placed on the outside ligaments of the knee joint and the inside of the carpal bones.

CUT OUT UNDER THE KNEES

Animals with this defect have a dished-out appearance below the knee joint on the front of the leg when observed from the side. It is a weak conformation.

TIED-IN KNEES

Horses with tied-in knees have the tendons at the rear of the leg pulled in closely behind the knee joint. This conformation may keep the animal from moving freely.

STANDING UNDER IN FRONT

Animals who "stand under in front" will stand with both front legs placed behind where they should be when viewed from the side; they appear to be too far under the body. If the animal persists in standing or traveling this way, it will result in an increased load on the front legs as they carry a larger portion of the animal's weight. The forward phase of the animal's stride may be shortened because of the abnormal weight-bearing. Each leg returns to the ground sooner with the animal making more and smaller steps. Because the foot arc is low to the ground, the horse may be prone to stumbling and even falling.

CAMPED IN FRONT

An animal who is camped in front stands with both front legs farther forward than normal. This is the opposite of an animal who stands under in front. This attitude is commonly seen with founder and is sometimes seen with navicular disease. The horse is trying to reduce the weight and pain on his front feet.

LONG SLOPING PASTERNS

Animals with long, sloping pasterns put excessive strain on the tendons and ligaments at the rear of the leg. They commonly have sesamoiditis or sesamoid fractures, as well as strains and other problems with the flexor tendons and the suspensory ligament.

LONG STRAIGHT (UPRIGHT) PASTERNS

Horses with this conformation tend to have problems with the fetlock joint, as well as navicular disease. This is because the fetlocks do not absorb shock as well as those with normal angulation in this area. If the shoer trims the animal's heels short to attempt to bring the hoof wall to a normal angle, this will cause an abnormal angulation of the foot, resulting in the deep flexor tendon being pulled tightly against the navicular bone. This can result in navicular bursitis or navicular disease.

SHORT UPRIGHT PASTERN

This conformation increases concussion throughout the foot because of its lack of shock absorption. Both the fetlock and pastern joints are jarred excessively, as is the navicular bone. These animals are prone to ringbone and navicular disease.

HIND LEGS

Check the hind legs by viewing them squarely from a short distance behind the horse. The hind legs should be well muscled, again according to breed characteristics. The hocks should be relatively large to carry the animal's weight, and smooth. The horse should have good muscling down the inside of the gaskin. Inside muscling is especially important in Quarter Horses who are expected to do reining, cutting, or similar strenuous movements. The hind legs should be straight with a vertical line dividing them into equal halves.

When viewed from the side, a line dropped from the hindmost point of the rump area below the tail should fall vertically down the rear line of the cannon bone. The upper leg muscles should blend gradually down into the thigh and hock area, rather than bunching up and stopping abruptly.

The stifle joints should show no signs of locking, stiffness, or abnormal swelling. The hock joints should be smooth and clean, without large soft swellings (bog spavins) or hard, bony swellings (bone spavins). Perform a spavin test on the horse (see Spavin Test).

CONFORMATIONAL DEFECTS, HIND LEGS

COW HOCKS

"Cow hocks" is the term for hocks which are closer together than the feet below them. The feet are rotated outward. The animal may also be sickle-hocked. This combination can be a severe defect and may result in bone spavin because of excess strain on the hock joint. Most horses are slightly cow-hocked; animals having this defect without any others may stand up to long and fairly hard usage without problems.

Cow hocks must be differentiated from the outward turning of the hindlegs that commonly occurs in Arabians. The Arab's hocks will appear to be turned toward each other as with cow hocks. Careful observation will reveal that NOT just the hocks are turned but the WHOLE LEG, from the hip on down. When viewed separately, each leg is straight with itself—the two of them are just not straight with each other. While this is definitely NOT an ideal conformation and does not occur in better representatives of the breed, there are many Arabians who have been used hard all their lives and not had any hock problems despite this defect. Check the animal's way of going—if he travels normally, this particular conformation may not cause him any difficulty. Some animals who turn their feet outward when standing seem to get them lined out and tracking straight when moving—look at the animal's tracks on dirt to see if the hind feet are landing straight or at an angle.

SICKLE HOCKS

Horses with sickle hocks have an excessive angle—the foot is farther under the body than it should be. This may cause bog or bone spavins due to strain on the hock joint. Curbs are another problem common in sickle-hocked animals. Sickle hocks are often referred to as a "curby conformation." Animals with sickle hocks who are also cow-hocked have the worst possible combination of hind leg defects and are almost sure to have problems if they are used much at all.

Sickle-hocked animals start with their legs more under them than the normal animal. A nationally famous reining horse trainer told me that he looks for animals that are a bit sickle-hocked because it enables them to get their hocks under them easily. Now, they may not last for a long time, especially under the stress of reining training, but if these animals could stand the stress, they were winning for him. There is no good correction for horses with the wrong angles in the hock and stifle joints; shoeing will not fix what the horse's mother and father didn't make right in the first place.

POST-LEGGED (EXCESSIVELY STRAIGHT HIND-LEGS)

If the hindlegs are too straight (often called post-legged), the horse is prone to upward fixation of the patellas (kneecaps) and to bog spavins in the hock joint. Post-legged horses also have problems getting their hind legs under them. They are poor athletes and do not make good barrel, reining, or cutting horses because they cannot bring the legs far enough forward to drive off of them well. These animals would also perhaps make poor jumpers because of this lack of spring action. Overly straight legs may, however, cause fewer leg lameness problems than sickle hocks.

BASE-NARROW

This conformation may be seen in the hindlegs as in the forelegs. It is most common in heavily muscled animals. The end result is often excessive strain on the tendons, ligaments, and bones on the outside of the leg. It is often accompanied by bow legs, with the hocks farther apart than the feet. This defect may result in interference between the hindlegs and forelegs. Some horses may have straight legs with the feet turned outward, resulting in a base-narrow stance, again placing strain on the structures on the outside of the leg.

BASE-WIDE

This is most commonly seen with cow hocks, where the feet are placed outside the vertical line down the rear leg.

CAMPED BEHIND

The entire leg may be placed well behind the vertical line. This is frequently seen with pasterns which are too straight.

UNSOUNDNESS

What is an unsoundness? An unsoundness is a problem which affects the animal's usability and durability (longevity of usage). In some states, certain unsoundnesses will disqualify a stallion for a breeding license. In some foreign countries, government inspectors evaluate all prospective stallions. In those countries, unsoundness will not only disqualify the animal for breeding, but will REQUIRE his castration so that he will not reproduce!

And just which problems are unsoundnesses? The list may be long or short, depending on the use to which you are going to put the horse and what you are willing to tolerate and care for. An example of this is a parrot-mouthed gelding who is going to be kept in a stall all his life; the fact that he is parrot-mouthed will not harm him because he will not be expected to graze. The fact that it is hereditary is of no consequence because the animal cannot reproduce. So, for this beast, it may be considered a blemish. Another example is a well-bred broodmare who has become blind because of an injury. She may produce many fine foals with a minimum of extra care, and more than repay any trouble needed to care for her. Again, this would be more of a blemish than an unsoundness. If, however, you're going out to buy a riding horse, blindness should be considered an absolute unsoundness.

Now let's discuss some specific unsoundnesses which may be problems. These are not all the ones which are possible, but merely a list of the most common.

UNSOUNDNESSES

1) PARROT MOUTH

The parrot-mouthed horse has his upper teeth lapping over the lower ones, much like a parrot's beak (rather than meeting each other squarely as they normally would). Due to its hereditary nature, this problem should definitely rule out an animal as a breeding mare or stallion.

It should also eliminate the animal from consideration if you wish to put it out on pasture, as the animal is unlikely to do well there. As a nonreproductive animal who is kept in confinement for a using animal only, such as a jumper, this may not be a serious handicap. This is a decision that only you can make.

2) UNDERSHOT JAW

The mechanism of this problem is the same as the parrot mouth, but in reverse. The lower teeth stick out past the uppers, much like a bulldog. The concerns with this problem are the same as those for parrot mouth.

3) BAD BACK TEETH

When the large, important cheek teeth—the ones that do all the major grinding and chewing of the horse's food—are defective, the animal will usually be a poor keeper. He may be impossible to keep in a normal condition. Wave mouth is an instance of bad back teeth, as is having one or more of the back teeth missing. This is especially a problem when the animal has not had enough

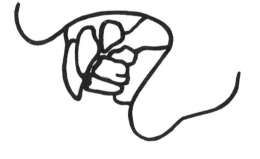

Parrot mouth.

care to keep the remaining teeth in as good a condition as possible. Bad back teeth can lead to abnormalities in chewing which are severely detrimental to the horse.

4) CRIBBING

Animals who crib may be observed in the act. Or, they may have the front edges of their front teeth worn off at an angle. Hair may be worn off the throatlatch area from the use of a cribbing strap, or there may be a white spot (similar to a saddle spot on the withers) in the mane or on top of the neck (see Cribbing). Cribbing is an unsoundness; however, if the animal is well-trained and usable, it may be an unsoundness you can live with. Because a mare may teach it to her foal, it should be considered an unsoundness in a broodmare.

5) BLINDNESS

Whether this makes the animal unsound for you depends on the cause of the blindness and the use to which the animal is put. Hereditary blindness observed in a foal should be considered an absolute unsoundness. The animal should be humanely euthanized rather than being allowed to grow up to take its place in the horse world and perhaps reproduce the problem.

Acquired blindness is usually an unsoundness for a riding animal, although this author has ridden a horse who was totally blind from the age of ten. At the time, he was 21 years old. The animal responded completely to voice commands and rein cues. However, an animal who is totally blind should not be trusted in the mountains or with an inexperienced rider who could not tell him what to do.

Blindness in one eye may cause the animal to shy and may be a hazard to the rider. This is a judgment that only the owner can make about a particular animal. If the horse has been a good rideable horse and becomes blind through injury, he may continue to be rideable for limited, light usage. One of the best-known competition trail horses some years ago was blind in one eye and traveled a great many miles in that condition, although there was a rumor some years later that he had eventually gone off an embankment with his rider.

If you are choosing the animal for a breeding animal and the blindness is not hereditary, then his or her suitability depends on the conditions and facilities that you are prepared to provide. A horse who is blind in one eye may be perfectly happy in a small pasture or corral. A broodmare who is totally blind may produce a good many foals if kept in simple surroundings with easily available food, water, and salt. Blind horses learn their surroundings by memory just as do humans, and are usually no more trouble than a sighted horse when kept for breeding purposes.

6) PERIODIC OPHTHALMIA

This disease tends to recur in an affected animal. While the intervals between attacks may be as much as a year, they tend to get worse with each recurrence, finally resulting in cataracts and often in blindness, as well as considerable pain to the animal. As the cause is not known for sure, it should be considered an unsoundness under all conditions.

7) CATARACTS

If due to periodic ophthalmia, these are an unsoundness. Cataracts may also be hereditary; if so, they should be considered an absolute unsoundness in the breeding animal. If they have occurred later in life, the considerations are the same as for blindness, above.

8) ROARING

A horse who roars is much less useful than a normal animal because of his reduced respiratory intake. Surgery to correct the problem is not always successful and is often expensive. Check into the cost of repairs and the likelihood that the animal will ever be usably sound before you purchase a roarer.

9) HEAVES

Horses with heaves are like humans with smoker's cough. The problem is chronic and usually progressive. An animal with heaves may be suitable for light use—say as a child's horse. They are rarely suitable for heavy usage without continuous medication. In addition, they need special care and feeding to keep the problem from getting worse. Decide whether you wish to be bothered with this for the rest of the animal's life or if you would be better off to keep looking for another horse without the problem. It may be a minimal problem in the breeding mare or stallion—if NOT combined with laminitis.

10) WRY NECK (CROOKED NECK), EWE NECK

These animals may have a crooked neck with one or more abnormal curvatures. "Ewe neck" is the term used to describe a neck that sinks rather than rises between the shoulders and the head. It looks like it was put on upside down. Either problem is a defect, cosmetically, and either one may adversely affect the animal's way of going. They are also frequently passed on to the animal's offspring.

11) CHRONIC COLIC

Like an animal with heaves, a horse with chronic colic may be a lifetime problem. They usually require special feeding, care, and attention to help insure that they do not colic again. They are often a source of continuous worry about whether they are going to colic when the owner is gone to work or on vacation and often live a shorter lifespan than the animal without chronic colic. Colic kills horses by its complications (for instance, rolling and twisting an intestine from the pain when the owner is not there). In my opinion, one of these animals is not worth the bother and headaches that accompany it. They also require more frequent worming and will often require several veterinary calls per year to treat their colic—both expenses that could be avoided by buying an animal without the problem.

12) CRYPTORCHIDISM

Having one or both of the horse's testicles up in his flank or retained in the belly is a hereditary problem. This should absolutely rule out the animal as a prospective stallion. In addition, tumors often occur in the testicle(s) which are retained in the abdomen. For this reason, castration is definitely recommended. A normal castration is a fairly routine procedure. A cryptorchid (ridgeling) castration is a major abdominal surgery with all its inherent risks in the horse. There is a greatly increased risk of losing the animal from the surgery or from complications after it.

Having a cryptorchid stallion castrated costs a LOT more than having the same type of surgery on a normal horse. If you are buying a colt, check to see that both testicles are in the scrotum. Often people put cryptorchid stallions up for sale when they find out what the surgery will cost and the unsuspecting (or unwary) buyer is stuck with the price of the surgery. In a recent year, this author examined one colt for four different buyers (AFTER each one had bought him and then called me) before one of them finally decided to put the money into him to do the surgery. Look before you purchase!

13) CHRONIC LAMENESS

The horse who is chronically lame should be considered unsound. It is one thing to stick band-aids on a horse you have owned for years trying to get a few more miles out of Ol' Dobbin. It is entirely another matter to buy an animal with a chronic problem and to keep trying to fix him from there. You're better advised to just keep looking for another animal.

If the chronic lameness is due to conformational factors, this should rule out the animal for breeding purposes as well. The breeding animal should be chosen with as much emphasis on correct conformation and good legs as with a working animal. Indeed, since he or she is going to be the parent of several offspring, it is MORE important that they should be good animals than a working individual. Now, let's discuss some specific foot and leg lameness problems.

14) POPPED KNEES

This is the common name given to a multitude of knee problems due to chips inside the knee joints, stretched ligaments, and other damage. These show up as various knobs and knots, usually rather soft, on the knee surface. These are an unsoundness in the using horse, although they may be something that you can live with under certain circumstances if they cause little or no lameness. They can even be tolerated in a broodmare, IF they are not due to an underlying conformation problem that she might pass on to her offspring.

One example which comes to mind is a superbly trained veteran cutting horse named Scissors. This gray horse was 28 years old the last time this author saw him work. His knees had so many lumps and knots as to resemble small cabbages. However, he has trained a multitude of riders because of his skill. The old guy knows what he is supposed to do when placed in front of a cow. He does his end of the work, leaving the rider to more

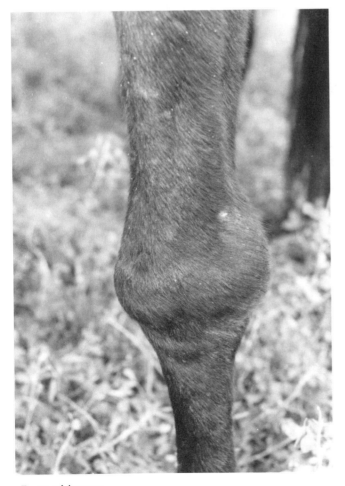

Popped knees.

easily learn how to ride a cutting horse. When a rider outgrows him, he sells him to someone else who learns from him.

There are plenty of fine animals like this in jumping, roping, and other fields as well. With careful warmup, good food and diligent care, they can give a certain number of miles of moderate usage without serious problems, and can often pass on a valuable education.

15) SPLINTS

Splints are an unsoundness when accompanied with lameness or poor conformation. If they are old, completely healed, and without lameness or involvement of vital structures, they are considered a blemish.

16) CAPPED ELBOWS

Capped elbows are also called shoe boils because they may occur from the horse hitting his elbow with his shoe while lying down. They are rarely accompanied by lameness, but are an unsoundness if lameness is present.

17) CAPPED HOCKS

Capped hocks may be a blemish or an unsoundness. They may be due to stall kicking. The horse may only do this at night so it may go unnoticed by the owner. If the blemish or unsoundness is combined with this vice, you should not buy the horse. He could possibly teach it to your other horses, and he will certainly continue to aggravate his own condition of capped hock. It may also be an unsoundness when accompanied by curbs, especially if poor conformation goes along with the two problems.

If capped hocks are unaccompanied by poor conformation or lameness, they may merely be blemishes. They may result from the horse being roughly thrown around while being hauled in a trailer or some similar situation which was not the animal's fault.

18) STRINGHALT

This is a spasmodic condition of the hindleg in which the hock is drawn rapidly toward the belly when the horse takes a step. The foot may then be returned to the ground with abnormal force. It may occur in one hindleg or both. Its cause is not known. Surgery occasionally helps, but many cases show no improvement. Animals with this peculiarity of gait should be considered unsound for either use or breeding because of the uncertainty about its cause.

19) KNOCKED DOWN HIP

These animals have one hip which is very obviously lower than the other when viewed from straight behind.

This condition usually occurs when two horses try to go through a narrow door or gate at the same time. One of the wings of the hip bone is broken and the animal will have a lopsided appearance for the rest of his life. Lameness may be seen soon after the problem occurs, but usually subsides after the fracture heals. At this point, it becomes more of a blemish than an unsoundness.

20) DISPLACED PATELLA

Horses whose kneecaps pop in and out of place are unsound. The problem causes both functional problems and a certain amount of pain for the animal. Since the problem is usually due to hereditarily faulty conformation, horses with it should be considered unsound for both performance and breeding.

21) BOG SPAVIN

Most authorities consider bog spavin to be an unsoundness. At least, a horse with this problem is certainly not perfectly normal. However, it depends on how the animal got the problem as to whether he is usable or not (unsound or merely blemished). Some cases of bog spavin occur due to overwork in the young animal. These horses will have swollen joint capsules for the rest of their lives, and yet may never take a lame step because of them.

If the problem is due to poor conformation in the hock joint, bog spavin should be considered an unsoundness. In older horses, bog spavin may be due to arthritic changes in the hock joint and should be considered an unsoundness. In any case, it is at the very least a blemish.

22) BONE SPAVIN

Bone spavin is definitely an unsoundness. The pull of the cunean tendon over the bony growth that forms the spavin causes the horse severe pain and may result in a visible lameness. The lameness may come and go, but is still hanging around to haunt the owner. Cutting the tendon may relieve the pain for some horses, but, in other cases, does nothing at all to make the animal more comfortable and usable. The spavin test will usually show these animals to be noticeably lame.

23) CONTRACTED FEET

When one or more feet are smaller than usual or the heels are contracted in relation to the toe, the horse has a severe problem which may take a year or more to correct. If it's due to a problem such as navicular disease, it may not be possible to correct. Bear in mind that some horses have feet that are more oval than round and that most horses' back feet are more narrow and long then their front feet. The problem is especially noticeable when it involves only one foot. It may be hereditary or it may be

due to injury. In general, contracted feet should be considered an unsoundness for both using and breeding purposes.

24) CORNS

Corns are often caused by improper shoeing. They also may be due to laminitis (founder). In either case, they can easily become chronic and may lead to osteitis (infection) of the coffin bone. Unless you know for sure that the corns are very recent and not due to laminitis, pass this animal up.

25) FOUNDER (LAMINITIS)

A horse with founder must be considered unsound. How badly unsound he is depends on how severe the founder was and how many complications have occurred because of it. Sequelae such as dropped sole, corns (which may become pedal osteitis), and abnormal hoof growth patterns may cause continuing problems.

Special shoeing may correct the problem enough to allow the horse to be usable, but bear in mind that the

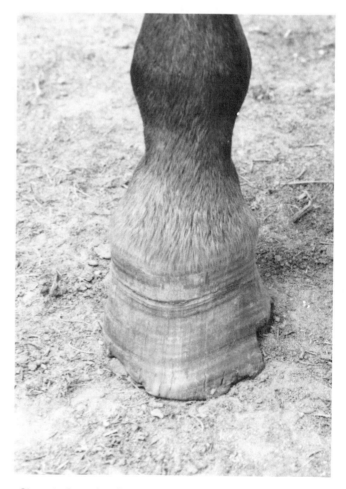

Chronic founder (laminitis).

horse could get worse at any time. Do not buy a known foundered animal for a using horse. A foundered brood-mare may not be a bad buy—if you are willing to give her the care she will need and if she does not have a case of the heaves so that she cannot eat hay. If she has both, keep looking for another animal.

26) NAVICULAR DISEASE

Navicular disease is a progressive and, at the present time, incurable problem. There are some methods which can help to make a horse with navicular disease usable, but none of them are sure cures. Don't buy a horse who already has the disease.

27) GAIT PROBLEMS (BAD WAY OF GOING)

Horses with gait problems are unsound because of them. This category includes horses who stumble (you can get killed by a horse klutz, especially in the mountains) and those who weave or otherwise travel abnormally. One of my clients had a mare who brought one back foot across the inside of the other back foot, tripping herself and falling to her knees when cantered. This horse fell about twice a week. Luckily, no one was hurt riding her, but that is an easy way to get killed.

28) NEURECTOMY ("NERVED")

A horse with a posterior digital neurectomy (as is done for navicular disease) must be considered less than totally sound—both because of the navicular disease and because of the neurectomy—but may still be rideable under certain conditions.

A horse with the nerves cut higher up in the leg (as is used for ringbone, or mistakenly, for navicular disease) will feel much like we do when we cross our legs for too long and our leg falls "asleep." He does not know quite where he is placing his foot. This animal may be usable as a breeding animal, but should not be considered at all sound for a working horse. On the other hand, do you want to breed what might possibly be a hereditary predisposition toward navicular disease into your herd?

29) RINGBONE

Ringbone is caused by damage to the ligaments and joint capsule attachments of the coffin and pastern joints. It is essentially a wear-and-tear disease, and is usually seen in older animals. If it involves the joint, it is definitely an unsoundness, and is incurable except by fusing the joint; this surgery is not always successful.

If the ringbone is not in the joint, it is still an indication of the wear and stress that has been inflicted on the foot and should be considered a warning of possible future trouble within the joint. It is a definite unsoundness in either case. It may be necessary to have x-rays taken to see exactly how bad the problem is. In general, it's not a good idea to buy a horse with ringbone for a using animal. You might buy one as a breeding animal if you are sure that the problem was due to trauma (as with a jumper).

30) SIDEBONE

Lameness due to sidebone is rare, unless the problem is in the acute stage and the cartilages have just begun to be replaced by bone. Usually lameness that appears due to sidebone is due to another cause, such as navicular disease. When you see a lame horse with side-bone, look further for another cause(s) of the problem.

31) QUITTOR

This is a chronic infection of the lateral cartilage of the third phalanx—the same one that turns to bone in a case of sidebone. The horse usually ends up with permanent damage to the cartilage and permanent lameness. Since quittor is often incurable, it must be regarded as an unsoundness.

32) CURB

A curb is a thickening of a ligament on the rear of the hock. It may be due to injury. It is a definite unsoundness if accompanied by cow hocks or sickle hocks.

33) SHIVERING

This disease is primarily seen in draft horses. Its cause is unknown, but it is thought to be a hereditary nervous disorder. Animals with this problem should not be used for breeding. When the animal is backed, the tail twitches upward and the muscles of the hindquarters become tense and trembling. The horse jerks one hind-foot from the ground and pulls it outward and upward. The leg shakes violently as the tail pulls upward and quivers. As the horse continues to be moved backward, he becomes less and less able to move and may fall over backward.

If the horse is allowed to stand, the muscles slowly relax, but the problem will reappear if the animal is again pushed backward. Some animals may flicker their eyes and ears and pull their lips backward. Occasionally the forelegs will be affected. The leg will be raised and pulled outward as the knee is flexed and the muscles above the elbow will quiver. Shivering is usually a progressive problem. Jumpers who have the disease gradually become unable to clear obstacles. No cure is known. Test the animal for this by backing him up for fifteen or twenty steps.

34) WOBBLER

The wobbler syndrome is usually considered to be due to a defect in the vertebrae of the neck. The animal moves peculiarly and may lift one or both hind legs in a jerky, outward movement when led forward. The horse may drag his toes or knuckle over at the fetlocks. It usually is seen in the hindlimbs first, but may progress to the forelegs. These horses are often unable to back. Since the disease is chronic and progressive, it is an unsoundness and the horse should be euthanized, not purchased. Some attempts have been made recently to stabilize these animals surgically, but since it is felt, at least in some cases, to be hereditary, the ethics of such repairs are questionable.

35) WOUNDS, INJURIES, OR SCARS

Any wounds, injuries, or scars that cause lameness or involve deep structures (as opposed to just surface injury) should be considered to be unsoundnesses.

36) HERNIAS

Umbilical or scrotal hernias should be considered unsoundness in a breeding prospect due to their hereditary nature. If the animal is under consideration for a riding animal, the cost of the repair should be considered as well as the possibility of losing the animal from the surgery.

37) CONTAGIOUS DISEASE

The presence of a major contagious disease must be considered an unsoundness. A Coggins test to check for the presence of swamp fever (equine infectious anemia) is well worth the price paid for it. A tick-borne disease called piroplasmosis is known to exist in Florida and appropriate tests should be run for it.

UNSOUNDNESSES OR BLEMISHES?

There are conditions which may be unsoundnesses under some circumstances. If they are severe enough to cause lameness or affect the animal's usability, they are unsoundnesses. Otherwise, they may be considered minor problems which are correctible or blemishes (such as an old, healed, bowed tendon which no longer troubles the animal). Some of these conditions are:

1. Sand crack
2. Bowed tendon
3. Dropped sole
4. Thrush
5. Malignant tumors
6. Sweeny

7. Windpuffs (when due to arthritis—it usually takes an x-ray to determine this)
8. Broken and decayed teeth
9. Conformation which predisposes the animal to lameness but where lameness has not yet occurred (such as an animal with curby conformation).

Some conditions may be considered to be an unsoundness on one horse and a blemish on another. The distinction between them usually depends on whether they are causing the animal serious difficulty and whether they are accompanied by lameness or otherwise incapacitate the horse. Examples of these conditions are:

1. Thoroughpin
2. Firing marks
3. Saddle sores, especially with severe scarring underneath
4. Sit fast. This is a term used to describe a sore which has been caused by an ill-fitting saddle. It has been allowed to continue draining and become chronic. If it can be healed without excessive scar tissue forming under it, it should be considered a blemish. If unhealed or there is excessive scarring, it may be an unsoundness.
5. Crooked tail
6. Corneal scars due to injury which are healed and not too large. Corneal scars may be unsoundnesses to jumpers who depend heavily on their eyes to determine when to jump. These scars may make the animal's vision much less accurate and can actually endanger the rider.
7. New bone growth (especially if of large size on the lower leg).

BREEDING UNSOUNDNESSES

If you are considering horses as breeding prospects, you must first eliminate any animals with hereditary problems, such as parrot mouth and crooked legs. Animals should also be palpated in the umbilical area to check for scarring which would indicate that the animal has had surgery to repair an umbilical hernia. Genital problems must be evaluated as related to the animal's fitness to reproduce.

MARES

Mares being considered for breeding should be examined by a veterinarian familiar with reproductive problems. This checkup should include examination with a vaginal speculum in addition to rectal palpation to determine the condition of the cervix, body of the uterus, and ovaries. Some problems which should be considered breeding unsoundnesses are:

1) Perineal Tears or Fistulas

These are openings between the rectum and vagina. Your veterinarian will check for these with a vaginal speculum when he does the soundness examination. He may also find one of these on rectal palpation.

2) Tipped Vulva

This conformational defect may cause air to be sucked into the vagina as the mare moves. It may also allow juices from the manure to run into the vagina. Until this problem is corrected, the mare will have a continuing vaginal and/or uterine infection and will rarely settle. After its correction, she may require special care at breeding time in addition to needing to be watched carefully and opened at foaling time. All of this adds up to extra bother and expense.

Check the mare for scars or evidence of stitch marks which indicate she has previously been sutured (Caslick's operation). While these mares can be bred and settled by being sutured and treated with antibiotics, we are still perpetuating the problem by continuing to care for them and to breed them resulting in more little horses with the same defect. Mares who are very old or very thin may be tipped because of this, not because they have a hereditary conformational defect.

3) Your veterinarian may find other problems on rectal examination which may be breeding unsoundnesses. These may include: ovaries that are hard, fibrous, or otherwise abnormal: ovaries which are exceptionally large; ovarian tumors (this author has palpated one the size of a small watermelon); abnormalities in the cervix or uterus; and adhesions which indicate previous tears or other damage. Any of these conditions may affect the mare's ability to produce a usable foal and should be evaluated in that light.

STALLIONS

As with mares, stallions being considered for breeding should be evaluated by a veterinarian familiar with breeding soundness examination. This examination should include rectal examination for scrotal hernia (which should be considered a breeding unsoundness if it is present). The veterinarian will also determine whether the internal glands of the reproductive tract are normal.

It is important that the horse's testicles are of a normal size, shape, and texture. In the absence of a semen examination, large, evenly matched testicles are the best single indicator of good libido and high semen quality.

A semen evaluation should be carried out if at all possible, unless you are absolutely convinced that the horse is a good breeder. Some stallions will mount and mate vigorously; all this activity comes to naught if he is "shooting blanks." A breeding soundness examination is imperative if the stallion is older (say, over 12 years) or is an expensive horse. This type of stallion should either be examined before purchase or purchased with a written

contract stating that the sale is not valid of the horse is found to be sterile upon examination by the buyer's veterinarian within a reasonable length of time.

A stallion who has not been used for a period of time may have large numbers of dead and abnormal sperm cells. For this reason, it may be necessary to check him several times over a period of a week or so to be fair to the horse. If the horse is your own and you are making a decision as to whether to keep him or get rid of him, it may be advisable to check him over a period of about 60 days. It may take him this much time to recover normal semen quality after a high fever or illness. Recently, one of my clients sold a 19-year old stallion who, when tested, showed adequate numbers of live sperm showing that he would make a good breeding stallion for the new owner. Some breeding unsoundnesses which may be encountered are:

1) Poor Semen Quality. If he doesn't have good semen, you don't have a breeding stallion no matter how perfect he is.

2) Undescended Testicles. Both testicles should be in the scrotum when the horse is born. No matter how hopeful you are, they only rarely come down into the scrotum later if they are not present at birth. The hereditarial nature of cryptorchidism makes it a breeding unsoundness.

3) Abnormalities of the Penis. These are especially seen in screwworm areas. Your veterinarian may wish to tranquilize the animal to allow him to be examined more easily and with less discomfort.

4) Scrotal Hernia, as mentioned above.

5) Lack of Libido. Some stallions have adequate semen quality, but do not have a desire to breed mares. This can be a serious problem and may be due to a combination of hereditary and learned factors. It is frequently seen in horses with small testicles.

If the stallion has good semen, but will not mount a mare because he doesn't care, he will not be a good breeder. Animals with little interest in breeding are also difficult to collect semen from so artificial insemination is rarely a cure for this problem. Stallions who masturbate may show a lack of interest in mares. These animals may need to have a stallion ring kept on during the breeding season.

6) Soundness of the Legs. If the horse is being bred naturally, he must be able to mount a mare and stay there long enough to get the job done. Hindleg soundness is very important in a breeding stallion because he must carry his whole weight on his hindlegs during breeding. Some stallions with hindleg injuries may be bred by artificial insemination after they are trained to mount a dummy with sideboards to support their front feet and to help keep their weight off the hind feet. Some nonhereditary foreleg lameness may be tolerated if it is not so severe as to decrease the animal's libido or make it difficult for him to mount the mare. However, you should consider carefully

what the lameness is and why he has it. Does his conformation predispose him to it?

VICES

Vices are bad habits which can make the animal undesirable. They may range from mere nuisances to those which are truly dangerous. Some vices, such as an animal who is hard to catch, are not a problem if you will be keeping him in a box stall. It may be intolerable if you have him in a hundred-acre pasture. You have to decide for yourself whether or not you can live with the animal's vice or vices. Bear in mind that vices are often contagious: one cribber may teach his vice to the whole barn. And once it is started, it usually cannot be stopped (not permanently, at least). A mare with a vice often teaches it to her foal before he is weaned. You have to decide if you want an animal with this sort of habit spreading it to any others that you might own. There are very few perfect horses. The question is, can you live with his problems?

1) Biting. Remember that a horse's bite can easily break a person's arm. A cute nibble from a hundred-pound foal can easily remove a hand when coming from a full-grown stallion. The best cure for this is prevention. Avoid playing with a horse's head. Handle his head only to groom or bridle him. Especially do not play with his mouth and lips. This actually teaches the animal to chew or bite. Discipline the young foal promptly for biting behavior so it does not become a habit. His mother won't put up with it—why should you?

2) Bucking. Some young horses buck before they are well trained. If the animal continues to buck after he is trained, it may become a habit which can cause serious injury and make the animal less saleable. Unfortunately, most horses who habitually buck are just bad enough to be dangerous—they are not good enough at it to be rodeo broncs. They generally end up in that in-between category called "Alpo" (or whatever other dog food you favor).

Bucking can sometimes be avoided by having a good rider work the horse the first few times—a rider who is capable of pulling the animal's head up if he begins bucking and who can ride the horse if he really throws a fit. Often if the rider wins the first few rounds, the horse will never challenge him again, except for maybe a crowhop or two on a frosty morning.

If a well-trained horse suddenly bucks, examine your tack. Have you changed anything? One of my own horses bucked me off when a new bit pinched her mouth. Other animals will buck if a different saddle pinches their withers.

3) Charging. Horses who habitually charge at a human who enters their stall can easily kill someone. If this vice cannot be cured, the animal should be put in that "in-between" category, as above.

4) Cow-kicking. Some horses tend to cow-kick when saddled. One of my own mares did, but only when she was in heat. Injury can be avoided by standing by the horse's shoulder when saddling, working with him, or mounting. It is easy for the animal to break a kneecap if the rider forgets to watch.

5) Cribbing (also called stump sucking, wind swallowing). Animals who crib stand in the stall, pen, or pasture, and suck on the top of an object such as a fence post or the door to their stall. The horse then pulls his neck muscles up and back as he takes in a gulp of air; he will usually make a grunting noise at the same time.

Some horses crib by resting their incisors on a fixed object without grasping it; others may rest their chin on some object and swallow air. Still other animals move their lips, close their mouths, flex and arch their necks (often with a jerk), swallow air, and grunt without grasping a fixed object with their teeth. Some horses move their lips, often licking the fixed object before grasping it with the incisors, and flex and arch the neck in a gentle rocking motion of the whole body without swallowing air or grunting. This last practice should probably not be considered true cribbing.

The major damage due to cribbing occurs in the digestive tract. The incisor teeth may be badly worn. Depending on the animal, this wear may occur on either the front or rear of the teeth. In very severe cases, the front teeth may be worn away completely with resulting dental disease. The incisors may be so badly damaged that the animal cannot graze adequately if turned out to pasture.

Because the animal is constantly swallowing air and because he cannot belch it up to get rid of it, the air has to travel the length of the digestive tract to be released. This leads to a chronic gaseous (flatulent) colic or other digestive disturbances. The animal's abdomen may be distended from the gas. He may lose weight and appear unthrifty. Some animals' performance may be impaired.

The fact that some animals crib the worst at feeding time compounds the problem. Indeed, some animals crib only at feeding time. Others crib only when fed treats by hand or while being groomed and saddled for work. Cribbing in response to food is most likely to be a display of pleasure or excitement. Some animals crib only when away from their home environment. Horses who begin to crib during enforced rest because of an injury may be doing so because of anxiety and apprehension as much as boredom.

Cribbing is seen throughout the world in domesticated horses and ponies. It is not, however, reported in feral horses or ponies. My research has not found any evidence of cribbing in mules or donkeys.

It is thought that the horse first acquires the habit of grasping an object and then quickly proceeds to learn to swallow air. A confirmed cribber will go to great lengths to continue the habit. Some habitual cribbers on pasture will ignore good grazing to suck on the top of a fence post or gate. Horses may suck their lips or knees; foals may use their dam's hocks. Most horses develop the habit after weaning. Cases are reported, however, where foals began cribbing during the first few weeks of life.

Some people feel that the habit is learned by one horse watching another. More likely, perhaps, a horse in a stable will begin cribbing because he is subjected to the same triggering factors which initiated the habit in other horses. Confinement without enough work or exercise may accentuate the vice. A lack of suitable roughage may also be an inciting factor.

At any rate, once cribbing is learned, it quickly becomes a chronic behavior and will be performed in many situations unrelated to the original cause. Thus, a conditioned cribber may crib whenever he is not otherwise busy, giving the impression that he cribs because of confinement or boredom.

Control of cribbing has been attempted by removing all objects from the horse's environment upon which he might crib. This is occasionally effective with animals who have just begun cribbing. Animals kept in crib-proof stalls have been observed to crib within seconds of being allowed into an area where they could do so.

Old remedies include putting substances, such as red pepper, on the cribbing surfaces to make them unpleasant. These generally do not work. Electric shock treatment (aversion therapy) has been tried, again with variable results.

Perhaps the simplest and most effective way of controlling the habit is the use of a cribbing strap. This strap is placed around the animal's neck. A metal plate on the bottom presses into the throat as the animal arches its neck making it both difficult and unpleasant to swallow the air. When the horse is swallowing normally, the plate hangs loosely and does not interfere with eating. An ordinary leather strap may be tried, but is not as effective on a confirmed cribber as the strap with the metal plate.

The use of a cribbing strap to prevent the horse from sucking air only works when the strap is in place. It usually must be left on a cribber at all times except when he is being worked. When looking for a horse to buy, it is worth checking the throatlatch area for signs of wear from a cribbing strap. Also, check the top of the mane for a worn area that indicates the constant use of a strap. In long-term cases, there may be a white patch of hair in the mane area, much like those seen as saddle marks on the withers of horses who have been ridden for a long time. These clues will tip you off that the animal is a cribber—a fact that you might otherwise determine only when you got the animal home.

A surgical treatment which has had some success is to cut the nerves to the muscles which flex the neck. If this is not successful, surgery may be done to cut the muscles which allow the horse to pull his neck up and back. This operation is a last resort. Most surgeons feel that the surgery has a greater chance of being successful if the animal is as young as possible when it is done—not over two to three years old at the latest.

6) Fence Chewing. Some horses get into the habit of chewing on fence posts and rails, the doors to their stalls, or any available wood. This is NOT the same as cribbing. A cribber goes through the whole range of neck-pulling and air-sucking motions, while the wood-chewer merely munches on wood. Horses who chew on wood rarely become cribbers. One of my clients had a mare who chewed a hole about $1 \times 1\frac{1}{2}$ feet in the side of a shed. She started at a windowsill and went downward, doing all this damage in two nights!

Wood chewing seems to be mainly a boredom problem, although, in some cases, it may possibly be related to a mineral deficiency. One horse often teaches others and a wooden stable can soon look like it was attacked by a herd of beavers. These animals may develop colic because of the swallowed pieces of wood and may get splinters in their tongues and lips.

7) Fighting Other Horses. This may be a real vice if you have a broodmare in a pasture who routinely kicks and bites other mares, running them through fences and otherwise injuring them. How a horse acts with humans is no indication of how it will act with other horses. The best mare this writer ever owned was so kind an animal that she

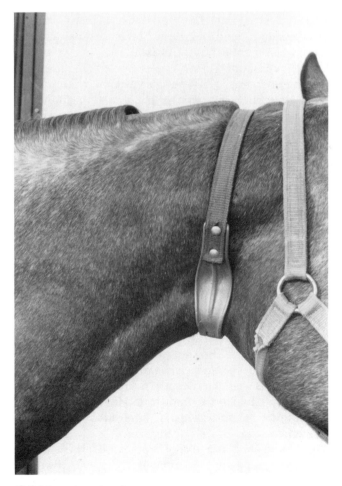

Cribbing strap in place.

would never have thought of harming a human. However, it was impossible to leave her with another horse because she would kick it. This is perhaps less of a problem if you have the animal stabled by himself and intend to keep him that way. If the viciousness if so bad that you can't work the animal with other horses, he's probably not worth keeping.

8) Halter Pulling. Some animals cannot be left tied. The problem usually begins when the horse is halter broken. If the owner used a weak halter which broke the minute the horse sat back and pulled on it, the animal began to learn a bad habit. If he did it a couple of more times and got away with it, he was well on the way to having a lifelong habit of pulling. These animals may be tied up with a belly rope (see Restraint). Often, you can do anything with the horse EXCEPT tie it. These animals can often be pregnancy checked, wormed, and shod by having someone hold the lead rope instead of tying them hard and fast.

9) Kicking. A horse may kick at other horses, at humans, or both. If he or she tends to kick other horses, this can be a very damaging habit in a pasture. If he takes aim at humans, it can be downright deadly. The animal may also kick the barn. This results in damage to the barn and may cause the animal to have capped hocks or a fractured coffin bone. Having one kicker in a barn can start other horses kicking their stalls. Some horses kick only at night when there is no one around.

10) Masturbation. This habit is one that many owners find embarrassing—especially when it occurs in the show ring. A stallion who is masturbating during the breeding season may have a significantly lowered desire to breed mares.

There are several devices made which allow the horse to drop his penis to urinate, but cause him discomfort if the penis becomes swollen with an erection. One of these is a stallion ring can be purchased in a size appropriate for the stallion. This is a plastic ring which slips over the end of the penis and sets behind the swelling at the end. If the animal becomes erect, it causes discomfort and he quits masturbating. These are good for use in show animals if needed. Both the ring and the stallion's penis must be kept scrupulously clean. The ring should be removed and washed daily at which time the horse is checked for any irritation that might be present.

11) Pawing. Some animals perpetually paw the ground when tied. They may also paw in the stall, ending up digging a deep cavern in the middle of a dirt floor. The only cure this writer has heard of is to tie a stick of wood to a string and put it on a strap around the horse's leg. The stick bumps the horse when he paws and is supposed to make him stop.

12) Rearing or Striking. Both of these vices are especially a problem with stallions. They are downright dangerous in any horse! They are part of the animal's natural defense against another horse, and if not man-

aged carefully, can be deadly. My great-grandfather died when a stallion reared up and crashed down on his head. These are habits which, like biting, may be cute when a stud colt is a month or two old. They aren't even a little cute when he is grown, weighs 1200 pounds, and is fast as a mountain lion. Prompt discipline and careful training of the colt will avoid or minimize rearing. Older animals who rear or strike should be handled with the utmost caution. The handler must be even more careful than usual not to stand in front of the animal or get within striking distance of the front leg. If there is any chance of mixing one of these horses with inexperienced handlers, riders, or children—GET RID OF IT—before someone gets badly hurt or killed.

13) Running Away. This is a severe vice of saddle horses. It often begins with a child or unsure rider who allows the animal to race toward home, out of control. Or, it may start with a rider who is simply unable to hold the animal to a safe speed.

It can occasionally be cured, if it is dealt with firmly the first time the animal tries it, before it becomes a habit. One of my clients had a four-year old filly who ran away with him in an 80-acre pasture of oat stubble. Because he had plenty of room and safe footing, he let her run. When she wanted to slow down, he used the end of the reins to encourage her to run some more. When he finally let her stop, the animal was more than glad to quit running. She has not run away since.

Sometimes the older animal who runs away may be stopped by a more severe bit or by having a rider strong enough and confident enough to pull the animal in a circle with one rein until he stops by himself. Like most other vices, once the animal learns it well, it is nearly impossible to totally eliminate.

14) Shying. This often begins with a horse shying and getting his rider off balance so that the rider no longer has control or totally dumping him altogether. Like bucking, it is learned and the better it works, the worse the animal gets with it. If the animal is truly afraid, patience and walking the animal carefully up to the object it fears may help. If it is being done as an excuse to unseat the rider, prompt discipline by a good horseman may nip the problem in the bud. If it is totally ingrained in the animal, it is probably not correctible. The only solution then is to hang on tightly or trade the horse in on a new model!

When a mature, nonshying horse begins to shy, look for changes: have you used a new bridle, bit, or saddle which may be pinching and making the horse uncomfortable? If the problem continues and no cause can be found, call your veterinarian and have him check the animal's eyes. Vision problems can cause the horse to see things peculiarly and shy because of his altered perceptions of the world around him.

15) Stall Walking. Some horses will walk continuously in their stall or pen. This problem usually starts either from boredom or it is learned from another horse.

Once it is firmly ingrained in the animal, you are unlikely to cure it. Exercising the animal will help to a certain extent. Stallions will often walk their pens during breeding season, but usually stop when they are no longer being used on mares and their hormones calm down in autumn. Exercise is doubly important for the stallion during breeding season to give him something to do besides pace the fence and think of mares.

16) Stumbling. If you have eliminated other causes of stumbling, such as improper shoeing or conformation, then it is often left in the category of a habit or a vice. More attention on the part of the rider to urge the animal into the bit and keep him actively involved in being ridden may help some horses. Others benefit when the rider is alert enough to catch the reins and "support" them as they start to go down.

Regardless of the method used, the problem is rarely cured and the animal is a hazard to ride. No matter how alert the rider is, there is always the danger that the animal will fall if the rider lets down his guard. A narrow mountain trail next to a thousand foot drop is NOT a place to ride one of these "stumble bums." One of my clients was riding her mare when the animal stumbled, going down far enough that she had dirt down the bridge of her nose from her ears to muzzle. Needless to say, the client didn't have much confidence in the horse after that. Perhaps the best cure for this problem is a different horse.

17) Tail Rubbing. Some horses will rub their tails on the stall or corral fence. Eliminate reasons, such as pinworms, sores, or skin problems on the tail or rear end. Check stallions and geldings to see that their sheaths are clean. Examine mares to make sure that they are clean between the halves of the udder. Wash the animal if necessary. If you have eliminated these causes of tail rubbing then, that leaves it as a vice—you're probably stuck with it.

18) Tail Wringing. This is a problem in show horses. It often starts as a response to the horse's being stuck with spurs and sometimes ends up being a reaction to any cue with rein, foot, or spur. It is especially a problem in cutting and reining horses, who let the judge know they have been spurred by cranking their tails, and in western pleasure horses who express their displeasure in the same way.

Attempts have been made to cure the tail wringing by cutting muscles on the upper side of the tail. This prevents the animal from lifting it to wring it. However, the American Quarter Horse Association has come out against horses with "dead" tails. These tails hang limply and without expression and are disqualifyed from being shown in AQHA competition. The best cure is to not let the problem get started during training by spurring the horse moderately or not at all. It may also help to give him a variety of work outside the ring or arena to help keep his mind fresh and relaxed. Once established, this habit is probably impossible to cure.

19) Viciousness. A horse who is vicious and wishes to attack people is a hazard and should be handled with the utmost care. The best cure is not to own or be around an animal like this, no matter what his bloodlines.

20) Vicious to Shoe. Occasionally, an animal is seen who is good to ride and work, but impossible to shoe. If you cannot come to an agreement with this horse through training, it may be necessary to have the animal tranquilized before shoeing. You can have your veterinarian do this or you may be able to get some tranquilizer granules to put in the feed an hour or so before the project begins. If this is a perpetual problem, your veterinarian may give you an injectable drug to use on the animal.

21) Weaving. Like stall walking, weaving often begins with boredom and/or a lesson from another horse. The animal will stand in the stall and sway from side to side. Once the habit is firmly established, there is usually no stopping it. This habit is seen as a caged animal behavior in many species in zoos, especially large cats, elephants, and bears.

22) Wolfing food. The horse who gulps his food so rapidly as to cause indigestion has a genuine vice. If you can't get him to slow down and eat properly, be prepared to deal with unthriftiness and digestive problems, such as colic.

Chapter 7

LAMENESS

History
Observation and Examination
   Hoof Testers
   Flexion Tests
   Wedge Tests
   Palpation
   Nerve Blocks
   X-Rays
   Other Diagnostic Tests
The Horse's Foot
   Chestnuts and Ergots
   Functions of The Foot
Malformed Feet
Contracted Feet
Keratoma
Gravel
Sand Cracks
Thrush
Corns
Sole Bruising and Abscesses
Punctures (Hoof)
Seedy Toe
Low Heels
Sheared Heels
Laminitis (Founder)
Azoturia (Monday Morning Sickness, Tying-Up)
Navicular Disease
Fractures of the Navicular Bone
Fractured Coffin Bone
Windpuffs
Ringbone
Rachitic Ringbone
Epiphysitis
Sidebone
Quittor
Sesamoiditis
Sesamoid Fractures
Contracted Tendons
Ruptured Flexor Tendons

Bowed Tendon
Splints
Splint Fractures
Bucked Shins
Fractures of the First or Second Phalanx
Hygroma of the Carpus
Popped Knee (Carpitis)
Fractured Carpal Bones
Crooked Legs
Upward Fixation of the Patella
Spavin
Curb
Wobbler Syndrome
Cast Horses
Radiographs (X-Rays)

What is lameness? It's one of those things that we all picture in our minds, but find hard to put into words. It could perhaps best be defined as a disturbance of the normal gait of any particular limb. It may vary from an animal who is "a little off" to one who is unable to move due to a severe problem, such as a fracture. A horse who is so lame as to not wish to walk at all should NOT be moved if it can be avoided until he is examined by a veterinarian. Lameness is often due to pain. Horses, like people, try to avoid pain by limping or moving oddly.

An animal who has been used hard may show general soreness and stiffness which is not localized in any particular limb. This is especially true if the animal was not in condition for the work he had been asked to do. A horse with laminitis may not wish to move at all. A horse who is lame in two limbs may show less soreness than an animal who is only sore in one. This seems to be especially true of problems such as navicular disease and spavin.

Animals may show apparent lameness due to pain not located in the feet at all, such as when their ribs are injured or when they are affected with pleurisy. Apparent lameness may originate in the spinal column due to narrowing of the tunnel through one or more vertebrae through which the spinal cord passes with pressure on either it or on the nerves coming from it. This condition is similar to a "slipped disk" in humans. This type of problem may be hereditary or it may be due to a vitamin deficiency in the mare before foaling. It may also be due to repeated concussion or injury or even sore back muscles.

Older animals tend to lift their legs less high than do younger horses. This often cannot be traced to any particular limb being sore, but to a general wear and tear on many leg joints throughout the body and the cumulative effects of this change.

A horse who is lame may show pain. He may be unable to move the limb. Or, he may show both lameness and pain. Lameness may be caused by falls, collisions, kicks, or other blows which cause bruising or splintering. Wounds and punctures may cause lameness, especially when they involve cut tendons or punctured joint capsules. The problem may be due to injury to muscles, tendons, or ligaments in the leg. Sometimes it may be due to damage to a nerve which makes it impossible for the horse to move the limb in a normal manner. Stumbling, sharp turns, and stepping into holes may cause lameness, as can slipping on poor footing. A strain or sprain may occur with slipping even if the animal does not fall. Collisions between horses can cause severe damage, as in the course of races or games such as polo.

Lameness may appear suddenly and disappear just as quickly or it may become chronic and result in permanent damage. A good example of sudden lameness is when a horse strikes the inner surface of the fetlock or cannon bone with the other front foot. This may also occur when a horse brings up a hind foot and steps on the bulb of the heel on the front foot. The horse may be so suddenly and acutely lame that the rider thinks that he has broken a bone. The pain lessens within a few minutes (although the horse is still definitely lame) and is gone within a week or two without any further signs.

Lameness may come and go from day to day or week to week and will often vary considerably in severity. An example of this is a horse with a developing spavin who may be almost unable to walk, but improves with a few minutes of exercise until he is normal or nearly so. This is called "warming out of a lameness." Horses with lameness due to joint problems may be very lame, become slightly better with a little exercise, and then be in severe pain after an hour or so of continued exercise.

It is said that the horse "warms into a lameness" when the problem becomes worse as the animal is exercised. This is especially seen with some of the more painful lamenesses, such as navicular disease. It is also seen with soft tissue problems, such as bowed tendons. Lameness is often improved by turning the horse out to pasture, allowing the animal to exercise and move freely, but at his own pace. Horses who are chronically lame may be more comfortable when exercised moderately than when rested.

Any examination for lameness should begin with the foot. Well over 75% of lameness problems are located below the knee, and of those, more than 75% are below the fetlock. It is worth checking "down low" to be sure that there is no problem there even if you are "almost sure" that the problem is higher in the leg. Shoulder and hip lamenesses are, in overall numbers, extremely rare. (41)

Lameness may not be visible at the time an injury occurs, but may become obvious later. A nail puncture, for instance, may cause only temporary acute lameness at the time it occurs. The animal may be nearly unable to walk a week or so later when the infection has had time to build up inside the hoof and cause severe pain.

Lameness may occur in young horses due to overwork. This especially seems to produce splint problems on the front legs and bog spavins on the hind legs. Windpuffs may be seen on the front feet, or on all four feet. Bog spavins and windpuffs occur because the joint surfaces are damaged by overwork. They may be aggravated by overweight if the animal is being fed into "show condition." Excess joint fluid is produced causing the joint capsule to bulge. They are usually accompanied by lameness.

Excessive jarring to the front legs may irritate the interosseous ("between the bones") ligament which lies between the cannon bone and the splint bone. This can cause considerable pain and may lead to the permanent blemish of "splints."

Similar problems may occur from other hard "work." One of my clients took a yearling Arabian colt from Wyoming to Florida. He was hauled in a large stock trailer with the idea of giving him room to move around. Unfortunately, this was the first time the animal had been in a trailer and only the second or third time he had been handled at all. The colt charged around the trailer both while it was moving and when they were stopped at night, despite the fact that he was tired and had adequate room to lie down. By the time he had journeyed the 2000 miles to Florida, he had raised huge splints on both of his front legs. The prospective buyer refused him and the animal had to be brought home. Here is an animal who would have been much better off in a small trailer where he would not have been able to move around.

HISTORY

Knowing your horse is the first step for you or your veterinarian in finding out why your horse is lame. It can make a world of difference in being able to make an intelligent diagnosis of lameness. How old is the horse? Young horses—say, those under three years old—who are overfed and/or worked beyond the capacity of an animal that age may show problems due to excess stress on the joints with abnormal fluid production, resulting in problems such as windpuffs and bog spavins. Old horses (those over 15 years of age) begin to show the effects of wear and tear—problems such as ringbone. Whether the animal is a mare, stallion, or gelding may predict a tendency toward certain injuries or lamenesses.

Knowing what breed the horse represents is also important. Quarter Horses have considerable trouble with navicular disease. They may also be more prone to hock problems and ringbone. Thoroughbred race horses often show bone and soft tissue abnormalities. High-stepping gaited horses may injure themselves by striking one front foot against the other leg. While other horses would hit themselves inside the fetlock or the lower end of the cannon bone, these animals may do the same injury to themselves, but at the upper end of the cannon bone or inside the knee. Finally, as stated in the section under soundness exam (which see), the intended use of the animal has a large bearing on whether a lameness matters or not. An injury that would be crippling to a barrel racing horse or racehorse may be a minor problem to a lightly used children's horse or a broodmare.

A good history should include anything that you know about the horse from previous problems you have had or from former owners. What happened to the animal, what was done to fix it, and how did it turn out? What medications were used or what surgery was done? If the horse has been lame before, how long ago did it happen, and how long did it last? It is very important to know if the animal has been turned out to pasture or otherwise rested recently. Is he on any medication or other treatment right now (such as heat, ice, forced exercise, etc.)? How well has the treatment been working? If the animal had recently been given painkillers or had a period of rest, he may show no signs of lameness even though it has occurred previously. Knowing whether the horse was resting or working when the lameness began is very important. If he was working, what was he doing? Turning, stopping, running, jumping, or what? Did he slip and fall or hurt himself in the middle of a gallop? How recently has he been exercised?

OBSERVATION AND EXAMINATION

Begin the examination by viewing the horse in his corral or stall. Stand back and look at the whole animal. What is his overall attitude? Is he standing normally? Does he hold one foot cocked at an angle? Horses will normally cock their hind feet alternately when relaxed. They do not usually hold their front feet tipped unless they are in pain. If the hind foot is hurting, it will be cocked in a different way than if the animal is merely resting it. One front foot may be "pointed"—that is, set out ahead of the other one in an extended, resting position. This relieves the pain of some lamenesses—especially navicular disease—or problems affecting only one of the front feet.

In problems such as laminitis, the hind feet may be brought well under the body to support its weight, while both front feet are extended ahead of their normal position. Some animals may put their front feet so far forward with this problem as to be nearly squatting. Horses having either both front legs or both hind legs afflicted with a painful lameness may constantly shift their weight from one foot to the other.

Are there any obvious swellings, lumps, or draining sores? You should already know about any conformational problems the horse has which may predispose him to problems—either from a soundness exam when you bought him or from one that you completed in the course of determining how correct and sound the animal is and when learning what normal is for your individual animal.

Look at the horse from a distance without touching him. You are looking for differences from one side to the other. Are both legs the same size and shape from the shoulders down? Look closely at the feet to see if they are exactly alike. Are both feet squarely on the ground or does the horse tend to lean in one direction or the other? Are the feet flat or upright? Do they have good heels or are they so flat that the bulbs of the heels are touching the ground.

Observe the animal from the rear, at a distance of 10 to 12 feet. Look to see that the hips are level and symmetrical. Check the muscles of the hindquarters to see that both sides match. If the animal has been lame for a period of time, the muscles on one side may be shrunken or withered. This is called atrophy.

Next, have someone walk him slowly and quietly—on a flat, hard surface if possible. Flat ground without gravel is good, as is concrete or asphalt pavement. Walking the horse on this type of surface avoids confusion because of the horse stepping on pebbles or into irregularities in the ground. Hard surfaces help to show up minor lamenesses. It is also easier to hear small differences between the various feet or diagonals when they hit the ground. Keep a lame animal off slick surfaces, such as mud or wet grass. If he is not moving well, he may easily slip and add to his existing problems or cause others.

How does the animal move? When does he show pain? These are two general kinds of lamenesses: supporting leg lamenesses and swinging leg lamenesses. A swinging leg lameness is one that interferes with the movement of the leg or causes it to move abnormally. Paralysis of the radial nerve is an example of this type of problem. Damage to the radial nerve keeps the animal from extending the front leg forward as it would normally and results in the toe being dragged along the ground.

A supporting leg lameness, on the other hand, is one that causes the animal pain when he puts weight on the leg or stands on it. The worst supporting leg lamenesses are noticeable when the horse is standing still. These are caused by problems like nail punctures in the foot, fractures, and similar injuries. Less severe supporting leg lamenesses become very obvious as the animal moves and his weight comes onto the injured foot or leg. They

LAMENESS

may show up as a limping or wincing step when the animal places that foot on the ground.

Less obvious supporting leg lamenesses may be seen by a bobbing of the horse's head—it goes up when the injured foot hits the ground and goes down when the weight comes onto the sound foot if the lameness is in a front foot or leg. In this manner, the head acts as a lever to help lift weight from the painful foot or leg. Observe which leg takes most of the horse's weight. The horse's neck and shoulder, as well as the rest of the leg, will sink more when the sound leg hits the ground than when his weight is sinking onto the lame leg.

A different picture in weight bearing and head bobbing between the sound and lame sides may be observed with hindleg lameness. The horse sinks into the sound leg, while raising the pelvis on the side of the painful limb. He raises his head as weight goes onto the sound hindleg, and lowers it to help take weight off the injured hindleg. Look at a particular point, such as the hipbone or the point of the buttock, to see which side rises the highest. This is the side on which the animal is lame. Observe how the animal is moving from the front and back as well as from both sides.

If the pain occurs in both forelegs, as with navicular disease, the animal may not nod his head at all. The weight is borne for an equal period of time on each foot, but the stride will be shortened. The gait is peculiar, and appears "choppy." A few lameness problems, such as wobblers, will become worse when the horse is backed up.

As the animal is led, check to see that he is moving in a straight line. Some lamenesses, such as certain neck injuries, stiffness from various causes, and true shoulder lameness often lead to an animal who is tracking diagonally. With shoulder lameness, this is because the injured shoulder is brought forward more slowly than the sound one.

Very old horses may develop an arthritis in the elbow joint which restricts movement. The foot is barely lifted from the ground and the horse may crouch a little as he moves. These animals seem to shuffle along rather than to step out. Excessive head-nodding may be seen with this problem. If both elbows are affected at once, the animal may be mistaken for one with chronic laminitis.

Bear in mind that some lamenesses may involve more than one leg, and the fact that one leg hurts more than another may make it appear as if there is only one lame leg. Lamenesses may also not be what they at first seem. Careful examination, observation, and thought are necessary to figure out what really is happening.

One of my clients had a mare who provided an example of "it isn't what it seems." The horse was being galloped on a race track. She was accustomed to the workout, as she was being galloped three days each week. They came around a turn on the third lap at a smooth hand gallop when the animal nearly fell out from under him, dropping hard on the left front foot. He immediately

pulled her to a stop and jumped off. The horse was holding up her left front foot. He checked for obvious problems, feeling for a fracture, but could find nothing. He had to walk the animal about a hundred yards to where he could get to a phone to call for help.

By the time he had gotten that far, the mare was using the leg, although she was still showing considerable pain. He walked her about a block to the clinic and we began an examination. The horse was trotted out as we observed her. She had been holding up the left front leg, but on a trot, she was showing severe lameness on the RIGHT front leg! Further examination showed a severely bowed tendon on the right side.

The farrier had not shod her the way that the owner wanted her done for an overreach problem, preferring to do her his way. As we reconstructed it, she had reached up in mid-gallop with the left hind and clipped the bulb of the left heel with her shoe. The pain caused her to get off stride. Then, the right hind foot came up and clipped the right leg in the middle of the tendon, causing a bow that took over six months to heal. In this case, the left foot hurt more than the right, but the severe injury was on the right. So, bear in mind that sore horses are not always what they first seem.

If you have watched the animal led at a walk and the problem leg is not evident, the next step is to have the person leading the horse trot him in a small circle (say, 20 or 30 feet in diameter). Be sure that they give the animal about two feet of free lead rope between the halter and their hand. Otherwise, it is easy to pull an animal off stride and cause him to appear lame even though he is not. Or, it may alter the appearance of the gait in an animal who is lame. The person leading the horse should stay to the inside of the circle. The person watching him is usually most easily able to observe the animal from the middle of the circle. Circle the horse first in one direction and then in the other, observing which direction causes him to appear most lame. The lame leg will be the one on the inside of the circle in whichever direction in which he shows the most lameness. This is because the inside leg is carrying the body weight for a longer period of time.

If the animal is something other than a trotter (a Foxtrotter, Paso, or other gaited horse, or a pacer), have him led at whatever gait he has that is equivalent in speed to a trot. You are still looking for irregularities in gait which will help pinpoint the problem. If you have a gaited horse in an area where they are uncommon, you may have to help your veterinarian with a lameness problem by pointing out exactly WHERE in his gait he has a problem. Many veterinarians are simply not accustomed to looking at these animals, and are not familiar with how they should move. If YOU don't know how the animal should move, it will be hard to tell anyone where he is going wrong.

Check the animal's way of going. Does he move his legs an equal amount and distance on each side? Is he hitting one leg or foot with another?

Look at each leg separately when analyzing a lameness. Look at the length of stride, how high each foot travels, and whether the arc is regular or higher at the front or back of the flight path. Then, look at each pair of legs, front and back, and compare them to each other. Even lameness experts are usually not able to concentrate on all four legs at once.

Sometimes your veterinarian will want to see a lame horse ridden or longed. He may want you to ride the animal up or down a hill or work him in an arena. Some lamenesses may not show up except when the animal is doing his normal work. Standardbred race horses are usually examined hitched to a cart and trotting or pacing as they would in racing or training. Some veterinarians will on occasion ride or drive a horse themselves to help identify a lameness.

Now that you have looked the animal over and decided which leg is lame (or at least, which of the legs is worst), it's time to look deeper into the problem. Begin at the bottom and work up, even if you are convinced that the lameness is higher. It's really embarrassing to say that a horse is lame in the knee and later find a nail in his foot. Remember that there may be more than one problem present and in more than one leg!

Clean the foot with a hoof pick. Scrub all dirt from the sole and frog with soap and water and a stiff brush. Next, take a hoof knife and scrape the whole surface of the sole. You are trying to get a fresh, clean surface over the entire sole so you can see if there are any punctures or defects.

Take the point of the hoof knife and press as hard as you can on the sole. If you find any tender spots, pare deeper into them. Try to determine the center of the painful area and then scrape down carefully, in a spot about an inch in diameter. Now you are looking for the track of a nail or for an abscess or bruise. If there is a sole bruise, you will come to a reddish or brownish area. An abscess will ooze pus as you dig deeper. If you find an abscess, don't quit now, but pare carefully until it is completely opened.

HOOF TESTERS

If you have not found an obvious foot problem while paring out the foot, a hoof tester is a very valuable tool. Begin by testing the "normal" foot so that you have a comparison when you get to the problem foot. Because the majority of lameness is due to problems in the foot, this tool will help to diagnose ailments, such as punctures, corns, sole abscesses, and fractures.

When using hoof testers, hold the horse's hoof yourself. This will allow you to feel him pull back or flinch as you press and find a painful area. Small people like myself can feel free to push hard on the hoof tester. Large men should use a moderate amount of pressure. Any horse can be made to flinch if you mash on his foot hard

enough! You are not trying to CREATE sole bruises with the tester.

Use the hoof testers between the hoof wall and the frog, between the sole and the wall, and across the heels. If you find a sore spot on the sole, pare down deeper into it to see if there is a problem with a false sole, abscess, puncture, or corn that was not visible with your earlier paring.

Pain when the tester is used across the heels is most commonly seen with navicular disease; it can also show up problems such as navicular fractures. Indeed, hoof testers will pick up some cases of navicular disease which look completely normal when x-rayed. If your horse is sensitive on this examination, the next step is to get your veterinarian to x-ray the animal to see if the problem can be positively identified.

FLEXION TESTS

If you've decided that there is not an obvious hoof problem, go on to test the flexion of joints in the affected pair of feet. "Flexion" refers to bending the joint as it normally bends or flexes. Flexion tests, on any joint or set of joints, are done in an attempt to stress the joint and the

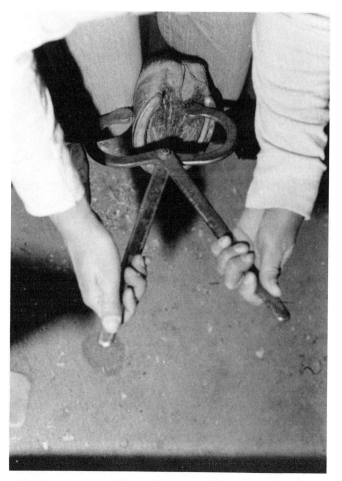

Hoof testers used from frog to wall.

hard and soft tissues around it bringing out evidence of pain if the problem is at that joint.

Begin by testing flexion in the fetlock joint. This will put stress on the coffin, pastern, and fetlock joints, as well as the soft tissues in that area. Flex the fetlock joint of the normal foot while keeping the knee as straight as possible (we'll do a flexion test on it later). Hold it tightly up for a minute. Then have the person leading the horse trot him smartly out in a straight line. Look for any evidence of lameness or soreness, especially in the first half-dozen steps after the animal's foot is released. Now, repeat the same test on the other side.

All flexion tests are done in the same order: good side first, then the lame side. This is so that you can compare the two sides. Now, do the same test with the carpal (knee) joint, this time holding the horse by the cannon bone and allowing the fetlock to hang freely so that the knee is flexed by itself.

If you are dealing with a hind leg lameness, perform the spavin test in place of knee flexion. This is the same sort of flexion test as has just been described for the front legs. Have someone hold the horse's lead rope, giving the animal about a foot and a half of slack. This person should be facing forward and ready to move out. Lift the horse's leg and cramp it upward toward his body, being careful not to pull it outward at the same time. Hold it in this position for 1–½ to 2 minutes. Tell the person on the lead rope to get ready. At a count, drop the leg and slap the horse on the rump at the same time as the person on the lead rope trots the horse rapidly forward. If the animal goes noticeably lame for the first few steps, this is indicative of spavin-type changes in the hock joint. Repeat the process with the other hind leg. Again, you are looking for a lameness which is especially bad in the first few steps after the animal is released (see Spavin Test).

Since approximately 70 to 80% of hindleg lamenesses are in either the hock or stifle joints, the spavin test is good for confirming a high hindleg problem. Hock problems are by far the most common, followed by stifle problems. Injuries lower in the hindleg are uncommon, unless the animal has been kicked by another or has kicked into something hard (such as a barn or trailer wall) and fractured a hind coffin bone. This kind of problem will not be worse with a spavin test. After the spavin test, try a lower leg (fetlock) flexion test as described above for the front leg, again testing the good leg first.

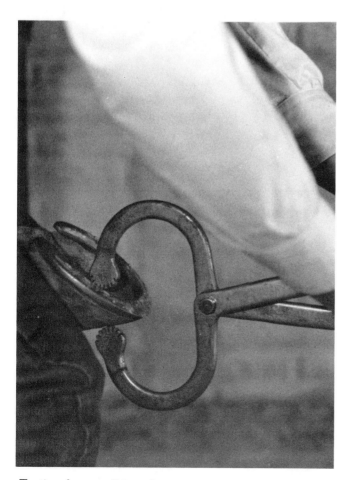

Testing from wall to sole.

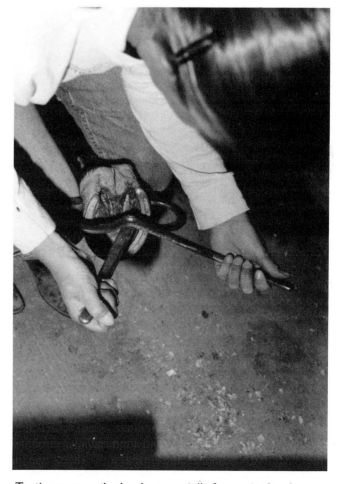

Testing across the heels, especially for navicular disease.

The shoulder joint can be checked by pulling the leg forward and upward. Then, rock it outward and back to see if the animal flinches.

After you have completed these tests, take the good leg and hold it firmly by the cannon bone. Grasp the hoof and flex it outward (away from the horse's body) and then inward. This twisting will put a strain on the fetlock and pastern joints, thus helping to pinpoint problems in those areas. Perform the same test with the knee joint, grasping the leg by the cannon bone and letting the hoof hang free. Rotate it inward and outward so as to put pressure on the knee joint. If the animal flinches when torque is applied, the test may point to a problem in that area. Again, the affected leg must be compared to the "normal" leg.

WEDGE TESTS

A wedge test is another type of stress test which will help to pinpoint problems below the fetlock. Stand the horse with the side of his hoof on a wedge approximately one inch thick. Then pick up the other front leg. This stresses the leg much as does the fetlock flexion test (above), but in different directions. Wedge tests are es-pecially good for ringbone and navicular disease, as well as for detecting sprains and strains of lateral ligaments of the lower foot.

PALPATION

Palpation should be used to determine if there are any obvious abnormalities in the foot or legs. This word means "touching" or "feeling." It refers to the use of your hands in diagnosing illness or lameness. Approach the animal quietly, calmly and confidently. Animals who are unbroken or nervous may not be able to be palpated unless they are tranquilized; this is sometimes necessary to examine them adequately anyway. Touch the animal firmly so that you do not tickle him. Determine if there are any swellings or bumps that should not be present. If you find something which you think to be a problem, check the opposite leg to see if there is anything like it there. If not, it is probably abnormal. This is a place where knowing what is normal for your animal is valuable; the ex-perienced horseman will know what scars and knots his animal has on its legs, so that he is not alarmed by suddenly discovering what are, in reality, old problems.

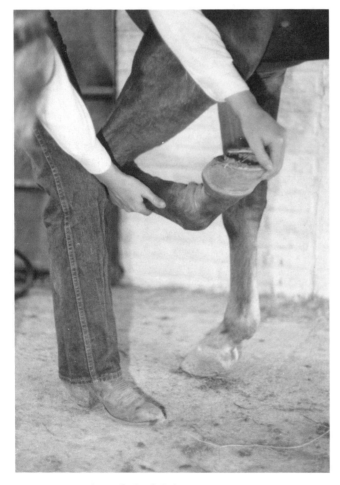

Flexion test, front fetlock joint.

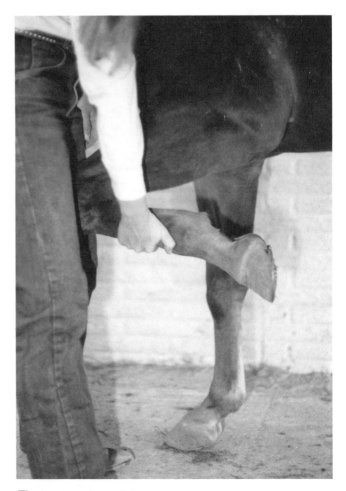

Flexion test, knee joint.

Some horses show a hypersensitivity upon palpation. Nervous horses or young ones who are not used to being handled may be very touchy and may give a false impression that they are in pain. Be patient and take your time with this portion of the examination. Often an animal who jerks his foot abruptly away from you when he is first handled will stand calmly and show no evidence of pain after you have worked with him for a few minutes. Animals who have been blistered may be overly sensitive to being touched, whether they are lame or not. The same hypersensitivity may also be seen in animals who have been treated for long periods of time. A few horses seem to be just plain ticklish.

Sensitive, experienced fingers can detect areas of heat. Heat indicates inflammation in the area and can be very valuable in pinpointing the site of a lameness or injury. A comparison can be made between different spots on the same leg, as well as with the opposite leg. It is especially valuable in detecting sprained ligaments in the lower leg.

The legs should be as clean as possible before any determination of heat is made—it is nearly impossible if the legs are caked with mud or dirt or if they are exceptionally hairy. If cleaning is necessary, the animal should be brushed rather than hosed down. Having the legs wet will make the test invalid. Use the same hand for all heat testing. Switching hands will often give false impressions of heat or coolness.

Palpation can often give a preliminary idea of whether a soft swelling is an abscess, tumor, or blood clot. An abscess often feels very hot in comparison to the surrounding area. Lack of heat hints toward a tumor, blood clot, or serum pocket. Of these, serum pockets and blood-filled cavities will feel soft and fluctuant, while tumors are often hard and well-rounded. "Fluctuant" is how a water-filled balloon feels when you poke it with your finger. Palpation can help to tell a tumor from a bony growth. Bony growths are always firmly attached to the underlying bone, while tumors may or may not be grown into the tissues under them. Of course, a bone tumor or infection of the bone would be firmly attached to it.

The presence of edema can also be determined by palpation. If you push your finger firmly into an edematous area, a dent will remain. You can then feel this by running your finger back over the spot. Severe edema may leave an animal's leg so swollen that it causes pain; the animal

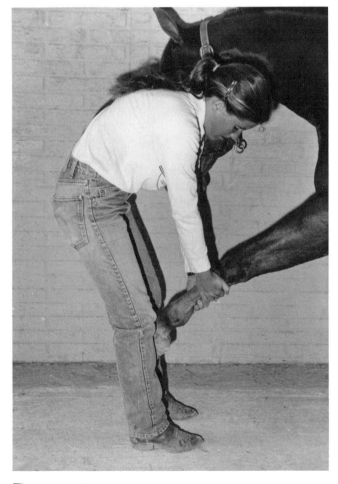

Flexion test for shoulder joint.

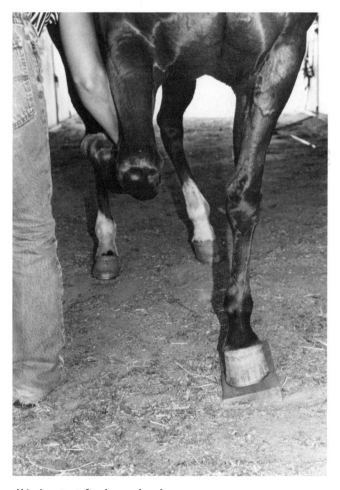

Wedge test for lower leg lameness.

may be unable to move because of it. Edema may occur because of disease problems, or because an animal has been standing very still, or not using one or more limbs because of pain.

Blood is easily pumped through the arteries to the feet. However, the feet are so far below the heart that venous return is either inefficient or impossible without help from the feet. Because of the important role of the feet in the return of blood to the heart, it is often said that the horse has "five hearts." The expansion and contraction of the structures of the foot as weight is placed on it and removed, acts on the blood vessels in the foot to create a pumping action. This action helps to force blood out of the foot and back up the leg on its return trip to the heart and lungs.

If the horse is not at least shifting his weight among his legs, the feet will not be acting to help return blood to the heart. Fluid from the blood will go out into the tissues and remain there, starting the swelling which we call edema.

Edema is not a disease, but a symptom of another problem. Fixing the edema does little good unless we can at the same time repair whatever is causing it in the first place. By the same token, it is often necessary to remove the edema before we can make any progress in treating the original problem. For example, the limb may be so swollen that it is impossible for the animal to move. Treatment to remove the edema will allow the animal to exercise which, in turn, will help to remove the fluid and reduce the swelling.

It is often helpful to palpate a swelling with weight off the affected leg. A swelling which may not be movable with the animal standing on it may move easily when you are holding his leg up. This is especially true of fibrous tumors which may occur over the hock joint in the same area as bone spavins. The bony growth will, of course, not be movable.

If there is a fracture and the animal is not in so much pain that he will not allow it to be moved, a peculiar grating sensation called crepitation may be felt. In some cases, the animal will be in so much pain that he will keep the tendons tight and no movement can be felt. A fracture may be suspected whenever the animal is severely, suddenly lame and is unwilling to move.

A sudden large swelling accompanied by severe lameness may also signal a fracture. If you suspect a fracture, immobilize the animal's leg and get veterinary help for him as soon as possible. In some cases, the veterinarian may come to the horse. It may be necessary for him to come and diagnose the problem and then make a decision as to whether the animal should be treated where he is or moved to a veterinary hospital for treatment.

Palpate the lower part of the foot, noting carefully any swelling, heat, or tenderness. Also check for cracks or a moist exudate. Check each part of the leg slowly and carefully as you move upward.

Examine the entire length of the flexor tendons on the back side of the leg. They should be flat and straight-edged. Feel carefully for thickening and whether the thickening is hard or soft. Observe whether their line on the rear of the leg is straight and vertical or bowed outward. Push your finger and thumb between the tendons and run down between them to feel for any abnormalities in this area. Check as they spread out under the fetlock area for swelling or heat.

Carefully check the inside of the leg for evidence that the horse may be hitting himself with his opposite foot. There may be small nicks or gashes, often oozing a bit of blood if they are fresh. Animals with a poor way of going often have a whole series of old scars, nicks, and small bony growths down the inside of the fetlock joint or cannon bone. Recent brushes may show up as small, roughened spots that look like a bit of hair has been clipped from them (which is exactly what has happened).

Palpate the splint bones down their entire length, noting any bony growths, pain, or hot spots. Feel the front of each knee. Here you are especially looking for swelling or fullness in the joint which will make the skin feel puffy or fluctuant rather than tightly joined to the bones underneath.

Observe the muscles of the foreleg for any signs of shrinkage or unevenness from side to side. Lift each foreleg and move it forward and back to check the movement of the upper joints. Be careful not to bend joints lower in the leg when doing this. Otherwise, a sore lower joint which is bent may cause the animal pain that will falsely appear to originate higher in his leg.

The hindleg is checked in the same manner as the foreleg, beginning at the hoof and moving carefully upward. While you are back there, palpate carefully into the scrotal or udder area to check for any tenderness. An animal who hurts between the hindlegs may appear to be lame.

NERVE BLOCKS

Your veterinarian may use local anesthetic blocks to isolate various nerves. This allows him to decide where the pain is and why it is occurring. It also gives us clues as to where to look further. It is silly to spend your money x-raying the whole leg on the off chance that we might find a problem in one of the joints without first isolating the problem more specifically. Occasionally, these blocks will even confirm a diagnosis without the need for further examination.

These are not tools for the horse owner because they require a very specific knowledge of anatomy in order to deposit the anesthetic exactly at the desired nerve so that it will take effect. It is also easy to put the injection into a blood vessel or into soft tissue where it will do no good. It could cause problems if you have not used good sterile technique. Leave this exam to your veterinarian.

Injections of anesthetic into the joint may be used to pinpoint the location of pain within the knee or other joints.

X-RAYS

Another diagnostic tool used by the veterinarian is the radiographic examination, often called "X-rays." While not technically correct ("radiographs" is the proper term), the term "x-rays" has been used throughout this book because it is so commonly used among horsemen—and veterinarians, for that matter.

With problems such as ringbone, fractured sesamoid bones, or navicular disease, x-rays can not only confirm the diagnosis, but can also give a good idea of the prognosis. They may indicate that surgery is needed or, conversely, that it is unnecessary. They may also tell you, as in the case of a severe ringbone involving a joint, that there may be little chance that the animal will ever get better. This will tell you that the animal may no longer be usable and should be retired to breeding, or that it's time for you to go looking for a new horse. It can save attempting to rest or treat a horse who would never have a chance of getting better no matter how long you care for him. It may also give a chance to a horse who might otherwise be thought hopeless or not repairable.

OTHER DIAGNOSTIC TESTS

In some cases, your veterinarian may wish to use synovial fluid analysis to help determine how badly the joint cartilage is damaged and how well the animal may respond to surgery or other treatment. He will carefully remove some fluid from the animal's joint and take it to a laboratory (or his clinic) for microscopic analysis. Chemical tests are sometimes run on this fluid, too.

This examination is very accurate in helping to show the amount of damage and degeneration that has occurred in a joint and for predicting the outcome of an injury or disease process. It can detect small amounts of damage which are not visible on radiographs. Conversely, it does not always show the presence of problems such as fractures.

Synovial fluid analysis is especially valuable in joints, such as the stifle, which are difficult to x-ray. While your veterinarian has a needle inserted in the joint to remove a sample of fluid, he may continue the examination by injecting a local anesthetic into the joint. By deadening the pain, this may prove conclusively that the animal's pain is coming from damage within that joint.

Arthroscopy is a technique in which a small incision is made into the joint capsule. An instrument called an arthroscope can then be inserted into the joint. Its fiber optics allow the operator to actually see the condition of the joint cartilages and tissues around the joint. In some cases, small chip fractures can be removed with this instrument.

THE HORSE'S FOOT

Before we go into specific lameness problems, let's begin by discussing how the foot is put together since this important structure is quite literally the foundation of the horse.

Deep inside the hoof are the bony structures which form the basis of the horse's foot. These include the coffin bone (third phalanx), the lower half of the second phalanx, and the navicular bone (distal sesamoid bone). The coffin bone is covered by a highly vascular modified dermis (tissue under the skin) called the corium. The hoof is an insensitive cornified (hardened) layer of skin (epidermis) covering the lower end of the foot; it corresponds to our fingernails and the layer from which the hoof grows (at the coronary band) corresponds to our cuticle.

The color of the skin at the coronary band determines the color of hoof which will be produced at this area and grow downward from there. Black hooves are generally harder and stronger than white hooves. White hooves tend to be brittle and may be "shelly" (thin and peeling).

The hoof wall is the portion of the foot that is visible when the horse is standing. The front is called the toe; the sides are called the quarters. The heels are the portion that turn sharply forward at the rear angle of the hoof, becoming the bars. The coronary band produces thousands of small tubules of horn which become the hoof wall; these extend from the coronary band toward the ground.

The periople is a thin layer of tubular horn which covers the hoof wall for a half-inch to an inch below the coronary band. It turns milky white when the hoof is soaked in water. This is normal and this area should not be trimmed or removed. It helps to prevent the hoof from becoming excessively dry. If it is rasped off, the hoof wall will become more brittle than it should. The laminar corium is a layer of tissue which adheres to the periosteum (tissue on the outside of the bone) over the surface of the third phalanx.

Front feet are almost round while hind feet tend to be more elongated and slightly pointed toward the front. The sole of the hind foot is usually more concave than that of the front.

CHESTNUTS AND ERGOTS

Chestnuts are normal, horn-like growths on the inside of a horse's legs. The front chestnuts occur above the knees, and the rear ones inside the hocks. They may be absent in some animals. They are considered to be the remains of one of the five toes that the horse had in prehistoric times.

Ergots are small, horny growths on the back of the fetlock. If the horse has much hair (often called "feathers") at the rear of the fetlocks, this may hide the ergot. This also is felt to be a vestige of one or more of the original five digits.

FUNCTIONS OF THE FOOT

One of the major functions of the foot is to resist wear and tear. The hoof wall grows as is needed to replace that lost by wear and tear. Increased wear will bring about increased growth. Much the same thing occurs when a callous forms on our foot or hand because of friction and usage. The outermost tubules of horn increase in length because more material grows from the coronary band. This wear is prevented in the shod horse so the animal's hooves must be trimmed periodically.

The hoof wall is very soft in foals because it has been immersed in fluid for a long period of time. The same situation occurs when horses stand in wet stalls or pastures or live in humid climates. Deterioration of the hoof wall may occur under these conditions. In dry climates or if there is interference with the blood supply to the foot, the hoof wall may become very brittle; it may crack or chip.

Hoof walls grow faster in warm climates and in summer. About eight months are needed for the horny material deposited at the coronary band to reach the ground under average conditions. After a disease, such as ergot poisoning, a new hoof will be formed. Care must be taken to avoid injury and infection as it grows out.

Support of body weight is another major function of the foot. The horse is adapted to traveling on hard or rocky ground. This is evident because of the large body mass which is supported on relatively small feet. If the horse were adapted to traveling on softer ground, he would have big, soft feet like a bobcat or snowshoe rabbit. In loose sand or mud, the hoof tends to cut in, requiring considerable effort to pull it out and advance it; compare this to the camel with his soft, expandable footpads.

The attachment of the tubules of horny material to the soft tissues underneath and then to the coffin bone down under it show that the animal does not actually

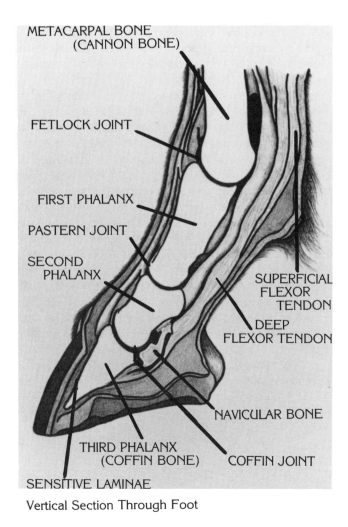

Vertical Section Through Foot

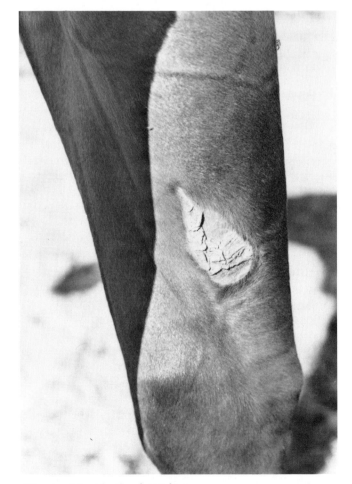

Chestnut inside the front leg.

"stand" on the hoof wall. Instead, his coffin bone is basically "slung" within the hoof wall. This laminar attachment distributes the weight over a far greater surface area and results in a better weight distribution. Because the sole is concave, it normally bears very little of the animal's weight. However, its "give" as the animal's foot hits the ground is an important part of the shock-absorbing mechanism.

For proper weight distribution, it is very important that the animal's feet be proportionate to its body. A 1200 to 1300 lb Quarter Horse standing on an 00 shoe is a case of navicular disease or other foot problems waiting to happen.

The entire foot is a sophisticated anticoncussion mechanism. When the hoof hits the ground, the initial impact is at the heel area. This puts pressure on the frog in a normal foot. Some of the shock is absorbed here; the rest is passed on to the digital cushion, which is a fibrous and fatty pad within the rear part of the hoof. The digital cushion transmits the force in all directions, helping to dissipate it. Part of the force is sent to the lateral cartilages. The bulbs of the heel are spread slightly which helps to expand the hoof wall in the heel area. If the lateral cartilages become replaced by bone (a condition called sidebone which is especially common in draft horses whose feet are subject to heavy concussion), the horse may become severely lame. This is due in part to the lessened flexibility of the hoof. From this point, the concussion is spread throughout the foot and passed to higher structures. The navicular bone acts as a pulley, helping to reduce friction of the tendons running over it.

For this concussion absorption mechanism to work, the horny part of the hoof wall must be somewhat flexible. Otherwise, it would be like having the inner part of the hoof encased in concrete—hard, painful, and not very efficient for absorbing shock.

The expansion that occurs in the hoof structures under weight is very important to circulation within the foot, and to helping to return blood to the animal's heart. The hoof has an extremely rich blood supply, especially considering the very small area which is involved. This is why the laminae of the foot are so sensitive to the presence of toxins which have been produced elsewhere in the body, resulting in laminitis. These toxins easily cause circulatory disturbances in the foot, although the original problem may have been in the uterus (in the case of a metritis) or the intestinal tract (as with a grain overload founder). Now, let's cover some specific foot problems.

MALFORMED FEET

Deformities in the feet may be hereditary. They may also be caused by neglect or injury. For instance, a foal may be born with a crooked leg which allows the animal to walk on the side of the hoof. If this is not promptly corrected, it may result in an animal who will walk on the side

of his hoof for the rest of his life. In these cases, the bones will grow crookedly, to help compensate for the foot deformity. The problem is unlikely to be correctable except in very young animals. These problems are often said by the owner to be due to injury. Unless you know that to be an absolute fact or see a scar to prove it, you should assume the defect to be hereditary and eliminate the animal from consideration for breeding.

Horses may have "odd feet" which do not quite match each other. The feet may be different sizes or shapes from one side of the animal to the other. Odd feet which occur naturally, as compared to those caused by injury or disease, will have normally rounded soles. They will have wide-open heels, and the frogs will make normal contact with the ground, rather than being recessed into a deeply concave sole.

The owner of an "odd-footed" horse may assure you that the horse threw a shoe and broke the wall or wore it away before the loss was noticed. While this may occasionally be true, other reasons are much more common—such as an old fracture or navicular disease which is particularly severe in one foot. The animal may not be lame at the time you examine him. Be suspicious of an animal with odd feet without an obvious cause (such as a wire cut with a noticeable scar) to the extent that you should not buy an animal with this problem.

One side of the hoof wall may be more concave than the other or it may be flattened. There may be an odd growth of hoof wall—a ridge or even a separate spur of hoof material that may be nearly unattached to the rest of the hoof. These problems are usually due to an injury to the coronary band above the hoof. There is often an obvious scar. If the problem is severe, the animal may be lame or almost unable to walk. Less severe cases may have no lameness, but could require special shoeing to protect the problem area.

CONTRACTED FEET

Long-term lameness almost always causes the foot of the involved limb to contract—even if the lameness is not in the foot. This is due to the fact that the animal does not put his usual amount of weight on that limb. This lessens the blood-pumping action that occurs with foot pressure at every step in the normal horse. The reduced frog pressure does not expand the heels as it would in a normal foot. A foot with this type of contraction always grows longer (or higher) than the other one. It will definitely be narrower than the other. It may look smaller and flatter than the normal foot.

Pick up the feet and look at the sole surfaces. The heels of the contracted foot will be narrower. The sole may b⁻ longer, but will not be as wide as in the sound foot. The wall may be a little higher. The sole of the contracted foot is usually more concave. The frog will be smaller and show less sign of wear. Contracted feet are more commonly seen in front feet than in hind feet.

A contracted foot is generally not a cause of lameness. Instead, it is a sign that lameness has occurred, or still exists, in that foot or leg. It is almost invariably present in cases of navicular disease in one front foot, especially if the problem has been present for a long time. Contracted feet may not be seen with horses who have navicular disease which is equally bad in both front feet because the horse cannot favor only one foot. Contracted feet are also seen in horses with chronic corns. Contracted feet are almost always present with ringbone, especially those cases causing signs of lameness. Some animals may show a degree of contraction in an unshod hoof on a leg which has had any severe lameness lasting more than a few days.

Lack of frog pressure caused by shoeing the horse when it is not needed, or by improper shoeing, may cause contracted heels. Hereditary causes have been proposed in some cases of contracted feet. When animals are kept in wet or swampy pastures and then moved to a dry pasture or corral, the foot may contract, especially if the weather is hot.

Contracted feet may be accompanied by a "dished sole." The sole appears to be more concave and farther from the ground than in a normal horse. If the hoof wall contracts far enough, the sole may put enough pressure on the coffin bone to cause lameness. This is called "hoof-bound."

Narrow feet should not be confused with contracted feet. Some breeds of horses naturally have feet that are more long and narrow than round. This shape, extremely long hooves, is also seen in Saddlebreds and Tennessee Walkers who are shod for show. These long feet contract because there is no frog pressure. Mules and donkeys normally have small, narrow feet; these are normal for the beasts and not a sign of defects or problems.

If the feet have been determined to be contracted and not just normally narrow or elongated, the contraction should be considered to be a serious defect. An animal who got that way in a month or two of disuse from a lameness or injury may take a year or more to get back to normal.

It is very important to determine the cause of a contracted foot. If it is due to navicular disease, it may not be curable. If it is due to improper shoeing, it may be corrected with time. The cause should be corrected whenever possible. If thrush is present in the frog, it should be treated. If the foot is hard and dry from disuse, the animal should be soaked in mud or damp sand for several hours two to three days before shoeing.

One of my clients purchased a Saddlebred gelding who was shod for show. He had been that way for some time; his hind feet were severely contracted, and the hooves were approximately six inches long. Rather than pulling the shoes, the seller cut them off in order to remove a part of the hoof wall and start the animal toward normal. The horse was trimmed every six weeks and left barefooted to get pressure on the frogs as much as possible. It took about six months to get his hooves back to a normal angle and length. The horse's feet were normal and sound, but still narrower than they would have been without the fancy shoeing.

KERATOMA

A keratoma is a growth of horn (hoof material) which begins at the coronary band. It extends gradually down the hoof causing pressure on the sensitive laminae as they are pinched between the hoof material and the coffin bone. It may produce localized atrophy and grooving of the coffin bone. Most keratomas grow in the toe area, although they are occasionally reported at the quarter. Those which occur at the quarters are usually due to injury to the coronary band. The cause of the usual type of keratoma which extends down the front of the foot is not known. It is apparently not always due to injury, but may just be due to an abnormal secretion of hoof material.

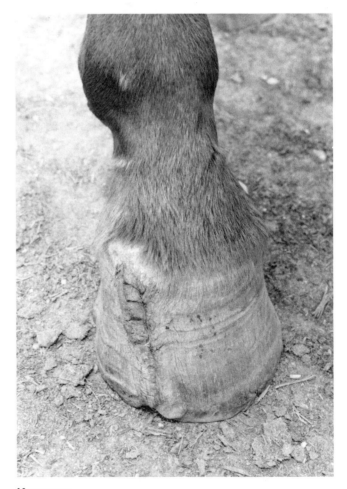

Keratoma.

Lameness due to keratoma comes on gradually. It may be due to injury to the coronary band, but often there is no evidence of cuts or scars. After a period of months, the growth will extend down the hoof. Consult your veterinarian, as surgical removal is the only treatment that seems to work. It does not always permanently correct the problem, but it may be worth a try.

GRAVEL

Old-timers considered "gravel" to be due to a piece of gravel which entered the white line on the bottom of the hoof and then migrated to the heel area and came out there. In reality what happens is that a defect in the white line allows bacteria to enter the sensitive tissues of the hoof, setting up an infection. Because it cannot drain there, it follows the path of least resistance and drains at the heel. This also occurs with infected puncture wounds which cannot drain out through the sole.

Feet which are too dry may crack and allow infection to enter at the white line or sole. Animals with chronic founder (laminitis) may have "seedy toe." This results in defects at the white line which allow infection to enter.

Horses with gravel are usually lame before the drainage is seen at the heel. Gravel may be difficult to diagnose until drainage begins. Black spots (like puncture wounds) may sometimes be seen if the white line is carefully pared out. Some may be pinpointed with hoof testers.

Treat gravel as for foot punctures. Tetanus treatment should be given. Gravels usually heal well unless they are occur in feet which are damaged because of chronic founder. In this case, they often recur. If the infection has been present for a long time, it may have involved the sensitive structures of the foot or even the coffin bone. These have an unfavorable prognosis.

SAND CRACKS

Also called quarter cracks or toe or heel cracks, these are cracks in the hoof wall which start at the ground surface and extend upward. Severe cases may extend to the coronary band. Occasionally, they originate at the coronary band because of a defect there and extend downward. They occur in both front and hind feet and are frequently seen in all four hooves of the same horse.

These cracks often start because the hoof wall is allowed to grow excessively long. It then begins to chip or break off, leaving ragged edges. The edges spread, becoming cracks which open upward as the animal puts his weight on them.

The coronary band may be injured causing cracks which begin at the top of the hoof and extend downward. These may also be caused by wire cuts, overreaching, or interfering. Cracks which begin at the coronary band are seen more frequently in the quarters of the front feet and the toe of the hind feet. They extend vertically down the hoof and through the whole thickness of the hoof wall.

Cracks in the hoof wall tend to spread open when the animal puts weight on the foot and close as he lifts it. Occasionally, they will do the opposite, opening when the foot is lifted and closing when it is put down. This pinching action produces pain. The pressure on the sensitive laminae will often bring on a laminitis and acute lameness.

Sand cracks may be caused in the beginning by severe drying of the foot which may be brought on by rasping the outer covering off the hoof wall. Some horses with dry, brittle feet may have a chronic problem with cracks. Neglected, sand cracks may become infected and cause extreme lameness. The infection may produce an abscess in the coronary band which may rupture and drain. Animals with thin hoof walls are also susceptible to these defects.

SIGNS

The cracks in the hoof wall are obvious. They do not usually cause lameness unless they extend into the sensitive tissues of the hoof. Lameness especially occurs with excessive hoof growth; large chunks may break out of the hoof wall, tearing directly into the sensitive tissues and allowing infection to enter.

Lameness may also be seen when problems at the coronary band are causing the cracks. These may cause a characteristic change in gait. The foot is lifted high and carried far forward. It is then brought to the ground heel first to avoid jarring the front of the foot. This movement may occur when the horse injures the coronary band by stepping on himself.

In the old days of horse traders, the cracks were often filled and the hoof carefully polished. It is well to closely examine the hoof surface of a horse you are planning to buy to be sure there are no cracks present.

TREATMENT

Cracks at the toe are treated by shoeing to protect the crack and keep weight off the area. This is done by cutting away the hoof wall so that there is a gap between it and the shoe. The gap between the hoof and shoe should be cleaned daily to keep pressure from developing on the area. Toe clips should be put on either side of the crack to keep the wall from expanding and making the crack worse. Tetanus antitoxin or a booster of tetanus toxoid should be given to prevent possible problems with this disease.

If the horse requires more drastic treatment, your veterinarian should be consulted. There are methods used by some veterinarians and farriers which involve undermining the crack with electric tools and filling in the area with epoxy or plastics during the healing period. Care must be taken so that the sensitive tissues inside the hoof are not damaged or killed by the heat generated during the plastic repair. Special supportive lacing is sometimes used to reinforce the damaged hoof. A similar type of repair may be used when a horse has lost a large chunk of hoof wall, as when a shoe tears off removing a piece of hoof wall from the nail holes down. A horse whose feet have been neglected and allowed to splay and break can also be helped in this fashion. A shoe is placed on the foot and the defect is filled with one of these materials.

Cracks at the quarter may be treated by cutting away the heel behind them, again to keep the shoe from pressing on the wall. This area should be cleaned daily as noted above. A shoe with a half bar can be used with the bar on the heel on the side where the crack occurs. If you are looking at the shoe from the side, the bar should be about ¼ inch higher than the upper surface of the shoe. This allows the frog to help bear some of the weight that would normally be carried by the hoof wall. Quarter clips may be used on each side of the crack to prevent the hoof wall from expanding. Cracks further toward the heel may not need the half bar.

It is important to balance the feet very carefully, as any slight difference in pressure may be harmful to a hoof which is already weakened.

In severe cases, the crack may be infected or may bleed when the horse is worked. With these animals or those who have cracks deep enough to expose the sensitive laminae, the area may have to be kept open and treated as an open wound. Antibiotic treatment may be necessary and the horse should have a tetanus booster as with any open wound.

Treatment of severe sand cracks is a job for your veterinarian, as the animal's foot should be blocked with a special nerve block to reduce the pain that the animal will feel from the treatment. It sounds rather drastic, but is necessary to keep the problem from continuing indefinitely. The hoof wall is divided horizontally through the crack, about ¼ inch below the coronary band (or at the top of the crack if it does not extend that high). This prevents further opening and closing of the crack which has been keeping it open as new hoof material is made. This may be done with a rasp or saw. Or, a flat iron heated to red heat may be used. A special clip is often inserted into the slit or burned spot in order to keep the crack from expanding.

In some cases, acrylic, plastic, or fiberglass materials are used to stabilize the hoof and hold it together until it heals. Your veterinarian may use sutures or screws to hold it together.

Sand cracks usually heal well if infection has not entered the area. Because the hoof only grows about ¼ inch per month, considerable time may be needed for cracks to grow out. If the crack is due to a defect in the coronary band, it may continue to be a problem,

necessitating corrective shoeing for the rest of the animal's life.

THRUSH

Thrush is a foul, black infection of the frog. In severe cases, it may penetrate the sole and involve vital structures within the hoof. It is thought to be caused by a type of bacteria or fungus. Many organisms are probably involved.

Thrush is most commonly seen in filthy stables, especially when the bedding is continuously moist or the animal is standing in manure or mud all the time. Lack of frog pressure due to poor shoeing or hoof trimming may be a contributing factor. Some horses seem to keep thrush going in their feet no matter how clean or dry their area is kept. These horses may have less individual resistance to the disease organisms than do normal animals.

Thrush is first noticed as a weeping, moist discharge along the sulci (grooves) of the frog. It has a very distinct, rotten odor. When the frog is cleaned, the sulci will appear deeper than normal. In severe cases, the horse may flinch when the area is cleaned or pressed with a hoof pick. This indicates involvement of sensitive tissues. In some cases, the animal may be lame and the foot may look like it has suffered a puncture wound.

Treatment begins by correcting stable conditions which may have initiated the problem. The stall should be cleaned thoroughly and good absorbent bedding should be provided. It may be necessary to dig all dirt out of the stall and refloor it to provide better drainage. Replacing the dirt is also helpful in removing some of the organisms which are causing the thrush. If mud is causing the problem (as with wet corrals during prolonged rainy spells), attempt to provide a dry, clean place where the horse can rest at least part of the day.

The feet should be cleaned daily. If there is still much black material left in the grooves of the frog, the foot should be scrubbed with a stiff brush and warm water. Pat it dry with paper towels or a rag. Soak the entire sole with medication. Strong (7%) tincture of iodine is one of the best products for treating thrush. Repeat daily until the infection is controlled.

Animals who continually suffer from thrush will benefit from treatment twice or three times a week with Kopertox (Fort Dodge, Fort Dodge, IA 50501) or a similar product after their hooves are cleaned. Strong iodine may be excessively drying if used on the hoof for long periods of time. It may be necessary to lower the wall to provide frog pressure; the normal hoof angle should not be changed.

Recovery is usually complete if the disease is treated before extensive damage occurs. If sensitive structures within the hoof are involved, the problem is much more serious and the outcome may be unfavorable.

CORNS

Corns are bruises resulting from pressure from the heel of the horse's shoe. They often occur only on the inner branch; if on both sides, they are generally worse on the inside. They occur at the angle of the sole between the main wall of the foot and the portion of the wall which turns in to form the bar of the foot. Corns are rarely seen in the hind feet. This is probably due to the fact that the front feet bear more of the horse's weight.

Conformational problems may contribute to the occurrence of corns. They are particularly common in animals with narrow, boxy feet. Flat, shallow feet without heels are also prone to corns.

Corns are, in the final analysis, usually caused by improper shoeing. When shoes are left on the hoof too long, the heels of the hoof grow out and around the heels of the shoe causing pressure on the sole at the angle of the wall and bar. This pressure bruises the sole and causes corns. Heel calks may make this effect worse. Shoeing the animal close at the heel which keeps the inner branch of the shoe well in to avoid hitting the other foot is also a common cause of corns.

If the foot is trimmed so the heels are too low, this will increase pressure at the angle of the wall and bar and may cause corns. Lack of frog pressure may contribute to the occurrence of corns. Horses with long, weak fetlocks and narrow feet may develop corns at the bars. Animals with wide feet more frequently have corns in the sole. Corns may also occur if a stone gets caught between the shoe and the sole near the heel. Corns are seen in animals with thin soles, as well as those who have been foundered.

SIGNS

Chronic corns may cause signs which look like navicular disease, sidebone, or low ringbone. The lameness which they cause may be severe and continuous or mild and intermittent. Pain may be quite evident when the heel of the affected foot is gently squeezed. Corns look different from one animal to another when the shoe is removed and the sole is pared to a clean surface. Their appearance depends on how long the corn has been in existence and whether the shoe is still causing pressure on the same spot. In an early case, there may be a reddened spot with heat present. There may be pain if the area is pressed with the point of a hoof knife. There may also be a damp oozing of yellowish serum.

To confirm the presence of a corn, it may be necessary to pare down into the sole at the angle between the bar and the wall. Trim as little as possible. Removing some of the material from the sole may help to relieve pressure, but sensitive tissues should not be exposed. Otherwise, you may introduce infection and turn a simple bruising into a serious suppurating corn. Where there has been an escape of blood from injured vessels, there will often be staining of the hoof material. When the bruising is recent, it may be red or bluish. Later, it may be brownish or yellow to copper-colored.

TREATMENT

When the corn is noticed before it becomes infected, it may be cured by removing the cause of pressure. Remove the shoe. Soak the foot in warm water to soften the hoof. Epsom salts may be added to help draw infection from the area. Leave the horse unshod until he is healed. If he must be used, reshoe the horse with a half-bar or full-bar shoe. This shoe will protect the area where the corn is located. It should exert about ⅛ inch of pressure against the frog to help prevent contraction of the heels (see Shoeing for Quarter Cracks, above). Later, replace it with one that has been widened a bit at the heels, or with a feather-edge shoe which does not put any pressure on the bar.

If the corn has become infected, the area will have to be drained. Treat as with a puncture wound in the hoof, including tetanus toxoid or antitoxin. The foot should be soaked daily in warm water with epsom salts.

PREVENTION

Corns may be prevented by allowing the frog to make slight contact with the ground, taking some of the weight off the hoof wall. Heels should be allowed to grow normally instead of being trimmed short. The toe should be kept short to avoid weight being thrown on the heels. Horses suffering from corns often turn the toe of the affected foot to the inside, thus putting more weight on the inside heel. Leaving a little more length of shoe on the inside branch may correct this problem. Corns are often caused by the farrier putting on too-short shoes. Make sure that shoes are adequately sized and properly fitted to the foot.

SOLE BRUISING AND ABSCESSES

Sole bruising may occur because the horse has hit his foot on a rock. It may also occur because of conformational problems. Horses with wide, flat feet are susceptible to bruising. Animals who have long toes and little or no heel area are susceptible to bruising at the heel. Attempts to correct feet which toe in or out (in the adult horse) by unleveling or unbalancing one or more feet may result in sole bruises by concentrating much of the hoof impact on a smaller area than normal. If a shoe becomes loose and shifts position on the hoof, bruising may occur. It can also happen when shoes are left on too long and the walls grow down over the edge of the shoe.

Bruising is more common in horses with thin soles, and in horses who have had laminitis. It may also occur when a farrier bends the inside branch of the front shoe to keep the horse from stepping on it and pulling the shoe. This allows the shoe to come into contact with the sole when the horse's weight is on it. Bruising can also occur if a lightweight shoe (such as a polo or racing plate) bends and puts pressure on the frog or sole. Overtrimming may leave the horse with little extra material on the sole and make him more susceptible to bruising.

Bruises may be dry or moist depending on how much damage has been done to the sole. Bruises may turn to abscesses if they become infected. The horse may rock back onto the heel if the bruising has occurred in the toe area. If the problem is in the heel area, the animal may land on the toe to protect the heel.

Sole bruises and abscesses are diagnosed much as are corns: by paring the sole to look for evidence of bruising and by the use of hoof testers to pinpoint the area of pain where further paring is needed.

If you cannot tell whether you are dealing with a sole bruise or an abscess, locate the affected area as well as you can with hoof testers. Then, soak the animal's foot in hot water with epsom salts several times a day. The horse who has an abscess will get more and more lame until the abscess finally breaks and drains. If it becomes apparent that you have an abscess, pare gently into the sole until you locate it. This is preferable to having it break at the top of the hoof wall. If the problem is a bruise or blood clot, it should get steadily better with soaking as the heat and moisture helps speed the absorption of the blood.

Treatment of bruises is similar to that for corns, as described above. Do not use pads to treat sole bruises if it can be avoided. Pads do give some protection to the sole. However, they do not eliminate sole pressure. They can also trap moisture and lead to further deterioration of the sole. This may further weaken the foot and lead to even more flattening of the sole. The horse should be rested until healed if at all possible and definitely should not be worked on rough ground. The prognosis is guarded with both corns and sole bruises, as they may become chronic; some of these lead to an infection of the coffin bone (pedal osteitis).

PUNCTURES (HOOF)

Puncture wounds are among the first problems the horseman should suspect when his horse is suddenly and acutely lame. Puncture wounds in the middle third of the frog may be quite serious, as they may injure the navicular bone or its bursa. Objects which go into the foot more toward the front may result in damage to the coffin bone or may even fracture it. Animals showing drainage at the coronary band or heel should always have the sole carefully checked. The drainage may be due to a puncture which occurred some time previously and only recently has built up enough pus to become obvious. Puncture

wounds of the frog may be difficult to locate because after the object pulls out, the spongy material closes the hole.

Nail wounds are especially likely if a horse is kept in a corral with old building materials or where barns are falling down. A veterinarian was called to examine a horse whose owner said that he had cleaned the hoof and checked it carefully. He was sure the horse had a shoulder lameness. The vet lifted the hoof and immediately saw the 3/8 inch diameter head of a roofing nail—a rather obvious cause when he noticed that the horse's barn was being reroofed and there were pieces of roofing everywhere (with, of course, the accompanying nails). Or, the horse may step on a board with a nail in it. The puncture occurs and then the board falls off his foot. The puncture may be covered by manure so that it is not easily noticed.

Begin checking an acutely lame horse by carefully cleaning out the hoof, removing all loose manure. Use a hoof knife to scrape a thin layer from the entire sole so that all surface dirt is removed, leaving a fresh, clean surface. At this point, a large puncture may be obvious. A smaller one which has closed after the object which made it has pulled away may only show up as a small, sharp black line or slit—perhaps only 1/8 inch long. It usually looks more sharply defined than other small, spidery lines which are visible on the sole. A small amount of reddening or blood may be present. If you suspect a puncture and cannot find it, hoof testers often allow you to localize the pain to decide where to begin paring out the foot.

Once a puncture is definitely located, pare down into the sole as deeply as possible to expose the punctured area. It may be necessary to pare quite a distance inward as you follow the tract made by the object. Make an opening at least 1/4 inch diameter into the sensitive laminae. Be sure to make the hole larger at the sole surface than at its deepest part so that it is cone-shaped and will not close over easily. When the wound occurs in the frog, it must be trimmed away until a hole large enough for drainage is made.

Saturate the area with strong (7%) tincture of iodine. Pour the liquid over the rest of the sole as well. Pack the pared-out hole (which usually ends up being a half to 3/4 inch in diameter) with cotton or gauze. Lay another layer of gauze, approximately 3/8 inch thick, in the hollow of the sole. Wrap over the hoof and gauze with bandaging material. Plain white adhesive tape is adequate, or you can use Elastikon or Vetrap. When you have the foot securely wrapped, saturate the sole of the bandage with strong tincture of iodine.

Keep the horse in a dry stall or pen and change the bandage promptly if it should become wet. Under dry conditions, changing it every other day is adequate. Use the same iodine bandage each time you change it. Continue to bandage the animal until the wound is well filled with new hoof material and lameness is no longer evident.

If the draining area is at the coronary band, the foot should be soaked daily in warm water with epsom salts.

When you have located and drained the tract in the sole, bandage and treat as above. Once healing begins, soaking every two or three days is sufficient.

Treatment should include a tetanus antitoxin injection or toxoid booster if the animal has not had one within the last month. The horse should also be given penicillin/streptomycin combination for a minimum of three days. If the wound is at all deep, it it best to continue the antibiotic for five to six days.

If you are on a hunting trip or otherwise away from help and must continue to use the animal, make a small temporary drain hole with straight walls and pack it tightly with cotton or clean, cotton string, saturated with tincture of iodine. When you get out of the back country, open up the drainage hole and treat as above.

SEEDY TOE

Seedy toe is a condition where there is a separation at the toe between the sensitive laminae and the wall. This area becomes filled with crumbly, disintegrated hoof material. When it is pared out, a hollow cavity is seen at the "white line" area because of the separation which has occurred there. Seedy toe may occur with laminitis (founder), allowing a thrush-like infection to penetrate the sensitive laminae. If severe, it may destroy all protection to the third phalanx and necessitate euthanasia of the horse. If it does not involve the third phalanx, seedy toe almost never causes lameness. Various products have been used as packing material, and nothing seems to work.

LOW HEELS

Horses with long toes and low heels may become permanently crippled because of this conformation. It is perhaps more common in Thoroughbred horses than in other breeds. This problem does not always cause lameness by itself, but should be corrected before serious complications occur. The extra toe length makes the horse work harder when he rolls forward and breaks over. Horses are often trimmed and shod this way on racetracks with the mistaken idea that this will increase stride length (and thus make the beast run faster).

Farriers on the racetrack often use shoes which are too small, to prevent the horse from pulling a shoe. Over a period of time, this way of shoeing causes the hoof to change shape, and can be very difficult to correct. Young horses may develop this foot shape by being allowed to go too long between trimmings so that the hooves get excessively long, especially at the toe. This often occurs in soft pastures where the hooves do not wear or break off by themselves.

Correction of low heels is relatively simple; use a larger-sized shoe and shorten the toe. If the toe is very long, it may have to be trimmed gradually over two or three shoeings so that the hoof angle is not changed radically at one time. This gradual change is especially important if the animal is competing or in hard use. (42)

SHEARED HEELS

Sheared heels result from imbalance over a long period of time which has resulted in overuse of one heel compared to the other heel on the same foot. This heel is overused to the point that shearing has taken place between it and the other heel. Animals with a severe difference between the two heels may be extremely lame on that foot. If the problem has been present for a long time, damage may extend to structures within the hoof and may be very difficult or impossible to reverse.

How do sheared heels occur? They generally begin when an owner or shoer trims one side of the hoof lower than the other in an attempt to straighten a crooked foot or feet in an adult horse. This is by far the most common cause. It can also begin from accidental trimming of the feet off level.

Conformational defects may lead to sheared heels if the feet are unequally loaded between the inside and outside walls. Some horses with conformational defects have feet which are level at the ground surface and contact it squarely. In that case, continue to trim them level, and allow the rest of the conformational defect to remain. It is nearly impossible to correct crooked legs or turned feet when the horse is much more than a year old. Beyond that age, all that can be realistically done is to trim the feet to be as level as possible. Use the animal if he is usable, or get rid of him if he is not.

Some cases of sheared heels occur when heel calks, "stickers," or other additions to the shoe concentrate the impact energy. This will exaggerate any differences in hoof length or balance which already exist, even if they are minute. Sheared heels are a problem also seen in gaited horses who have extremely long feet with heavy, special shoeing.

Horses with sheared heels will be lame when trotted on a hard surface and will be worse when turned sharply. Look at the heel area by grasping the horse's leg by the cannon bone. Sight along the cannon bone and see if the heel area lines up with it. The sole surface should be perpendicular (at right angles) to the line of the cannon bone. Both heels should be the same length.

In a case of sheared heels severe enough to cause lameness, the difference between the two sides is usually obvious. In some cases, it may be possible to grasp the two sides of the heel and move them independently of each other. This will nearly always cause pain. The division between the heel areas may be so deep that it appears to be an extension of the sulcus of the frog. The problem may also be mistaken for a case of thrush.

Treatment is aimed at returning the foot to a level and balanced condition. This will usually have to be done in a series of steps rather than all at once because sudden removal of the excess hoof would cause as severe a lameness as the one we are trying to correct. Remove as much hoof material as can be removed without crippling the horse or making his lameness worse. Then shoe him so as to leave a space between the shoe and the heel which will allow the problem heel to drop toward normal. It may take several months and several shoeings to get the animal back to normal. A full bar shoe may help remove the pressure and prevent movement in the heel area. (43)

LAMINITIS (FOUNDER)

Laminitis and founder are names given to a foot problem in which there is inflammation of the laminae in the hoof. These are delicate tissues, loaded with small blood vessels, that attach the hard shell of the hoof to the bone underneath. Laminitis is characterized by congestion of these laminae with blood. It may be caused by either infectious or noninfectious agents. By far, the most common cause is feeding problems. Whatever the cause, laminitis results in severe pain due to pressure on the sensitive laminae, since they are caught between the hoof wall and the hard bone below (between the proverbial rock and hard place). The front feet are nearly always involved and in really severe cases, all four feet may be affected.

CAUSES

Many factors cause laminitis. Some of the more common are:

1) Grain founder. This is caused by the horse eating larger quantities of grain than he can handle. A horse who is normally fed large amounts of grain will usually develop a tolerance, but may suddenly show signs of founder. Accidental founders are perhaps more common. Grain founder is due to inflammation of the gastrointestinal tract, probably associated with toxin production. Barley, corn, and wheat seem to be the worst offenders. Overeating of oats usually produces a more mild founder, or may not cause it at all. Any grain product can produce founder—it has been seen in horses who have eaten such items as rabbit pellets and hog feed.

2) Grass founder. This type is common in horses grazed on lush green pasture. Legume (alfalfa and clover) pastures are felt to cause it more commonly than grasses. Horses who founder on pastures frequently have large, heavily crested necks in addition to usually being overweight. This gives them a characteristic "founder type" or look. Ponies are more prone to grass founder than horses, and fat horses of all breeds seem to be more susceptible. It has been my impression that geldings are more often affected by grass founder than mares.

Grass founder can be seen in fat horses during the winter who are fed legume hays. While this is more common in horses that have been previously foundered on grass, it can also be seen in horses not known to have had prior problems. Grass founder is thought to be caused by hormones, probably estrogens, that occur naturally in the forage.

3) Water founder. Most of us know about the colic that may be caused when an overheated horse drinks cold water. Instead of colic, the animal may founder—another good reason for allowing hot animals only a few sips of water until they are well cooled. The reason this occurs is not understood.

4) Road Founder. This can be caused by concussion to the feet from hard work or fast work on hard footing. One of my clients ponied a young colt behind a pickup three miles at a hard trot on a ranch road of dried mud, nearly as hard as concrete, and foundered him severely. Road founder is also seen in animals given a long ride in a horse trailer over rough roads, or in a trailer with inadequate springs and/or cushioning.

Animals in poor physical condition are more susceptible to road founder. Excess work (work to exhaustion) may cause founder if the horse is not kept fit by regular exercise. (44)

Sole bruising may occur along with road founder if the original cause is not corrected. It is more common in horses with large, heavy bodies and slender legs, such as Thoroughbred/draft horse cross animals. It can be worse when they have long toes. Animals with road founder may show an acute lameness in one or both forelegs which subsides with rest and recurs when the horse is worked again.

5) Postparturient laminitis. This develops shortly after foaling due to retention in the mare's uterus of some or all of the membranes around the foal. It may also occur due to an infection in the uterus. This type of laminitis is very serious. Laminitis may also occur after a severe pneumonia or other major infection.

6) Miscellaneous causes. Hormonal causes may be involved in the production of laminitis. They are not well understood. Laminitis may occur in mares who are continually in heat. It may also occur, on the other hand, in mares without exposure to any of the above causes and cease immediately when the mare is brought into heat. This type of founder does not cause permanent foot damage as quickly as other kinds.

Viral respiratory disease has been incriminated in some sudden cases of founder in which rotation of the third phalanx and sole penetration occurs quite rapidly (within 10 days). Some of these animals may completely slough their hooves.

A substance is present in black walnut shavings which may cause a severe founder. This may even be seen in areas far from black walnut trees if this wood is worked by a local mill or cabinet shop and ends up in the resulting shavings. Black walnut should be immediately suspected if founder occurs when the shavings used for bedding are changed. If you use wood shavings for bedding, it is best to ask if there might be any black walnut wood in them. Don't use them if there is ANY black walnut present.

The administration of drugs, such as strong laxatives or corticosteroids, have occasionally been felt to cause founder. Overeating on feeds, such as beet tops, has been reported to cause founder. Ponies have a greater risk of occurrence of laminitis, but the most severely crippling cases invariably occur in horses.

Insufficient exercise may predispose an animal to laminitis as can feet which are too small to support the animal's weight. This problem is said to occur on sea voyages where the horse cannot move and has so little space that he cannot lie down. Seagoing horses must have their feed kept to a maintenance level and be exercised for a short period of time daily, if possible.

Horses who have one severely injured leg may place enough weight on one or more of the remaining legs that laminitis will occur.

SIGNS

ACUTE LAMINITIS

Acute laminitis most commonly affects the front feet, but, in severe cases, all four may be involved. If all four feet are affected, the animal may lie down for long periods. Or, the animal may be standing and in too much pain to lift a single foot. For this reason, he may not move even when pushed or pulled.

Early in a case of laminitis, the horse may not show lameness, but may have a short, stilted trot. Later, the gait may be stilted at a walk, and the horse may be reluctant to move without being forced. When the horse is standing, the hind feet will be pulled forward under the body to take much of the body weight off the front feet. The front feet are usually pushed far forward of their normal position. They may also occasionally be pulled backward, giving a very poor base of support. In any case, the animal will be unwilling to move and will vigorously resist any attempt to lift a foot.

An excessively strong pulse may be felt in the digital arteries over the fetlock joint, due to increased arterial blood pressure in the foot. Laminitis may also cause the feet to feel warm or hot. Swelling of the sensitive laminae can ultimately result in a reduced blood supply to the feet. Increased blood output by the heart and increased blood flow in the upper leg may be, paradoxically, associated with the reduced blood supply in the feet. Decreased levels of potassium, sodium, and chloride are seen in a blood sample, along with increased concentration of red blood cells and total protein. Plasma fluid content is decreased in horses but not in ponies. Acidosis has been seen in blood samples taken prior to the onset of lameness.

Anxiety and muscular trembling may be observed from the severe pain of laminitis. The respiratory rate is usually increased and the temperature is elevated. Muddy (brownish or mud-colored) mucous membranes may be seen. If you can even lift one foot to use a hoof tester, the entire sole area will often show tenderness. The tenderness may be more severe ahead of the point of the frog. Especially with grain founder, the horse may have diarrhea.

Signs of grain founder may be seen within a few hours after eating the feed, but frequently do not appear until 12 to 18 hours later. This time lag often lulls the owner into a false sense of security, thinking that the animal has eaten the grain but is not going to show any ill effects from it. Then, the diarrhea, pain, muscular tremors, and other signs appear as mentioned above.

Rotation of the coffin bone may occur in severe cases of founder within as little as 12 hours from the time the animal has ingested the offending feed or suffered injury. This makes it VERY important to treat any animal suspected of grain overload or other laminitis-producing problem IMMEDIATELY. If you wait until the animal shows signs of laminitis, the permanent damage may already have been done to his feet. Most veterinarians would rather treat early and have it be unnecessary rather than to wait and see what happens and have the horse suffer severe hoof problems or go into a chronic laminitis.

If the laminitis is due to a uterine infection after foaling, the mare's temperature may rise to 104 to 106 degrees F (40 to 41 C). Pulse and respiration rates may be increased considerably. An examination of the uterus may show large amounts of dark watery fluid and possibly pieces of fetal membranes.

Death from acute laminitis may be seen, but is not common. With any severe laminitis, the hoof may slough because of the separation of the sensitive and insensitive laminae due to infection or simple fluid accumulation creating enough pressure to force them apart.

Current thinking favors the following sequence of events in the development of laminitis: intake of excessive carbohydrates (sugars and starches) or other metabolic upset triggers excess growth of lactic-acid-producing bacteria (and a corresponding decrease in other types of bacteria). The bacteria increase the acid content within the intestine which dissolves the walls of one type of bacteria (called gram-negative bacteria), releasing a chemical called an endotoxin.

The high acid content also stops the intestinal lining from acting normally to keep out the toxins, allowing them to be absorbed and to affect the circulatory system. The result is a degeneration of cells in the liver which can no longer act to strain out the toxin. As a result, the blood may be carrying both excess acid and endotoxin products. Small blood vessels may be damaged throughout the body, especially in the feet. This impairs the circulation to the feet, depriving them of blood containing oxygen and nutrients necessary for the delicate laminae. The blood seeks shunts and bypasses the feet, leading to further accumulation of toxic products in the feet. The blood flow is decreased, preventing return flow to the heart and compounding the problem. If this shutdown is severe enough, the hooves will slough.

CHRONIC LAMINITIS

Radiographs show downward rotation of the third phalanx in chronic laminitis. If severe enough, the toe of the coffin bone may push out through the sole of the foot usually necessitating euthansia of the horse. This rotation may be started by the inflammation causing separation of the sensitive and insensitive laminae, as well as different growth rates of the hoof wall between the quarter and toe areas. The pull of the deep flexor tendon at its attachment on the rear part of the coffin bone may also help in moving the bone around to the abnormal position.

Once the coffin bone has rotated, it cannot be returned to its normal position without trimming the foot to make the bottom of the coffin bone parallel to the ground. Plastic fillers may be used to help restore the hoof shape to normal. Horses with chronic laminitis tend to land on the heel of the foot. The sole may be dropped and flat with excessive quantities of flaky material. Infection, such as thrush, may invade this flaky sole, destroying what little protection remains over the coffin bone. Severe laminitis may result in the hooves sloughing completely.

Chronic inflammation causes the hoof wall to grow more rapidly than normal, resulting in a long toe that curls up at the end. In ponies this frequently shows up as sled-runner feet that may be 12 to 15 inches long or more. Consequently, the animal may be nearly unable to walk. Heavy ring formation also occurs on the hoof wall and usually persists for the life of the horse. This is due to inflammation and changes in the coronary band.

Diagnosis of laminitis is usually easily made by clinical signs. The animal shows a typical stance, a heavy, strong pulse in the digital arteries, heat in the foot, and pain when tested with hoof testers. With chronic laminitis, typical rings are seen on the hoof wall and a characteristic gait or stance is often seen. It may be difficult or impossible to determine the cause of a case of laminitis.

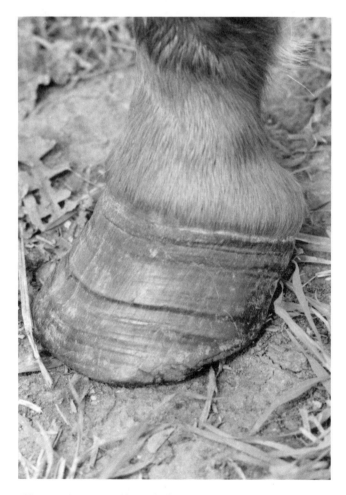

Chronic laminitis (founder).

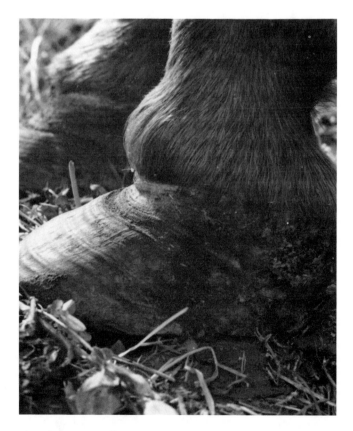

Another case of chronic founder.

TREATMENT OF ACUTE LAMINITIS

Acute laminitis should always be considered an emergency because irreversible changes have been shown to occur as early as 12 hours after lameness starts. Even then, permanent damage may be unavoidable. Call your veterinarian IMMEDIATELY.

Treatment varies with the type of founder. Grain founder is treated by attempting to counteract the effects of grain overload. Some type of laxative is usually administered to help speed the grain and toxins out of the digestive tract, as well as to help neutralize toxic products of grain digestion. Your veterinarian may use mineral oil or other laxative via stomach tube to help remove the grain from the digestive tract. He may give an injectable laxative to help move the oil through the horse. Don't mess around trying to give bran or other slow acting laxative to one of these animals. They work too slowly. Again, lack of immediate treatment may result in permanent damage to your horse.

Your veterinarian may administer other drugs, such as antihistamines, as well as medication to help control pain in the feet and make the animal more comfortable. Corticosteroids are usually not recommended because, in some cases, they have been shown to cause laminitis. Founder which has been caused by corticosteroids (as well as that caused by other drugs) generally has a poor prognosis. Oral antibiotics may be included with the laxative to help kill bacteria which are producing endotoxins in the digestive tract.

If the animal is in shock due to pain or dehydration, your veterinarian may administer intravenous fluids. Traditionally, the animal's feet have been soaked in cool mud or sand or in a running stream. While this temporarily relieves pain in the feet, it may be detrimental in the long run because it slows circulation in the feet at the time when it needs to be increased, not retarded. Warm soaks will help to dilate the blood vessels and improve circulation. (45)

Mechanical support for the soles of the feet helps to prevent rotation of the coffin bone. Allow the horse to lie down if he wishes. Horses are often stood in mud or a running stream, but this does not permit them to lie down. If the animal is wearing shoes, they should be removed if the horse's feet can be held up. If the feet cannot be picked up because of the pain, a sharp chisel may be used to cut the nails and allow removal of the shoes. This procedure is often easier if the nerves to the horse's feet have been blocked. Hammering on a foot afflicted with acute laminitis would be the most exquisite form of torture—a lot like bamboo slivers under your fingernails!

Current thinking favors forced exercise (after administration of appropriate painkillers) to help circulation in the feet. Normal circulation within the hoof is partially dependent on the pumping action created as the animal walks. Getting the animal walking helps to restore circulation and will often allow the horse to recover more rapidly with less damage. In some cases, it may be necessary for your veterinarian to block the nerves to the foot to allow the animal to be walked. The nerve block(s) may have to be done several times a day for a few days.

Mild exercise may also be helpful in providing sole pressure and lessening the chance of coffin bone rotation. Walk the horse slowly on soft ground for 10 or 15 minutes every hour for 24 hours, and then stop the exercise. Benefits from exercise are only seen with acute laminits; with less acute or chronic cases, exercise will not help, and may actually be harmful.

Oral administration of the amino acid methionine may help provide compounds necessary for rebuilding the bond between hoof wall and bone. One authority recommends removing salt from the animal's diet and replacing it with one ounce of potassium chloride per day in the drinking water. This idea is similar to that used in treating high blood pressure in humans. Immediate elimination of all grain from the diet and feeding high-quality grass and legume hay is recommended until the animal is well. Similar treatments may be used in cases of water or road founder.

Postparturient laminitis treatment begins by treating the metritis (uterine infection) which caused it in the first place. Your veterinarian will remove any membranes that have been retained in the uterus. He may place antibiotics in the uterus. Drugs to help shrink the uterus and encourage explusion of the infected matter may be injected into the mare. The mare is usually placed on injections of antibiotics for three to five days. Additionally, drugs to reduce both pain and inflammation may be given. The feet may be treated as above.

Grass founder is treated the same as grain founder. A crash diet may be necessary to get the animal down to a normal weight. Hormone treatments or thyroid medications are sometimes used to counteract the action of hormones in the grass and speed up metabolism in general. Put the animal on good quality grass hay (without any legumes if you can get it) until the animal is through the problem. Then, gradually put the animal back on legume hay (if that is what you have been feeding), stopping it immediately if he appears lame.

TREATMENT OF CHRONIC LAMINITIS

Rotation of the coffin bone may occur in severe cases of founder within days or even hours after the initial problem. In other cases, it may take some months or even years to occur. When it does happen, it is life-threatening. The reason for this is that if the point of the coffin bone penetrates the sole of the hoof, infection and damage to the bone usually follow. The damage can rarely be repaired. If it can be fixed, it is usually more of a salvage operation (where you end up with a breeding animal) than a return to usefulness. For this reason, every effort must be made to keep the penetration from occurring. Prevention means that we must deal with the tendency toward rotation and minimize it. In the worst cases of founder, the best treatment in the world may not work, and the owner may be lucky even to save the horse for breeding use.

When laminitis reaches the chronic stage, treatment consists mostly of regular and diligent hoof care. The hoof should be trimmed as nearly normal as possible. Horses who have been foundered usually need their hooves trimmed more often than the normal horse—often every six weeks. Hoof care cannot be neglected in the winter when many northern animals are turned out and not seen again until spring. This practice may result in loss of use of the horse or may even be a death sentence for him if his feet get in bad enough shape that he can't travel and care for himself.

Frequent trimming is needed to help keep the toe from growing too long and throwing the hoof angle off again. Excess toe length also contributes to the rotation that is occurring in the coffin bone; removing it helps stop the rotation. The heels may need to be lowered in order to bring the coffin bone back to a more normal angle in relationship to the hoof wall. Excess toe length should be removed at the same time. Sometimes acrylic or fiberglass material may be used by the farrier to build the hoof back to a more normal shape if it is deformed or badly changed. If this type of treatment is used, it must be modified approximately every six weeks until the foot resumes a more normal appearance and the coffin bone begins to go back to its normal position.

If your veterinarian has x-rayed the horse's feet, he can often give you a better idea of how much to lower the heels to coincide with the animal's needs. The horse's feet may (and often do) differ from each other in a laminitis case, and different shoeing may be needed from one to another.

Wide-webbed shoes may be used to help prevent further dropping of the sole. Additional protection may be given with rubber or leather pads or a sheet metal plate. Do not use the pad unless you need it. Remove as much of the old, dead sole as your vet and farrier feel is safe. If the coffin bone comes through the bottom of the foot, that is the worst possible thing that can happen and often makes it necessary to euthanize the animal.

It is often helpful to either square the toe or to round it off slightly more than normal to help the animal break over the toe more easily.

Combined with corrective shoeing, the hoof wall may be grooved, or the hoof quarters thinned by rasping to allow expansion of the quarters. The nerves to the foot may be ultimately surgically cut to relieve pain, but this practice is discouraged because a median or volar neurectomy is most commonly used (in contrast to the posterior digital neurectomy used with navicular disease). The median or volar nerves are higher or further forward

in the foot and cutting them presents a definite danger if the horse is ridden. It would be like having the animal's foot "asleep" all the time—he wouldn't know quite where or how he is placing it on the ground. Also, he would not feel any pain if the foot were to be injured (as by stepping on a nail). Severe damage or infection could occur before it is noticed.

Infection may penetrate the sensitive laminae of a foot with chronic laminitis due to separation at the white line, similar to the condition commonly called "gravel." An infection similar to thrush may invade the flaky sole and destroy all protection to the coffin bone. Thrush may also occur in animals who have flat, thin soles which become cracked or are softened because of too much soaking. "Seedy toe," resulting from separation of the sensitive and insensitive laminae, is usually present in chronic laminitis.

If infection is present in the sensitive tissues because of a defect in the white line, the defect should be opened to allow drainage. The foot should be treated with strong (7%) tincture of iodine and kept bandaged. A tetanus booster or antitoxin shot should be given if this occurs. Do not put pads under shoes until the infection is completely controlled.

Weight control is of the utmost importance in the foundered animal. Careful management may significantly increase the animal's chances of being usable. Many animals with chronic founder are "easy keepers," to say the least! It's often hard to say whether the animal became overweight after he foundered, or whether the overweight existed previously and contributed to the problem. In many cases, the chunky, heavy animal with a large, crested neck is more prone to founder than is one of a normal size and shape. In any case, the more weight the animal is carrying, the more pressure and strain it puts on the feet and the greater the degree of pain that it causes. Many foundered horses have to be put on perpetual diets for the rest of their lives.

PROGNOSIS

A foundered horse may or may not be usable. A horse with a mild case and few changes in the hoof may be useful for years with only a little extra care. If the symptoms persist for more than 10 days, the outcome is likely to be unfavorable. Some cases, such as those associated with hormone imbalance, may continue for months or even years without causing more than mild changes in the feet. Some cases may continue for a long time and then become sound, but with malformation of the hooves. These animals often show rotation of the coffin bone when radiographed. Rotation of the coffin bone is an unfavorable sign. If cracks appear around the coronary band, the hoof is likely to fall off, again making the outcome unfavorable. Any infection makes the outcome unfavorable.

The degree of rotation seen on x-rays gives a good

indication as to whether or not the animal will return to usability. Animals with a lesser amount of rotation (less than 5–½ degrees) usually regain their full athletic ability. Horses with more than 11–½ degrees of rotation usually lose their usefulness. Ponies tend to have more rotation of their coffin bone than do horses. (46)

Because of the changes it makes in hoof growth patterns, founder often causes rings to appear around the horse's hooves. They are typically about ¼ inch deep and run around the hoof parallel to coronary band. If you see these rings on a horse that you are thinking of buying, it might be best to have the feet x-rayed prior to purchase to see if there is rotation of the coffin bone which may give you serious problems in the future. Horses sometimes have shallow grooves running around the width of the hoof. These are different from founder rings and generally have no significance.

PREVENTION

Feeding a large amount of hay in relation to the amount of grain fed considerably reduces the risk of laminitis. Sudden changes in feed quantity, quality, and type should be avoided. Sudden changes in the amount of exercise, large amounts of cold water after hard work or on a hot day, and unrestricted grazing of lush grasses should be avoided. Make sure that all membranes are removed from your mare after foaling. Try to eliminate combinations of stresses which, when added together, lead to laminitis.

AZOTURIA (MONDAY MORNING SICKNESS, TYING-UP)

Azoturia is a an inflammation leading to destruction of the skeletal muscles. It is also called Monday morning sickness because it occurred in work horses who were fed the same amount of feed all the time, but were given Sunday or Saturday and Sunday off. These animals became ill with azoturia when they were put back to work on Monday morning. Similar problems may occur when unfit and overweight horses who are being fed at high nutritional levels are suddenly put to hard work. Azoturia may be more common in younger animals. It is also seen more frequently in animals with exceptionally heavy muscling, such as draft horses and some Quarter Horses. Nervous animals or horses who are exercised in cold, damp weather may also be more susceptible to azoturia. Tying-up (also called cording-up) is thought to be a mild form of the same problem.

IMPORTANT NOTE: Tying-up can occur in horses who are used extremely hard, such as on endurance rides. Many of these horses are in severe pain and may act as if they have a colic. An attempt to walk the horse with a myositis can result in permanent damage. Until proven otherwise, assume that the horse has a muscular problem and rest him until he has been examined by a veterinarian. Colics are much less common in this situation. When in doubt, do NOT walk an endurance horse who is in distress!

CAUSES AND SIGNS

Either azoturia or tying-up may be seen in a horse who is on a regular schedule of hard exercise and good feed, especially with grain being fed. The animal is then not used for a day to three or four days, but without the feed being reduced accordingly. The amount of work necessary to cause azoturia is often very small. Azoturia can occur after an animal is cast for a surgical procedure. For this reason, it is often advisable to withhold feed for 24 hours prior to surgery that will necessitate laying the animal down.

When the animal is put back to work after a day or two of rest, he may begin the workout by moving normally, but then become increasingly sluggish and unwilling to move. He may sweat profusely, often to the point of having sweat running down his body although he is standing still. The pulse rate will be elevated. The animal is stiff in the hindquarters, moves only when forced to, and shows considerable pain when he does move. The muscles over the rump are very firm and hard and the horse may show pain when this area is palpated firmly. Some animals become uncoordinated and may show muscle tremors.

In severe cases, the urine may be reddish (this is a deep wine-red, not a bright, fresh-blood-red) or brownish. In some animals, the urine will be nearly black. This color is due to breakdown products released from damaged muscle tissue. In azoturia, the animal may lie down and be unwilling or unable to rise. Some animals assume a "dog-sitting" posture.

Animals who "tie-up" usually show a milder combination of these symptoms. Some will show pain only in the back and may walk with the loin area held rigid. The back muscles are hard to the touch and the animal may show severe pain when they are palpated. These horses usually do not show the urine discoloration seen with azoturia.

Azoturia is thought to occur because a chemical compound called glycogen has accumulated in the muscles from the rich feed during the rest period. Normally, this is used to help fuel the muscles when the animal is worked. In azoturia, the glycogen is used so rapidly and in such large quantity that it forms large amounts of lactic acid (its breakdown product) in the muscles. The lactic acid destroys the muscle fibers. As the waste products from the muscle breakdown are removed, they are filtered out by the kidneys and passed in the urine, giving it the dark color. Occasionally, animals suffer kidney damage as these organs try to remove the breakdown products from the bloodstream. These horses may suffer permanent damage or even die.

TREATMENT

Nursing is of the utmost importance with these diseases. If you are out riding when this occurs, stop immediately and get off the horse. Get a trailer to the animal if at all possible and HAUL the animal back to the stable. Do not ask the animal to walk if there is any way to avoid it, as continued movement may make the problem immeasurably worse. If the animal is standing, he should be blanketed and kept warm and comfortable.

The horse should not be allowed any grain and should be fed only small amounts of hay. It is important that the horse have water available at all times. Rest should be continued for several days to several weeks after all signs of problems have disappeared, depending on the severity of the attack. Feed should be increased gradually as the animal recuperates. The animal should be gradually brought back into training, starting with hand-walking.

Horses who are down should have plenty of deep, soft bedding. The animal should be turned from side to side frequently to help his circulation and help prevent "bedsores." Avoid trying to get the animal up before he is ready to rise. Our instinct is to get the animal to his feet as soon as possible, but the animal who tries to rise before he is ready may cause further damage to the muscles and may become so injured that he will never rise. Be patient as the animal's muscles heal and keep up the careful, supportive nursing. When the animal is ready to get up, give him help if needed.

Most veterinarians treat these animals with a mixture of vitamin E and selenium. The recovery after the administration of this medication is often nothing short of miraculous. The animal relaxes immediately and shows pain relief. This combination of drugs seems to be a specific treatment for the problem and works in most cases. B-complex vitamins are also used to treat these problems. Drugs, such as phenylbutazone or other non-steroidal anti-inflammatory agents which both relieve pain and help treat some of the problems within the muscles themselves, may be given. A severely stressed endurance horse may also be given fluids to help restore his fluid balance and to aid the kidneys in flushing out the muscle breakdown products.

Animals who are severely affected may require intravenous medication to reduce the acidity and help stop the muscular damage. The animal may also be treated via stomach tube to neutralize the excess acid in his system. Corticosteroids are sometimes given, as well as antihistamines. Nervous or thrashing animals should be tranquilized or otherwise sedated to relieve their anxiety. If it looks as though the animal may be down for some time, your veterinarian may want to stomach tube him and administer mineral oil or other laxative to help keep the intestinal contents moving normally.

Horses who are showing only the back pain of tying-up are treated differently. Slow walking for 30 to 45 minutes will often relieve the pain and return the animal to normal. These horses can be medicated as for azoturia.

PROGNOSIS

The outcome of this metabolic problem depends on the amount of destruction of muscle tissue and scarring which has occurred. The outcome is better for animals which remain on their feet. It is also favorable for animals who go down (because they have lost the use of their hindquarters), if they remain quiet and do not thrash around and cause further muscle damage, provided that they are back to normal within 24 hours. Animals who come through a myositis may suffer from lameness. Occasionally, they will show prolonged or permanent shrinkage of the involved muscles.

The prognosis is unfavorable for nervous, high-strung animals who go down and cannot be calmed with tranquilizers or other sedatives. Severe muscle damage can be caused by forcing the animal to continue moving after the problem becomes apparent. If, after 24 hours, the horse is unable to at least roll onto its chest and remain upright, this is an unfavorable sign.

Animals who tie-up apparently have little muscle damage and do not get the scarring that occurs with azoturia. They are, however, prone to having the problem recur and should be managed accordingly.

PREVENTION

These problems are, for the most part, preventable. When the horse is being fed a considerable amount of feed (especially grain) and worked hard, reduce the amount of grain on the rest days. Unfortunately, once this problem has occurred, the animal may be susceptible to azoturia for the rest of his life. Some horses may need a preventive injection of vitamin E-selenium every 3 to 6 months for the rest of their lives, especially if they are in competition or otherwise working hard. Giving two to four ounces of bicarbonate of soda (baking soda) per day may help prevent myositis in animals who are especially prone to it. This is easily done by adding it to the horse's grain. Make sure the animal has access to as much salt as he wants to eat and to adequate water at all times.

Animals who are prone to tie-up should have their grain ration cut in half for 24 hours before they are used in performance or racing. As with azoturia, feeding baking soda with the grain ration may be helpful.

Keeping the animal on a careful feeding routine that varies little from day to day is helpful in preventing recurrences in some animals. The ration should be well-balanced and should be gauged to keep the animal a little on the lean side. A commercial grain mix is often a better feed choice than eyeballing a homemade mixture. The grain should be carefully measured, as should the amount of hay fed. If exercise varies from day to day, the amount of grain fed should be adjusted accordingly. Ideally, the exercise level should be the same from day to day. If the problem horse is only ridden on weekends, balancing feed and exercise may be impossible. It may, in some cases, be advisable to trade the horse for one who is less sensitive.

NAVICULAR DISEASE

The navicular bone is a small flat bone which lies inside the hoof. It is located between the coffin and pastern bones, where it acts as a pulley for the deep digital flexor tendon.

Navicular disease is thought to begin as a bursitis of the bursa (fluid-filled pocket) between the navicular bone and the deep flexor tendon. Navicular disease goes on to become a chronic inflammation of the bone. The cartilage may become roughened and pitted on its joint surface. Calcium deposits may organize themselves into new bony growth on the bone itself. This usually occurs on the sides ("wings") of the bone. There may be spots where the bone becomes thinner and pitted with a hole or holes, looking a bit like a section of Swiss cheese. This can weaken the bone and predispose it to a fracture at the weakened site.

The bursitis in the bursa which cushions the bone may be followed by adhesions between the bone and the deep digital flexor tendon. Calcification may occasionally be seen in the ligaments which suspend the navicular bone, especially those at the ends of the bone. In some cases, the tendon becomes so weakened that it ruptures. This complication is usually seen after neurectomy. The part of the navicular bone which adjoins the coffin joint may be involved, resulting in arthritis of the coffin joint. Ligaments attached to the navicular bone are almost always involved and may cause much of the pain seen with the disease.

Occasionally, only one front foot is affected. Nearly all cases of navicular disease, however, involve both front feet. Initially, it may appear that only one foot is affected. However, if the nerves to this foot are blocked, lameness is usually evident in the other front foot. The disease is not reported in the hind feet.

Heredity is felt to be involved in the development of navicular disease. It is more commonly seen in some families of Quarter Horses than others. Extra weight on the animal aggravates the condition. A good example of this is a 1200 to 1400 lb. animal who is standing on a 00 shoe. His feet are not big enough to adequately absorb the shock of the foot hitting the ground. This concussion is definitely a contributing factor in navicular disease. Horses doing strenuous work involving landing or stopping hard often develop navicular disease. Hunters, jumpers, cutting horses, reining horses, and rope horses are more prone to it than, for example, western pleasure horses who are used at slow speeds and not asked to stop or turn hard. Horses used for barrel racing can often be seen to have navicular disease in both front feet, but to have it worst on the side to which they turn two barrels. Here, the inside foot on the turn is taking a larger percentage of the concussion than the outer foot.

Conformation can contribute to navicular problems: horses with upright pasterns and straight shoulders have less shock-absorbing ability than horses with a normal angle to the shoulder and pastern. Each step they take has less cushioning, creating more concussion on the foot and its internal structures.

Many horses who have navicular disease have a long toe with a low, underslung heel. If the disease has been present for a long time, the feet may take on a characteristic "navicular disease look." This is a upright foot with a narrow, contracted heel. Since this change may occur in the feet after the disease is evident, it is sometimes hard to determine which came first, the foot shape or the disease. However, many long-term cases of navicular disease do not have this hoof appearance and may, indeed, look completely normal.

Wounds which penetrate the frog can contact the navicular bone or its surrounding structures and start navicular disease. A case of sidebone may occasionally extend to the suspensory ligaments of the navicular bone.

Improper shoeing may contribute to navicular disease. A farrier may trim the heel too short on an animal with upright pasterns. The short heel would throw the pastern and foot out of line with each other and result in increased pressure from the deep flexor tendon on the navicular bone.

SIGNS

The signs of navicular disease come on very gradually. For this reason, the disease is often well advanced by the time the owner notices it. Early cases may show lameness which comes and goes, becoming noticeably less when the animal is rested. The animal may be significantly worse the morning after he is worked hard. The horse improves when rested, causing the owner to think that he is getting well, but becomes worse when worked again.

In the early stages of navicular disease, the horse may point his feet, putting first one and then the other forward to take the weight off them. Moving them forward also helps to relieve pressure of the deep flexor tendon on the navicular bone. This foot-pointing is said by some people to be symptomatic of navicular disease. This is not true—the animal may point his feet with ANY discomfort below the fetlock joint simply in an effort to reduce weight on the foot.

The animal will not stride out normally, but will shuffle his feet and take short steps. The problem may be very noticeable when only one foot is affected. The horse tries to land on the toe to avoid the pain. The attempt to avoid hurting the heel area will hinder reining and roping horses who must stop hard. A racehorse will be slowed because the forward phase of his stride is shortened. Trying to land on the toe will make the horse more likely to injure the fetlock area, as well as making him more likely to stumble.

The toe of the hoof or shoe may be badly worn. The animal will appear more lame on rocky or rough ground because of the sharp pressure on the frog. Bruising on the toe because the animal is constantly landing there may be mistaken for a problem in itself. If it becomes bad enough, the animal may then try to walk on his heels, looking like a case of founder.

When both feet are involved, the horse may try to point and/or shuffle both feet and will be less dramatically lame. This shows up better on hard ground. The lameness is more evident when the animal is turned in a short circle. He may both wince and shuffle or drag the foot on the inside of the circle as he is turned. The horse may attempt to rotate on the foot rather than picking it up to take a step. The shuffling gait often leads people to think that the lameness is in the shoulder or shoulders. This gait, combined with the improper landing of the feet, give the rider of a navicular animal a jarring, unpleasant ride.

Hoof testers will show the horse to be lame when one tong is placed on the outside wall while the other is placed on the sole or frog. Pain is worst over the middle third of the frog. It will also be painful to the animal when clamped across the outside of the heels, approximately two inches forward from the rear of the foot. Response to the hoof testers should be compared to the other front foot (remembering that navicular disease may be present in it to a lesser degree) as well as to the hind feet on the same animal.

At the same time, the sole must be carefully checked to rule out sole abscesses, corns, and other hoof problems. The sole is often bruised in cases of navicular disease, especially on the less-affected foot. This may make it difficult to separate the amount of pain due to the sole bruising and that due to navicular disease.

Horses who have navicular disease may develop contracted heels. The hoof may become narrow and high in the walls. Horses with navicular disease which is worse in one hoof may have that hoof become upright and narrowed. The opposite foot, which is bearing most of the animal's weight, becomes widened and flattened. Strain on this foot is greatly increased, and the fetlock may be chronically swollen. The sole of this foot may have sole bruises and be highly sensitive to pressure because it is bearing so great a proportion of the animal's weight; it may be badly "run under" at the heel.

Severe cases of navicular disease may show atrophy (shrinking) of muscles in the forearm and shoulder muscles. These changes are not seen in all cases of navicular disease. Some horses may show clinical signs of navicular disease and be quite lame, yet not show visible changes in the hoof. One of my clients owned a good cutting mare who had had a mild clinical case of navicular disease for four years. It was enough to cause her to be unable to walk comfortably on hard or rocky ground and to stumble. This animal never developed any hoof changes, nor did she ever have any visible signs of navicular disease on x-rays. It is not unusual for the horse to have enough damage somewhere in the joint or around the bone to cause clinical lameness, but not enough to confirm by x-rays. Adams claimed that only 50% of cases showed damage on x-rays. (47)

DIAGNOSIS

If you have tentatively diagnosed your horse as having navicular disease, the next step is to take him to your veterinarian. He will use nerve blocks to see whether the animal goes sound when the pain is removed from the feet. Most veterinarians will then take x-rays. As mentioned above, about half of the animals do not show changes on x-rays. If x-rays do show changes, however, they will either be changes typical of navicular disease or a navicular fracture. We arrived at a diagnosis of navicular disease on the mare mentioned above by observation of her gait, use of hoof testers, and the use of nerve blocks. Incidentally, remember that lamenesses do not always come in neat packages by themselves: a case of navicular disease may be complicated by or accompanied by ringbone, arthritis in the coffin joint, fetlock injury (osselets), and numerous other problems. A few horses will show severe radiographic changes in the navicular bone, yet be clinically and usably sound; these, unfortunately, are in the minority.

X-rays of animals with navicular disease may show numerous small bony growths on the wings of the navicular bone. Pitting of the joint surface may be seen, as may be the rarefied holes in the body of the bone. X-rays should always be taken in a suspected case of navicular disease. They may not conclusively prove that the animal has the disease (as with the above mare). If, however, the animal is proven to have navicular disease, you may be able to get an idea of how severe the problem is and how it can be managed, as well as what you can expect from the animal in terms of a working future.

In any case, navicular disease reduces the animal's chances for a long, useful life. It is hard to imagine a circumstance under which one should purchase an animal with known navicular disease to be used for hard work or performance. The useful life of a horse is unpredictable enough without starting with a problem as incurable as this one.

TREATMENT

The best approach at the present time seems to be a combination of careful and conscientious shoeing, together with medication to relieve pain when needed. Neurectomy ("nerving") may be performed if necessary to relieve the animal's pain and, with luck, to get continued use out of him. How successful treatment is may be determined in part by how much may be expected of the animal after he is discovered to have navicular disease. Will he be expected to keep up a full schedule of work, or will he cut back to a lower level of activity? Obviously, the less work and stress on the feet, the longer the useful life of the horse.

One study reported on various types of treatment on 580 horses. The study included injection of corticosteroids into the navicular bursa, neurectomy, anabolic steroids, and several other treatments. Only 4.5% of the horses were reported sound a year later. The author concluded that no one treatment was more successful than any of the others. (48)

Another study reported that approximately 75% of the cases treated were returned to normal work as long as the shoeing was carefully maintained. This study also concluded that sufficient exercise was an important adjunct to shoeing. (49)

At the present time, there is no treatment for navicular disease that can permanently cure the problem. Treatment is totally aimed toward relieving symptoms and making the animal as comfortable as possible in an attempt to extend his useful life.

Shoe the animal with a rolled toe shoe to allow his foot to roll forward more easily. This shortens the amount of time that there is pressure on the navicular bone from the deep flexor tendon. Half-round shoes will serve the same purpose. Polo plates may be sufficient for animals early in the disease.

It is often good to use only three nails on each side of the shoe to allow the hoof to expand at the heel. This helps to prevent the contracted heels that can occur with navicular disease.

Do not use heel caulks if you can avoid them. Horses who have to turn and slide their feet (such as barrel racing and cutting or reining horses) should NOT have heel caulks used. The caulk will stick into the ground and grab as the horse swivels his body over the foot. This may result in a fractured bone in the foot. This type of horse should have carefully slippered (tapered, raised) heels on his front shoes.

Or, one of two types of bar shoe can be used. One is made by welding a tapered piece of metal across the heel, with the thin edge forward. This is easily cut from a piece of angle iron. It should be well blended into the shoe at the front so that it does not act as a grab to stop the foot. The other is made with a bar across the center third of the frog.

In either case, care should be taken that the bar does not touch the frog. If it does, it will make the navicular disease much worse.

Some animals may benefit from the use of pads. You can use either a tapered wedge pad with the thick part toward the back to help elevate the heel, or a flat pad. The pad material should be as stiff as possible to offer protection against the pressure of rocks, dirt clods, etc. on the frog. Have your farrier clean the foot extremely well before he puts on the pads and shoes. Saturate the sole with either strong tincture of iodine or Kopertox and then let it dry before putting the pads over the soles. This will help to prevent thrush, a problem that is all too common with pads.

Nail the pads and shoes on the hoof. Stand the horse on a hard, flat surface, such as pavement or a piece of plywood. Inject clear silicone caulking compound under the pad—between it and the sole of the foot. If you like, a bit of silicone hardener from an auto parts store can be mixed with the silicone. This product comes in a tube. A small amount will help the caulking to set up more rapidly, while still retaining its spongy texture. Fill each hoof with as much of the caulking or mixture as will fit into the void. Then, tape around the heel of the hoof with duct or adhesive tape. The kind of tape doesn't matter—it's just temporary protection to help hold the caulking in place until it dries. Let the horse stand in place for about an hour. He can then be turned loose in a stall or corral. Leave the tape on for four or five hours until the caulking is completely set. Remember that it will take longer to dry under the pad. After the caulking has set, remove the tape and, with a pocket knife, trim off any excess caulking which has oozed out from under the pad.

Horses with navicular disease should be shod more frequently than normal—every six weeks is good. They should not be allowed to go more than eight weeks, maximum, in order to help keep the hoof at a proper angle.

Whether pads are used or not, the foot should be trimmed with a short toe and a proportionately long heel. Do not use pads if you can get by without them, as they are a bother, and require diligent care as outlined above to help avoid developing problems under them. If care is used in removing the pads and shoes, pads can sometimes be reused.

Aspirin, phenylbutazone (one trade name is Butazolidin, Wellcome Animal Health, Kansas City, MO 64141), and other painkillers will get an animal through specific days when you need to use him. Butazolidin is now available in a paste (much like a paste wormer) which is quite convenient to use. Other medications such as naproxen (Equiproxen, Diamond, Des Moines, IA 50317) come in powder form and can be given with a bit of grain. These drugs are illegal in many shows, races, and other activities, such as competition trail rides. They are a means of extending the useful life of an animal who would otherwise be put down because of the navicular disease. They are perhaps most useful when the animal is used only intermittently, such as a rope horse who is used on weekends. Medication may be quite impractical (and prohibitively expensive) for the animal who is used on a daily basis, such as a ranch or school horse.

Posterior digital neurectomy is the treatment of last resort, when shoeing and medication do not control the pain. In this operation, the nerve which supplies the rear part of the foot is surgically cut. A section is usually removed to prevent it from growing back. This procedure leaves the animal with no feeling of where his heel is placed. It would be much like when we have our legs "go to sleep." The surgery does some good in a majority of cases where it is used. When it fails, it is thought to be due to a small branch of the nerve which cannot be located that takes a different route to the heel, leaving it with pain sensation after the main branch is cut. If this surgery does not work, you are basically at the end of the line. Surgery can be done to cut the nerve which supplies the whole foot. This makes the animal EXTREMELY dangerous to ride, as he has absolutely no idea where his foot is. That would be like having the whole of your foot "asleep" all the time. Animals who have had this surgery are barred, with good reason, from racing.

Several complications are possible following surgery to sever the nerves. Bear in mind that these are not common, but DO occasionally occur. Some horses will still show pain, as mentioned above. Other animals will have the pain decreased to where they begin to use the leg normally; those who have a severely weakened deep flexor tendon may put enough strain on it to rupture it. This may not occur for several weeks to a month after surgery. There is no treatment for this rupture.

Some animals may have the entire hoof wall slough after surgery. This problem was originally thought to be due to the lack of nerve supply to the foot, but has since been proven to be due to complications after surgery which cause sufficient damage and scar tissue formation to shut off the blood supply to the foot, leading to a gangrene. Or, the animal steps on a nail and gets an abscess in the hoof. Because the nerve is cut, he does not feel any pain and no symptoms are noticed until the hoof begins to slough. It is necessary to be extra careful when nailing shoes on a horse who has been nerved. If a nail penetrates sensitive tissues in the heel area, the animal cannot feel it. The resulting infection may become serious before it is noticed. The hooves should be cleaned frequently and thoroughly to keep an eye on their condition and to catch any nail wounds or punctures before they lead to complications.

Occasional horses have the nerves regrow after surgery. This generally occurs six months or more after the operation. You know this has happened because the animal begins to show the same pain and symptoms that he did before surgery. New surgical methods have eliminated most of these regrowths.

Other animals will form a neuroma. This is a painful growth at the cut end of the nerve and may lead to the animal becoming unusable. The lesion may also wrap around blood vessels and become extensive enough that it is nearly impossible to remove without causing damage to the vessels. As with nerve regrowth, new surgical methods are making neuromas less common.

Other treatments for navicular disease have been proposed. Most authorities feel that the changes in navicular disease are so irreversible that when it has started, it is a one-way street with no good end in sight. Some authorities also feel that when people work "cures" on navicular horses, they are not indicative of a cure, but of a wrong diagnosis. Cortisone-type drugs have been injected into the navicular bursa. They give the animal temporary relief, but do nothing to fix the problem. Certain iodine solutions have also been injected there; they cause the animal severe pain and do NOT repair the navicular disease.

FRACTURES OF THE NAVICULAR BONE

Fractures of the navicular bone are uncommon. They may occur after it is weakened by navicular disease, or may be due to injury. A sudden, violent pressure on the navicular bone can cause it to break. Navicular fractures usually occur at the weakest part of the bone, usually 1/3 of the distance from either side.

When the foot makes a hard landing from a jump, or a hard, foot-jamming stop, the bone is tightly squeezed between the tendon and the bones underneath. Imagine the pressure that is placed on it when one forefoot is planted solidly as in a stop, and the other forefoot comes by as the animal's weight rolls forward. The heel is being used as a brake, the toe is advanced as far as possible, and the tendon is pulled to its ultimate limit of tension.

Signs of a fractured navicular bone are identical to those caused by navicular disease, but will occur much more suddenly. X-rays (which should be taken in any case of navicular pain) will allow your veterinarian to tell whether it is navicular disease or a fracture.

The only treatment for a fracture which will allow the animal to move without pain is posterior digital neurectomy, as described in navicular disease, above. It does not allow all animals to be returned to use, but is worth a try if you wish to keep using the animal at all.

FRACTURED COFFIN BONE

Fracture of the third phalanx (coffin bone) is fairly common. It is more often seen in the front feet than the hind. This fracture is usually caused by injury, as when the horse's foot is firmly planted and his body weight rolls around in a different direction. It may also be broken when the animal steps on a nail. One of my clients had a stallion who fractured the coffin bone in his hind foot—he had kicked the wall of his stall. If the cartilages of the third phalanx have turned to bone in a case of sidebone, one of these "wings" may be broken off. This usually occurs at the side rather than through the middle of the bone.

The animal with a fractured coffin bone becomes lame very suddenly, and may refuse to even put his foot on the ground for as long as two to three days. The lameness may have occurred suddenly while the animal was being worked, with no apparent injury at the time. The entire sole will be painful when examined with hoof testers. Any horse with this sudden and painful a lameness should be immediately examined by your veterinarian. X-rays will confirm the presence of a fracture.

The animal is usually shod with a full bar shoe with quarter clips. The bar should be thinner than the shoe and welded toward the ground surface so as to keep from putting any pressure on the frog. The animal will need to have the shoe reset every four to six weeks, for a total treatment time of three to six months.

Six months to a year of rest are necessary so that the bone will heal properly and the animal will again be usable. If lameness persists after the bone is healed, posterior digital neurectomy may be necessary to make the animal usable. Fractures through the sides of the bone usually heal well if the horse is adequately rested and carefully shod. Fractures through the center of the bone may result in arthritis in the coffin joint; the animal may be unusable as a result.

WINDPUFFS

Also called wind galls, these fluid-filled swellings can occur on either the front or the hind legs; they are due to swelling of a tendon sheath, bursa, or joint capsule, and are caused by wear and tear. Windpuffs are most commonly seen above the fetlock, but occasionally may occur under the pastern. They are usually seen as soft swellings toward the rear of the fetlock (in front of and above the sesamoid bones). They vary from quarter to silver-dollar size. Old windpuffs may have scarring and fibrous tissue which make them feel quite firm. Lameness is rarely seen with windpuffs.

Windpuffs are common in old horses who have been used hard throughout their lives, especially rodeo and racehorses and gaited animals. They are an indication of the animal's usage, and should not be considered an unsoundness unless the horse is lame. Even then, the lameness is often due to arthritis or joint lesions rather than the windpuffs themselves. Once the joint capsule is stretched, it rarely returns to normal. Thus, when a young animal develops windpuffs, they do not usually go down much in size and become a permanent blemish.

Windpuffs occur in young horses who are worked too hard, and are especially prone to occur if the animal is also overweight for his age and stage of development. Overwork on hard ground or pavement can also bring them on. Working the animal in small circles, such as on a longe line or a hot walker, may put enough stress on the young horse to cause him to develop windpuffs even if the footing is soft and good. Nutritional imbalances may contribute to the development of windpuffs in young animals in heavy training.

If you notice the windpuffs right after they have occurred, treatment may be helpful. Soak the animal's feet in cold water or wrap them with ice packs. Do this intermittently the first 24 to 48 hours. Pressure bandages may be helpful—be sure to wrap them all the way down around the hoof to prevent swelling below the bandage. If swelling is still present after 2 to 3 days, call your veterinarian. He may wish to inject the swelling with a corticosteroid to help reduce the inflammation. As with a bowed tendon, rest is extremely important to healing. Older windpuffs do not require treatment, as nothing is effective in reducing them. Animals who have windpuffs and are lame should be x-rayed to rule out chip fractures, arthritis, or other problems.

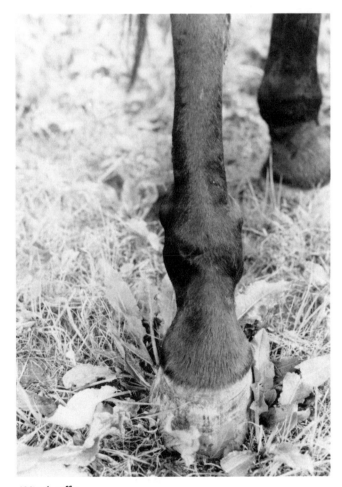

Windpuffs

RINGBONE

The term ringbone is commonly used to refer to disease and erosion of the joint surface of one or more joints from the fetlock down. An arthritis sooner or later occurs. This is followed by the development of small spurs of bone (called osteophytes) around the edges of the joint surface. Severe cases may have enough arthritis that the joint cartilage is destroyed and the two bones fuse across the former joint space.

Diagnosis of this problem is complicated by the fact that bones below the fetlock easily develop swellings of new bone growth which may be quite large. These are called "false ringbone." In false ringbone, the bony spurs are present, but the joint surface is normal.

Both true and false ringbone seem to have a hereditary predisposition. The nature and amount of work for which the horse has been used may also influence its development. Animals who have suffered concussion from being worked hard on pavement or on uneven, rocky footing may be more prone to ringbone. Some animals may be more susceptible to the effects of concussion than are others. Thoroughbreds, who tend to pull their front legs far forward and land more on their heels than on the flat part of the sole, rarely seem to have ringbone. Big draft horses with large flat feet and high knee action tend to hammer their feet onto the ground quite hard. It is in these animals that ringbone is quite likely to occur.

Ringbone may also result from damage, such as wirecuts or blows to the coronary band, as well as from faulty shoeing or rope burns. Animals suffering from ringbone from these injuries may remain lame for many months and later become sound. Ringbone may occur as a sequel to degenerative bone diseases, such as rickets and osteomalacia.

Some conformational problems predispose horses to ringbone. Animals who are base-narrow often have ringbone on the outside of the foot, while animals who are base-wide may show it on the inside. Horses with short, straight pasterns are susceptible to ringbone. Ringbone has been considered to be inherited by some authors. Any heritability involved is probably due to poor conformation.

In either true or false ringbone, the bony spurs from near the two joint surfaces may meet and fuse the two bones together, a process called ankylosis. It quite effectively immobilizes the joint, usually resulting in a reduction of the pain which the animal shows. Unfortunately, it is also accompanied by a lessening of flexibility in the joint, resulting in a change in gait. If your veterinarian anesthetizes the animal from the fetlock on down, the impairment in gait will remain.

Ringbone occurs in two locations. It is called high ringbone when it occurs on the lower end of the first phalanx and the pastern joint. It is called low ringbone if it involves the lower end of the second phalanx and the coffin joint.

SIGNS

Heat and swelling are usually present over the involved area, and the animal may flinch when palpated over an active ringbone. It is extremely difficult (if not downright impossible) to tell by running your fingers over a swelling whether it is true or false ringbone. If a severe lameness has appeared within the past few weeks, true ringbone should be suspected. At this point, the swelling may still be compressible and can be traced around the edges of the joint surface. At this early stage, x-rays will usually not show significant changes. The bony growth of false ringbone usually forms first around the shaft of the bone and later extends to the edges of the joint surface. The rate of growth of false ringbone is usually much faster and larger than in early cases of true ringbone. These generalities do not always hold true as there is considerable variation in the position and rate of growth of individual lesions.

The effects of concussion on the articular cartilage may be seen on the joint cartilage of an animal with ringbone. The cartilage does not contain any blood vessels, lymphatics, or nerves, but is nourished by a highly vascular (filled with blood vessels) layer under it. Concussion causes the bone under the cartilage to turn from pinkish-gray to a purple or dark blue color, looking very much like it is bruised. The inflammatory changes travel down the length of the bone to the vascular layer around the cartilage. Exudates form, isolating areas of the joint cartilage from the tissue underneath. Death of the cartilage occurs, followed by ulceration. Inflammation usually begins at the attachments of the collateral (side) ligaments of the involved joint. In high ringbone, it also occurs at the lower attachment of the superficial digital flexor tendon. From these starting points, the inflammation and growth of bony spurs proceeds around the bone.

How lame the animal appears is determined by how badly the bone growths press outward from under the extensor tendon on the top side of the foot or the deep digital flexor tendon below. The new bone growth also invades the involved joint and may lead to a solid fusion of that joint. High ringbones are slightly more common than low ones. Ringbone may occur in any of the four feet without preference.

Changes in the gait may help to locate the exact site of the ringbone. When it occurs on the front of the foot, the heel will often strike the ground first. When it occurs in the rear of the foot, the toe often hits first. The fetlock of the affected foot may be held rigid. This produces a hitch in the flight as the foot travels through its arc. These changes occur only in well-developed cases; they are not seen in early cases of ringbone. Lameness is usually evident at all gaits.

A high ringbone which has been present for some time will show a convex bulge on the upper surface of the pastern. Low ringbone will often cause a bulge or swelling just below the coronary band at the front of the foot. There is usually no heat present. Swelling is the result of underlying bony spur growth (calcium deposits).

Early in the course of ringbone, the animal will warm out of the lameness. As the disease progresses, the lameness becomes constant. It may even increase as the animal is worked. These changes are often seen before there is enough new bone growth to be felt with your hand. X-rays by your veterinarian can demonstrate the bony lesions of ringbone before they can be clearly palpated.

TREATMENT

Because of the arthritic changes in the joint which are involved in true ringbone, treatment does not work well. Animals with cases of false ringbone may recover in time, whether or not they are treated. Since there is little chance of permanent recovery in cases of true ringbone, a decision needs to be made weighing the chance of recovery versus the costs of providing for an idle horse for a prolonged period of time.

Left to themselves with adequate rest, the two joint surfaces may produce enough bony material to fuse the joint. Fusion leaves the joint as a solid rather than a movable area in the leg. Lack of joint mobility usually results in a shifting of the stresses which caused the problem to another site in the leg, which may, in turn, develop a lameness. Once the joint has fused, the animal may be usable to a limited extent until further joint changes occur.

Casts are sometimes placed on the foot from the hoof wall to just below the knee joint and left on for a month or more. This allows the joint to fuse more rapidly. When the joint refuses to grow together, the animal may secrete a huge growth of new bone around it. In some cases, surgery may be necessary to destroy the joint cartilage and to force the two bones to fuse together.

The animal should be given prolonged rest in as level a field as possible. The area should be smooth and free from rocks. The shoes should be removed and the animal rested until several months after all signs of lameness are gone. When returned to work, the feet should be shod so as to be perfectly level. Full roller motion shoes are often used. A thick rim pad between the shoe and the hoof wall will help to reduce concussion.

Some animals show swellings on the lower end of the first phalanges. If these are cold and no pain is evident, there may not be ringbone at all. X-rays may reveal that the animal merely has enlarged epiphyses (growth plates) on the lower ends of the bones.

The prognosis for continued usability of an animal with ringbone is poor to totally unfavorable, depending on the amount of joint involvement.

RACHITIC RINGBONE

Rachitic ringbone is a nutritional disease of young horses. It occurs most frequently in animals between 6 and 12 months of age, but may be seen in animals as old as two years. It occurs at the same site in the pastern area as does true ringbone, but is a fibrous tissue buildup rather than a bony growth. No arthritis or joint involvement is seen with this problem. Rachitic ringbone is caused by imbalances or deficiencies in vitamins A and D, as well as in the minerals calcium and phosphorus.

Usually more than one foot is involved. Many animals show swelling in all four feet. Some lameness and joint pain may be noticed. Other problems may accompany rachitic ringbone. The most common of these are bog spavin, swelling of the knee joints, and contraction of the flexor tendons causing the animal to stand much straighter on his legs than is normal. The new tissue growth is very firm and may be confused with bony growth on palpation. X-rays show that the swelling only involves the soft tissues.

In order to correct rachitic ringbone, it is necessary to analyze the animal's diet to see what the imbalance is and how to correct it. Blood chemistry tests may be needed to make this determination. One to two months are needed to see any significant change after adjusting the diet.

If the problem is caught and dealt with early enough, the swellings will get smaller and become less obvious as the horse becomes older. The animal may grow up to be a sound and usable adult. If not corrected in time, the rachitic ringbone may lead to permanent blemish or crippling.

EPIPHYSITIS

Epiphysitis is an inflammation of the epiphyses (the plate near the end of each long bone from which it grows in both directions). This causes swelling of the legs near the ends of the long bones. Epiphysitis is usually seen on the lower end of the cannon bones (both front and hind) in the foal and just above the knee in the yearling. These swellings are usually bony and hard. The afflicted animal may be lame.

Predisposing factors include poor conformation which puts uneven stresses on the epiphyseal plates, excessive work of a too-young animal on hard ground, and improper hoof trimming.

The most common cause is a nutritional imbalance. Epiphysitis is frequently seen in yearlings which are being heavily fed for halter showing and worked at the same time to increase the size of their muscles. High grain diets may not have enough protein. These animals may be lacking in vitamin A. Excess protein or imbalances in protein, vitamins, and minerals may also cause epiphysitis.

Treatment of epiphysitis begins with correctly balancing the horse's ration, if it is not already balanced. In severe cases, it may be necessary to feed the animal only hay and a salt/mineral mix, withholding grain until the problem is under control. Protein should be kept under 10% of the ration (on a dry matter basis).

The change in diet should be combined with an initial 4 to 6 weeks of stall rest. The stall should be well bedded with deep sand, shavings, straw, or other appropriate material. The feet should be carefully trimmed. If severe angular deformity is present and is not corrected by rest and diet, surgery may be necessary.

SIDEBONE

Sidebone is a partial or total replacement of the lateral cartilage of the third phalanx by bone. This ossification is common in certain breeds. It is more frequently seen in heavy hunters and heavy draft horses. In light horses, sidebones are seen less often, and the problem seems to occur with age. Sidebones are uncommon in Thoroughbreds.

Sidebones usually occur in both front feet. They are rarely found in the hind feet. Animals who are base-narrow tend to develop sidebones on the outsides of the feet, while those who are base-wide tend to have sidebones on the insides of the feet. There may be enough stress on the feet with both these types of conformation that all four cartilages are eventually involved. There are two cartilages in each foot.

Poor shoeing may increase concussion on the feet, resulting in sidebone; long heel caulks often cause them. Not having the horse shod level may change the concussion enough to initiate sidebones. As with quittor, injuries, such as wire cuts, can initiate the problem; here, the cartilage turns to bone rather than becoming infected and draining.

While heredity may play a part in the animal's susceptibility to sidebones, their development is felt to be mainly due to concussion which stimulates the ossification (turning to bone) of the lateral cartilages of the coffin bone. Laminitis can lead to sidebone, as can faulty shoeing which has led to contracted heels. If sidebones are seen in a young horse (say, under 12 to 15 years of age), they should be considered to be a hereditary unsoundness and the animal should not be used for breeding.

The cartilage attached like a wing to the side of the coffin bone begins to harden from the coffin bone outward and upward. In draft horses, this usually begins at about seven years of age. It continues until the cartilage has completely been replaced by bone, usually between 12 and 15 years of age. All four cartilages in the front feet do not turn to bone at the same time. The outside cartilages usually harden before the inside ones; one cartilage may become bone long before changes are seen in the other three. Bony growth may be so profuse that the entire lateral cartilage becomes hardened. The profuse new bone may extend to the pastern joint, forming a new bony growth around it similar to, if not identical to, low ringbone. There may be accompanying erosions of the joint surface. The lameness which accompanies this type of sidebone is largely due to the joint involvement (as with low ringbone) rather than to the sidebone itself.

When both lateral cartilages have been replaced by bone and there is no joint involvement (ringbone), there still may be interference with movement of structures within the foot. This is due to restriction of the normal expansion and contraction of the foot produced by pressure on the frog and plantar cushion. The ossification of the wings of the coffin bone keep this movement from occurring. This, in turn, restricts the pumping action which normally circulates blood out of the hoof.

On rare occasions, bony spurs develop on the cartilage after it has ossified; these cause lameness whether or not ringbone is present. These spurs are most likely due to the horse stepping on himself or being stepped on by another horse.

SIGNS

The horse may show lameness, especially when moved in a circle. The worst pain will occur when the leg with the sidebone is on the inside. In navicular disease, the horse is usually lame going either way in a circle. In sidebone, it is worse when the animal is going in one direction. If the horse is shod, the shoe may be worn on the outer branch showing that the horse is breaking over the outside of the toe. Observation may show that when the horse puts the affected foot down, the outer wall strikes first; then, the foot rocks to the inside wall. Many cases of sidebone show transient lameness which goes away when the cartilage has completely turned to bone. Some animals show no pain at all. Sidebones may also be present as an incidental finding (but not the cause of lameness) when they accompany problems, such as navicular disease.

If the ossification is advanced, pressure on the cartilage above the coronary band will usually produce pain. Heat is often present and, in some animals, there may be a visible bulge. The presence of sidebone is easily confirmed by an x-ray; deciding whether or not it is the cause of a lameness is considerably more difficult (even for your veterinarian) since the occurrence of sidebones is part of the normal aging process.

Early changes in the cartilage, when ossification has just begun, may be difficult to detect by palpation. Lift the suspected foot from the ground and support it with one hand. With the thumb and fingers of the other hand, follow the cartilage from back to front to test its flexibility. Also, feel the free edge of the cartilage and compare its flexibility with that of the opposite foot. Bear in mind that both cartilages may have some degree of abnormality.

TREATMENT

If the processes of inflammation and ossification have stopped, surgical procedures may be quite helpful. Posterior digital neurectomy (as is used for navicular disease) is usually the treatment of choice. In some cases, the quarters of the hoof may be thinned or grooved to allow extra expansion in this area to compensate for the lack of expansion in the lateral cartilages. This will help to relieve the pain. Shoeing the horse with a full roller motion shoe is also helpful. Small sidebones may not cause any further problem after the initial inflammation has subsided and the cartilage has completely turned to bone. Large sidebones may involve enough structures to cause lameness and render the animal unfit for use.

QUITTOR

Quittor is an infection which involves the cartilages which are attached like wings on the sides of the coffin bone—the same ones which turn to bone in sidebones. It is most common in the front leg.

Quittor is caused by injury. It was a common problem in draft horses in winter. The horse would step on one foot with the caulk of the shoe on the other foot. It is now more often due to a wound, such as a wire cut. Quittor may also be caused by a nail or other object having penetrated the sole of the foot, going deeply enough to involve the lateral cartilage. Animals who interfere may damage the cartilage on the inside of the leg.

The horse will show swelling just above the coronary band on the side of the foot. This will be accompanied by heat and pain. Often, the area will break and drain, heal over, and later break and drain again. Quittor may be accompanied by sidebone as the cartilage turns to bone.

Treatment of quittor usually involves surgery to take out the damaged piece of cartilage. This may be accompanied by treatment with drugs to cauterize the wound, killing the bacteria which are causing the infection. The infection may invade deep into the tissues and even into the underlying bone in some cases. Even if treatment is successful, it often takes a long time for the healing process to take place. For this reason, the prognosis with quittor is never good. It should be considered an unsoundness if you are looking at a horse to buy.

SESAMOIDITIS

The sesamoid bones are a small pair of bones which lie behind the fetlock joint. They act as pulleys between which the deep flexor tendon passes. The tunnel between them is formed by the intersesamoid ligament. The ligament is lubricated by the synovial (secreting) membrane of the metacarpophylangeal sheath. Inflammation and fluid filling of this sheath may result in sesamoiditis. The location of the sesamoids on the rear of the foot leaves them vulnerable to injury. Trauma or tearing of the attachments of the suspensory ligament to the sesamoid bones (caused by strain or concussion) can result in sesamoiditis.

Sesamoiditis affects both the front and hind limbs. Because the front limbs suffer most from concussion, more cases are seen in the front legs. X-rays may show new bone growth at the inflamed or injured areas.

Sesamoiditis is most commonly seen in lighter breeds of horses, especially hunters and steeplechasers. It is seen, to a limited extent, in horses that are raced on the flat. The lameness associated with it is constant and may increase with work. Old books mention the disease in Shire horses that were worked on hard roads, but this is mainly of historical interest.

SIGNS

Swelling is seen at the back of the fetlock joint. If your fingers are sensitive and you are familiar with what is normal for your horse, you may be able to palpate a fullness in the metacarpophylangeal sheath. The swollen area is painful, and the horse will protest if the hind part of the fetlock is gently squeezed between the fingers and thumb. This is especially true if the leg is held up so that there is no weight on it while it is being examined.

When the animal is standing, he may hold the fetlock slightly flexed with the heel of the foot raised slightly off the ground. When moving, he will attempt to keep the fetlock from dropping to its normal position.

At a walk and trot, the animal will show difficulty starting, making several uncoordinated, sloppy steps using the toe of the foot without placing much weight on the foot or heel. Some thickening of the flexor tendons may be felt, especially between the sesamoids. This thickening may lead to shortening of the tendons with some knuckling at the fetlock. Advanced cases may show adhesions between the bones of the fetlock and the sesamoids with fusion and total stiffness of the joint.

The prognosis for sesamoiditis is never good; if the condition is diagnosed early enough, it can sometimes be stopped or slowed. Some of the pain may also be due to problems in the suspensory ligament, complicating healing and making the prognosis worse.

TREATMENT

Cold water or ice packs may help to reduce inflammation early in a case of sesamoiditis. Corticosteroid therapy may be useful early in the disease. Another treatment that may be used with cold water or steroids, or by itself, is a thick bandage, called a Robert Jones bandage. It acts much like a soft splint, supporting the leg and keeping the animal from moving it in order to permit rest and healing. Some veterinarians immobilize these animals with a solid cast, leaving it on two to three weeks.

Shoe the horse with heels or with a bar welded across the heels of the shoe to raise the heels ½ inch off the ground. Raising them relieves pressure on the intersesamoidean ligament and the underlying sesamoid bones. If the animal returns to normal, the heels should be gradually lowered to a normal angle. After the acute stage is over and the heels are back to normal, the animal should be turned out to pasture without shoes for three months or more. Rest is perhaps the most important part of the treatment, and it's better to err by resting the horse too long than by trying to use him too soon.

If the animal shows much new bone growth and/or damage to the suspensory ligament, the outcome may not be favorable.

SESAMOID FRACTURES

Sesamoiditis often causes weakening of the sesamoid bone, causing the bone to become porous. It is then easily fractured, especially when the horse is galloping. Each sesamoid bone has to withstand the pull of the suspensory ligament above and the ventral (lower) sesamoidean ligaments below at the moment when the full weight of the horse rolls over the fetlock joint. In the normal animal, the attachments of the superficial digital flexor tendon onto the second phalanx and the deep digital flexor tendon onto the distal phalanx provide a margin of safety and prevent overextension of the fetlock joint. The degree of safety depends on the degree of coordination between the flexor and extensor muscles. If the flexors do not contract at the proper time, the extensor muscles will pull the toe forward, overextending the fetlock joint. At this point, the first phalanx is in danger of being shattered. A sesamoid weakened by sesamoiditis may give because it is the weak link in the chain of support.

Sesamoid fractures often occur at the end of a long race. Some cases have occurred from something as minor as the animal stepping on a small rock.

SIGNS

Sesamoid fractures may occur either horizontally or vertically. Horizontal fractures are by far the most common. If both sesamoids fracture horizontally, the fetlock will drop toward the ground. If the flexor muscles function in time, the fetlock will not drop all the way to the ground and the foot will remain in a normal position with the sole flat. If the deep digital flexor tendon ruptures at the same time as the fracture occurs, the fetlock will drop toward the ground and the toe will turn up. If the fracture occurs vertically through the bone, the fetlock may not drop.

The prognosis for sesamoid fracture is poor if any disease is present in the fetlock joint at the same time. If the fetlock has dropped, the prognosis is unfavorable because of the accompanying damage to the tendons or ligaments.

After the fracture has happened, severe inflammatory changes will occur in the sesamoid area. The animal will show severe pain on palpation. The swelling may be so severe as to make palpation difficult. If the animal is palpated carefully shortly after the accident and before the swelling becomes pronounced, it may be possible to feel the separation between the bone fragments. Heat may also be felt. The animal will show severe pain when the fetlock drops. When moving, the animal will attempt to keep the fetlock rigid so that this pain is lessened.

X-ray examination will confirm the diagnosis of sesamoid fracture. Radiographs should be taken on any animal who has a badly swollen fetlock joint and shows pain when pressure is applied over the sesamoid bones.

TREATMENT

Keeping the fragments of a horizontal fracture of the sesamoid bone together long enough to heal is nearly impossible, especially if the bone is already weakened by previous sesamoiditis. Your veterinarian may advise you not to even try to repair the damage.

If the fracture is vertical and the fetlock has not fallen, the horse should be strictly confined to a stall. The heel should be raised with a special shoe. The fetlock may be given additional support with a plaster or fiberglass cast. Bone screws are occasionally used to hold the fragments together. After two to three months, the horse should be shod with wedge heels. The heel height can be reduced at each successive shoeing. If a small fragment is present, surgical removal may be the only way to keep the detached fragment from undergoing avascular necrosis. This condition occurs when a small fragment is broken off a bone and left without a blood supply. It dies and then acts as a foreign body, and will cause problems until it is removed.

Prolonged treatment may result in a weak fibrous union rather than a solidly healed bone and the horse may be of little use. This union may break down at a later time. After stall rest and special shoeing, another 6 to 12 months rest is necessary before the animal can again wear a normal shoe. Few horses with fractures dividing the sesamoid bone in half ever heal well enough to run again. If the broken fragment is small and can be surgically removed without complications, the animal may return to full function. If the fracture has been left a long time without treatment or surgery, the prognosis is dim at best. In general, the smaller the fragment is broken off the main body of the bone, the more favorable the outcome will be.

CONTRACTED TENDONS

Contracted tendons are almost entirely seen in young horses—from birth to two years of age. The problem usually occurs in both front legs, especially in the newborn animal. It is considered by some to be hereditary. Many dystocias (difficulties in foaling) are caused by foals whose tendons become contracted while still in the uterus.

In older animals, the condition is felt possibly to be due to imbalances of calcium, phosphorus, vitamin D, and vitamin A. Contracted tendons are often seen in phosphorus-deficient areas of the country, especially east of the Rockies. Horses who are fed excessive protein may also show contracted tendons. Slightly older horses may show it in only one leg.

Recent research at Cornell University has demonstrated that young horses who have a period of restricted growth due to poor nutrition or a heavy parasite load can show knuckling at the fetlock, excessively straight pasterns, and a more upright conformation than normal. This occurs when the marginal nutritional status is followed by good feeding. Animals who were kept on a constant plane of good nutrition did not show this problem. It has been speculated that these animals had a spurt of bone growth unmatched by a corresponding lengthening of the tendons. Lack of exercise may contribute to the deformity, as it is more often seen in animals confined in small pens or stalls.

Foals with contracted tendons in the forelimbs may be born to mares who have eaten excessive amounts of inorganic iodides during pregnancy. (51) Contracted tendons have also been reported in foals born to mares who have excessive zinc intake, or when the foals themselves are exposed to excess zinc. (52)

Foals with contracted tendons have been born to mares who have ingested woolly locoweed (Astraglus mollissimus). In some mares, this has apparently caused abortion, while others have live foals with limb contractions. Some angular deformities were also seen in these foals. Limb deformities are common with locoweed toxicosis in sheep and cattle. (53)

SIGNS

The horse will stand with one knee flexed more and more frequently. The pastern will be held nearly vertical, and the ankle may be twisted to the outside. If the problem has been present for a long period of time, the hoof may be severely deformed. In some cases, the horse may walk on the front of his fetlock as the foot knuckles completely over. He may lie down much of the time due to pain caused by spasms in the muscles because of the increased tension.

TREATMENT

If the problem occurs in a newborn foal, massage and pull the leg straight, gently stretching the muscles and tendons. You may be able to lengthen the tendons enough that the animal may stand. This should be done every two hours day and night for the first three or four days. It may be necessary to milk the mare and bottle feed the foal if he is unable to stand.

If the foal is only a week or two old, casts or splints may be used to help straighten the legs. If no improvement is seen within a short period of time, surgery to partially or totally sever the tendons may be necessary. The surgery has a high success rate if done early in the course of the problem, before permanent damage has been done.

When the problem occurs in the yearling to two-year old animal, it may appear suddenly. Some animals may be so crippled that they have trouble getting up and down or moving around. The animal may stand with a humped back and quickly become thin and slab-sided. These horses may have muscle tremors in their legs because of pain and weakness. The animal's overall health quickly declines. If the problem is allowed to continue too long, it may be impossible to correct and the animal may have to be euthanized for humane reasons.

Begin treatment of contracted tendons by having the animal shod immediately. Have the farrier correct the foot to a normal shape and angle as much as possible. Lower the heel as much as possible to help pull the tendons straight. Keep the toe as long as possible. Reset the shoes every three weeks and retrim as above. You are trying to prevent the tendon from shortening even more by putting a gradually increasing amount of tension on it. Straightening the foot also helps to minimize joint damage.

Phenylbutazone may be used to reduce the pain and help the animal to use the leg. At some point, the animal may be in severe pain from the shoeing and may have to be returned to the abnormal angle for humane reasons. However, when he is shod this way to reduce the pain, the contraction may then occur again. The prognosis for cure of these cases is never good.

Dietary management is important in a case of contracted tendons. Any imbalances in the horse's diet should be corrected, paying close attention to calcium, phosphorus, vitamin A, vitamin D, and protein levels. Many animals may be helped by being placed on a diet for 1-½ to 2 months which limits the growth rate. This is particularly helpful if the animal is under a year of age. (54) Stall rest with a near-starvation diet will often give dramatic improvement. Grass hay with little or no grain frequently gives remission of symptoms within a few weeks. Stall rest should be continued for at least two months after remission. Then exercise can be gradually increased. Grain can be gradually added to the ration in proportion to the amount of exercise. (55)

The outlook for a horse with contracted tendons is generally favorable if the animal does not require surgery. Surgery is occasionally necessary on older animals. If the leg cannot be pulled down to a normal position after the tendons are cut, the outlook is unfavorable. The outlook is very poor if infection and arthritis have occurred in the fetlock joint due to the damage caused by the animal walking on it.

Contracted tendons are occasionally seen in older horses. These cases are usually due to imbalanced nutrition, overwork or abuse, or severe stress and speed work early in the animal's life. Some may be due to problems when the animal was 1–½ to 2-years old, but were very subtle at that age, only developing into serious problems later in life. Contraction of the superficial digital flexor tendon can contribute to problems, such as cocked ankles or animals who are "over at the knees." These problems may or may not be correctable by surgery on the tendons or ligaments.

Occasionally, horses are sold who have one severely twisted foot. It is always said that the animal was "injured when he was little." Unless you know this to be absolutely true, the problem should be considered to be a hereditary defect. Many of these animals will walk on the side of the hoof for the rest of their lives. They are often sold cheaply and used for breeding stock. Since the problem is considered to be hereditary, to use them for this purpose is asking to have more side-walking horses. This author would not personally use one of these animals for breeding stock even if it were given to me, much less sold cheaply to me.

RUPTURED FLEXOR TENDONS

If both the superficial and deep flexor tendons on one front leg rupture while the animal is at a gallop, the animal nearly always falls; he may turn a somersault. If one of these tendons ruptures, the horse may pull up on three legs, showing severe pain as he holds the leg up and shakes it. If the superficial flexor tendon is ruptured, the fetlock will near the ground while the foot remains flat. When the only deep flexor tendon is ruptured, the toe will turn upward, and the back of the fetlock may rest on the ground.

When you suspect ruptured tendons, contact your veterinarian immediately. Two treatments are most commonly used. Surgery is sometimes done to unite the severed ends of the tendon. Or, the problem may be treated by resting the animal in a sling with the leg supported by very thick bandaging or a cast. Special shoes may be constructed to support the leg to allow the tendon to heal. Healing time is quite long, and can involve considerable trouble with nursing and bandage changes. The animal may or may not be usable after he has healed. In most cases, they heal well enough to be usable for light work or as breeding stock.

BOWED TENDON

Bowed tendon is the term used to describe a severe strain of one or both of the flexor tendons. The tendons are not completely severed as in the preceding problem—only some of the tendon fibers have torn. How severe the bow is depends on how many of the fibers have broken. The blood vessels supplying nutrition to the tendon may be ruptured, allowing bleeding and serum drainage to occur in the tendon as well as within the tendon sheath and under the skin. Adhesions may form between the tendon and its sheath and even between the deep and superficial flexor tendons. Other ligaments in the area may be involved in the formation of adhesions, resulting in pain and lameness.

The problem is called a "high bow" if it occurs near the knee, and "low bow" if it is closer to the fetlock area. The bow is often seen as a bulge or long, lumpy area on the rear of the cannon area.

Long, weak pasterns may contribute to the development of bowed tendons. Sudden, excessive exercise may also be a factor in its development, especially if the animal is not in condition for the work being asked of him. Muscular fatigue at the end of a long race can also be a factor. It may occur when the horse bucks or suddenly turns hard or accelerates. Toes which are too long may contribute, as can excessive body weight for the strength of the animal's tendons. Muddy tracks can lead to the development of a bowed tendon. The condition is also occasionally seen with animals who are worked in deep sand or in bogs or similar areas, especially if they get into poor footing, and panic and thrash around. Improper shoeing may be a contributing factor. Bandages which slip and bunch or are excessively tight while the animal is being worked may make the animal more susceptible to this injury.

SIGNS

If the animal has caused the bow by hitting the tendon with a hind foot, he may come to a sudden stop during a workout, showing severe lameness. The same signs may occur if the bow is due to a strain, with or without tearing of the ligamentous fibers. There will usually be heat over the tendon. The animal may point the toe and attempt to hold the heel up to ease the pain. The knee may be pushed forward as the animal is standing. He may try to keep the fetlock from dropping when he is forced to move.

The tendon may feel thickened when palpated. Palpate the tendons both with the horse standing on the leg and with the leg flexed so that you can feel their whole length. Heat and swelling may be found and the animal may flinch with pain as you palpate the problem area. If the fetlock is dropped below its normal position, there may be damage to the suspensory ligament; this is a much more severe problem than a bowed flexor tendon by itself.

TREATMENT

Immediate treatment involves cooling the leg as soon as possible. Use water from a hose or ice packs for the first 24 to 48 hours. A gentle pressure bandage will help to lessen the bleeding within the tendon. Corticosteroid injections are often used early in the treatment and may be continued for as long as 10 days. Your veterinarian may, in some cases, inject corticosteroids directly into the tendon.

Consult your veterinarian immediately if you think your horse may have bowed a tendon. Prompt treatment may mean the difference between a usable animal and a permanent cripple.

When 48 hours have passed since the injury, the animal may be soaked with warm water with epsom salts in it, once or twice daily. A whirlpool boot, if available, may be used to help stimulate circulation and relieve pain in the area.

The horse should be rested completely and confined to a stall or small corral so that he will not move around. If the animal is bothered by being alone, he may be more calm and quiet if given a companion with whom he is familiar. The importance of complete rest cannot be overemphasized. If you continue to use the animal, or even to walk him a little, you are encouraging continued bleeding within the tendon sheath thus adding insult to the injury. You are also helping to keep the torn tendon fibers from growing together. Six months is usually a MINIMUM rest period. Due to the healing process involved in mending a tendon, a year is often a more realistic time frame. Using the animal before healing has completely occurred may result in re-injury of the area and permanent damage. Cut the animal's feed so that he is not high and restless and to reduce weight if he is heavy.

A cast may be used to immobilize the horse. This should be applied by your veterinarian. Some people prefer a cast-like bandage such as a Robert Jones bandage. It should be applied from just below the knee down to the hoof. Use this bandage until there has been no heat in the leg for 7 to 10 days. Then, remove it, still keeping the animal strictly confined. Watch the leg for swelling or heat in the bow. If these recur, rebandage the leg immediately.

Many other methods of treatment have been used for bowed tendon. Some veterinarians perform surgery to remove the blood clot from the tendon sheath. Surgery does not seem to return more animals to usefulness than does plain old rest. Ultrasound and other therapies have been tried. In the long run, the animal must still be rested at least six months. It is my opinion that the rest is what heals the damage, not all the other things that we use or do. So, why bother with all the other work? Do what is necessary early in the problem to ease the pain, make the animal as comfortable as possible and prevent further bleeding so that the bow does not get worse. After that, give him the rest he needs so that he can heal himself.

Firing and blistering have been used in the past to treat these problems. Again, the healing factor is not the firing, but the rest which the animal is forced to have after he is fired. In 98% of the situations for which firing is used, it is absolutely barbaric and medieval. Some veterinarians fire animals because they cannot get the owner to rest him any other way. Save your animal the pain and give him the rest without having to heal burns in addition to his strained tendon.

Because of peculiarities of the healing process, a tendon which has been bowed is never as strong as it was before the injury. Some animals will become sound after a prolonged period of rest. Others will have a chronic lameness which usually does not show up when the animal is walked or trotted, but becomes evident when he is worked hard. If the bow has become chronic and heavy scar tissue is present, the prognosis is unfavorable.

SPLINTS

The horse walks on one toe which has remained out of the five that he had when he was a beast the size of a dog a few million years ago. Partial remains of the second and fourth toes form the splint bones. These lie on each side of the cannon bone, just below the knee, toward the rear side of the leg. They actually form part of the carpal (knee) joint, with their top surfaces carrying some of the horse's weight. The same is true in the rear leg, where they are part of the hock joint.

Since these bones are not complete, they only go a short way below the knee or hock joint; they do not rest on anything at their bottom end. They are attached to the cannon bone by a ligament called the interosseous ("between the bones") ligament. When excess strain is placed downward on the carpal joint, it is transferred to this ligament. This is primarily a problem in the front legs because they bear so much of the animal's weight. Later in life, splint problems are uncommon (unless the horse hits himself with the opposite foot and injures or breaks one of these bones) because the ligament turns to bone, permanently joining the splint bones to the cannon bone.

Splints, like many windpuffs and some bog spavins, are primarily a disease caused by overwork or excessive work on too-young bones and ligaments. The concussion of a horse being worked on a hard surface can start a case of splints, as can excess weight on bones which are not mature enough to carry the load. Splints in very young horses can be caused by mineral imbalances. When horses were running free on the soft sand of the plains and not worked on hard surfaces, overfed, or used too young, the fact that there was a small amount of movement between the splints and the cannon bone was not a problem. Now, with horses in hard training, the pressure on the joint above and the concussion from the ground below join to cause "splints."

Bench-kneed conformation contributes to the development of splints on the inside of the leg. This conformation puts more concussion on the inside splint bone and less on the outside one.

Splints may also occur in a horse who suffers severe leg strain from other reasons. One example that comes to mind is a yearling who was loaded in a stock trailer for the first time in his life and then hauled from Wyoming to Florida. He was upset and walked and ran around the trailer, as well as jamming his legs hard into the bedding to maintain his balance with the unaccustomed movement. By the time he reached Florida, he had developed huge splints on both front legs.

Horses with thick legs, such as heavy hunters, suffer more cases and more severe splints than do lightweight horses. Arabians and Thoroughbreds, with their thin, lean legs and comparatively lightweight bodies, have less trouble with splints than do heavy horses.

Splint lameness is most common between 2 and 5 years of age. If the splint bones have not completed a bony fusion with the cannon bone, the disease may occur at any time in the animal's life. More commonly, splints in older horses are seen as a re-injury of an existing splint problem. Splint lameness is rarely seen on the hindlegs.

SIGNS

Lameness is often seen when an animal is placed into hard work. That can mean anything from ten minutes jogging around a horse walker for an overweight yearling to galloping a young racehorse during training. It is more common when the animal is worked on hard ground.

Because more weight is carried by the inside splint bone, it usually shows more pain when palpated, although the problem usually occurs, to a degree, in both splint bones. The inside ones are also more prone to injury from the opposite foot. Any bony swellings that develop are usually closer to the knee than lower in the leg. There may be one small, prominent lump, or a large one, which may extend the whole length of the splint bone. There may be a series of small lumps, sometimes called "chain splints." These do not all become active at once. Any one or more of them may be causing pain at a given time.

The pain caused by splints is not consistent; its intensity may vary from day to day. The lameness may be seen for several days before a tender spot can be found. The animal's movement somewhat resembles that seen with lameness due to foot problems. Mild cases may not show lameness at a walk, but will when trotted. The lameness is more evident when the animal trots downhill or on a hard surface. Small splints may be more difficult to detect than the large, obvious ones, but they may produce more pain. When first seen, splint lameness is often intermittent. It is not present when the animal is resting or cold, but becomes obvious as the animal is worked. Occasionally, a horse with a developing splint will appear to

twist the lower leg to the outside when the leg is brought forward. When the condition has caused the splint bone to fuse with the cannon bone and the inflammatory process is no longer active, the location of the lesion will determine how much unsoundness is caused. Some cases of splints never cause lameness.

After the splint has been active for a few days, a prominent swelling or lump may be seen. It will be tender to the touch and heat may be felt. Smaller splints are most easily detected by flexing the knee, holding the cannon bone parallel to the ground. With the leg in this position, palpate the splint bones, feeling both sides of each bone. Animals with early splints usually show pain when pressure is placed on the injured area. Splints which occur at the back of the splint bone or on its inside surface will cause more persistent and obvious lameness because there may be damage to the flexor tendons and suspensory ligament. Splints which occur right under the knee joint may cause enough new bone growth to invade the carpal joint, resulting in arthritis. Or, the bone may put pressure on the suspensory ligament, causing lameness. If the lameness persists or the swelling is large, a splint

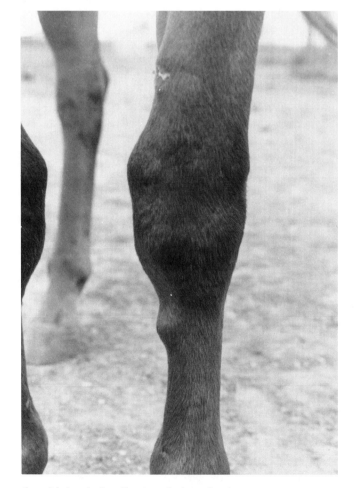

An old, healed splint just below the knee.

fracture should be suspected and x-rays taken to confirm or deny it.

TREATMENT

Veterinarians and horsemen have a running debate about whether recovery occurs more rapidly with rest or with exercise. Pasture rest is perhaps the best treatment as it allows the animal to exercise when he is feeling better and rest when the splint is hurting. Light, regular exercise seems to help the bones fuse together, thus helping to end the pain. About 30 days rest is a good beginning toward healing in many animals. In any case of splints, examine the animal's diet and correct any mineral deficiencies or imbalances.

Firing has in the past been a standard treatment for splint lameness in racehorses. It is, however, usually not the firing, but the rest which must accompany it that causes (or allows) the healing to occur. The same healing would occur, in about the same amount of time, if the animal were merely turned out without being tortured by firing. Many racehorse owners or trainers are reluctant to accept the fact that the animal cannot stand up to the work being asked of him, and will not rest him unless the animal is subjected to firing. How many of these people would fire themselves or their teenage offspring for the same sort of problem? My bet is they'd prefer rest! Blistering is in the same category of treatment: it merely irritates the skin and forces the owner to rest the animal.

If the overwork is continued, excessively large bony growths may occur. Extremely large ones may press on the digital nerve or interfere with the function of the flexor tendons and suspensory ligament. They can also invade the carpal joint. Large growths may have to be surgically removed in order to allow the animal to function normally.

Special shoeing should be used after large splints are removed. Use a shoe with the inner branch filed or pounded thin on the top side, from the toe to the quarter. Nail the shoe closely at the outer toe and caulk. Use only two nail holes on the inner branch, near the heel.

Splints which occur when the animal is younger usually heal totally and do not cause further lameness unless they are injured again later, as when hit by a horse who interferes. They do, however, usually leave a blemish which may be detrimental to the show horse. They may become smaller as the years pass, but almost never go away entirely.

Surgery to reduce the size of a splint can be done after the splint has totally healed. This is sometimes attempted with halter-class horses where the owner feels that judges may count the blemish against the animal. Surgery is successful in about half the cases. The other half have enough scarring and new bone growth after surgery to create as large or larger a blemish than the original splint. Splints really should not be counted against

the animal unless he is bench-kneed, or base-narrow and toe-out.

Prevention is the best cure. If you never cause the animal to have splints, you never have to worry about curing or getting rid of them. They are almost totally preventable with proper management, weight control, and training.

SPLINT FRACTURES

Fractures of the splint bone are caused by injury. They usually occur because the animal has hit one front leg with the opposite front foot, often during a turn or interference. For this reason, they are most commonly seen on the inside splint bone. The bone may be broken anywhere along its length, but fractures are most commonly seen in the lower third of the splint bone. Occasionally, a break may occur just below the knee joint. Fractures of the outside splint bone usually occur from a kick or other trauma.

The horse will show typical splint lameness as described above. The swelling, which is usually present, is larger and less definite than with an ordinary splint. It may extend the entire length of the splint bone. The lameness often becomes much worse with exercise, being most noticeable at a trot.

The swelling from a broken splint may extend far enough to cover the whole area over the bone. It will be hot and often is quite painful under palpation. Any splint that does not show relief within, say, a week, should be x-rayed to rule out the possibility of a fracture, as should all splints with severe swelling and pain. A few horses will show a fractured splint on x-rays which is not causing lameness and never has caused it. This helps emphasize the importance of a thorough examination to make sure that a fractured splint is actually what is causing the lameness.

If the fracture is seen soon after it occurs, nonsteroidal anti-inflammatory agents (such as phenylbutazone) may help to reduce swelling and heat in the area. Cold water therapy is often useful. Drawing agents (if the skin is unbroken) and DMSO may help. A support wrap is used on the animal for about a month. Recommended treatment usually includes resting the animal until the inflammation goes down. Simple splint fractures can heal well in 30 to 45 days of rest and the prognosis is favorable.

When x-rays show that the splint fracture is healing or has healed, the fragment is usually not removed. If the injury persists for some time without showing signs of healing, your veterinarian may surgically remove the fractured end, thus allowing healing to occur more rapidly. He may do this with the animal standing, or anesthetize him and do surgery with him lying down.

If the fracture has been present for some time, one of the bone fragments may have died. A draining tract will form to the outside that will remain until the dead bone is surgically removed. As with a nonhealing fracture, surgery is the only cure. In many cases, the wound can be sutured after the fragments are removed. In others, the area will have to be left open and be flushed or swabbed daily until it finally heals. This may take 2 to 3 weeks.

Aftercare following surgery usually consists of careful bandage changing to maintain constant pressure on the healing area. Follow your veterinarian's instructions to the letter for best healing. It does no good to pay to have the surgery done and then have complications because of inadequate aftercare. The animal will probably be confined to a stall for one to two months. It is better to have him in for a longer period of time than to let him out too soon and have him re-injure the area.

With good recovery, the animal may be back to training or use approximately three months after surgery. Consult your veterinarian before starting the animal back to work to be sure that the horse is ready for use. If the animal is not allowed enough time to heal, large amounts of new bone growth may occur. Fractured splints usually heal quite well and return the animal to usability unless there is enough new bone growth to cause problems with the flexor tendons, the suspensory ligament, or the carpal joint.

BUCKED SHINS

"Bucked shins" is the term given to a tearing of the periosteum (the membrane covering the bone) on the front of the cannon bone. The common digital extensor tendon is very loosely attached to the cannon bone here, and is held in place by fibrous bands. Hard pulls caused by this tendon attachment result in small stress fractures on the front of the cannon bone. These lesions are similar in cause and result to the "shin splints" that occur in teenage athletes. (56)

CAUSES AND SIGNS

Bucked shins is almost entirely a disease of young running horses. They are rarely seen in animals over three years of age. The small stress fractures are caused by excessive physical demands on a horse who is not mature enough or well-enough conditioned to handle them. Some Thoroughbred trainers, especially, seem to feel that every horse must "buck his shins." A few even seem to feel that they need to force the animal to do this before his training can proceed. This is unfortunate, because they are almost entirely preventable. Bucked shins may be due, in part, to hard track surfaces, as they are less commonly seen in horses who are worked on turf. In horses who are exercised and raced counterclockwise, the problem is more commonly seen in the left front leg since it is the inside leg on turns and carries more of the animal's weight.

The horse will show tenderness along the front of the cannon bone, about midway between the knee and the fetlock. One of the best ways to test is to run the back of your finger down the front of the cannon bone from below the knee, pressing firmly. The animal will flinch sharply when you touch the area of the shinbuck. The animal will show some lameness and his gait will usually be short and choppy. Heat and swelling are often evident. The animal may show increased lameness when worked. If only one leg is involved, the animal will tend to rest the affected leg. If both legs are affected, he may constantly shift his weight from one leg to the other.

TREATMENT

Cold water and anti-inflammatory agents such as phenylbutazone, will help the animal to be more comfortable when used shortly after the shinbuck occurs. He will then need limited exercise for three or four weeks, until the problem becomes less acutely painful. This gradual return to exercise will allow the fractured area to recover without becoming worse. If the horse is completely rested, the remodeling of the bone will not occur as rapidly. A few

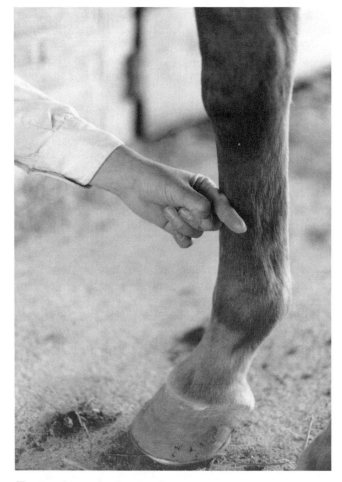

Testing for a shinbuck.

animals may take six months or more to return to normal. Periodic x-rays are valuable to assess the animal's condition and guide his return to training.

Bucked shins are almost unknown among Standardbred horses. These animals are trained at least as hard as a running horse (or maybe more so). However, they are generally brought into condition more slowly and carefully than running horses, which suggests that application of the same training methods to running horses would sharply reduce the incidence of this injury.

FRACTURES OF THE FIRST OR SECOND PHALANX

Fractures of the first or second phalanx are not common, but do occasionally occur. They are most frequently seen in animals who do hard turning work, such as barrel or cutting horses. They are more often seen when these animals are shod with caulks. The animal puts his foot on the ground and pivots his body over it. In this position, the front leg acts as a post, being completely locked and inflexible as the body rolls over it. If the body turns while the foot is firmly fixed to the ground, a fracture may occur.

A horse with a fracture in this area is reluctant to put any weight on the leg at all and may even hold it up. Swelling may be seen in the pastern area. It is common for these bones to shatter into many small pieces. You may be able to feel these if the break has just occurred. When you palpate the area, there is a peculiar crunchy-mushy feeling called crepitation. Stabilize the animal's leg and get him to a veterinary facility as soon as possible for x-rays to confirm the diagnosis and get an idea of what may be expected from repairs.

The fracture may be anything from a split or crack in the bone, to one that is shattered into a large number of pieces. One or more of the breaks usually extend into either the fetlock, pastern, or coffin joint. These may heal, but often leave the animal crippled and unusable. If the animal is to be salvaged for breeding, it is often advisable to surgically fuse the joint or joints which are adjacent to the break. This makes the leg more stiff, but avoids much of the pain that may otherwise result.

Chances of salvaging an animal with one of these fractures as a using horse are remote. X-rays will show your veterinarian how bad the break is and allow him to give you some estimate of the chances of healing. If you don't feel comfortable with his diagnosis, get a second opinion before you decide to put the animal down. Often, you can do that just by taking the x-rays to another veterinarian, thus sparing the animal the pain and discomfort of being transported. When these fractures are treated, a plaster or fiberglass cast may be used. If there is one major fragment or just a few large ones, they may be surgically wired together, or put together with screws or pins.

HYGROMA OF THE CARPUS

Also called "water on the knee," this problem occurs for the same reasons as capped hocks and elbows, and is the same type of lesion. Like those problems, it is due to injury. It may be caused by the horse getting up and down on hard ground. It is often seen in summer with horses who have concrete or other rigid feeders; the animal stamps his feet to get rid of flies and in the process hits his knee on the feeder.

A large, soft swelling is seen on the front of the knee area. The size varies with the amount of damage and the structures which are involved.

Consult your veterinarian for treatment. If the problem is fresh, he may wish to use an injection of a corticosteroid (done under sterile conditions to prevent infection in the joint). This may be followed by bandaging for a period of time. Occasionally, surgery is used to remove the lining which is secreting the fluid.

Hygromas which are treated early may have a favorable outcome. Those which are old may have enough scar tissue that they will never return to normal. The problem often results in a permanent blemish, but only rarely is there functional impairment.

POPPED KNEE (CARPITIS)

Carpitis involves many structures around the knee, including the joint capsule, ligaments, and bones. It is an arthritis that begins because of injury, and is commonly seen in racehorses. Later, the problem may have enough bone involvement that the animal is severely lamed or permanently crippled.

Conformational defects, such as bench knees or calf knees, contribute to the development of carpitis. It may be caused by the animal hitting his knee on a wall, as with hygroma, but this is rare.

New bone growth commonly occurs and the cartilage of the joint may be severely damaged. Lameness varies from slight to severe, depending on the location and degree of injury and involvement. Chip fractures of the carpal bones may be present; the extent of these problems can only be determined by x-rays. Corticosteroid injections often give relief. However, they may also mask and relieve the pain, allowing the animal to be used before healing has occurred, resulting in more damage than was originally present.

If carpitis is treated early and no fractures are present, satisfactory healing may occur. If bony growth occurs, the prognosis is far less favorable; when this growth involves a joint surface, the outcome is likely to be unfavorable. If the animal's conformation is poor, the prognosis is poor. If you get this episode repaired, the animal is likely to re-injure the area again. Sooner or later, this process results in permanent damage.

FRACTURED CARPAL BONES

Fractures of the carpal bones may be small chips, often called "joint mice." Or, they may be larger, slab fractures. They are often due to stress, especially when compounded by muscle and tendon fatigue. When these are accompanied by poor conformation, such as calf knees, they are even more likely to occur. Carpal fractures are especially common in racehorses.

While these fractures may seem to occur suddenly (such as during a race), they are, in all likelihood, due to an accumulation of stress and damage over a period of time. Repeated injections of corticosteroids into the joint may permit continued usage, while masking signs of developing arthritis (degenerative joint disease).

As with cases of carpitis, the animal often shows swelling, pain, and heat in the knee joint. Horses with fractures usually show pain both while standing on the leg and while moving it. The animal may hold the knee slightly flexed to rest it and relieve the pain when he is standing still. Knee problems should be x-rayed to determine whether fractures are present. It does no good to treat the

problem as a simple carpitis and then find that a fracture is present.

Surgery is the only satisfactory treatment for carpal fractures. The joint is opened with the animal fully anesthetized and under sterile operating conditions. If the chip is small, it is removed. Larger slab fractures are often stabilized and reattached to the bone from which they have fractured by one or more screws. About 80% of the horses treated return to useful work after this type of surgery.

If x-rays have shown a small fracture, your veterinarian may choose to use an arthroscope rather than to do surgery. A small incision is made in the skin and joint capsule and a fiber-optic instrument is inserted. This procedure allows the surgeon to see the chip and remove it. At the same time, he can evaluate the joint to see how much damage has been done by the chip, and whether other problems are present. This can give the veterinarian a much better idea of what is going on in the joint, as well as allowing him to remove the chip.

Healing may occur on rare occasions without surgery. However, the irritation caused during this healing period often results in severe arthritis and damage to the joint surface, causing more problems than if surgery had been done in the first place.

CROOKED LEGS

Crooked legs are often seen in newborn foals. In fact, most foals are born with some sort of leg deformity. It may, in some cases, be due to the position of the foal in the uterus. This especially seems to be true in horses such as the Thoroughbred, where the legs of the newborn foal are very long. It may be due to pressures exerted while the foal was delivered or to actual injury during delivery. These sorts of deformities usually correct themselves if the mother is a good milking mare and the foal gets normal exercise within the first two or three weeks.

Other cases appear to be due to inadequate nutrition of the mare during pregnancy. One of my ranch clients had all his foals born with crooked legs. We were beginning to think there was something wrong with the stallion and that the condition was hereditary. Finally, we analyzed the diet and found that the animals were on a phosphorus-deficient pasture. The next year, the mares were supplemented with phosphorus during pregnancy and the problem was no longer seen. In some cases, however, hereditary causes are undoubtedly involved.

The front legs seem to be affected more often than the hind legs; some foals may show severe curvature in all four legs. The deviation may affect only the knees, or it may involve more than one joint. The legs may bow outward or the animal may be knock-kneed. Others foals will have legs that are partially straight and turn inward or outward at the fetlock or pastern joints.

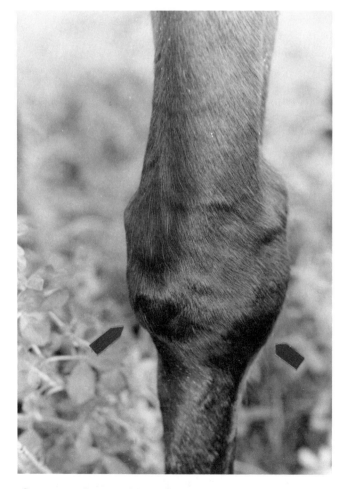

Carpitis or "popped knee."

Some foals have both hind legs curved in the same direction. This condition is sometimes described as "windswept." Many of these will straighten if given normal exercise (not too much!). If the condition has not significantly improved within a couple of weeks, or if the animal is getting worse, splints may be applied to straighten the legs.

In foals who are several weeks old when the problem occurs, the curvature is usually due to disproportionate growth somewhere along the limb. Some foals may have angular limb problems because of necrosis and partial collapse of the small bones in the hock or knee joint. These can be straightened surgically, but this does not fix the disease which caused the bone damage in the first place.

Occasionally, limb deformities straighten out by themselves within a few weeks. If they have not become obviously better within ten days to two weeks, consult your veterinarian. When crooked legs are allowed to go uncorrected for a long period of time, the deformity may become permanent. Damage to the joint cartilage or the growth plate of the bone (the epiphysis) may result in a leg which continues to grow in the wrong direction. Enough arthritis may occur to cripple the animal for life. Or, one of the feet may turn enough that the horse walks on the side of the hoof, again leading to permanent deformity.

While the foal is young, it may be possible for your veterinarian to anesthetize him and put a lightweight splint on the leg to help straighten it. In many cases, one or two changes of the splint will result in a straight leg. Animals who are older when treatment is started will often require surgery.

One of the most common types of surgery is called epiphyseal stapling. The foal is anesthetized and a surgical incision is made over the epiphysis on the OUTSIDE of the curvature. A staple is placed vertically so that it bridges across the growth plate. This keeps the stapled side from growing. Meanwhile, the other side grows normally, gradually straightening the leg. The leg must be watched closely and the staple removed at exactly the right time. Otherwise, it will result in the leg becoming curved in the opposite direction! Another variation of this treatment is to put screws in the leg above and below the epiphysis and joining them with wire. This procedure gives the same basic result as stapling. Like splints, this correction must be done before the deformity has resulted in damage to the joint surface.

Another technique cuts a slit in or removes a triangular piece of the periosteum (the membrane which covers the bone). This is done on the INSIDE of the curvature and apparently relieves a tension or tightness of this membrane, allowing this side of the leg to "catch up" with the other.

In some cases, it is possible for the surgeon to remove a wedge-shaped piece of bone from the affected leg and then put one or more bone plates on it until it heals. This is the equivalent in humans of "rebreaking" the leg. This surgery is usually only done on animals less than four months old who have no lameness due to their crooked leg and have no evidence of arthritis (degenerative joint disease) in the joints. This surgery is only used on horses with severe deviations; more conservative methods are used to try to correct lesser angulations.

The prognosis for a crooked-legged foal is good if corrective measures are started early and the defect is treated as intensively as necessary. It is poor when treatment is inadequate, is started too late, or if damage has occurred to the joint surfaces or epiphyseal plates because of the angulation. The presence of any arthritis due to the angulation is also an unfavorable sign.

UPWARD FIXATION OF THE PATELLA

"Patella" is the technical name for the kneecap. In the normal horse, it rides in a groove in the lower end of the femur exactly like your kneecap or mine. An affected horse has the kneecap slide upward and "catch," causing his leg to lock straight rather than being able to bend normally. This problem is considered to be hereditary because it is more common in animals with overly straight, upright hind legs. They inherit the conformation which brings on the displacement. Occasionally, fixation occurs because the animal is injured while the leg was overextended. Animals who are weakened and thin are more prone to it than are animals in normal condition. Fixation generally is seen in only one hind leg at a time, but often occurs in either hind leg in susceptible animals. It is common Shetland ponies.

The animal's leg is locked in the extended position, stretched out behind him. The animal cannot flex the stifle and hock, but can still move the fetlock. The leg may unlock and then catch again in a few steps or it may stay locked for hours or days. Some horses have the kneecap catch as they move, giving a rough, jerky gait, without its ever locking and staying locked. If the animal is forced to move while the patella is locked hard and fast, he may drag the front of the hoof on the ground. A snapping sound can sometimes be heard as the kneecap pops in and out of place without locking.

If fixation happens to your horse suddenly and does not relieve itself shortly, first-aid to get the kneecap popped back into place may be in order. Put a sideline on the affected side. Pull the leg forward. At the same time, push the kneecap toward the horse's body. This will often push it back into place. Other animals benefit by being backed while someone pushes inward and downward on the kneecap. It has been recommended that the horse be startled sharply so that he will jump forward. In some cases, this will release the kneecap.

These are JUST first-aid measures. If the problem recurs, have the animal checked by your veterinarian to confirm the diagnosis as the condition can be confused with several other problems which are uncommon and hard to tell apart. At the same time, you can consult with him about surgery to remedy the fixation. Your veterinarian will surgically cut a ligament, allowing the kneecap to return to its normal position rather than getting caught out of place. This repairs the problem permanently. Both legs can be done at the same time without difficulty. Approximately six weeks should be allowed for healing after the surgery.

When intermittent catching is seen in yearlings, it may be advisable to wait until they are two to three years old, as some animals grow out of the problem. If, however, the kneecap locks in place or bothers the animal continuously, surgery should be done without delay. Delay under these conditions can lead to permanent damage of the knee joint.

Animals who have patellar luxations because of poor conformation should not be used as breeding stock because of the tendency to just breed more foals with the same problem.

SPAVIN

Spavin is a general term for disease of the hock joint. This lameness problem may or may not be accompanied by bony enlargement. A horse with a large bony swelling may be sound because the bones have fused together, while a horse with no bony signs may be lame. Some horses with a spavin may recover and lead useful lives, while others are permanently crippled. Horses with spavin tend to alternate between sound and lame days. Let's discuss some different types of spavin.

BONE SPAVIN

This is an inflammation of the cannon bone at its upper end and of several of the tarsal bones in the hock joint. It is often brought on by poor conformation, specifically sickle hocks and cow hocks, which are often seen together and are frequently hereditary. An animal with narrow, thin hocks is more likely to have problems than one with full, well-developed hock joints. It can also be seen in horses with excessively straight hind legs. Animals with poor conformation may develop bone spavins before they are old enough to be more than started at work.

CAUSES

Trauma, such as quick stops, may help to cause bone spavin. For this reason, it is more common in animals used for roping, reining, and cutting. It may also be seen in horses that jump. Another cause is working the horse on a hard surface.

Rickets, other nutritional deficiencies, or vitamin and mineral imbalances may predispose the animal to bone spavin. Animals developing spavin for these reasons usually get it between four months and three years of age. Pushing very young horses for rapid growth can lead to bone spavin. It may also occur during a period of heavy feeding following a period when the animal has been lacking good nutrition. Exercise throughout the growth period may help to prevent development of the disease. Shoeing a horse with the outer heel higher than the inner heel can throw his weight to the inside, thus placing unequal strain on the ligaments of the hock joint and increasing the tendency to bone spavin.

This condition may also start with a sprain that tears the ligament where it attaches to the bone. The resulting bony growth fuses the cannon and tarsal bones, resulting in a loss of hind leg flexibility. There is usually arthritis in the involved joints which causes pain.

SIGNS

Bone spavin is characterized by a bony swelling on the front inside of the hock joint. X-rays readily confirm it. The horse experiences pain when he flexes the hock joint; often this is the first sign of a bone spavin. The pain causes a marked change in gait by lowering the height of the foot arc and shortening the forward phase of the stride. The foot lands on the toe. Over a period of time, the toe wears short, leaving the heel too high.

If the horse is shod, the toe of the shoe will show excess wear. Excessive wear may also occur on the outside branch as the horse tries to put weight on that side to relieve the pain.

Reduced flexion in the hock joint results in an exaggerated hip action, giving a kind of rolling motion. As the spavined leg goes forward, the hip on that side rises and the opposite hip drops.

The problem is often worse when the horse is first used and, in mild cases, the horse tends to warm out of it. In severe cases, exercise makes the lameness worse.

Most horses with bone spavin react positively to the "spavin test." This exam requires two people, one of whom holds the horse by the lead rope. In most situations, it is recommended that the person holding the horse stand on the same side of the horse as the person working on the animal. However, for this test, it is often best for the person holding the horse to stand on the left regardless of which side is being worked on by the other person. This is because most horses are accustomed to being led from the left side and will move out more freely.

The other person picks the suspect hind leg straight up (with the foot under the belly, not out behind or to the side of the horse) so that the hock joint is flexed. Hold it tightly for one to two minutes. Then drop the leg and slap the horse on the rump while the other person leads the horse at a smart trot for at least 100 feet. A horse with bone spavin will be noticeably more lame for the first few steps than before the test. To be accurate, this test must be performed on a hard surface with good footing. Otherwise, the animal may stumble from unevenness of the ground or wince from stepping on a rock. If in doubt as to the horse's reaction, repeat the test once or twice. Test both hind legs so as to be able to compare them. A horse with spavins in both hind legs will show the lameness on both sides.

TREATMENT

When spavin occurs in horses four years old or younger, begin by resting the animal (turning him out to pasture) for four to six months. If excessive or imbalanced feed intake is a factor in the development of the disease, the diet must be corrected. The horse should be brought back into condition gradually when work is resumed and may only be usable for lighter work than that for which he was previously used.

Older animals should be shod so that the hoof lands level. The toe of the shoe may be rolled for easy breakover, and an outside trailer without a caulk may be used. Phenylbutazone or other nonsteroidal anti-inflammatory drug may be used. This might be needed on a daily basis for many animals in order to relieve pain and allow them to be used. In some horses, these drugs do not give relief.

The prognosis for complete recovery from bone spavin is poor. Surgery, in which a portion of the cunean tendon is removed, may or may not help. This surgery is very much a matter of personal opinion and experience. Some veterinarians find it to have some success, while others feel that it gives little or no relief and have stopped doing it. Another surgical procedure destroys the joint surfaces, thus shortening the time needed to fuse the bones together and eventually relieves the pain due to the arthritis (after the pain from the surgery finally stops). Some animals take a year or more to recover after the surgery is done. Others will be usable in four to five months. Firing has been used, but is not considered effective. Anyway, you already know what I think about firing!

Which treatment is used depends on the individual horse and must be determined by your veterinarian. With luck, the horse may become usable after treatment, although he may always be slightly lame until warmed up, especially in cold weather.

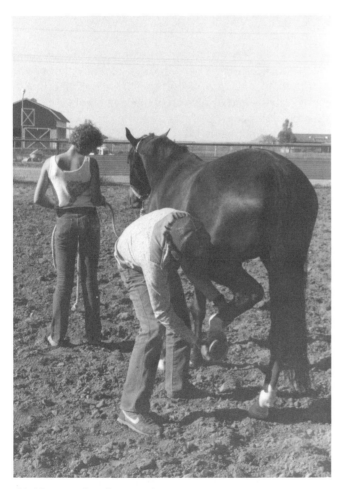

Holding up leg for spavin test.

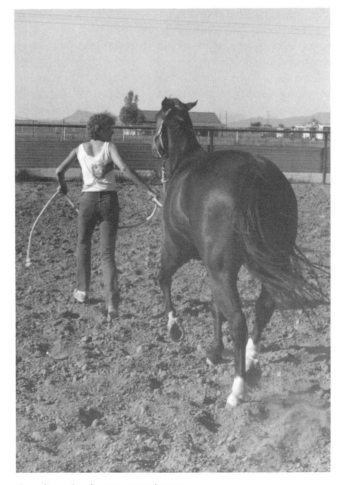

Leading the horse, spavin test.

BLOOD SPAVIN

This is an old term for enlargement of the saphenous vein where it crosses the front and inside of the hock joint. Since it occurs directly over the point where a bog spavin appears, it may be confused with the latter. It is a varicose vein just like some people get in their legs and does not cause any problems. There is no lameness associated with a blood spavin by itself.

BOG SPAVIN

This is a swelling of the joint capsule of the hock due to excess fluid which is usually caused by a weakness of or strain on the hock joint. It often results in a permanent blemish since once the joint capsule is stretched, it rarely returns to its original size.

It is important to determine what produced the bog spavin in order to establish the prognosis. If it's caused by a nutritional imbalance or conformational defect, it could be a serious problem.

Being too straight in the hind legs is a conformational fault that often predisposes a horse to bog spavins. If they don't occur when the horse is young, they may develop when he enters training.

Trauma—hard stops and quick turns—can result in bog spavins, especially in a horse that has less-than-ideal conformation. They can also be caused by hard or excessive work on a young horse, especially if he is overweight for his size, age, and stage of development. This spavin is perhaps more of a problem in horses subjected to a lot of circular work, such as with longeing and hot walkers.

Rickets due to imbalances or deficiencies of vitamin A, vitamin D, calcium, or phosphorus may cause bog spavin. This is most common in horses six months to two years of age. The swelling may (but does not always) disappear four to six weeks after the diet is corrected and the horse dewormed to remove parasites.

SIGNS

The most obvious sign of bog spavin is a soft swelling on the front inside of the hock joint. There may also be smaller swellings on the sides of the rear of the hock joint. These rear swellings are located just below the level of the point of the hock, whereas thoroughpin swelling is slightly above this level. Pressure on any one swelling causes the others to become larger and more firm. Bog spavins often do not cause lameness. When these spavins are caused by injury, lameness may be seen and will frequently be accompanied by heat and pain. No bony changes can be felt, nor are any seen on x-rays. If the animal is very lame, x-rays are often necessary to rule out a chip fracture in the hock joint.

TREATMENT

It is almost impossible to treat bog spavins caused by conformational defects. Because the strain on the joint capsule caused by faulty conformation can't be changed, any reduction in the swelling is usually only temporary. The swelling may be regarded as a safety valve. If the bulging did not occur, the horse would be lame. Spavins due to nutritional problems may or may not improve when the diet is corrected as noted above.

Treatment may help with bog spavins caused by trauma. If the spavin has just occurred, cold packs may lessen the size of the swelling. After two or three days, warm epsom salt soaks will improve circulation in the area and help speed healing and fluid removal. A whirlpool boot is great if you have access to one. Your veterinarian may inject corticosteroids into the joint to help reduce inflammation. Elastic bandages will provide gentle pressure and perhaps limit the amount of swelling. They should not be wrapped too tightly. Tight elastic bandages are known as tourniquets!

Stall rest is essential, especially if any lameness is present, and should be continued for three to four weeks after all lameness disappears.

OCCULT SPAVIN (BLIND SPAVIN)

This is a term used for problems in the hock joint which cause lameness typical of spavin, but without bony changes. Most cases of occult spavin are probably due to injury. Arthritis and ulceration of the joint cartilage may be involved. Joint capsule thickening may be present. Many cases of what appear to be occult spavin may, in reality, be stifle problems.

Signs of occult spavin are like those of bone spavin; the horse reacts positively to the spavin test, and moves the affected leg in the same manner. Radiographs and nerve blocks are necessary to distinguish between the two.

Treatment of occult spavin is difficult. Occasionally, a temporary response is seen with corticosteroid injections. The problem usually persists for the life of the horse, and chances for a cure are very low.

CURB

Curb is an enlargement at the rear of the hock joint due to inflammation and thickening of the plantar ligament. Horses may be predisposed to curb because they have sickle hocks or cow hocks. Sickle hocks are often called "curby hocks" because of this tendency.

Curb may be due to injury from violent exertion, such as digging out of a roping chute, or from kicking a wall or trailer. The horse may strain the ligament in a strenuous attempt to extend the hock. These types of trauma can cause curbs in horses with normal conformation.

If a curb is noticed shortly after it occurs, the swelling on the rear of the hock will be obvious. It is usually 2 to 4 inches below the point of the hock. There will usually be both pain and heat in the area. The animal may stand with his heel held off the ground at rest as he attempts to relieve pressure in the area. He may have a short, clipped gait.

Exercise may make an acute curb noticeably worse. Severe curbs may result in new bone growth in the area. Scar tissue often forms, resulting in a permanent blemish. Animals with severe blemishes may not show any lameness. Some animals will have an enlarged upper end of the splint bone on the outside of the leg which must be distinguished from a curb. X-rays may be necessary to make this distinction.

Treat an acute curb with ice packs or cold water soaks, changing to warm water after two or three days. The animal should have stall rest. Your veterinarian may wish to inject a corticosteroid into the area of the curb. In some cases, this will reduce the amount of scar tissue which forms and lessen the size of the final blemish. Do not attempt steroid injection yourself because if the drug is injected into the wrong area, it may cause far more harm than good.

The outcome of curb is favorable when it occurs due to injury in a horse with normal conformation. The blemish will persist for the life of the horse, although he will probably be serviceably sound. If the curb is due to poor conformation, the stresses which caused the original curb will still be present, and chances are good that it will recur, especially if the animal is used for strenuous work, such as reining or roping.

Gradually increasing work to allow the plantar ligament to strengthen and toughen before maximum work is asked of it may help to prevent curb in animals who may be susceptible to this injury because of their conformation.

WOBBLER SYNDROME

Also called equine incoordination, ataxia of foals, and wobbles, wobbler syndrome disease is characterized by varying degrees of incoordination. It is felt to be due to deformities in the vertebrae of the spinal cord in the neck area. These, in turn, lead to pressure on the spinal cord with resulting clinical signs. A genetic predisposition for rapid growth to a large size, combined with excessive feed intake, may combine with external forces to cause abnormal bone metabolism and growth.

One study considers the problem to be inheritable, although the exact mechanism of inheritance is not known. It is seen in about three times as many males as females, and seems to skip generations. Wobblers are often found in the same family lines, but a wobbler rarely sires another one. Some people feel it to be due to injury, but the current concensus is that the injury just aggravated the wobbler lesion which originally existed and made it obvious. If the condition were due entirely to injury, some animals would be likely to recover, whereas wobblers only get progressively worse.

A wobbler syndrome occurs in dogs with abnormalities in the cervical vertebrae similar to those seen in horses. Experiments have been done separating littermates and feeding different diets. Wobblers were produced in those fed a high-protein growth ration, suggesting that overfeeding foals on a growth ration may bring on the syndrome. This is thought to occur due to excessive protein and phosphorus levels in the ration.

Wobblers may be seen any time from birth onward. It is most common in animals under two years of age. Signs may appear suddenly. Incoordination of the hind legs is often seen first. It always involves both hind legs. As the disease progresses, the front legs may become involved. The horse's condition gradually changes for the worse.

Some horses become so incoordinated that they fall when attempting to turn. Others drag the toes of the hind feet and seem to have problems controlling their hind legs

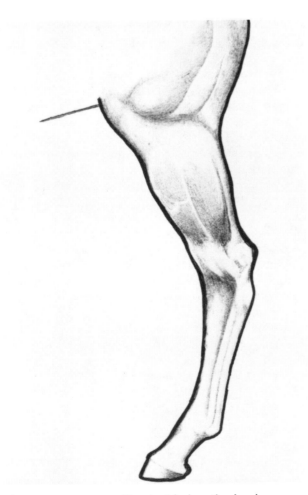

Curb appears as a swelling just below the hock.

in an organized manner. If backed, the horse may stumble or fall. Upward fixation of the patella may occur because the muscles are relaxed. Most animals will swing the hind leg outward when they are moved in a small circle. The horse otherwise appears completely normal. Most horses change rapidly within the first two or three weeks after the problem is noticed; they then stabilize and may stay at that point indefinitely. If the animal recovers from an apparent neck problem or injury, chances are very good that it was not a wobbler.

There is no sure treatment for wobblers. Vitamin and mineral supplements are said to have helped in some cases. In most cases, nothing works, and the animal will remain in whatever state he is in six to eight weeks after the problem is first seen. Surgery has been attempted on some young horses. In some cases, these are successful, while little improvement is seen in others. If you have a wobbler and breed it, even one that has been "cured," you risk getting more of them—not necessarily in the next generation, but almost certainly after that. The ethics of having surgery done on the animal and later selling him as a breeding or using animal are surely questionable. Most insurance companies recognize wobbles as a legitimate reason for euthanasia.

CAST HORSES

A horse is said to be "cast" when he is down in his stall or pasture and is unable to stand. This may be because he has rolled over and trapped his legs against a wall, or he may have them caught in or under a fence. He may have rolled into a ditch or up against a tree or rock.

If the horse is against something, loop a rope or strap around the BOTTOM legs. You can use one rope under both legs, or a separate loop around each one. Be careful not to get kicked while placing the rope. Many horses who are down and trapped will become excited when someone approaches them. It often helps to talk quietly to the animal. After the rope is in place, go to the side away from the wall or fence and pull the horse over. At this point, most horses will stand if they have not been down too long. If the horse can rise, allow him to stand quietly until he feels like moving.

If the horse cannot stand, or can stand but looks ill and battered, call a veterinarian IMMEDIATELY. A horse's circulatory system is such that he cannot lie on his side or upside down for long periods of time without circulatory

distress. Also, many animals struggle to rise and, in doing so, can batter the eye on the bottom side as well as inflicting all sorts of bruises and cuts. Shock is often a serious problem. In many of these cases, prompt veterinary care means the difference between saving and losing the horse. Some of these animals require extensive care before they are able to function. The horse may take several weeks to recover from being down for several hours. Delaying treatment for even a few hours may result in death of the animal due to shock. Note: the term "cast" is also used to refer to forcibly pulling the horse to the ground with ropes or other devices. The process is called "casting."

RADIOGRAPHS ("X-RAYS")

Radiographs (or as they are commonly called, "x-rays") are one of our most valuable diagnostic tools. When used on horses' legs, they can give information as to how bad a problem is and whether or not it is repairable. Problems involving soft tissue and those involving bone can be distinguished. Good quality x-rays can be worth literally thousands of dollars if they allow us to repair an animal which might otherwise not have been considered repairable. Conversely, they can save the same sort of money if they keep us from attempting to repair something that is not fixable.

There are, however, some things that these miracle examinations cannot do. They often cannot distinguish between similar problems in soft tissue. For instance, it may not be possible to differentiate between scar tissue and a tumor. They are nearly useless for chest and abdominal examination on adult horses. This is because the x-ray machine must be extremely powerful and put out a large amount of radiation to get through that much tissue. Even then, the radiation is scattered and absorbed by the animal mass, resulting in a foggy, indistinct film. There are only a few x-ray machines in the world capable of taking a reasonably clear picture of a grown horse. This type of examination can, however, be quite practical in a foal or younger horse. If your veterinarian has only a small machine made for x-raying horses' legs, and x-rays are needed of the body of a foal, sometimes arrangements can be made to take the animal to a small-animal veterinary clinic which has a larger and more powerful machine. This can sometimes be used to diagnose impactions and other chest or abdominal problems.

Chapter 8

BACK PROBLEMS

Back Conformation
Examining the Back
Causes and Cures of Back Problems

"No foot, no horse" is a favorite adage among horsemen, and there's no doubt feet are important. However, many owners don't realize that the back is as important as the feet and legs when it comes to comfort and utility. While judging two North American Trail Ride Conference (NATRC) rides in California, this author noted a surprising number of horses troubled by back problems. At the Mt. Diablo ride on a Labor Day weekend, there were 23 incidents of back pain among 41 animals, and two animals were removed from the ride after the first day because of back soreness so severe it would have been cruel to allow them to be ridden another day.

At the Cuyamaca ride two weeks later, 24 horses showed 28 incidents of back pain (considering withers, midback, and loins to be separate areas of pain). Two horses came into this ride with large saddle sores, but were allowed to compete because the sores were healing, the riders had them adequately padded, and they rode carefully. Interestingly, one of the sores showed definite healing from the time it was checked on Friday to Sunday afternoon when it was last examined. This demonstrates that a sore can heal even while a horse is being ridden if it is given proper care and attention.

First, this section will discuss how the back of a horse is constructed and how it works. Then, we will discuss some causes of back problems and cures for them.

BACK CONFORMATION

The horse's back is a chain of bones, cartilages, ligaments, and muscles all working together to give strength and flexibility. The vertebrae of the back are individual bones separated by pads of cartilage, called discs, which allow for some movement between the bones. The total spinal column is therefore very flexible even though there is little movement between the individual bones.

Strength is as important as easy movement. The bones are held together quite firmly; the rounded head of one bone exactly fits the cavity of the one immediately before it. Between the bones are ligaments of great strength. In addition, ligaments run along the undersurface of the bones and between the side or transverse processes of the bones. A continuation of the strong ligament of the neck runs along the back, forming a powerful union between the bones.

The withers are formed by the upright processes of the vertebrae, giving an elevated area at the beginning of the back. High withers are often associated with good and high action, and thus are especially desirable in gaited horses. High withers give a large surface for attachment of the muscles of the back and front legs. They also help hold the saddle in place and keep it from turning, often allowing the rider to cinch the horse more loosely.

The back should be hollowed a little immediately behind the withers and then continue in almost a straight line over the loins. Horses with a considerable hollow behind the withers are said to be "saddlebacked." These animals are often easy goers, having more play in the joints of the spine. Their backs are also weaker and more liable to sprain. An excessive curvature is called a swayback and is common in older horses, especially broodmares who have carried a number of foals.

A few horses have a curve outward (upward) in the spine. This usually occurs around the junction between the loin and croup, but may occur anywhere in the back. This conformation is called "roach-backed," and is a very serious defect. It is also called "jumper's hump" because it is frequently seen in these animals. Aside from detracting from the animal's beauty, the saddle does not fit well, the elasticity of the spine is destroyed, the rump is badly set on, and the hind legs are carried too much under the animal. He may continually overreach and his head is often carried awkwardly low.

The loins should be broad and muscular—they contribute greatly to the overall strength of the back. A depression between the back and loins often shows faulty construction in the spine and is regarded as an indication of weakness.

The muscles of the back are extremely thick and heavy and tie the bones firmly, but flexibly, together. This musculature gives protection to both the back and the structures underneath, especially the kidneys and internal organs. Fractures of the bones of the back rarely occur because they're so firmly tied together by ligaments and covered by strong, heavy muscles.

The length of the back is an important consideration. A long-backed horse will generally give a smooth ride because of the greater play and spring in the back. A long-backed horse is sometimes felt to be better for work at speed because there's more room to bring the hind legs under him at the gallop. However, a long-backed horse will be comparatively weak in the back and will be more easily strained by weight. The weight of the rider is farther from the extremities and is more likely to cause strain. It is rather like comparing a long bridge to a short bridge.

Short-backed horses are better suited to carry heavy weights; they often have greater endurance. The comparative advantage of a short or long back depends on the use for which the horse is intended. For general purposes, the horse with a short back is often preferable.

EXAMINING THE BACK

There are several different ways of checking the back to determine its soundness. The first method is to merely look at it. Observation will show any gross deformities, such as a roach back or saddle sores. Spots which may later become saddle sores can often be seen by noting spots where the hair is worn short or ruffled in several directions, indicating wear on the area. These areas may feel hot to the touch, indicating inflammation. Often, a sensitive hand can feel a slightly raised area under the hair in time to avoid a saddle sore by resting the horse for a couple of days.

Note any areas which sweat when the rest of the back is dry, or conversely, are dry when the rest of the back is wet. Odd areas, such as these, often indicate saddle pressure spots which bear careful watching to make sure they do not become sores (see also Saddle Sores).

Palpation (firm touching or pressure) is the next step. Several methods may be used here. One is to press firmly down with one hand while moving it along to check various areas of the back. You can also press down with both hands, one on top of the other.

My preference is to run my hand down the back with fingers on one side of the backbone and the thumb on the other. For me, it works best to use the left hand on the left side and the right hand on the right side, facing to the rear of the horse.

Press down lightly at first and then apply more pressure on subsequent passes. Initially, some horses will drop down, wince, or ripple the skin. This is a normal reflex or ticklishness. Most horses will relax after a couple of passes, when they become accustomed to your touch.

Run from the withers to the croup several times, slowly, noting any spots where the horse continues to flinch or react to a hard touch. If you suspect that the horse may be very sore, it is well to start palpating gently; a horse with a sore back often reacts violently—somewhere between laying his ears back and cow-kicking or taking a vicious bite toward you. Some people perform this examination from the left side of the horse, reaching over the top of the horse when practical to check the other side. Later, return and examine more closely any sore spots.

Examine the withers by pinching your fingers and thumb firmly together on opposite sides, pushing hard. This will often pick up soreness not detected by the overall examination.

A sore horse must be distinguished from a ticklish

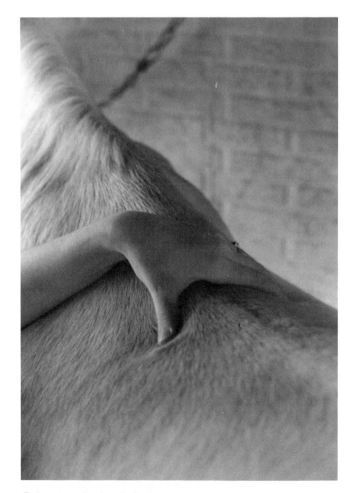

Palpating the back for soreness.

horse. Knowing your horse and his normal reactions will help you determine whether or not he is sore and whether a soreness is getting worse or improving. This is part of the reason for a thorough physical examination at the check-in prior to a NATRC ride. It helps the judges get to know the individual animals—which horses are ticklish, and which horses are sore coming into the ride. Careful palpation can often detect potential saddle sores before any skin rub or other outward signs are present, allowing corrective measures to be taken before the horse develops a problem.

CAUSES AND CURES OF BACK PROBLEMS

WITHERS

Inadequate clearance at the gullet or pommel will result in the saddle resting on the withers. The saddle is actually lying on the tips of the vertebral spines; it can cause pain and damage to the horse. Problems here start with rubs and saddle sores, going on to bursitis and necrosis (death) of the bone on the tip of the vertebral spine. A saddle with little or no clearance can occasionally be used by taking a thick saddle pad and cutting a notch out of the front to allow the withers some clearance. It may also be padded for a short period of time with a pad of hospital acrylic material or sheep's wool.

The cutback saddle used on many park and gaited horses is notched in front to allow for prominent withers and is a good example of building a saddle to fit the animal. Any saddle, English or western, should allow about three inches of clearance at the withers when placed on the animal so that it will not be touching the vertebral spines when the rider's weight is on it. When you are trying a different saddle on a horse, check the fit in the gullet area before you mount. Check it again when you are mounted to be sure that it will work. When in doubt, get a saddle with more clearance than you think necessary. Too high a clearance doesn't hurt anything. Too little may cripple your horse.

A saddle too narrow at the front of the bars or tree, such as a saddle suitable for a high-withered Thoroughbred, will often result in pressure spots on each side of the withers on wide-shouldered Arabians or Quarter Horses. With the rider's weight on top, the horse is literally being pinched by the saddle. These animals will show spots on each side of the withers which are extremely sore when pressed. They may also show the wet or dry spots mentioned above. Pinching at the withers should also be suspected when a well-trained horse suddenly bucks, balks, or otherwise acts abnormally. If a different saddle is being used, pressure in this area may be causing the dispositional problem.

When the blanket or pad is not pulled up into the gullet, it stretches tightly over the top of the withers. This results not only in a lack of air circulation under the saddle, but also causes a weight transfer to the tops of the vertebrae. This can happen even with a well-fitted saddle as the rider's weight pulls (or pushes) the blanket tight under the saddle. It is easily remedied by placing the left hand vertically under the pad or blanket after setting the saddle in place. The left hand then pulls up on the blanket while the right hand rocks the saddle gently from side to side.

A rider who consistently rides too far forward will cause soreness of the withers, as will a rider who bounces limply on the pommel while riding downhill.

MIDBACK

Problems in the midsection of the back can also be caused by poor saddle fit. Using a saddle with narrow tree bars on a Quarter Horse or flat-backed individual of any breed is an example.

A horseman who rides heavily can also cause problems. The person who lands with a thump at every trotting stride can cause soreness. So can a rider who sits in the saddle regardless of the pace or terrain, rather than rising out of the saddle and absorbing some of the shock with his feet and legs. Also included are people who get tired while riding and throw a leg over the saddle horn, or slouch to one side, with all their weight in one stirrup, thus pulling the saddle off center. Instead, the rider should get off and walk for a while. This helps prevent injury to the horse's back and works the kinks out of the rider's body. It is my understanding that the cavalry dismounted and walked 10 minutes out of every hour during long marches; whether this is truth or fiction, it's not a bad idea for those who get a bit stiff when riding and need to limber up.

LOINS

Poor saddle fit can also cause rubbed spots or soreness in the loins. Occasionally, a broad-loined horse is seen with a saddle that is too narrow. When used on short-backed horses, the very large square-skirted saddles can also cause rubbed spots in the loin area.

The rider can cause soreness by riding heavily on the loins. It is especially hard on the horse when he's ridden in the mountains where everything is either up or downhill. In competition trail riding, the rider is expected to take hold of the mane or saddle horn when going uphill, and to pull himself forward off the cantle, carrying his weight mostly in the stirrups.

Severe pain in the loin area is often seen in young racehorses who are ridden in very small (almost invisible) saddles by heavy or indelicate riders who bump along on the horse's loins. One of my clients had a racehorse who was returned to him because of "hock problems." Careful scrutiny showed no leg problem at all, but a terribly sore back. In many cases, these horses would do much better if a larger saddle were used to spread the pressure, despite the slightly greater weight. Pain in the loins is often mistaken for kidney disease. True kidney disease in the horse is so rare as to be practically nonexistent.

OVERALL PROBLEMS IN THE BACK

A clean back is important in preventing back problems. Dry grooming is best—curry comb and brush and lots of elbow grease to remove old hair, dirt, and mud. This helps prevent physical irritation and helps fluff the hair so that it can act as natural padding. If desired, rinse the horse's back with water. Do not do this if the animal is extremely hot; he should be cooled out thoroughly before being sponged to avoid sudden chilling. If a shampoo or soap is used, it should be one made especially for horses. It must be rinsed out completely. The hair should be completely dry before the animal is saddled. Liniments and braces should not be used on a horse's back because there is considerable danger of blistering. Medication causes the hair to stick together so use it sparingly and only where needed.

Dirty blankets, pads, or saddle lining can definitely irritate the back. Hay, weeds, burrs, and other foreign material can quickly cause sores. The practice of feeding grain from a saddle blanket, often done in hunting camps, can result in enough oats and chaff being left in the blanket to cause problems if the blanket is not carefully cleaned after use. Use a washable blanket next to the horse's hide, washing it as often as necessary with a minimum amount of soap in the washing machine and rinsing carefully. If you are using one of the acrylic pads, these are generally washable—check the instructions. It is often necessary to take them to a laundromat with large front-loading commercial washers to get them clean. When the pad is dry, use one of the wire-toothed doggy brushes or a sheep card to fluff the lining.

Saddle fit is perhaps less of a problem than it may seem. Most of the back problems seen at trail rides are due to poor horsemanship rather than fit of the saddle. If a horse is being ridden hard (i.e. daily) and if the rider owns or has access to more than one saddle, it may be beneficial to switch saddles occasionally. The difference in saddle fit will often relieve pressure in many areas of the back. Changing from English to western tack occasionally will accomplish the same thing. It's a lot like changing to different shoes so that your feet get a change and don't hurt.

If you're convinced that poor saddle fit is the culprit, it's advisable to borrow different saddles and use each for a few days before rushing out and buying a new saddle. Sometimes a saddlemaker can modify an existing saddle and can be of considerable assistance in deciding what type of saddle is needed for a given horse. Take your horse along when you're shopping for a saddle, or make arrangements to try the saddle on the horse before making the final purchase. Use a piece of old bed sheet or plastic when you're trying the saddle, not a saddle blanket. If the saddle fits without a pad, it will fit well with one.

Sometimes a saddle that fits poorly can be used with a heavy pad or several blankets. Hospital acrylic-type pads are very good for ill-fitting saddles and also for use on horses with saddle sores. A saddle sore can often be healed if the animal is used with one of these pads. It is well worth buying the best. Most pads are washable and can thus be cleaned. Brush or comb off hair and dirt between washings. Hang blankets or pads after use to allow them to dry. For a horse, having a dry saddle pad is much like our having dry socks—it makes a world of difference in comfort and avoiding sores.

A rider who is too heavy for the animal, such as a large man on a very small horse, can cause back problems, as can a rider who rocks from side to side as the animal travels. This sort of motion is especially damaging if the horse is going downhill at the time. Upper-body sway by the rider contributes significantly to back problems for the horse. Each time the rider allows his body to wobble, it causes wear and tear on his animal. Try to ride centered in the saddle, with a minimum of sideways sway. A well-balanced rider who works a little harder to save his horse is, in the long run, miles ahead.

Saddle sores, if not treated carefully and promptly, can develop thick scar tissue and become permanent problems. They can be caused by chafing, such as a rusty cinch ring rubbing on the skin. However, pressure is the most common cause; the blood supply to the cells of the skin is decreased and if enough cells die, a sore results. A breast collar or crupper, if allowing the horse to be cinched more loosely, may help prevent both saddle and cinch sores.

Excessively thin horses are back-problem prone. A horse needs reasonable padding at the sides of his withers, the top of his shoulders, around his backbone, and over his ribs. A horse who is excessively thin because of health problems, lack of feed, or severe overuse cannot help but be more affected by a saddle and rider than a horse with normal flesh. On one of the competitive trail rides which this author judged, there were several horses who had been on 100-mile endurance rides during the summer and/or ridden hard on competitive trail rides the previous two weekends. These horses were gaunt and thin—tucked up in the belly and excessively thin all over. They had literally been beaten to pieces by miles and miles of work. When a long-distance horse (whether endurance, trail ride, or just a hard-working using horse) has been put into good condition, less work is needed to keep him at a peak and allow him to compete in hard rides. When he's in shape, a horse should be fed according to how hard he is being worked and how he looks. More feed may be needed to keep him up and give him some natural padding.

Chapter 9

HORSE RESTRAINT AND SAFETY

Equipment
Leading the Horse
Holding the Horse
Tying the Horse
Restraint Facilities
   A Good Solid Post
   Crossties
   Stocks
Hand Restraints
   Earing the Horse
   Shoulder Roll
   Stick in the Shoulder
Twitching the Horse
Leg Restraints
   Front Leg Restraints
   Hobbles
   Hind Leg Restraints
Other Methods of Restraint
   War Bridles and Lip Chains
   Neck Cradle
   Side Sticks
   Blindfold
   Foal Restraint
   Slings

So now you've figured out why your horse is lame, and it's time to treat him. This book dwells at length on restraint and safe horse handling. It's easy to get seriously injured or even killed by the critters and you only have to be careless once!

The importance of forming good habits when working around horses cannot be overemphasized. It's even more important to teach the best of habits to your children. Your horse may be the gentlest one in the world, but if children are sloppy and careless, the same approach to a friend's or neighbor's horse may get them killed. Don't be afraid of the animal—just have a proper respect for his size, strength, and speed. If you are in the right position and are working in a safe manner, you are less likely to get hurt.

Safe habits around horses are important in routine matters. They are even more important when the animal is hurt and frightened. Pain may make the animal irrational and he may behave much differently than he normally would. In any case, use the least amount of restraint that will allow you to do the job you have to do, yet use enough to be safe. Good restraint may also keep the horse from hurting himself by fleeing blindly or otherwise going berserk from pain and fright.

Judgment is needed with any restraint. Do not use one which will make a horse's injury worse, such as tying up a leg which is already cut. In many cases, it is necessary to have the animal tranquilized in order to proceed with bandaging or suturing a wound. It may save much fighting and upset on both sides, and be better for everyone in the end.

It is important to understand that the horse thinks in terms of fight or flight when he is upset. This type of thinking occurs from the wildest bronc to the best trained show horse. It is perhaps more predictable in the bronc—you know that chances are, he is either going to try to get away from you (usually his first choice), or try to attack and disable you so that you are no longer a threat. The tamed, trained horse may or may not do these things. Under the influence of pain and fear, the best-trained animal may react quite the same as a bronc—you never know! Finally, the fact that a horse handles an injury calmly one time does not mean he will do so the next! So, be alert, be aware, and either stay out of his way or stay close enough so you cannot be hurt.

Because of their size and strength, horses have the ability to severely injure or kill a person. They can kick hard enough to break a leg or strike with enough force to kill. Some vicious animals may deliberately press a handler against a wall. Something so seemingly minor as being stepped on by a horse can easily result in broken bones in the foot. Foals, although small, can still injure a handler by striking or stepping on him.

Mature horses, especially stallions, can bite with enough force to break bones, and can even lift a person from the ground and shake him severely before letting go. When a horse bites, it is said that he cannot let go until he completely closes his mouth. This can result in severe bruising; in some cases, chunks of flesh may be torn from a person's arm or leg.

Horses often kick directly backward, with one foot, or with both hind feet at once. However, they have all sorts of variations on the kick. There is the cow kick, in which the horse reaches forward toward his front leg, or outward to the side, with one of his hind legs. There are rare animals, who, like the yearling who flattened me last year, lunge forward while kicking sideways with both hind feet.

It is easy to be kicked in the head and killed while working on a horse's legs. Try to keep your head above hock or knee level at all times when working around horses. Stay in close physical contact with the animal so that he cannot get a swing at you and make contact at the end of the swing. Being close also helps you to feel the animal begin to move. Either get very close, or get completely out of reach. The in-between distances are deadly.

Horses can strike with one foreleg from a standing position. Or, they can rear and strike out with both front legs. A blow from a striking horse can easily cause severe injuries, often fatal. The safest place to stand is next to the left (near) front leg, close to the animal's body. This puts you out of reach of a strike by the front legs and reduces the danger of being cow-kicked by a hind leg.

A horse should be approached with respect, but not with fear. They are good at sensing nervousness and fear in people around them and they tend to react badly to its presence. Horses are startled by sudden movements and loud noises; they respond well to quiet voice commands. Speak firmly, but do not shout. The animal may possibly pick up signs of fear from your voice, so if you are afraid, keep quiet.

Before you approach a horse of whom you are afraid or uncertain, stop and take a deep breath. Then approach him slowly and calmly. Make firm contact with his shoulder or lower neck area, touching him firmly and talking to him to let him know that you are there. If you touch him very lightly, it will be much more like tickling, and will not convey the feeling of confidence that you wish to convey. Also, some horses ARE ticklish, especially in the flanks and around the ears and eyes. Light touches in these areas may cause the animal to kick or strike you. From this point of firm contact, you can work smoothly forward or back as you need to in order to handle or work on the animal. Abrupt movements may startle the animal and make him feel threatened, resulting in danger to you as he reacts to either attack or flee. Handling a horse seems to let him know that there is nothing to be afraid of, and that

he is in no danger (or maybe, that you and he are in it together?).

It is often helpful to talk continuously to the animal as you work around him. This is especially true with young or fearful animals. It also helps the horse keep track of where you are, making it less likely that you will be kicked. Talking continuously with the animal helps to reassure and soothe him; it doesn't matter what you say. One of my clients is an old rancher who continually cusses his horses as he works on them. But he does it in such a low, soft voice that they are instantly calmed. It's not what you say, it's the way you say it!

Begin by handling any unfamiliar horse from the left (or near) side, as most animals are accustomed to being led, mounted, and otherwise handled from this side. Your own animal should, of course, be trained to be worked from either side.

Adjust the restraint to the animal's temperament—use as little and as mild a restraint as you can to get the job done. Don't assume that since a horse needs to be trussed up like a turkey one day, he will always need that much restraint. Begin with a moderate amount each time and add what you need to handle him on a given day.

EQUIPMENT

Let me begin by making a plea for buying the best quality, stoutest tack that you can afford. It's better to have one expensive, reinforced nylon halter with good quality hardware than a bushel of silver-mounted show halters when it comes to working with any horse. Get a good lead rope with the very heaviest snap available. Even better, have a halter with a lead rope braided or spliced onto it, so there is no hardware to break. Halters with only nylon rope and no hardware are better yet—they are nearly indestructible. One-inch cotton lead ropes are the most comfortable to hold, but nylon lasts longer.

The animal who sets back and breaks a halter when he is tied learns that he can do it. It may become a habit that will last the animal's lifetime. Conversely, one who never breaks anything will not get the impression that he is strong enough to do so, and you will never have the problem of owning a puller.

On the subject of halters, it is never a good idea to leave one on the animal while he is loose in a pasture or stall. Halter accidents can severely injure or cripple the animal; in some cases, they may be fatal. The sad thing is that they are totally preventable—just don't leave a halter on an unattended horse. He may catch it on a fence post or nail. Or, he may scratch his head with a hind foot and get it caught under a loose shoe. These accidents can easily lead to an animal with a broken leg. These accidents are much worse with good halters, because they don't break when the animal gets hung up.

When you're getting equipped, buy a good pair of leather gloves. It's hard to hang onto an animal while the rope is zinging through your hand creating a rope burn. Wear the gloves until you know that an animal is not prone to pull or jerk the rope away from you. Wear them while breaking young colts. And, use them when you are holding the animal for a veterinarian or farrier until you know what your horse will do in these unfamiliar circumstances. Sometimes an animal who would never pull under everyday conditions will jerk away when he smells the combination of other animals and medication odors on the vet's clothing.

LEADING THE HORSE

A halter and lead rope (also called lead shank) is usually used to hold and lead the horse. It is often easier to put the halter on the horse if you place the lead rope around the animal's neck first, and then proceed to put on the halter. The rope around his neck makes him think he is already tied and cannot jerk away—if he's been trained properly!

Most horses are led from the left side, but they should be trained to allow leading from either side. This training is especially valuable when the animal is being checked for lameness. Do not face the animal when you are leading him. This is often intimidating enough to the horse that he will not move, or will follow only irregularly. Lead a horse from the left side by having your right shoulder opposite his left shoulder.

Give him enough slack that he can move freely. If he wishes to pull out ahead of you, tugging harder on the lead rope is not the answer. If it comes to a tug of war, the horse will usually win. He is in need of some training to get him to walk alongside a human without any noticeable pull on the lead rope.

If you allow the horse to tag along behind you on a slack lead rope, there is always the chance that the animal may be startled by something and jump on top of you. Or, he may step on your heel or on the back of your leg. This can occur even if he is the most docile beast in the world, and has been led this way for years. It only takes once for you to end up crippled for life. If he's walking beside you, you know where he is at all times, you know what he is doing, and you can take measures to control him or push him away from you if anything goes wrong.

Carry the extra lead rope or strap folded in loops, but not coils, in your left hand if you are leading the animal from his left. This is very important. If you have the rope in coils, a sudden jerk of the horse's head may tighten the coils around your hand before you can react. You may be dragged if the animal panics; if you're lucky, you'll just end up with a crushed hand out of the wreck. Learn to avoid the problem in the first place.

A lead shank with a piece of chain on the halter end is often used for animals who need more restraint than is provided by a lead rope. The chain may be placed under the animal's jaw, but this often causes the animal to throw his head, making the restraint problem worse rather than better. The chain should never be placed under the jaw of animals less than two years old. In these animals, the pain may be so acute if you pull on the lead that the horse may flip over backward in shying away from the pain. This may result in serious injury to the animal, permanent damage to the neck, or even death. It is usually better to place the chain over the animal's nose. Used reasonably in this manner, it can actually be a training method and can help to gently lower the animal's nose and educate him to keep it there.

A chain over the nose can also be used to pull down a stallion who rears. In this instance, do not engage in a tug-of-war with the horse. Pull down sharply to discipline him and then give him slack until he misbehaves again. In this way, you reward him for suitable behavior. If you pull and fuss at the animal all the time, you only encourage him to fight and resist you.

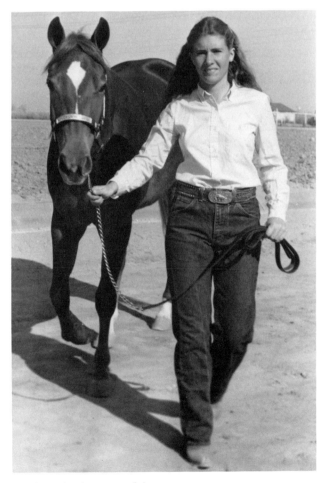

Leading the horse, safely.

For animals who are extremely unruly, the chain can be placed in the mouth where it will act somewhat like a bit. However, if you injure the animal's mouth while using the chain like this, he may later fight and resent all bits because he thinks he is going to be hurt.

HOLDING THE HORSE

Keeping the horse in one place for examination can sometimes be a real project. Stay on the same side as the person who is working on the horse. This is so that if the horse throws a fit, you can pull his head toward you, and thus get his hind end away from the examiner to keep him from being trampled. When the examiner switches sides, the person holding the horse should do the same. This is also a good practice when holding a horse for your farrier.

Stay alert when you are holding a horse for someone else. If you squat down to see what is happening, you may not be able to control the horse if something goes wrong. Remember that the person working on the horse is depending on you to protect his life. If you are alert to the horse's movements, you can often take a lot of weight off your farrier by turning the horse's head to take weight away from the leg on which he is working. He will greatly appreciate your doing this for him.

TYING THE HORSE

Having tack that will bear any strain that might be put on it is half the battle when tying up a horse. Then, you need to use a knot that is safe, and that can be undone when it is under strain if the animal should happen to set back and tighten the knot. And, you should carry some sort of pocket or belt knife at all times when you are working around horses so that you can quickly cut a halter or rope if an animal throws himself, chokes, or otherwise gets into trouble.

When tying a horse because you wish him to stand for a period of time, allow about 12 to 14 inches of rope between the post to which he is tied and the ring of his halter. If you leave the rope too long, the animal may step over it and get tangled, resulting in severe injury to himself. Or, he may become angry and pull back. When he has a lot of slack, he really gets a run at the post and can severely hurt himself. If he is closely tied, he will usually only bump his nose or scrape himself slightly. Tie him approximately at nose level.

While we're at it, let's discuss what to tie the animal TO. A good stout post is probably my first choice. Something the thickness of the average telephone pole is ideal. If you're tying to a steel post, it's usually easier to get the rope loose from the post if it is four inches in diameter or larger. The post should be tall enough that the animal cannot pull the rope off over the top, or hit himself on the top of the post if he gets excited and fights or if something spooks him. There should not be any projections which might cut or tear the animal, or perhaps put out his eye.

If you are tying the animal to a fence, be sure that you are tying to the side opposite to where the rails are nailed. One of my clients tied a horse to the inside of a fence rail. The animal panicked and pulled back, jerking the rail from the post and causing a severe concussion to the owner as the rail hit her in the head. Luckily, the mare was on the inside of the pen at the time where she could not go anywhere. It is not uncommon for a horse, when "pursued" by a rail tied to his halter, to run in terror through fences or other obstacles and injure himself severely.

Where do you walk around a tied horse? NEVER walk under a tied horse's neck, no matter how reliable you think he might be. If he spooks at anything, you are between the horse and a hard spot, and maybe getting hurt or killed in the process.

One of my clients was nearly killed by her own horse. She had snapped the lead rope around the animal's neck, without putting a halter on the mare. She tied the rope hard and fast to the fence, rationalizing that she was not going to ride the horse, but was merely going to put insect

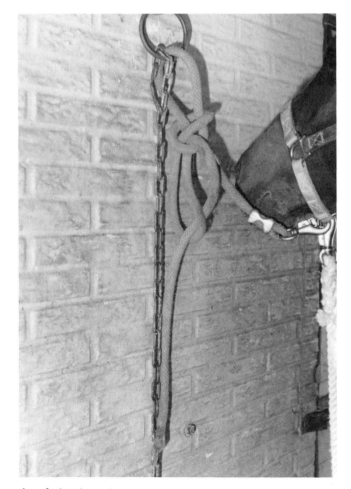

A safe hitching knot.

repellent on her. The horse spooked—she never knew at what—and pulled back, promptly choking as the lead tightened around her neck. My client ran around behind the mare and slapped her rump as hard as she could, trying to get her to jump forward and get unchoked. The horse would not move forward. Not having a knife (mistake #2), she yelled at some children who were nearby to run in the house and get one. They brought her a knife. Not wanting to see the animal rewarded for pulling back, she decided to hold onto the rope with her left hand as she cut it with her right, stepping in front of the horse, between it and the fence (mistake #3). At this point, the horse was so short air that when the rope was cut she went straight up, gasping, and lunging forward, came down on top of the woman. This client was lucky to live through the accident and spend only a few days in the hospital with a severely crushed vertebra which will continue to plague the woman for the rest of her life.

Now that you've resolved NEVER again to step under a tied horse's neck no matter how much you trust the animal, where else should you be (or not be)? When walking behind a horse, either stay close to his hind end and touch his tail firmly as you pass—or pass behind him completely out of hindleg reach. The intermediate space is where the animal gets part or most of a swing at you, and can really do some damage. Veterinarians and horsemen alike refer to this intermediate distance as "the kill zone."

When you are near the front of the horse, stand close to his shoulder. This protects you from being bitten, or knocked over by a swing of his head. He may be swinging at you, or he may only be trying to get at a fly on his belly—the results are the same. One of my friends had her nose broken that way. Being by the shoulder also keeps you out of range of a strike with a front foot—or a cow kick with a back one. If you are beside the horse's hind end, get in close and touch him firmly. As with walking behind him, either stay close enough that a kick will merely push you away, or get far enough away so that you will not be in striking range.

RESTRAINT FACILITIES

A GOOD SOLID POST

If you do not have any other form of restraint facility, please have at least ONE good, solid wooden post. This should be a thick post—eight to twelve inches is a good size. It should be set FOUR feet into the ground, and firmly tamped or else set into a good pad of concrete so there is no possibility that it will give or come loose. The area around it for eight to ten feet in all directions should be free of obstacles or trash upon which the animal could injure himself or upon which you or someone else could stumble. The post should have at least six to seven feet

showing above the ground; it should be free of any projections which might cut or tear the animal or put out his eye.

Veterinarians have treated many horses with no more to restrain the horse than an electric company power pole. Restraint can be a real problem if not even that much is available. One of my clients had two unbroken two-year colts with colic—and corrals made of 2 × 4 posts with 1 × 4 crosspieces. There was nothing solid to tie to, and several people were rather battered before we got the colts treated. So, set a pole for your veterinarian if you don't do anything else.

CROSSTIES

Crossties are a very useful restraint. They are often placed in an alleyway or in the aisleway of a barn. A rope or light chain is attached securely to each side; each of these has a super-heavy snap on the end. Use the best snaps that you can buy. Many horsemen prefer crossties made of rope rather than those made of chain because there may be less chance of permanent eye injury if one side breaks and snaps back toward the animal (or toward the

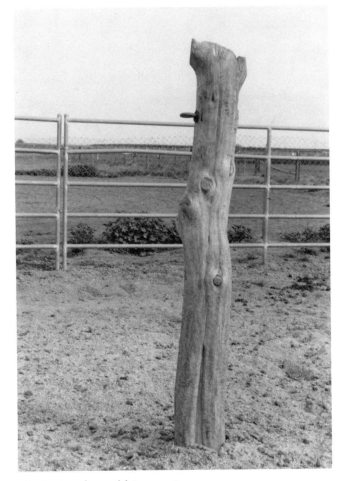

A stout, safe snubbing post.

owner). If you use chain, make it heavy enough (within reason) that it would not be expected to break.

Each rope or chain is snapped to the SIDE ring of the animal's halter. Needless to say, the halter should be stout and large enough to fit the horse's head without having any slack to allow him slide out of it. The horse is held securely between the crossties. This restraint is good for many procedures. It is especially valuable for shoeing. Some stables use crossties for all grooming, trimming, and saddling. Once accustomed to the setup, the horse will usually stand quietly without complaint.

STOCKS

Stocks are a narrow, short alleyway where a horse can be safely restrained. Many types of stocks are in use, from simple, homemade ones made of posts and poles to sophisticated veterinary restraints with a multitude of panels that open to allow access to various parts of the animal's body. Stocks are perhaps the ideal restraint and are indispensable for farms or stables with large numbers of animals.

Simple, inexpensive commercial stocks are available which are especially suited to breeding operations where a minimum of restraint is needed for mares who are being cleansed or treated. These may be set with a stout post about three feet in front to allow for tying the animal. A pad of concrete around the base of the pipes holds them securely and serves to keep the area around it from becoming a mudhole. A reasonably priced set of stocks of this type is marketed as a "wash rack" by Port-A-Stall (P.O. Box 1627, Mesa, AZ 85201). The horse should be pulled snugly to the front of the stocks before tying to the post. This helps keep the animal from getting enough of a "run" at the front of the stocks to hurt himself. It also prevents him from getting a leg over the front or side of the stocks if he fights them.

A homemade working area can be made by lining a section of fence with solid material, such as plywood, on the side toward the horse to provide a smooth surface. This panel should be eight to twelve feet long. Set a stout post about three feet away from the center of the panel. This will allow the horse to be pulled snugly against the panel. This arrangement is mostly good for working on the head and neck. It can be used for your veterinarian to stomach tube horses, for vaccinating, and for checking

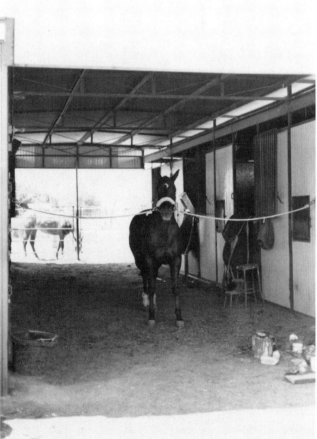

Crossties.

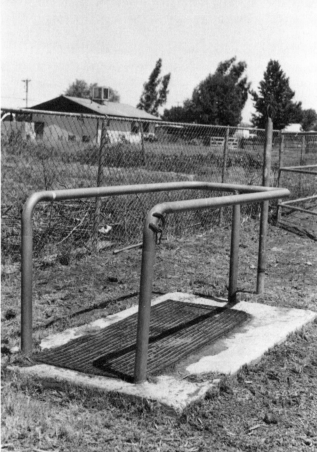

An inexpensive set of stocks made by Port-A-Stall.

and floating teeth. Because no side bars are present, the animal can still swing his hind end from side to side, which makes this restraint minimally useful for working on the rest of the body. A wooden set of stocks or a narrow alleyway (chute) will allow many procedures on difficult animals.

HAND RESTRAINTS

We often use pain to take the animal's mind off what is happening elsewhere. For instance, the application of a twitch to the horse's nose will make him think about his nose and ignore the fact that the veterinarian is sticking a needle into his cut leg, injecting anesthetic so that the area can be sutured.

We divert the animal's attention with pain to avoid having to use more severe restraint measures. We could, for example, totally anesthetize the horse and have him lying on the ground asleep before we suture his leg. However, if his disposition is halfway decent (or can be made that way by a bit of tranquilizer), it is safer for the animal to be awake rather than risk total anesthesia for a minor cut.

EARING THE HORSE

This is a common method of restraint but should not be used if other methods will work as it is easy to make the animal headshy. When you ear a horse, do it carefully. Move your hand up the animal's neck to the top of his head. Cuddle your hand around the base of his ear if possible. Then, slide the hand forward and outward to grasp the ear. This gentle approach tends to leave fewer bad memories than if you make a mad, direct grab for the animal's ear.

To ear the animal, squeeze the ear as you pull it straight down the side of the horse's face. If you are standing on the left side of the horse, you should be facing forward, holding the halter in your left hand, so that you can keep track of the animal if he moves, and holding the ear in your right hand. Try to be on the same side as the person working on the animal if at all possible. Keep hanging on if the horse jerks his head. As long as you have his ear, he usually will not strike, as he is concerned with trying to get away from the pressure on his ear. Of course, you should be standing beside him rather than in front of him so you are well out of range if he strikes. If added restraint is needed, you can rock the ear from side to side and up and down slightly at the base.

It is not a good idea to twist the ear. Occasionally, this will result in broken cartilage and may leave the animal permanently blemished. Some old-timers bite the edge of the ear. This probably wouldn't cause any long-term damage (unless you bite a chunk out of it), but is a good way to lose a few teeth if the animal jerks his head suddenly.

When the person who is working on the horse is finished, release your hold on the ear gradually and then rub the animal's ear for a few seconds. Try not to just let go and get out of the way. A fraction of a minute spent here is an investment in good memories for the animal because the horse tends to remember the last thing you did to him. If he remembers you rubbing an ear that is for some reason uncomfortable, it will help to guard against his becoming headshy.

Tall persons can often ear a horse by standing by his neck, facing forward. They can then reach over the animal's neck, taking the right ear in their right hand and the left ear in the left hand, pulling down on both at the same time. This also forces the horse to lift the person's whole weight if he tries to rear or pull away.

It is said that the ear restraint is never used on mules as they are quite violently opposed to it, and may become so headshy as to be unusable if handled this way.

SHOULDER ROLL

A shoulder roll is a good method for taking an animal's mind off his problems elsewhere. It can be used, in

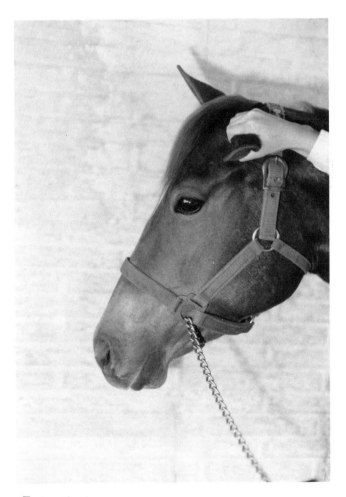

Earing the horse.

general, to get his attention and help restrain him, or it can be specifically used above a front leg which is being treated. If you are right-handed, take the roll with your left hand and wield the cotton swab, scissors, or other instrument with your right hand. Be sure to stand clear of a possible cow kick as you do this. Some animals will also reach around and try to bite you if they are not crosstied or held by someone. This method is extremely tiring to your hand if used for a long period of time, but it is a good trick for a quick procedure. Make a shoulder roll by wrapping the loose skin just in front of the elbow around your fingers.

STICK IN THE SHOULDER

This is used mainly when an animal is being branded. The horse is first tranquilized and restrained. Most people brand horses standing, but will use a stick even if the animal is lying down. A short, stubby, but slightly pointed, wooden stick is pushed firmly into the shoulder just ABOVE where you are going to place the brand. This diverts the animal's attention and helps avoid the blurring or blotting of the brand that can occur when the animal

twitches his skin just as the hot iron is touched to it. The same restraint can be used on the horse's rump.

TWITCHING THE HORSE

Using a twitch is one of the oldest and most commonly used methods of restraint. A twitch works by producing a certain amount of pressure (and therefore, pain) on the sensitive nerves of the upper lip. This takes the animal's mind off a painful or annoying procedure being done elsewhere on his body.

If a twitch is used too tightly or for too long, it may break the skin or otherwise injure the lip. Circulatory damage or injury to the nerves may occur. When used prudently, the twitch is one of our best and least harmful methods of restraint. It is inexpensive (as compared to chemical methods), and can be quickly applied and just as quickly removed when no longer wanted. Care is needed, however, because done improperly, you have just given the animal a club with which to beat you.

The twitch should be placed about midway on the fleshy part of the nose. If placed too high or twisted too

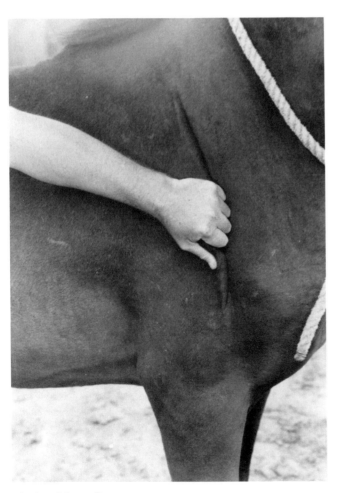

A shoulder roll.

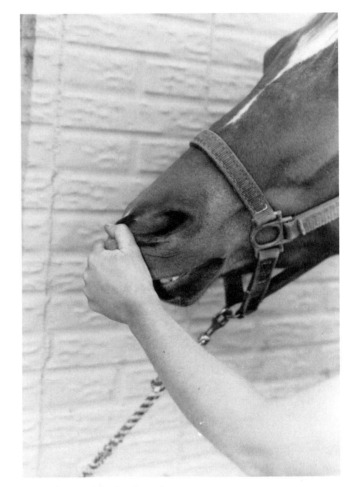

Twitching with the hand.

tightly, it may interfere with the horse's breathing and cause him to panic. He may lash out violently, rearing or striking. If placed too low, it only includes the thin front part of the upper lip and may cause more pain than is necessary.

Horses occasionally get harder to work on when they are twitched as they become angry or otherwise excited. One of my clients has a mare who throws herself over backwards when she is twitched. Needless to say, chemical restraints work much better on that sort of animal.

A horse can be twitched by hand; this is useful for short procedures when only a quick restraint is needed. You can either grab a handful of the end of the nose and twist or can just dig your fingernails in as you pinch from side to side. This procedure is also convenient when you don't have a twitch handy.

Various twitches can be used. These range from a piece of hammer handle with a hole in the end of it and a piece of nylon cord run through to sophisticated mechanical gadgets. Twitches with a long wooden handle and chain on the end are very effective and are safer because you can hold them with both hands. The only problem is that the halter and twitch MUST be handled by someone reliable and strong enough to hang on no matter what happens. If the horse jerks loose, he will fling his head wildly until he gets rid of the twitch. In the process, the flying instrument may injure (or possibly even kill) the holder, the person who was working on the horse, or an innocent bystander. Twitches made with stick and rope are more gentle on the horse, but are slower to twist into place.

A popular sort of twitch is made like a nutcracker. It has a cord and can be snapped onto the animal's halter. This is useful when you have inexperienced help who can hold the animal by the lead rope, but cannot handle a twitch at the same time. It also works well when you are trying to do a procedure by yourself.

Most twitches are best applied by first hanging the twitch over your left hand. Hooking it over the little finger will keep it from sliding down your arm and out of reach. You can then hold the halter with your right hand as you slide your left hand down the bridge of the horse's nose. If you do not put the twitch over your hand first, you are left with a handful of nose and the necessity of changing hands or removing your grip to apply the restraint device. As with earing the animal, try to work gradually down the side of his face until you reach his nose, rather than making a grab for it from a distance away. If you do it that way, immediate evasive action is usually taken by the animal, who either ducks to the side or raises his nose far out of reach. Besides, I don't know of a horse that isn't easier to work on if he isn't excited or scared. A sudden grab for his nose certainly won't improve his disposition.

Once you get hold of the lip, hang on firmly. Often, it is relatively easy to put a twitch on a horse if you get it done on the first attempt, and nearly impossible after that when the horse is wise to what you want. So, hang on tightly with your left hand and work the twitch off your hand and onto the animal's nose with your right hand. Twist the nose enough to maintain a grip. Then tighten the twitch enough to restrain the animal as needed. Do not twist it so tightly that the animal reacts to the pain by striking or pulling away. The twitch should twist on the nose, not pull on it; it should not be used as a lever.

If you are using one of the nutcracker-style twitches, pull the handles tightly together with your left hand to put pressure on the animal's nose and get his attention. Then, wrap the cord around the handle one or more times to take up some of the extra cord and keep pressure on the nose. Drop the cord between the handles and proceed back to hook it on a convenient halter ring. These twitches seem to work best (as do most others) when applied to put pressure from side to side on the lip rather than up and down.

If you are using a twitch with a handle, it should be twisted snugly as soon as it is in place, both to get a grip on the animal's nose so that it does not slip off, and to exert the force necessary to control the horse. Let the animal tell you by his actions how much pressure he needs. If he is

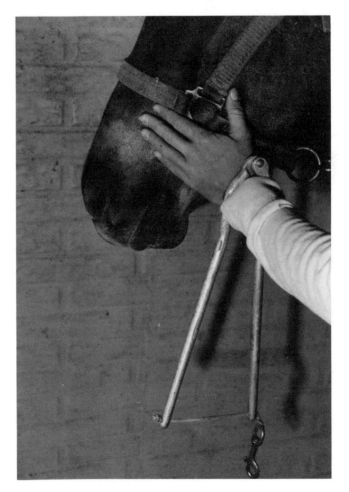

Sliding twitch along the horse's face.

still fighting you, he may need to have the twitch twisted tighter. If he is relaxed and standing for the necessary procedure, moderate pressure is enough. When the person working on the animal comes to a critical point in the procedure, it may be necessary to rock or jiggle the twitch to take the animal's attention off the work being done elsewhere. Good teamwork is essential.

Stand next to the animal's left shoulder as you hold the twitch. Use the lead rope to keep the animal's head pulled around to the left so that you will not be struck by the front feet if the animal "blows up." NEVER STAND IN FRONT OF THE HORSE.

Do not let the horse "go to sleep" while twitched during a long procedure. Some animals will get so "tuned out" that their heads droop lower and lower. They are no longer feeling the pain. The danger here is that if the person working on the horse hits a particularly painful spot in the procedure, the animal may suddenly wake up and kick or otherwise injure them. If the horse seems to be going to sleep, relax the tension and let the feeling come back to his nose. If there is a break in the procedure, it is often good to back off a turn or two on the twitch. You could take it completely off for a few minutes to let circula-

tion and feeling come back to the area so that the twitch will remain effective when needed later.

On rare occasions, a twitch is used on the lower lip. The only occasion which comes to mind for using this technique is to restrain a horse so that a cut on his upper lip can be injected with local anesthetic to get it ready for suturing.

What you do when you are finished twitching the horse will have a considerable bearing on how easily you can do it to him again. Loosen the twitch slowly until it is free of pressure. Then quickly take it out of the way so that you do not get hit by the free end. Some animals will pull away or strike when it is removed. While the animal is still thinking about his nose, rub it vigorously with the flat of your hand. This helps to restore circulation and will make the animal feel better. He will be much more inclined to let you twitch him again if you will do this every time you take a twitch off.

Some people are in the habit of twitching horses by the ear. This is not a good idea if you value your animal. The nerves around the base of the ear may be injured quite easily, resulting in a horse that is flop-eared for the remainder of his life. That's too high a price to pay for a few

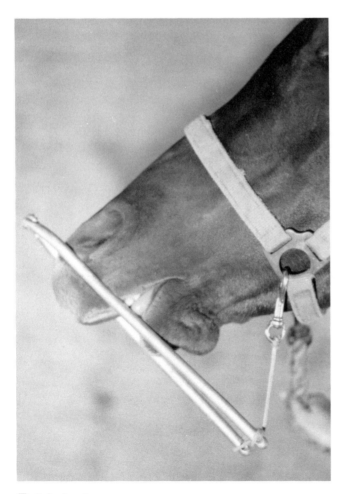

Twitch, in place.

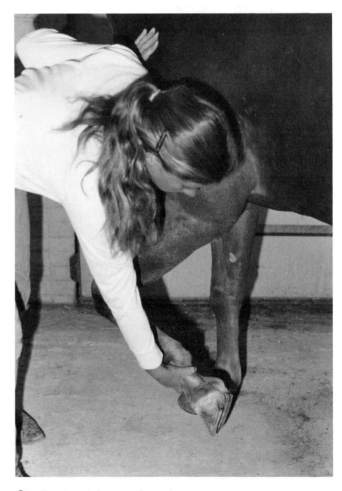

Starting to pick up a front leg.

minutes' restraint. It also tends to make the animal headshy.

LEG RESTRAINTS

All horses from foals on up should be trained to allow their feet to be handled, both with the foot on the ground and with it picked up. Many people teach their animals a cue, such as pinching the tendons when they want the horse to pick up his leg. This particular cue can be very annoying as it makes it nearly impossible to keep the animal's leg straight and on the ground when you wish to examine his tendons. One of my clients teaches his horses to pick up their feet when he bumps or nudges them with his shoulder while he has a hand on the horse's foot. Most horses, fortunately, will allow their legs to be held up.

When picking up an animal's foreleg, it is usually best to face to the rear. For the left foreleg, put your left shoulder against the horse's left shoulder. Then push into him just a little—more of a pressure than a shove. At the same time, reach down and cup your left hand inside the animal's cannon bone or fetlock area. Now it is easy to hold the foot with your hand for examination or treatment. If you need to keep the foot up for a while, or to hold it for cleaning or shoeing, it is easy to place his leg inside yours, and hold the foot against the inside of your leg.

Try to keep the animal's leg as much under his body as possible. If you pull it too far outward, it will be uncomfortable for many animals and they will try to pull the leg away from you.

When you have the animal's leg held up, it is important to hang on firmly, and only allow the animal to put it down when you are finished. Otherwise, the animal may get into the habit of trying to pull the leg away as soon as it is picked up. This habit is annoying and, in the worst cases, can be dangerous. Conversely, if you are doing a lengthy procedure, such as shoeing the horse, it is only considerate to allow him to put his foot down from time to time to rest and relax for a minute or two. This will make him much more cooperative and willing to stand on three legs when you want him to do so.

It is occasionally necessary to pull the animal's leg forward. This can be done by picking up the foot as above,

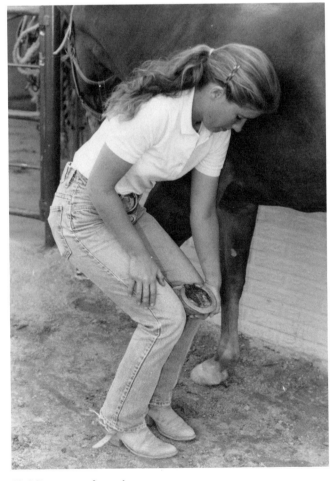

Holding up a front leg.

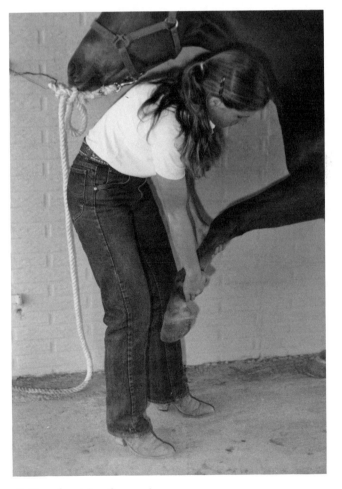

Pulling front leg forward.

and then turning around and pulling the foot out forward. Or, the leg can be grasped at the knee and moved upward and forward. This is a good procedure after you have tightened the saddle cinch, as it helps to pull out any skin wrinkles which may have occurred under the cinch, and will help prevent cinch sores.

Hind legs are picked up by facing the rear of the horse and placing the hand nearest the animal on his hip. For the left hind leg, the left hand stays in place on the hip bone. This allows you to feel what the horse is doing, and allows you to push him away from you somewhat if the animal becomes upset. Then you can pat the horse's rump with your right hand, then gradually move the right hand down the leg. This tells the animal that you are going to do something with his hind leg. If he is going to kick, he may try to do so at this point. Better he kick now than when you are bent over toward the lower part of the leg! Be careful not to tickle the flank area. Move the right hand down until it is about the middle of the cannon area. Now you can pull the leg forward and upward. If the horse kicks at this point, you will still be in a relatively safe position and not likely be injured. Now you can place the left arm over the hock and step under the leg pulling it slightly to the

rear of the horse. The leg can be supported by your legs, leaving your hands free to work on the foot. If you have any questions about lifting or holding a horse's legs, have your veterinarian or an experienced horseman show you how it's done and help you to do it yourself.

FRONT LEG RESTRAINTS

One of the animal's front legs can be held up to allow examination of the other foreleg. This is effective with many animals. It can also be used to keep a hind leg on the ground for treatment. Do not underestimate the athletic animal, however—there are some horses around who can have one leg held up, balance on two, and kick with the remaining one. If you are alone, you can tie the front leg up with a belt or other wide leather strap or a loop of thick rope to allow treatment of the other front leg or hind leg. It is not totally effective to keep the animal from kicking with a hind leg, especially if he is leaning against a wall or post, or is an exceptionally coordinated and balanced animal. Don't get careless and rely totally on one leg being tied up.

A rope with a loop in the end may be placed around the front pastern, or a hobble may be placed on the front

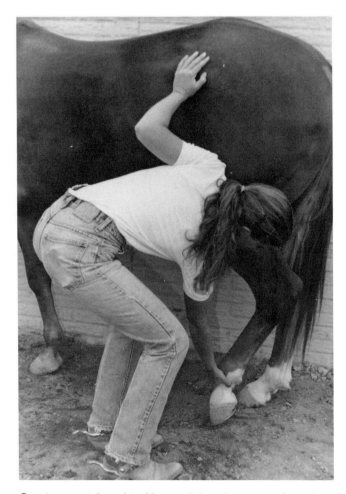

Starting to pick up hind leg, with hand on rump for safety.

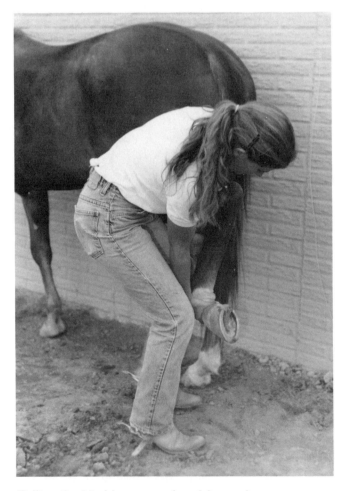

Pulling the hind leg upward and forward.

pastern and a rope attached to it. The rope is then run up over the animal's withers, down the opposite side of his neck, and then back through the first piece of rope. This will allow the animal's front leg to be held off the ground. This method can be used to hold up a front leg for examination, or to restrain the animal for work on the hind end. The end of the rope should not be tied off, but should be held by someone so that if the animal starts to become tired or fall, it can be released to prevent damage to the animal's knee.

HOBBLES

Also called hopples by some, this form of restraint can be used to hold both horse's front legs together. The wider the hobbles are, the less likelihood there is of rubs or abrasions on the front legs. Hobbles are useful in helping to immobilize an animal who persists in walking off or otherwise trying to leave the country and who will not stand tied. It sometimes works well on an animal who strikes. Be aware, however, that an occasional horse will still attempt to strike with both front legs hobbled together. Hobbles are also made for use on a single front foot. These are often used to picket animals for grazing.

HIND LEG RESTRAINTS

TYING UP A HIND LEG (SIDELINING)

Inch-thick cotton rope is useful for tying up a horse's hind leg. If you do not have it, do NOT use a lariat down around the animal's pastern, as it will almost invariably cause a rope burn, which may be much more difficult and time-consuming to treat than the original problem. Take the cinch off a saddle and loop it once or twice around the pastern area. Run the lariat through the rings and pull the animal's foot up with this. Or, a one-foot hobble with a large ring can be used. A piece about 15 inches deep can be cut across a burlap bag. This can then be rolled downward to form a doughnut of cloth. This loop can be used around the pastern area, and the lariat threaded through it.

Pull the horse's leg forward until the foot just bears a little weight. The horse will fight harder if the leg is pulled as far forward as possible and he is left standing on three legs. Sidelines are especially valuable as breeding restraint for a mare. She can be sidelined on one side, with the leg pulled just far enough forward so that she cannot kick, but not so far that she is unbalanced. Then, have the

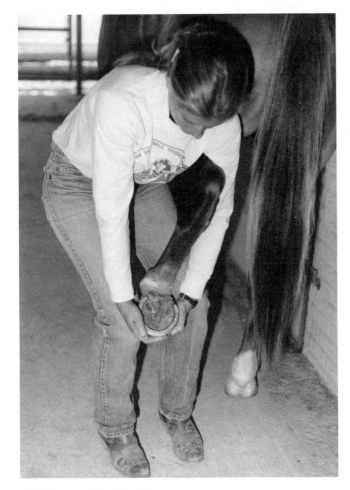

Holding up the hind leg.

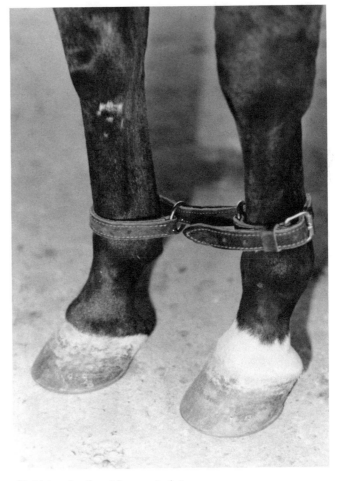

Hobbles for front leg restraint.

stallion approach and mount from this side. When he is finished with the breeding, pull him off and take him away from the same side. Sidelining is occasionally a useful restraint for treating an animal.

BREEDING HOBBLES

Breeding hobbles are a kind of ready-made sideline. They usually have a leather or web neckband which goes around the lower part of the animal's neck and ropes made to restrain one or both hindlegs. Some breeding hobbles have special double web slings which go over the hocks. Breeding hobbles are useful (and generally well worth the money you spend on them) if you are hand-breeding large numbers of mares. They work much like the sideline mentioned above.

FOUR-LEG HOBBLES

Sets of hobbles hooked together with chain in an x-shape which have a band for each leg are made. It seems to me that if you can get close enough to put all that hardware on the animal, you can probably figure out an

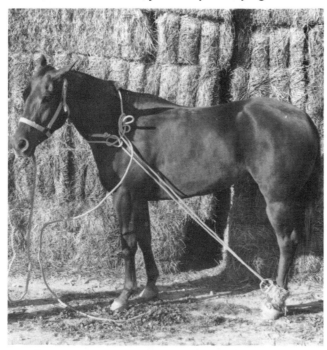

A safe way to sideline a horse with a lariat. Begin by tying a large loop loosely around the lower part of the neck, using a bowline knot. This is the lower of the two knots in the photo. Then wrap a saddle cinch twice around the fetlock area. Run the long end of the rope through both cinch rings. Then take it back through the neck loop and tie with a safe knot. Most horses fight a sideline less if the hoof is left resting on the ground so the horse can partially use it for support. If the leg is pulled up to the belly, the horse may throw himself while fighting to keep his balance.

easier and simpler way to get him to stand still for the necessary treatment.

CASTING HARNESS

Regular casting harnesses are made for pulling horses down and tying them up. The same setup can be made from an eighty-foot length of inch-thick cotton rope. The need for these has been much reduced since chemical restraints have been developed that allow us to lay an animal out flat with three to five cc's of a drug. If the animal is either so injured or so intractable as to need to be trussed up like a Christmas goose, it's better to tranquilize him or use some other form of chemical restraint, thus saving anxiety and injury both to the animal and to the handlers.

Animals may be severely injured by casting because of the struggle and fight that they put up. Occasionally, they will fracture a tibia in the course of the battle. Broken backs have also resulted from use of a casting harness. Also, when the animal is fully awake and being fought in this way, he may hit his head on the ground and damage the facial nerve, resulting in facial paralysis.

Casting also has the disadvantage of requiring several stout helpers. It must be done on a soft surface or on good bedding in a level place. Throwing an animal to the ground on a hard or rocky surface may result in severe abrasions and injury to the animal's skin.

All in all, casting is a method of restraint not worth using in these days of easy, safe chemical control. If the animal is that bad and you need him on the ground, it should be worth a call to your veterinarian to give him an injection to get him there, sleeping quietly and with no injuries.

OTHER METHODS OF RESTRAINT

WAR BRIDLES AND LIP CHAINS

War bridles and lip chains have their place in equine restraint. They are not methods that are used as a first choice, but definitely come in handy at times when nothing else works. In most cases, they are best replaced by chemical restraints because they can be quite severe, painful, and can sometimes cause permanent injury.

An example of lip chain usage is an extremely large horse with an injured eye whose owner had to put ointment in the animal's eye daily in order to help save his sight. The animal was about 17 hands tall, long-necked, and headshy. We did not wish to tranquilize or otherwise sedate him every day because that would not have been good for him, as well as being expensive. The owner wrestled with him for several days before deciding in desperation that a lip chain might work. He had already tried a chain under the jaw, and then one over the nose, with no results. The third day, he slid the chain under the animal's upper lip, after having hooked it to the right ring of the halter and running it out through the left ring (he was treating the left eye). When the horse pulled upward, the owner came down with all his weight (which isn't much). The horse came back to the ground immediately. The horse made one more halfhearted attempt at rearing, and then stood to be treated. The owner kept a snug, but not heavy, pressure on the chain while working.

The second day of lip chain usage, the gelding only reared slightly. The third day he did not rear at all, and stood quietly. While he stood quietly, the owner was extra careful not to pull on the chain and to reward him by petting and praising him. At the end of two weeks, the horse would stand quietly for treatment and ALSO to have his head handled—something he would not previously do for his owner.

Many kinds of war bridles are available, or they can be homemade. They work on both the extremely sensitive nerves on the horse's upper gums as well as on the nerves of the poll which are also quite sensitive. Some of these were the basis of famous horse training "systems" in past years. War bridles are minimally useful for treating horses;

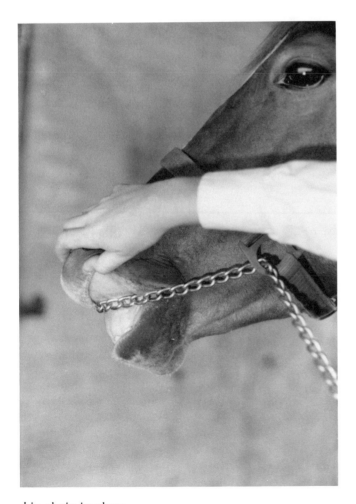

Lip chain in place.

if the animal is intractable enough to necessitate using one of them, most veterinarians will give him a tranquilizer rather than fight the horse.

NECK CRADLE

Neck cradles can be made of wood or metal. They prevent the animal from or turning his head and neck. Cradles are great for keeping horses (especially those of a nervous nature) from chewing bandages or otherwise damaging themselves. A cradle may be homemade from 15 or 20 pieces of splinter-free wood, such as doweling, with holes drilled through each end. They may then be strung together on light nylon cord with fat wooden beads between them for spacers, or they may be separated by knots tied on each side of the wooden bars. They should be about two inches apart at the neck end and three inches apart at the shoulder end. Feed and water must either be raised to the height of the animal's mouth, or the cradle must be taken off when the animal is fed.

SIDE STICKS

These are used for the same purpose as neck cradles, but are often more effective in keeping a horse from irritating a hind leg injury. They allow the animal more freedom of movement than does a cradle, and he can either eat from the floor or graze fairly normally. A girth or surcingle is placed around the animal. Then, a stick is run from there to the animal's halter to keep him from reaching around to the side where the injury has occurred. A sidestick will not keep an animal from reaching his front legs—a cradle is necessary for foreleg injuries which need protection.

A similar sort of restraint can be made from a piece of plastic pipe and a piece of rope. The pipe is slid over the rope. In cold weather, the end of the rope can be tied to a hole punched in the bottom of the front part of the horse's blanket. In hot weather, a loop of rope around the animal's girth area will keep the pipe in place.

BLINDFOLD

Blindfolds are occasionally useful in working with horses. One can be improvised from almost any piece of soft cloth which will not irritate the eyes. Jackets and towels are often handy and work well. One of my clients loaded a severely ill and incoordinated horse in a trailer by blindfolding him so that he quit fighting and would allow himself to be pushed in to the trailer. Some horses will become crazed when blindfolded; other methods of restraint must be used with them.

FOAL RESTRAINT

Foals can struggle amazingly strongly for animals no larger than they are. Small foals are best held front and rear, with the handler's arms around each end, or with one arm under the neck and the other hand grasping the tail. The foal's tail may be pushed firmly forward over its back to act as a twitch. Occasionally, a foal will reach around and bite when held in this manner. If restrained for a long period of time by the tail, the foal may attempt to sit down.

If you wish to lay the foal down, this can be easily done by pulling the tail between the hind legs and keeping a steady pressure on it. Soon the foal will relax and droop to the ground. He can be kept down by pulling the tail in front of the stifle and putting downward pressure on the neck.

Never use a lip or chin chain on a foal (or any horse much under two years old, for that matter) because it may flip over backwards at the pain. This may result in severe injury which will never heal, or, in some cases, may even be fatal.

It is not advisable to stand directly behind a foal facing his hind legs, as he may kick out unpredictably. It is much safer to stand sideways, to prevent a kick into the groin or abdomen.

SLINGS

Slings are used to help support a horse who is unable to stand by himself. They can be used to reduce the pressure on a broken leg. They lessen the strain on the opposite leg and help to prevent it from breaking down. They can help a weak animal to stand. Some horses who are down for a long period of time give up; a sling can help one of these to become upright and get both his confidence and strength back. The horse cannot hang totally supported by a sling for more than a few minutes; for this reason, the horse must be conscious and able to partially support his weight.

The animal's disposition must be such that he will work with the sling. An animal who fights it may further damage a broken leg or other injury, necessitating euthanasia for humane reasons. The ideal patient is one who has enough gumption to try and make it, yet is docile enough to tolerate the boredom and restraint of the sling.

An illustration of a sling shows the belly and rump straps which help keep the horse from sliding forward or backward. The animal will need to be haltered with the

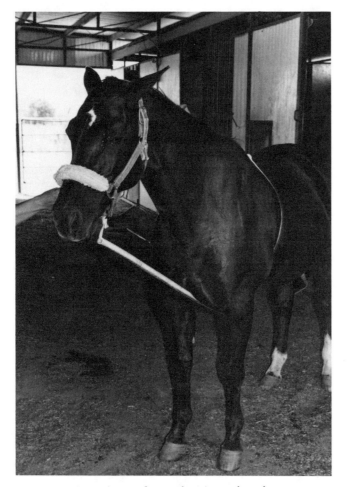

Device to keep horse from chewing a bandage.

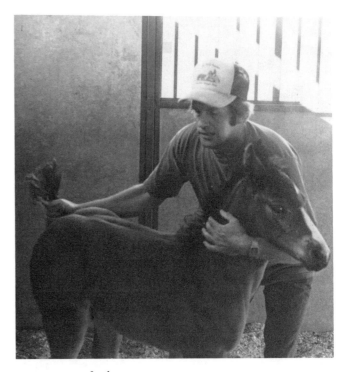

Restraining a foal.

halter tied to the side of the stall to keep him from swiveling around the block and tackle which are used to lift him. Rope slings may be made to lift an animal out of a ditch or bog. These are only for temporary usage, as they may cause severe disturbances with circulation if used for prolonged support.

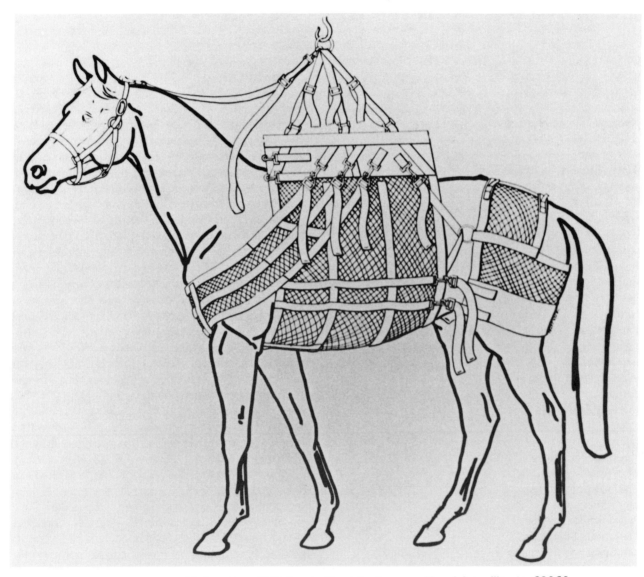

Example of a sling, courtesy of Liftex, Inc., 250 South Shaddle Avenue, Mundelein, Illinois, 60060

Chapter 10

TREATMENT METHODS

The Importance of Nursing
Cold
Heat
Soaking Solutions
Massage
Rest
Exercise
Acupuncture
Electrical Stimulation
Blistering, Firing, and Counterirritation
    Blistering
    Injectable Counterirritants
    Firing
    Liniments
Oral Medications
    Drenching
    Boluses and Tablets
    Pastes
Stomach Tube
Enemas
Injections
    Anaphylactic Shock
    Local Reactions
    Legal Complications
Route of Injection
    Intramuscular Injections
    Intravenous Injections
    Subcutaneous Injections
    Intradermal Injections
    Intra-articular Injections

THE IMPORTANCE OF NURSING

". . . grant me the serenity
To accept the things I cannot change,
Courage to change the things I can,
And wisdom to know the difference."

These comments by Reinhold Niebuhr seem particularly applicable to the field of veterinary medicine. There are those problems that we can change, such as suturing a wound, splinting a broken leg, injecting the proper antibiotics to help kill infection-causing bacteria, or helping a mare to give birth to a malpositioned foal.

The rub comes with problems that we cannot directly relieve—those that leave veterinarian and horse owner alike feeling helpless. If you are cursing your veterinarian's inability to affect the course of a virus respiratory infection or a case of sleeping sickness (a virus encephalitis) in your favorite horse, stop and consider how little human medicine can do for the common cold! Medicine has not developed to the point where we can influence, and certainly cannot cure, most viral diseases. Problems, such as laminitis and heaves, can be largely prevented by careful feeding and management. But when we have a horse with one of these problems, or something like navicular disease, we are again left feeling helpless. While cures will probably be found for some of these problems within our lifetimes, there are, at present, no specific treatments that work once the animal has the disease or condition.

It is in the area of no specific treatment where the owner can make his influence felt on the outcome of the disease through good and diligent nursing care. We cannot heal these problems directly—we can only help the animal have the most resistance and best conditions possible, hoping that his immune system and bodily defenses are strong enough to overcome the problem. Here, nursing does make a difference. The day-to-day nursing care and help supplied by the owner quite often mean the difference between life and death. Let's discuss some specifics about nursing the sick horse:

1) Shelter. This is often more important than any other consideration. One case that comes to mind is a mare dying in a western Nebraska field with the air temperature about 20 degrees F (−7 degrees C), wind blowing and snow falling. The veterinarian suggested that the rancher begin treatment by getting the animal to the barn.

The owner recited a long string of excuses as to why he couldn't, then proceeded to ask the vet to give her a shot of antibiotics "to make her well." All the antibiotics in the world wouldn't have saved the animal—her immediate problem was that she was dying from exposure!

Begin treatment by considering what kind of shelter is needed to help improve your animal's chances of survival. He may need nothing more than a tree or shed in spring or fall in a mild climate. If it is winter, or a cold rain is falling, treatment must certainly begin by getting the animal in out of the weather. Conversely, when it's 110 degrees F (44.4 C) in Phoenix in the summer, shade is the first requirement to keep a sick horse from dying of heatstroke or suffering complications on top of the problems he already has.

Keeping the temperature as comfortable as possible may involve heaters in winter if it is extremely cold. When using heaters or heat lamps, make sure you don't cause a fire hazard. A chilled foal may be warmed by placing plastic gallon jugs filled with hot water around him like hot water bottles. In an emergency, an animal who is still standing can be placed in a horse or stock trailer overnight. Remove the dividers if at all possible.

When no shelter is available, coverings can be improvised. Horse blankets are nice if you have them. If not, regular blankets, canvas, or burlap bags can be used to cover a chilled animal. In rainy weather, garbage bags, plastic, irrigation dams, or anything waterproof can be placed over a horse blanket, and then covered by another blanket. The top blanket gets wet, but the plastic barrier keeps the blanket underneath dry. A burlap bag with a couple of holes cut in it makes a fine emergency blanket for a newborn foal.

In summer, a fan will help move air and make the animal more comfortable. If the animal is in a hot climate and is lying down outside, it may be necessary to build a shade for him if he cannot be moved into shelter. Lacking this, sponge the animal with cool (not cold!) water several times a day to help keep his temperature down to normal.

2) Feed. Feed should be of the best quality that is available so that it is easy to digest. It needs to have adequate nutritional content to provide materials needed for healing damaged tissues. The animal who is ill may not be eating as much as normal, making it doubly important that the feed give as many nutrients as possible in a small amount. On the other hand, avoid sudden changes to over-rich feed that may add digestive problems on top of the existing illness. Use your judgment or ask your veterinarian any questions regarding feeding your ill horse.

3) Water. Water is very important to maintain fluid balance within the body in order to aid healing. Your doctor often advises, "Take two aspirin and drink lots of fluids." Especially with virus diseases, it is important that the body not become dehydrated because this can cause serious complications for an already-sick horse. The water should be fresh and clean and be changed frequent-ly. Try to keep it cool, but not cold, in summer. In the winter, it should be heated so that it is available at all times and is neither frozen nor icy-cold. Water once or twice a day is not enough for any horse, and especially not for a sick animal—he should have it in front of him at all times. Shut off the automatic waterer, if you have one, and water the sick horse from a bucket so you can tell how much he is drinking.

4) Bedding. Bedding should be deep, warm, dry, and be cleaned frequently. In the western states, horses are often bedded on sand or on tamped dirt floors. These are neither soft enough nor warm enough for a sick animal. It is well worth buying straw (if the horse does not eat his bedding) or shavings and putting them 8 to 12 inches deep to give a cushioned floor that will encourage the sick animal to lie down and rest which he may be unwilling to do if the floor is cold, damp, or hard.

5) Freedom from insects. Can you imagine lying in bed with a cold and having flies sitting all over your body? A sick horse surely can't enjoy it. A light sheet or fly net will protect most of the animal. Spraying the stall or corral will often control flies so they are no longer a nuisance. Be sure that the fly spray used is not toxic to horses. Poisoned baits may help to reduce fly numbers in the area—make sure they are set safely outside the horse's reach.

Insect repellent may be used on the horse. When using a new insect repellent, try a small spot on the horse's neck and let it set for 12 hours or so. One of my clients raised welts about an inch high on a horse, from one end of the animal to the other, by using a repellent to which the animal was allergic. So, try a small patch and see if that works; if it does, then apply it according to directions. The stick-type repellents will help keep insects away from the animal's nose and eyes without getting repellent in the eyes or nose.

6) Grooming. Don't overdo it, but a sick animal should be brushed to help remove dirt, stimulate circulation in the skin, and just generally help the animal feel better. Cleaning the feet out helps prevent thrush in the stabled horse. Sponging drainage from the eyes and nose will make him feel better and reduce the number of flies that are attracted. If it is an extremely hot day and there is no shelter, sponging cool (not cold) water over the entire animal will help reduce fever, keep the animal comfortable, and help prevent heatstroke.

7) Exercise or rest? The decision to exercise or rest the horse depends on the illness and your veterinarian's instructions. If you don't understand or agree, ask the veterinarian why he is recommending the rest or exercise. One good example is exercising a horse following castration. It is no kindness to let the animal stand still and swell and get sore. This can lead to serious and often life-threatening complications. So, if the vet says to exercise your horse for two hours, do it!

8) Medication. Pills or injections should be given as close to prescribed times as possible. The vet may tell you

to give a shot every 12 hours because the drug only stays in the blood for 14 hours. If you go much past this time interval, the animal may be without adequate levels of antibiotics in his body which may give bacteria a chance to get growing again and maybe get ahead. Bandages should be changed or wounds cleaned according to your veterinarian's instructions.

If you have any questions about treatment or progress, don't hesitate to call your veterinarian. Most of us would rather get an extra call than to have an owner treat the animal in a way that would be harmful to healing in the long run. Regular medication or bandage changes will result in faster healing than treatment by fits and starts. Thus you save time and money on medications, bandaging materials, and extra vet calls.

9) Miscellaneous. Some animals do best with a companion in the same corral, while others are just as content to be by themselves. If you have a horse who is going to go crazy when separated from others, ask your veterinarian if it would be okay to pen him up with a companion. On the other hand, you don't want the sick horse bullied or pushed around by other horses, so separation is often the only way to allow the animal to get some rest and relaxation. Sometimes another kind of animal, such as a goat, will provide companionship without bullying.

Speaking of rest, don't worry the animal to death—groom him enough so that he is comfortable, but don't fuss with him all day long. That's why hospitals have visiting hours—so that sick people can get some rest! Strangers may be upsetting to a sick animal—think before you call all your friends to see Ol' Dobbin. Last, but not definitely not least, hang in there. Many problems can be cured if we just keep after them long enough to give the animal a chance to heal himself.

Now that we've discussed some important points about nursing, let's cover some treatment methods which may be used.

COLD

Cold therapy is often valuable with injuries, such as bruises, sprains, muscular strains, and similar problems which have JUST occurred. Cold therapy is also good for animals who have been burned. Cold helps relieve pain. This is important with an animal as sensitive to pain as a horse. The sooner an injured limb can be restored to normal function, the less wear and tear there will be on his other, sound legs.

Cold helps to reduce the inflammation which is occurring in the freshly injured tissues. It can help reduce swelling, probably by slowing circulation in the injured area and lowering the amount of fluid which leaves the blood and lymph vessels and pools in the damaged tissues. It can also help stop bleeding by constricting

capillaries in the area; the less blood that gets out of the blood vessels and into the tissues, the less has to be removed in the healing process. Look back to the times when you have had a severe, large, purple bruise—and remember how long it took to heal! If you can avoid some of this blood pooling in the first place, it will make healing quicker and easier. In this way, prompt application of ice or cold water may significantly reduce healing time. If you use ice, be sure to wrap it in a towel or some other barrier to avoid freezing the skin.

Cold is often used in addition to pressure bandages, especially with problems such as bowed tendons.

Cold is most valuable when used during the first 24 to 48 hours after the injury has occurred. After this time, it is of little or no value. By slowing circulation, it may even hinder resolution of the problem.

Ice may be used to chill an injured area if it is available. Ice cubes can be placed in an ice bag or plastic sack, and then wrapped in a towel or rag. This may be held over the injury by a loosely applied elastic bandage. This works best if the animal is placed in a set of stocks or otherwise restrained so that he cannot wander around while being treated. The refreezable, artificial-ice bags are convenient, and often stay frozen longer than ice made with water. They can also be shaped around a box of frozen vegetables or package of meat so that they approximate the curve of the animal's leg.

Another handy way to make an ice container is to take an old inner tube and cut it so that you have a long tube. Then, roll the bottom end a couple of times to hold the ice. Slip it up over the horse's leg and fill with ice. Tie it loosely over the withers with string or baling twine. Or, make an elastic band from another strip of inner tube (but make sure it's not too tight).

Cold water may be run directly onto the area with a garden hose. In an emergency, an inner tube may be used to hold cold water instead of ice. The leg may be wrapped with strips of old blanket or other bedding or burlap sacks, and these can then be soaked with cold water. If you are near a river, stream, or irrigation ditch with good footing on the bottom, the animal may be soaked there. Stand the animal in the cold water for an hour or so every three or four hours. Be sure to allow him some time out of the water. There is no advantage in standing most injuries in cold water continuously for 12 to 24 hours. Use the cold water off and on for the first 48 hours or so after an injury.

If you are using cold water on an animal who has been burned, do not use it for an excessive length of time as it may contribute to the shock that the animal will be experiencing. In general, if the animal is in shock, large amounts of cold water or ice should not be used. Treatment with cold should also not be used if infection is present.

When water is put on an open wound, the horse's tissues tend to absorb it. This may carry in infection as well as swelling the tissues, and may drastically slow the healing process. For this reason, cold running water should not be used on open wounds—use an ice bag instead. Again, be careful using ice so you don't freeze the skin, as that will severely retard healing. You don't need frostbite in addition to a cut!

Cold should not be used for an excessive period of time, as it may then cause the blood vessels to open up and increase circulation to the area—just the opposite of what you want. Using it in addition to a compression bandage will help to prevent this problem.

Heat and cold may be used alternately in some problems after 24 to 48 hours have passed. This treatment is often used on sprains and similar injuries.

HEAT

Heat may be used to warm a chilled animal, such as a very ill horse in a cold climate, or a foal born in a snow or rainstorm and suffering from exposure. Plastic gallon jugs or similar containers may be filled with hot water and used as hot water bottles to help warm the animal. A chilled foal may be warmed in a tub of lukewarm (NOT HOT) water. He should then be carefully dried. A good way to do this is to first dry him with towels or other cloths and finish the job with a hair dryer. Be careful not to get him too warm with either the water or the dryer. He can be returned to his mother after he is warmed and dry.

A grown horse who is down and suffering from cold may be warmed with water bottles as above. Or, an electric blanket may be placed over the animal and turned on low. Someone should be present to be sure that the animal does not roll or thrash and become tangled in the blanket or wire, or that it does not start a fire. Electric blankets should NEVER be left on an unattended horse. Infrared lights may be used to warm foals or grown horses. They can burn the animal if the distance is not exactly right, and they carry considerable danger of fire if they get near bedding or other flammable materials. The animal may knock the bulb down and break it and then injure himself on the glass. In general, infrared lights and electric blankets are not good heaters for horses. With a bit of ingenuity, you can find a substitute method which is at least as effective and much safer.

Heat is used on injuries after 24 to 48 hours have passed. At this point, it helps to stimulate circulation in the area. This aids the body in removing toxic products from the area and makes healing more rapid. Heat also helps the body's circulation to remove blood and other fluids from the area. This, in turn, leads to a reduction in swelling.

Heat should not be used if infection is present in an area—or even suspected! In this case, it may cause the infection to spread. It can also cause problems because of increased absorption of toxins into the body. Increased circulation in the area may lead to severe edema and swelling which may further complicate the injury. If heat is used on a fresh injury, it may make the problem worse than it would have been without it.

Hot water can be used from a hose (if you have a large water heater), or it may be applied to bandages or wraps as mentioned above for cold. Hot towels are useful for mares with udder edema. Make sure they are not so hot as to scald the animal or the problem may get rapidly worse instead of better. Begin with lukewarm water and gradually make it hotter as the animal becomes accustomed to it. If the animal keeps trying to remove his foot from the hot water, you may have it hotter than is comfortable for him. It's sometimes a struggle the first soak or two; after that, most animals come to enjoy the process.

Hot water may be put into an inner tube as described above for cold therapy. If you're really lucky and have access to a whirlpool boot, these are an even better way of applying hot water. These boots have a small air compressor attached to the boot by a piece of hose. The compressor pushes bubbles of air through the boot and has a stimulating action—a miniature Jacuzzi for the horse's legs! Try turning on the compressor at a distance from the horse before you attach it to the boot to see if he will tolerate the noise and not panic and hurt himself or someone else. Like the hot soak itself, some horses seem to actually enjoy the bubbling action after they become accustomed to it. A vacuum cleaner can be used to blow air into the soak water for a whirlpool-like effect. Be sure to keep the vacuum itself well out of the way so that there are no electrical problems if the horse spills the water. Soak a horse for 30 to 45 minutes twice a day for most leg problems requiring soaking.

Deep heat and diathermy have been used to produce heat in tissues. These should be used only under the direction of your veterinarian, as damage to bones and other underlying tissues can occur with improper usage. Like other forms of heat, they should not be used for at least 48 hours after an injury has occurred, nor should they be used when ANY infection is present.

Infrared light has been recommended as a way of producing heat in horse tissues. It is not a good idea because of the very considerable danger of skin burns. Like a sunburn, these burns may not show up until some time after the treatment which caused them. If the animal's injury needs heat, it's probably going to benefit from being soaked as well.

SOAKING SOLUTIONS

Epsom salts (magnesium sulfate) can be added to help draw swelling and fluid out of the area. One or two cups may be used per gallon of water. It can be used with either hot or cold water. Commercial soaking solutions are often available. These are mainly based on epsom salts, with menthol and other aromatic substances added.

It's much cheaper to just buy plain epsom salts. It is usually available from a drug store. Many horsemen keep two to five pounds on hand at all times; you might even end up using it on yourself, for soaking aching muscles, sprains, or other similar injuries!

MASSAGE

Massage is often used in addition to heat treatments to help healing of sprains and similar problems. It often helps to lessen swelling and reduce pain. Many people like to use liniments, "braces," and other products, rubbing them into the skin over the injury. They may produce some reddening and irritation in the skin over the injury, but don't do anything for the underlying tissues. Improvement is due not to the product used, but to the massage. For best effect, massage should be repeated three or four times a day. Massage often helps to keep scar tissue from forming adhesions between the skin and the underlying tissues.

REST

Rest is often used to help keep leg injuries from getting worse or becoming further irritated. It is helpful with problems such as bowed tendons. If the animal continues to move around and use the leg, more fluid and blood may leak from the injured area, causing more swelling and pain, and lengthening the time necessary for healing. Make sure what your veterinarian wants in the way of rest. He may want the animal totally confined to a small stall (say, 16 × 16 feet or less) or may merely want him in a small corral. He may allow the animal to be turned loose in a small pasture to graze and to move as the animal wishes. He may want the animal rested most of the day, but taken out for a few minutes exercise. Check on this matter and follow his instructions. This author prescribed strict rest for one client's horse. When the animal did not heal, the owner consulted me. When I asked about the rest, I found out that they were feeling sorry for the animal because he was "cooped up all day" and were taking him out and walking him for an hour every evening. Hardly what I had in mind when I prescribed strict rest!

EXERCISE

Exercise is used in treating several lamenesses. For instance, it may be used to help the circulation in the feet of a freshly foundered horse. If the animal's feet are hurting him badly, it may be necessary to administer appropriate painkillers before the animal can be moved. Exercise may be used to help remove swelling from infections,

gunshot wounds, or abscesses. It is VERY important after castration.

Exercise may be used to build up an animal's muscles and tendons after prolonged confinement. Horses who are being built up gradually should be worked very slowly and carefully. If turned loose in a corral or pasture and allowed to do as they wish, some animals feel so exuberant that they will overwork and reinjure themselves. An hour's time out may undo months of massage, soaking, and rest. This happened with one of my own horses after a bowed tendon. Lead the animal by hand for several days until the novelty of being out has worn off, then turn the animal loose. This gradual start into exercise is especially important to animals recovering from fractures.

Swimming is excellent exercise for building up horses who have had leg injuries or surgery. It helps the animal to build up both lung and cardiovascular capacity without jarring his legs. Swimming can strengthen the animal so that when he begins work in the arena or track, he will not re-injure his previous problem (see Swimming).

ACUPUNCTURE

Acupuncture has been touted as a cure-all for anything and everything that ails horses; it has also been debunked as being total quackery. As with many disputes, the truth probably lies somewhere in between. No one knows how (or for sure IF) it works in the horse (or in the human!). There are probably some cases where this technique will help an animal by relieving pain. If you've tried everything else and someone is available who is experienced in it—why not give it a try? This author will be the first to encourage any treatment which works.

ELECTRICAL STIMULATION

This technique has had much the same history as acupuncture. It is likely that the best use of this technique is for pain relief. It has been widely used for pain therapy in humans following muscular injury. It is far less likely that it will build up a horse's muscles or help him to run faster, judging from experiments which have been run on humans.

BLISTERING, FIRING, AND COUNTERIRRITATION

BLISTERING

Blistering is the name given when irritating substances are applied to the animal's skin. The theory is that chronic problems will be converted to acute problems and thus be healed. The animal suffers the same irritation and pain as if he had been burned; this is because you are actually causing a chemical burn when you put this type of substance on his skin. Skin treated by blistering may develop blisters which ooze serum and weep. The process can go so far as to cause sloughing of patches of skin. In my opinion, there is little or no indication for blistering an animal. Put yourself in his place. If you had a sore tendon, would you burn the skin over it until it fell off? It doesn't make sense. Most of the effects of blistering are due to the rest that the animal must have after this procedure is done. In that case, why not just rest him in the first place and not put him through the extra pain?

In addition, there are some aftereffects of blistering that can cause more problems than the original one. Horses have been known to chew at the blistered area because of the pain, removing skin, tendons, ligaments, and even chunks of bone. When that happens, you REALLY have a problem. Horses who rub their heads against a blistered area have been permanently blinded because of corneal burns. Also, once signs of the severity of the blister have appeared, there is no practical way to stop its action. Like a sunburn, damage has already been done and cannot be reversed; all you can do is to stand by and watch as it becomes more severe.

INJECTABLE COUNTERIRRITANTS

These are much the same as blisters, only they are injected below the skin, into muscle or other deeper layers of the body. They cause the same sort of damage as they would on the skin—the only difference is that the tissue destruction is not happening where you can see it. Excessive scar formation may occur that can be permanent, causing stiffness or loss of function in an area.

Abscesses and sloughing can also occur—large chunks of tissue may be lost in this manner. Like a blister, once the caustic agent has been injected, there is no way to stop its action. On the rare occasions when this type of medication is used, it should be injected by a veterinarian; he is familiar with the anatomy of the area where he is putting the drug, and can avoid injecting it where it will cause damage. Even then, there is a risk of undesirable scarring or side effects.

FIRING

Firing was used a lot in the old days with chronic problems, such as bowed tendons. The person doing the firing would use an electric iron, much like a soldering iron, or one fired by ether or another chemical. He would use this to make a pattern of burns over the problem area, going deep into the tissues. The animal was bandaged for a few days, and then turned out to pasture for, usually, "a minimum of six months." That was how long it took the

burns to heal and the animal to feel like doing anything again. And lo and behold, by that time, he was cured!

The only problem with firing is that the same progress would have been made with the same six months' rest without the firing. It is the rest that makes the difference, not the firing. For that reason, firing rates as a rather barbaric form of torture in my opinion. Unfortunately, some horsemen, especially racehorse trainers and owners, will not turn the animal out to rest without some excuse to do so. Therefore, the trainer or veterinarian will fire the poor beast in order to "buy" him the rest that he needed. It's not 1894 any more and we would hope to see horsemen abandoning this barbarism in favor of enlightenment, modern medicine, and consideration for the animal without torture. We need to face the fact that there are times when nothing but rest will make the animal well, and times when nothing at all will fix him.

LINIMENTS

This author is rather neutral about the use of liniments. As long as they stop short of blistering the animal, they probably don't do any harm. On the other hand, they probably don't do a whole lot to help the horse, either. Liniment companies probably make a lot of money by helping the horse owner's head, first and foremost. We all like to feel that we are doing something to help our injured horse, and rubbing liniment on him is surely doing something! A good deal of the beneficial action of liniments comes from the fact that the directions usually tell the horse owner to rub them in for 10 to 20 minutes. This massage and the stimulation it provides probably do more for the animal than all the gunk in the world pasted on the outside of his skin. Skin, after all, hardly absorbs anything that is placed on it, let alone permitting the material to reach the deeper structures where the injury is.

ORAL MEDICATIONS

DRENCHING

Drenching is the name given to the old-time practice of pouring medicine down a horse's throat. Some people used a wine or pop bottle, while others used specially made "drenching bottles" which were covered with leather, or similar devices made of metal. Unfortunately, many drenchings were followed some days later by the animal coming down pneumonia (from the medication which he had inhaled into his lungs) and later dying.

About the only reason we have to drench a horse nowadays is to give small amounts of antidiarrheal or vitamin mixtures to a foal. Be careful when giving these not to raise the animal's head too high. It is better to lose some medicine rather than to get it too high and have him inhale some with his next breath. In an emergency, this method can be used to give a foal small amounts of milk or milk replacer until you can get a bottle with a nipple.

Liquid products can also be given with a dose syringe. This is like an injection syringe, but a LOT larger. Most dose syringes are calibrated in ounces. The principles and problems are the same as those with drenching the animal, namely, the danger that the animal may inhale some of the medication.

If you must drench a horse, hold the animal's mouth only slightly above level. Holding or tying it high up may cause the animal to inhale the medication. Mineral oil should NEVER be given orally because of the chance that the animal may inhale it because he cannot smell or taste it.

BOLUSES AND TABLETS

Occasionally, boluses (large tablets) may be given to a horse. These used to be a common method of treatment. However, some of these boluses were prone to lodge in the animal's esophagus, causing a choke. They occasionally caused death of the lining of the esophagus, sometimes with subsequent death or the need to euthanize the horse. For these reasons, boluses are rarely used now. When we do use them, they are usually crushed and fed with a bit of grain. Small boluses are often used for foals with diarrhea. These are more likely to slide down without lodging if you first lubricate them with butter or salad oil.

Tablets may be given for some diseases, especially for foals. They are often fed, either crushed or uncrushed, with some grain. If the animal is not eating, they may be crushed and mixed with a bit of water. They can then be given with a dose syringe or spooned into the animal's mouth.

PASTES

Paste medications are becoming widely used. Paste formulas available commercially include many worming products, nutrient and intestinal bacterial pastes for foals, and phenylbutazone (Butazolidin). These products are easily administered by the owner.

Make sure the animal's mouth is clean before giving a paste product. If there is any feed in the animal's mouth, it will make a large enough wad that he can easily spit out both feed and medication. Rinse the mouth with a dose syringe filled with water. Some animals will tolerate having a garden hose gently inserted into the corner of the mouth to cleanse it. When it is clean, squeeze the paste into the corner of the horse's mouth. The horse will wallow it around and try to spit it out. Most of these products are sticky enough that, like peanut butter, they "stick to the roof of your mouth." They stay in place long enough for the animal to have to swallow them rather than spit them out.

It is occasionally useful to make your own paste for an animal who will not take pills or other medication. Crush the pills or run them in a blender until they are finely powdered. Then, mix with peanut butter or jelly to make a sticky paste. This can then be placed in the horse's mouth.

STOMACH TUBE

Medication is often given to the horse via a tube which is passed through the nose into the stomach. In this way, we can give a horse medication that he would never take willingly. We can also treat an animal who is not eating, feeding him electrolytes and nutrients. We can give drugs, such as mineral oil (paraffin oil), which cannot be given orally because the animal cannot smell or taste it and may inhale it, causing a pneumonia which is nearly always fatal. And, we can make sure that he gets the WHOLE dosage without spitting or dribbling it out.

Passing a stomach tube into a horse is a highly technical procedure. If the tube is accidentally passed into the trachea, administration of medication through it may result in the animal's death. For that reason, this procedure should be left to your veterinarian.

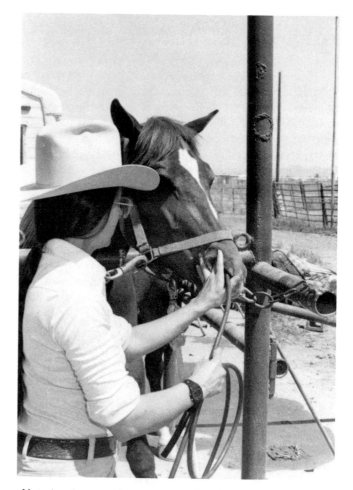

Veterinarian passing a stomach tube.

ENEMAS

Enemas are used routinely in young foals to prevent or treat meconium impaction. These should be given with an enema can and soft rubber tube, or a soft rubber infant syringe. About a pint or pint and a half of lukewarm water is enough. Alternatively, you can use a commercial human enema from a drugstore (see also Meconium Impaction).

Enemas are all but useless in the adult horse. Some old-time books recommend their use for colic. A horse's digestive tract is more than 100 feet in length, and greatly twisted. Even if large quantities of water are used, they will almost never get far enough forward to do any good. All they do is increase the discomfort and straining for an animal who is already miserable. Don't inflict this kind of cruelty on your horse!

INJECTIONS

This is the general name given to the process of putting a vaccine or medication into the animal's body with a syringe and needle. Injections may be placed under the skin. These are known as subcutaneous (S/C or Sub-Q for short) injections. Injections made into the upper layers of the skin are called intradermal injections; some of the older sleeping sickness vaccines are examples of this method of administration. Injections into the muscle are called, logically enough, intramuscular injections. Those into veins are called intravenous injections. Specialized injections may be made into joints; this route is called intra-articular.

Before we go into different types of injections and how to give them, I would like to discuss the problems and liabilities of giving them. If you are giving an injection to your own animal, you are obviously assuming the risk of doing so. By giving your own vaccinations and antibiotic injections, you may save considerable time and money as compared to having your veterinarian give them. You can give the injections when they are scheduled, without waiting for anyone but yourself. If your animal requires a prolonged course of antibiotic injections, your veterinarian may PREFER that you give these "shots" yourself.

NOTE: If the horse is insured, the policy may REQUIRE that any immunizations or injections be given by a veterinarian, and the policy may be voided if you treat the animal yourself—be sure to check this before giving the animal ANY medication.

On the other hand, you are taking the responsibility for any reactions that may occur. Reactions are of two types: local and systemic. Systemic reactions are the most serious and life-threatening. Fortunately, they are also extremely rare. One which may occur is:

ANAPHYLACTIC SHOCK

Anaphylactic shock is the name given to the most serious systemic reaction that may follow an injection. It occurs most commonly after injections of vaccines or antibiotics. Normally, it does not occur the first time the animal is given a drug (although in exceptional cases it may occur the first time). Most of the time it follows more than one exposure to the product. This is because anaphylactic shock is basically a very acute, powerful allergic reaction; the body usually requires some previous exposure to become allergic. Incidentally, anaphylactic shock can occasionally occur because of allergy to something the animal has eaten. This is even rarer than anaphylactic shock in general.

What happens in anaphylactic shock? This problem usually occurs within a few minutes to four or five hours after the offending material has been injected. The animal may begin to gasp and show trouble breathing. This comes on very suddenly. The animal may shiver and appear very upset. Lung sounds may change to a bubbling or gurgling sound. Some animals may show severe edema (fluid accumulation) in the legs and lower belly.

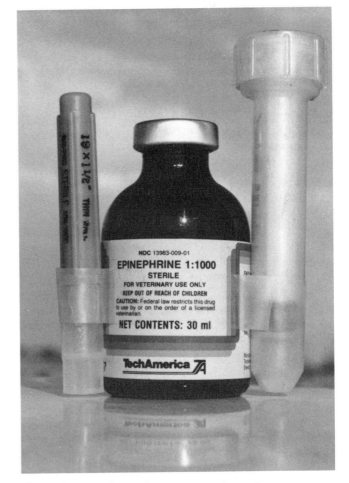

Epinephrine with sterile syringe and needle.

The "shock" part of the problem may cause the animal to be very pale and weak. This is caused by disturbances to the heart and blood vessels. Laminitis may also be seen. If the problem is not treated promptly, the animal may DIE. Death can occur within minutes. If the animal survives until you can call a vet and he can get there, it will probably make it anyway. It will be important for the vet to know that you gave an injection within the preceding few hours.

Treatment must be immediate and sure. Epinephrine (also called adrenalin) is the drug which is used. An approximate dosage is 4 to 8 ml. of a 1:1000 solution, given subcutaneously or intramuscularly. Check the bottle which you have to make sure of the dosage and method of administration BEFORE you need it. Chances are good you will never have to use it. But if you do, there will not be time to stand still and read the label. Put the medication intravenously if you can hit the jugular vein. Otherwise, put it intramuscularly or subcutaneously, depending on the instructions on the bottle.

A bottle of epinephrine and suitable syringe and needle (say, a 12-cc syringe and a 20-gauge, 1–½ inch needle) should be handy WHENEVER you give an injection. It need not be right on your person, but should never be more than a few yards away in your medicine kit. It is often convenient to tape a sterile syringe (still in its plastic case) and needle (same) to the bottle so they are always convenient—and so you are never tempted to use them when you are short of supplies.

If epinephrine is not available, prompt administration of an antihistamine solution according to the directions on the label may save the animal's life. Epinephrine is usually preferred if you have it (and there is no excuse not to have it).

Occasionally, hives (also called urticaria) may be seen as a systemic reaction following an injection. Your veterinarian should be consulted if they are numerous or do not go down within 12 to 24 hours.

LOCAL REACTIONS

Reactions may occur at the injection site itself. They do not usually show up right away, but may be seen a few hours to as much as a week later. The swelling may range from a mere bump an inch or so in diameter to a blob half the size of a football or basketball. These are from several causes:

An allergic reaction may occur at the injection site; it will usually occur within a few hours after the injection is given, and will go down in several days (with or without treatment).

The swelling may be due to an infection. This may be because bacteria were carried in with the needle when the injection was given. Or, it may be due to bacteria being brought by the bloodstream to tissues which were damaged or weakened by the injection. Abscesses tend to feel hotter to the touch than the surrounding areas. After

several days, the abscess may come to a point, getting a soft area—usually in the middle—at the highest part of the swelling. At this point, it is necessary to drain the abscess.

An abscess may affect the animal's general well-being, causing him to go off feed and appear generally "droopy." An abscess on the neck may keep the animal from turning or cause him to rein stiffly. He may simply fight to keep from turning to the sore side. Because of the chance that the animal may be sore after an injection (even if he does not develop an abscess), it is not a good idea to vaccinate an animal right before a show or other workout.

The possibility of an abscess makes it important to utilize injection sites that will drain well if an abscess occurs. One of the worst injection abscesses this author has ever seen occurred when an owner gave an injection in the top of the rump. The site swelled enormously and eventually required drainage. Even though it was opened to the outside, the tendency was still to drain inward and downward because that is the way the muscles in the area run. The problem threatened the animal's life for a time until it was finally brought under control with massive doses of antibiotics and other treatment measures. This would have been a minor problem if the injection had been given in the lower part of the hind leg. An abscess there would merely have drained to the outside, and healed after a minimum of time and treatment.

Some soft-tissue swellings have been seen with the injectable horse wormer, invermectin (Eqvalan, MSD Agvet, Inc., Rahway, NJ). They may be brief local reactions, or life-threatening infections caused by the bacteria called Clostridium. This product has been removed from the market, but some unused supplies may be remain. They should not be used.

A swelling called a "sterile abscess" is another of the problems which may occur after an injection. This looks much like an abscess, but does not get hot or come to a point. The animal may get a hematoma at the injection site. This is a blood clot which occurs because you have punctured some small (or large) blood vessel in the process of giving the injection. Because it occurs either under the skin or deeper in the muscle, it is impossible to prevent a hematoma from occasionally happening. But, by utilizing good injection techniques and giving injections in the proper sites, hematomas can be minimized.

LEGAL COMPLICATIONS

If you are treating your own animal, you are obviously taking the risk of anything that might happen. It becomes another matter entirely if you are treating an animal belonging to a friend or neighbor. Several things happen if a reaction occurs, whether it is an anaphylactic reaction that causes the animal's death or "merely" an abscess or other "minor" complication. The first is that you feel horrible, and will probably lose a friend. The second is even worse. There is a good possibility that the other person may sue you for the loss of his animal—and stand a good chance of winning.

Finally, YOU may be charged with practicing veterinary medicine without a license, which is a serious crime in some states—enough to get a stiff fine or a jail sentence. It usually doesn't matter whether the other person is paying you. What seems to matter is that you were practicing medicine on someone else's animal.

How do you avoid this problem? Easy. Just don't work on other people's animals. Period. If someone wants you to help them and you know how to give injections, that's fine. Show them how to give the injections themselves (and, make sure you're right or that could be another possible liability) or suggest they ask their veterinarian to show them how.

Some veterinarians are reluctant to teach their clients how to give injections because of the problems which may occur. However, if you offer to pay them for the time it takes to teach you, it will be money well spent, and will often change the resistance to cooperation. This is because many of us get so tired of being milked for free information by clients, who then misunderstand or misuse it, that we get a little gunshy about dishing it out. If, however, you make him understand that you are aware of the dangers, and that you would like to learn anyway, he may change his mind.

Now that we have discussed some of the advantages and dangers of giving your own injections, let's talk about the hows and whys of technique.

ROUTE OF INJECTION

It is very important that injectible drugs be given in the manner prescribed on the label. To use a drug which is meant for intravenous injection and give it in the muscle may cause the animal severe pain, and cause a large chunk of muscle to slough. If a drug meant for intramuscular use is injected into the animal's vein, carriers and other agents in the medication may cause a severe reaction and/or death. Vaccine which should be given intradermally may not develop a good immunity if it is given subcutaneously or in the muscle. Read the label and respect it. The horse you save may be your own.

INTRAMUSCULAR INJECTIONS

Most of the injections given in the horse are placed in the muscles (intramuscular). There are several reasons for using this route of administration. The animal's muscles are large and provide plenty of space for injecting materials with relatively little discomfort to the animal. In contrast, the only major veins which can be used for injection are the jugular veins; there is one on each side of the neck. When they are damaged, you're out of luck for

further injections into them. Thus, many drugs for horses are specifically formulated so that they can be injected intramuscularly. The muscles have a good blood supply, giving a rapid absorption of medication into the circulation which will spread it throughout the body. And, last but not least, intramuscular injections are easier than any other kind for most people to give.

What drugs are given in the muscles? Probably the most common is the antibiotic combination, penicillin/streptomycin. Other drugs, such as tranquilizers, some corticosteroids, and many vaccines are made to be given intramuscularly.

When should medication be given intramuscularly? Vaccines should be given intramuscularly when so directed by the labeling or package flyer. Like any other medication, it's very important to read the label to see where the drug is supposed to be given. Just because you have been giving a drug in a certain manner, don't forget to read the label occasionally for good measure. The manufacturers sometimes change formulas (and recommendations for their administration) in midstream. Do not automatically assume that since you gave the medication intramuscularly a year ago, that a new bottle is necessarily still the same. Read the label to make sure. Any medication that your veterinarian prescribes to give in the muscle should be given according to his directions and dosage.

Where do you give intramuscular injections? Sites for injections into the muscles should be chosen with an eye to avoiding bones, main blood vessels, and areas, such as the nuchal ligament, where the absorption would be poor. The site should cause the animal as little discomfort as possible. It should be in an area which will allow good drainage if the worst possible side effect, an abscess, should follow the injection. While abscesses are a rare complication, if you give every injection in a site which would not cause problems if one occurred, you are protected. The injection site chosen should allow the person giving the injection to be safe from being kicked or struck by a patient who objects to being treated.

The most common and easiest site for intramuscular injection in the horse is the middle third of the neck, measuring from top to bottom. The top part of the neck (the crest) is what is called the nuchal ligament. This heavy ligament helps to hold the animal's head up and has very little blood supply. Injections should not be given there. In the lower third of the neck, the jugular vein lies in a hollow called the jugular groove or jugular furrow. Giving a medication meant for intramuscular use into the jugular vein may result in severe reaction or even death of the animal. It is necessary to avoid that area. The spinal column snakes down through the neck, and it is necessary to avoid the bones which stick out from the side of it. This site is often avoided in working and race horses because of the possibility that the animal may be stiff or may not turn normally to the side where an injection has been given.

An equally good or even better site (considering efficient absorption of the medication) is the muscle of the lower hind leg. It's been listed as a second choice because it may be totally unusable in some horses if their disposition does not permit it. Use the large muscle at the rear of the leg. Give the injection so that it is below the hindmost point of the animal's rump, where the muscle is curving back in toward the leg. This allows for good drainage if anything should go wrong and an abscess should occur.

When giving an injection in the hind leg, it is important to stand close to the animal. If you are standing away because you are afraid of getting kicked, that is probably just what will happen because the animal has the room to take a good swing at you. If you are close, he usually cannot do much more than push you away.

The third choice for injection site is the pectoral muscles, those two bulges between the animal's front legs. They are made of muscle, fat, and connective tissue and allow less efficient absorption of the injected material than do the muscles of the neck or thigh. They work well, however, with animals who are headshy (where you cannot give an injection in the neck) or animals who kick if their rear end is approached.

The pectoral (chest) muscles seem to be less sensi-tive than some others—many animals seem to feel no pain at all when injections are given there. These muscles are often used for injections for performance and race horses where it might impair the animal's action to have him stiff in the neck, and it might also cause him some soreness to give them in the hind leg. One disadvantage of giving injections in the pectoral muscles is that they can sometimes develop seromas or other soft, puffy swellings. Sometimes these don't go away, and the animal is left with a baggy, floppy pouch of skin between the front legs.

A fourth choice, if you must, is the large muscle of the front leg. This is definitely not my first choice, but if you have an animal who cannot be injected in the neck or hind end and you've put so many injections into the pectoral muscles that they will not take any more, the front leg muscles can be used.

Whatever site you use, alternate sides from day to day. If you give a shot in the right side today, use the left side tomorrow. Then, come back to the right side again. If the animal will allow injection in more than one site, move around the animal in a pattern: left neck, left hind leg, right hind leg, right neck, and back again. Or, you can use any other pattern—just so it gives each site as much time

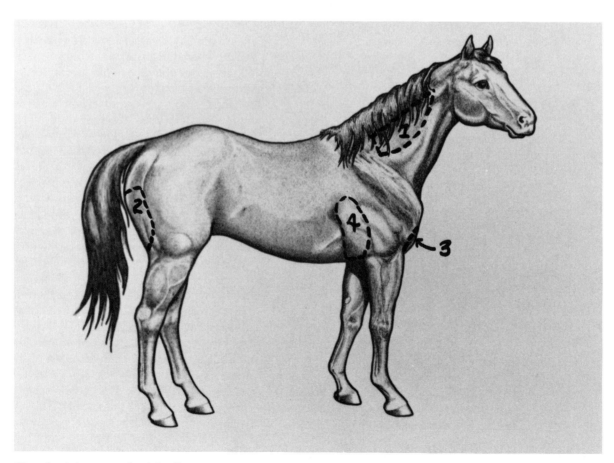

Sites for intramuscular injections.

between injections as possible. Also try to alternate between sites in the same area. For instance, if you give the injection high in the neck today, try to give it a couple of inches further back the next time around.

When you are repeating injections of a drug like penicillin into a muscular area, you will sometimes hit a pocket of the drug which you have given previously. When you pull out the plunger on the syringe, you get penicillin instead of blood or nothing. No problem—just pull the needle out and move to another site. This happens because the body has not absorbed all the previous dosage. Just be aware that it occasionally happens.

What do you need to give an intramuscular injection? You need the medicine which is to be injected—make sure that it is labeled for intramuscular use. You need alcohol or other disinfectant for the skin. You can apply it with a cotton ball or just spray or flood it onto the skin. If the animal is very dirty (muddy or bloody), it is good to curry the dirt from the skin before beginning the injection. In warm weather, the area can be washed or hosed off first. This is unnecessary when the animal is reasonably clean.

Syringes should be sized according to the injection that is being given. Syringes are sized in cubic centimeters, also called cc's. A cubic centimeter is the same, for practical purposes, as a milliliter (ml). So, if someone gives you a dosage in milliliters and your syringe is calibrated in cubic centimeters, they are the same thing. A 3-cc syringe is adequate for most vaccines. A 12-cc syringe is convenient for smaller dosages of antibiotics and other medications. The largest syringe many veterinarians routinely use on horses is a 20-cc syringe. The horse may receive 40 or 60 cc of penicillin/streptomycin, but you should not put more than 20 cc in any one spot. This is because larger amounts cause considerable pressure and pain, and probably slow absorption as compared to spreading the same dosage in smaller amounts. A maximum of 20 cc is a suitable compromise among sticking the animal the least number of times, causing him the least possible discomfort from pressure, and getting the most efficient drug absorption.

Syringes come with two different types of tips. Luer-lock syringes have a threaded end which you have to screw onto the needle. These are not my favorites; the animal always seems to jerk away when you are putting needle and syringe together, pulling out the whole thing so that you have to start over. Luer-slip ends, which merely slide into the end of the needle with a snug fit, are much easier for me to use. Syringes have the business end either centered or offset to one side. For most injections, it doesn't matter which you use. For intravenous injections, the offset ones are easier to use than the centered ones.

The size of the needle depends on what medication you are giving. Most vaccines, for instance, are best put deep into the tissues because they cause less reaction when administered that way. They are given in small quantity and are usually liquid enough that they flow

through a needle well. For this reason, a small needle can be used which will cause the animal less discomfort. My preference is a 20-gauge needle, 1–½ inches long for intramuscular vaccines.

Penicillin-type products are thicker and given in larger quantity. In fact, some penicillins inject about like Jello! If you gave it through the above needle, it would take forever, it will require considerable pressure to force it in, and the animal would probably not stand still for the whole operation. For this reason, use a larger needle—either an 18-gauge or a 19-gauge thin-wall needle. The 19-gauge thin-wall has the same size opening in the inside as the 18-gauge, but a thinner wall so that it has a smaller outside diameter which makes it less painful for the animal. These needles should be 1–½ inches long.

A selection of the two above needles will allow you to give any necessary injections to a horse. These may be purchased individually in sterile plastic containers. My preference is for needles and syringes made by Monoject (Monoject Division, Sherwood Medical Industries, St. Louis, MO 63103). Others are made which are less expensive, but are not consistently sharp and are more subject to breakage.

There is no excuse for using anything but disposable syringes and needles in horses today. The old-fashioned needles could be sharpened, but it seems no one ever bothered to do so. Using a dull needle on an animal as sensitive as a horse causes him considerable pain. Pretty soon, you have a rodeo each time you give an injection.

No method of cold sterilization (such as soaking in alcohol) will kill the virus which causes swamp fever 100% of the time. Boiling the needles and syringes also does not always kill it. The ONLY sterilization method which kills swamp fever virus is sterilization with live steam under pressure, such as your veterinarian does with a contraption called an autoclave to prepare instruments for surgery. Most owners do not bother with such sophisticated methods. So, don't try to save a few cents and then maybe lose a horse because you are using a needle which is not sterile. Use a separate, new, sterile needle for each horse.

If you are treating the same horse day after day with a medication, such as penicillin, you can just throw the syringe in the refrigerator along with the penicillin. This will keep the penicillin in it from spoiling. Then, take the syringe out the next day, put a fresh needle on it and give the injection. You can use the same syringe for three or four days in this manner if you have not drawn any blood into it in the process of injection. If you do draw blood, start with a clean syringe for the next injection.

Now it's time to fill the syringe with the medication or vaccine. Let's assume that you are starting with a new bottle of the product. Take the tip of a fingernail or sharp knife and remove the small flap of metal covering the center of the bottle cap. It will usually have one or more raised edges which make it easy to remove. Take your syringe and draw in air, an amount equal to the amount of drug you are going to remove from the bottle. This need not be an exact measurement. Shake the bottle well. Wipe the center of the rubber top with a cotton ball moistened in alcohol. Rubbing alcohol from the drugstore is fine for both this and for wiping the horse's skin.

Hold the bottle of medicine upside down and insert the needle (attached to the syringe with air in it) into the center of the rubber top. Inject the air into the bottle. This equalizes the pressure and prevents a vacuum from occurring in the bottle, allowing you to remove the medicine more easily. Draw out the amount of drug which you need. If there is a bubble of air in the top of the syringe or hub of the needle, merely inject it back into the bottle and draw out enough of the product to fill the syringe to the required amount. Now, you're ready to give the injection.

How do you give an intramuscular injection? Begin by having the animal properly restrained. If you have him tied, the halter and lead must be stout and solid and he must be tied short, in a safe manner. Make sure that you can get away from him if he throws a fit when you give the injection. If you have help, it is often best to have someone hold the horse rather than tying him. Most people give the first injection in the animal's left (near) side, as most animals are more accustomed to being handled from that side. This gives you an indication of what the animal will do when an injection on the other side is necessary the next day. If the animal does not wish to stand still, it may be necessary to have someone hold up the opposite front leg or to twitch him. This extreme is uncommon. Most animals can be accustomed to accepting injections without too much protest if you use sharp needles and handle the horse carefully.

One of the biggest causes of problems while giving injections is the owner's attitude. If you are upset or anxious about having to give your horse a shot, you are probably going to communicate this to the animal. He will then become upset and will dance around and protest. If it bothers you too badly to give an injection, it's probably best to get your veterinarian to do the dirty work. Get your own mind under control before you approach the horse. Take a deep breath and let it out, and RELAX! You're just giving the horse a shot to help him, not facing a firing squad! Now that you are calm, cool, and collected, approach the animal.

Pick the site where you are going to place the needle. Cleanse a spot two to three inches in diameter with disinfectant. Having a large area disinfected allows you some leeway. If you don't hit the exact spot you have in mind, you still can hit a cleansed area.

Remove the needle from the syringe. You are going to put the needle into the animal separately. This way, you do not have to control the weight of the syringe while you are placing the needle. Also, if the animal moves or jumps, the needle will stay with him rather than being pulled out as you hang onto the syringe. Grasp the needle with your thumb, butted against your index finger. This allows you to

use the full force of your hand to put it into the animal's muscle. Do not merely hold it poked out with the thumb and forefinger. This technique will result in weakly placing the needle or dragging it back out after you have put it in and does not work nearly as well.

Take a firm, short swing at the neck. Placing a needle is a wrist motion rather than a whole-arm arc. If you swing from a long distance, the animal will probably duck. As the needle goes into the neck, remember to LET GO! The first time or two you do it, you will probably pull the needle back out. Most beginners seem to forget to let go. Don't worry about it, because it happens to most everyone, even me from time to time. Just take a deep breath, relax, and try again. If the needle is sharp, it doesn't bother most animals to be stuck more than once—if you're not so nervous that you make them nervous. It may help to think in terms of "following through" on your swing rather than "stopping" at the horse's neck, much as you would do with a bowling ball or golf club.

It is useful to divert the horse's attention before you give the injection. If you have someone holding the horse by the lead rope, they may be able to shield the eye on the side where you are working. It is also helpful to pinch a small fold of skin upward and forward from an injection site on the neck. This causes a short, sharp pain (much like being twitched), taking the animal's mind off the sting of the needle that follows shortly after. Firm contact seems to help with some animals. As you take the pinch, push slightly into the horse's neck. His natural reaction is to push back. He thinks about pushing back rather than expecting the needle to hit. These subtle controls are enough to allow many horses to be injected who would otherwise object to the procedure.

Now you have the needle in the animal's neck—what next? Grasp the base of the needle with one hand and attach the syringe with the other. If you are right-handed, it will probably be easiest to hold the needle with the left hand and attach the syringe with the right. If you do not hold the needle, it will wiggle as you attach the syringe. This is painful to the animal and he will often jump or jerk, perhaps pulling the needle completely out. Push the tip of the syringe into the hub of the needle until it is firmly seated.

Now, pull gently OUTWARD on the plunger. At first, it is helpful to hold the syringe with one hand and pull on the plunger with the other. As you become more experienced, you can pull out on the plunger while steadying the end of the syringe barrel with the same hand. This procedure is done to make sure that you are in the muscle and NOT in a blood vessel. Injection of drugs meant for intramuscular use into a blood vessel may be harmful or even fatal. If you suck blood into the syringe, don't panic. Pull the needle out and place it an inch or so away from the first site. It is not a good idea to just push the needle deeper or to pull it out to a shallower position along the same track. Reactions or infections are more commonly seen when drugs

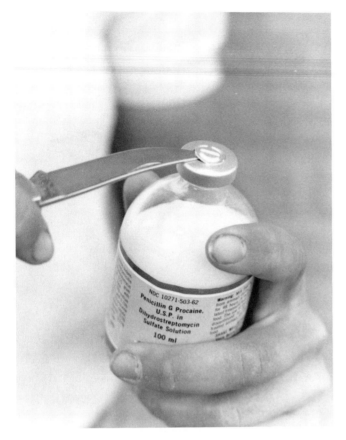

Removing top from bottle.

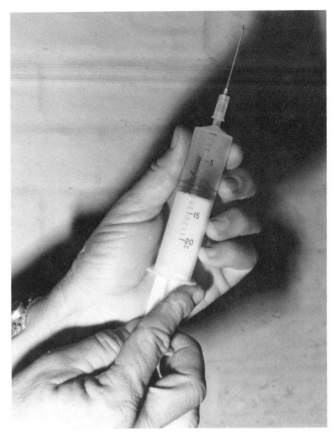

Drawing air into the syringe.

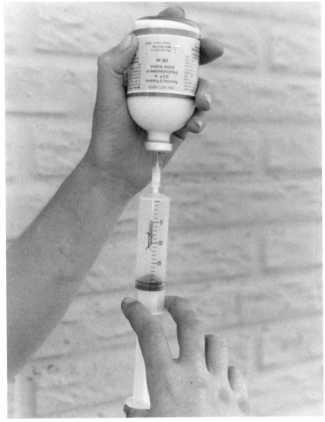

Injecting air into the bottle.

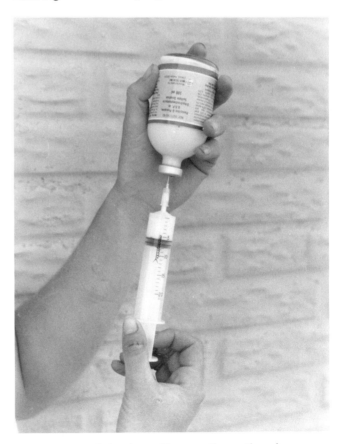

Draw out medicine by pulling gently on the plunger.

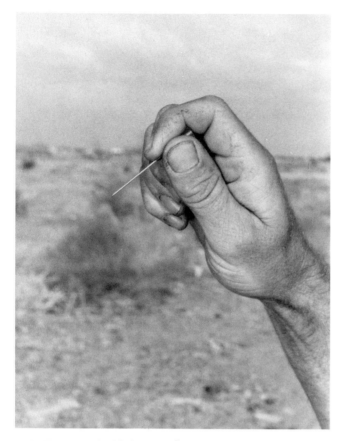

RIGHT way to hold the needle.

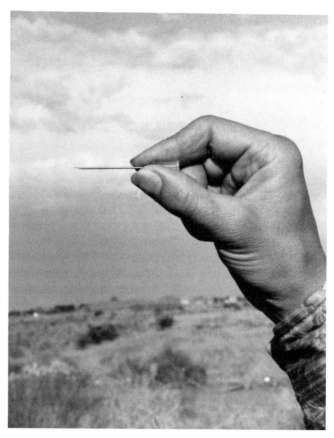

WRONG way to hold the needle.

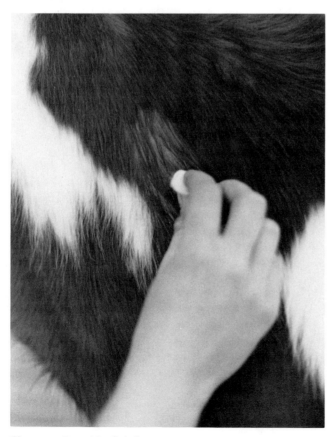

Cleanse site with disinfectant.

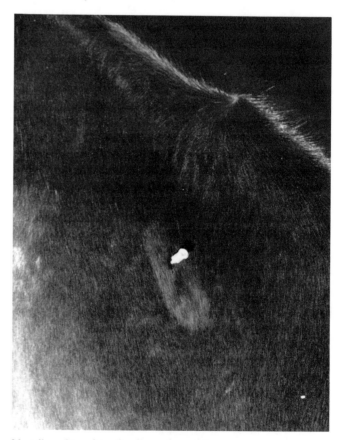

Needle, placed in the horse's neck.

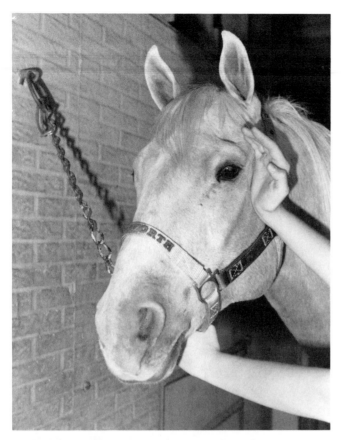

Helper shielding the horse's eye.

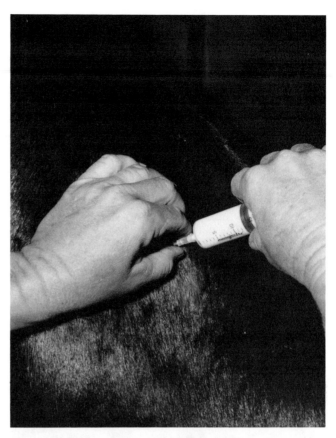

Attaching the syringe to the needle.

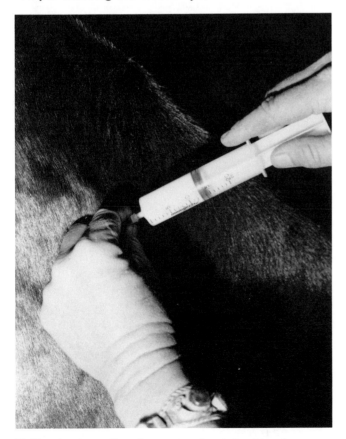

Pulling back on the plunger to check for blood.

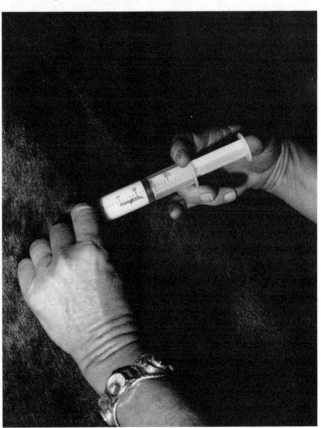

Injecting the medication.

are placed in an area where bleeding has occurred, especially if vaccines or oily solutions are used. Pull back the plunger at the second site and check for blood. There will be a little in the hub of the needle from the last puncture, but that is no problem. No more blood should rush into the syringe. If you do not get blood the second time, go ahead and inject. It does not hurt to inject the small amount of blood which is in the syringe. It's just going back into the same animal.

You can inject the medication as fast as you can comfortably push. It is probably no less painful to do it very slowly. The longer you take, the more chance there is that the animal may pull the needle out, forcing you to start over. Most people find it easiest to hold the hub of the needle with one hand and inject with the other. This helps keep the needle and syringe coordinated together. Occasionally, if you do not do this, the needle will pop off the syringe and medicine will spray all over you. If the drug is chloramphenicol, for instance, it's so bitter that you will spit for hours (experience speaketh).

When you are finished, don't be in a hurry to get free. Place the fingers of one hand against the skin at the base of the needle and hold it toward the horse as you slowly

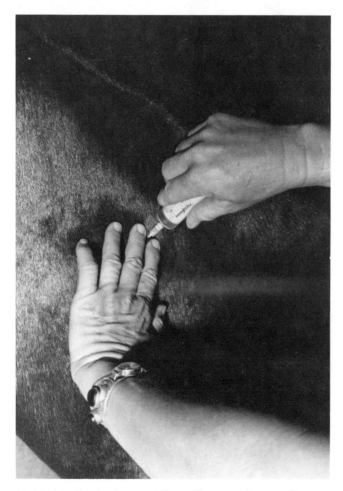

Hold skin firmly down while pulling out the needle.

withdraw the syringe and needle. This helps avoid pulling the skin away from the underlying tissues as you remove the needle. If not done this way, air will sometimes be sucked into the tissues. After you are have removed the needle, don't forget to handle the horse. Praise and pet him and tell him that he was good. Any goodwill you can create will make it that much easier the next time you have to give a shot, whether it is tomorrow or next year. Try to leave the animal with a good feeling about the whole procedure, as horses tend to remember more about what happened last than what happened in general.

INTRAVENOUS INJECTIONS

Some drugs are given by the intravenous route. They may be given this way so that they will take effect within a short time, rather than having to wait several hours as with intramuscular injections. Anesthetics are commonly administered this way. Certain antibiotics may be given intravenously in severe infections so that they can begin working immediately. Other medications are given intravenously because they are very acid or very alkaline or otherwise severely irritating to tissues. It is possible to give these products intravenously because the bloodstream dilutes them as soon as they are injected. The same products, when injected into the muscles, will damage or kill the tissue and may cause large areas to slough. A good example of this is when phenylbutazone is given and the person administering it misses the jugular vein. Or, the animal may move and pull the needle out of the vein, resulting in the drug being deposited in the tissues surrounding the vein. Intravenous injections with some drugs must be given very slowly to avoid reactions or having the animal collapse because of a large amount given suddenly.

Because of the possibility of severe complications during and after intravenous injections, this technique will not be described in this book. If it is necessary to treat your animal with these injections for a prolonged period of time, your veterinarian will either treat the animal or hospitalize it, or show you how to give the injections. They are definitely not "read and do" procedures.

SUBCUTANEOUS INJECTIONS

These injections are given into the loose tissue right under the skin. They are often used in the dog because they have so much loose skin. The horse's skin is firmly attached to the underlying tissues over most of the animal's body. This makes it unhandy to give injections subcutaneously. The one exception to this is treating foals with fluids. These are sometimes administered subcutaneously to foals with diarrhea or other problems which are causing dehydration.

For this treatment, the foal is restrained on its side, and held gently to the ground to avoid struggling and thrashing. The skin is swabbed with alcohol as for intramuscular injections. The fold of skin may be picked up with one hand and the needle placed with the other until you get the feel of where the needle goes. Be careful not to stick the needle through the fold of skin and into your other hand! The animal is treated with fluids which are in a large bottle or plastic bag connected to the needle by a long, flexible plastic tube. Put enough fluid into one spot to form a lump about half the size of a baseball. Then, move the needle to a new spot several inches away and repeat the procedure. After you have moved the needle, go back to the previous spot and gently massage the hole made by the needle to help it close as the skin may not be healthy and elastic enough in a dehydrated, sick foal to close and seal.

Several days after fluid has been given in this manner, you may notice large amounts of it hanging in pouches of skin under the foal's belly. Gravity has pulled it down into that area before it could be absorbed. This only occasionally happens and is not a problem unless an abscess should form in the area. If the pockets of fluid are cool and soft, there is no problem. If they should become hot and more firm, consult your veterinarian immediately about possibly draining them, and the foal's possible need for antibiotic treatment.

INTRADERMAL INJECTIONS

These are made into the upper layer of the skin. Some sleeping sickness vaccines were given in this way. Most companies are getting away from this method of administration because it is tricky. They are going to intramuscular injections instead.

Intradermal injections are made high up on the neck (say eight or ten inches below the ears) and often just two or three inches below the mane. It is helpful to clip the hair from a small patch of skin—an inch or inch and a half in diameter is enough. Swab it with alcohol. These injections use a very fine needle—usually 25 gauge and only about $3/4$ inch long. The needle, rather than being perpendicular to the skin, is held at a very low angle. The needle is inserted BARELY under the skin—only about $1/16$ to $1/8$ inch into it. The trick is to get it in far enough that the vaccine doesn't drip out around it when it is injected. When the needle is inserted correctly, a small bump (called a bleb) should appear ahead of the tip of the needle. This bump is usually about a half inch in diameter and should stand up sharply. If you get the needle in too deeply, the vaccine will spread out subcutaneously rather than making a sharp bump and may be less effective.

INTRA-ARTICULAR INJECTIONS

This is the name given to injections into the joints. Several serious complications may follow injections into the joints. Infection may occur if sterile technique is not used. The point of the needle may penetrate the joint cartilage, damaging it and starting an arthritis. Bleeding may occur because a small blood vessel in the joint capsule has been punctured; the blood which leaks into the joint may cause severe problems, including arthritis, at a later date. For these reasons, joint injections should be left to your veterinarian. Again, these are not "read and do" procedures.

Now that we have discussed methods of treatment and how to give injections, Chapter 11 talks about some different types of medication which are commonly used on the horse, both those given by injection and others.

Chapter 11

MEDICATIONS

DMSO
Nonsteroidal Anti-Inflammatory Agents
Corticosteroids
Anabolic Steroids
Sulfa Drugs
Antibiotics
    Penicillin
    Tetracyclines
    Chloramphenicol
    Other Antibiotics
Oxytocin
Epinephrine
Disinfectants and Antiseptics
Insect Repellents
Liniments and Lotions
Wound Medications
Colic Mixtures
Antidiarrheals
Cough Mixtures
Tranquilizers
Anesthetics
Products for Immunization
Home Cures and Herbal Remedies

Medications which are commonly used to treat horses will be discussed here—some of which should be in the horseman's medicine chest, and some of which should be avoided like the plague. The list is by no means complete, but is meant to give an overview of some of the more common ones. Let's begin with drugs which reduce pain.

DMSO

This drug is really in a class by itself. The technical name for it is dimethyl sulfoxide. It is currently manufactured by Diamond Laboratories (Des Moines, IA 50317). This is a medical-grade product, containing 90% DMSO. It comes either as a liquid or an ointment. Other

DMSO is on the market, sold by feed stores and roadside stands. This is usually only 50 to 70% pure and may contain unknown contaminants. This less pure form is the one used as a paint thinner and solvent and should be avoided for animal or human use.

DMSO is recommended by the manufacturer and licensed by the Food and Drug Administration to reduce acute swelling due to trauma. At the present time, DMSO is the only product known which will carry other products through the skin. Cosmetic ads notwithstanding, the skin is a very efficient barrier against most substances. DMSO can be mixed with antibiotics, corticosteroids, and other drugs to allow them to be carried through the skin. For this reason, it is very important to clip the hair off the area you are treating. Then, wash the skin carefully (several times) with an antiseptic soap (such as pHisohex, Winthrop Laboratories, New York, NY 10016) and water. Dry the water off and rinse the area with alcohol. Allow it to dry. Then go ahead and apply your DMSO mixture.

Because DMSO tends to absorb water, it should be kept in a tightly closed container. Otherwise, the next time you use it, you may find that it has absorbed enough water from the air to be more water than DMSO. When adding other substances to it, a convenient way to mix them is in a clean glass fruit jar with a wide mouth. This allows you to use a paintbrush to apply the mixture to the animal's skin. Use only natural-bristle paintbrushes. Over a period of time, the DMSO may dissolve both plastic bottles and nylon paintbrushes. If you are applying DMSO with your hands, use rubber or disposable plastic gloves to keep it off your skin. If you get some on your skin, you may experience an unpleasant, garlic-like taste in your mouth. This means that the drug has penetrated your skin and is circulating in your bloodstream.

DMSO is often mixed with nitrofurazone solution and a corticosteroid to paint on bowed tendons, bog spavins which have just occurred due to overusage, and similar problems. Some people tout the drug as a cure-all for whatever ails your horse. It's not THAT great, but does have some use in reducing acute swellings. It is used to help reduce hematomas, seromas, and other non-infectious problems where the skin is not broken. It is also useful when drugs, such as phenylbutazone (which must be given intravenously), have been deposited in the tissues outside the jugular vein. Used twice a day for several days, it may help to reduce the tissue irritation and reduce the chance that sloughing will occur from the phenylbutazone.

This drug should not be used on open wounds. DMSO should never be applied after blisters or similar drugs have been put on the skin, as it will carry them right into the tissues, causing a severe reaction.

NONSTEROIDAL ANTI-INFLAMMATORY AGENTS

This is the name given to a class of anti-inflammatory drugs which are not related to cortisone. One of the best known of these drugs is aspirin. Aspirin (Mallinckrodt, Inc., Paris, KY 40361.) can be used in horses. As with the same drug in people, it is relatively safe, and has few side effects, especially when compared to other pain-killing drugs. Horse aspirin are huge pills, in keeping with the size of the beasts we're using them on.

Phenylbutazone is the generic name of the drug most commonly used to reduce pain in horses. Its best-known brand name is Butazolidin, otherwise known as "bute" (Wellcome Animal Health Division, Burroughs Wellcome Co., Kansas City, MO 64141). This drug reduces inflammation in a manner similar to aspirin and can help to lower fever. It is used to help reduce the pain in animals who have arthritis and helps to relieve pain due to colic.

The injectable form of phenylbutazone MUST be given intravenously and it can cause a severe reaction if some gets outside the vein. If enough is placed outside the vein, a large area of tissue may slough from the animal's neck, or an abscess may form. Tablets are available. They should be crushed and fed with grain. Several companies make phenylbutazone powder in premeasured packets, to be mixed with the horse's feed. A paste form similar to paste wormer is available (also from Wellcome Animal Health Division).

Full doses of "bute" should not be given with full doses of corticosteroids. These drugs have similar actions and may have adverse side effects when used together at full dosage; partial dosages of each, given together, are permissible.

Horses should usually not be treated more than five consecutive days with "bute" because of the possibility of side effects. The most severe of these is a blood disorder called aplastic anemia. This disorder lessens the number and quality of red blood cells available to the animal. In the most severe cases, the body may not resume normal production of these cells and the animal may become severely ill. Other side effects include digestive upsets and liver problems. The latter may show up as icterus (a yellowing of the membranes of the eyes and mouth).

Drugs such as "bute" and other anti-inflammatory agents (new ones appear frequently) are valuable for keeping animals with chronic problems in use, when it is used sparingly and only as needed. Flunixin meglumine (Banamine, Schering Corp., Kenilworth, NJ 07033) is another of these.

Naproxen (Equiproxen, Diamond Laboratories, Inc., Des Moines, IA 50317) is a relatively new anti-inflammatory agent. It comes in packets of powder which are given to the horse with his grain and can be used in much the same manner as phenylbutazone.

One good example of use for these drugs is a rope horse with ringbone who was used in high-school rodeos. There is no treatment for the ringbone. The horse was 15 years old and it would be easy to tell the people to put him down. But why waste the animal's years of training and experience and the fine disposition which made him a champion? Better instead to have the owner give him "bute" paste before the weekend rodeos and rest and coddle the old fellow in between. In this manner, they may get several more years of usage without causing the animal excessive pain.

If a horse is being kept on a nonsteroidal anti-inflamatory agent for a long period of time, or is given the drug at intervals, as with the horse mentioned above, it is often worth trying more than one of these drugs. One may work much better than another for a given animal. Also, it may be helpful to alternate between them to keep the animal from building a tolerance to the medication and to keep side effects at a minimum.

IMPORTANT NOTE: Giving painkillers, such as phenylbutazone, or drugs such as corticosteroids to relieve an animal's pain is NOT a substitute for finding out what is actually wrong with the animal. Using these drugs in this manner is as smart as putting a band-aid on a broken leg and hoping that it will heal. If the animal does not respond to rest and the passage of a little time, consult your veterinarian for an accurate diagnosis.

CORTICOSTEROIDS

"Corticosteroids" is the general name given to a group of hormones manufactured by the adrenal glands (which are found near the kidneys). These chemicals are produced by the body in response to stress. When normally produced, they help the animal to adapt to his surroundings. As manufactured chemicals administered by the veterinarian or owner, these drugs may help the animal to overcome insults to his body. Improperly used, they can render the animal helpless to defend himself against disease.

Horse owners and veterinarians often refer to this class of drugs as "steroids" or "cortisones." Both terms are shorter and simpler than saying "corticosteroids." Generic names include drugs such as dexamethasone, prednisolone, hydrocortisone, and flumethasone. Azium (Schering Corp., Kenilworth, NJ 07033) and Flucort (Diamond Laboratories, Inc., Des Moines, IA 50317) are perhaps the best known trade names. Other drugs, such as Depo-Medrol (Upjohn Co., Kalamazoo, MI 49001) and Betavet Soluspan (Schering Corp., Kenilworth, NJ 07033), are injected into joints.

WHAT CORTICOSTEROIDS DO—AND DON'T

These drugs help to reduce inflammation and the body's responses to it. They often give considerable relief in acute problems. They may or may not help chronic problems by temporarily reducing inflammation and allowing the body to heal itself.

Steroids affect nearly every system of the body to a greater or lesser extent. They work on the brain, giving an increased tolerance to pain and often true pain relief. They give the animal a sense of well-being and help him to feel better. They also stimulate the appetite. Steroids increase acid production in the stomach; this may be harmful in horses who are not eating. They reduce mucus secretion in the intestinal lining causing decreased lubrication and digestion.

Steroids stimulate potassium loss from the circulatory system which may cause muscular weakness. They help maintain blood pressure and avoid fluid loss. This aids in shock by keeping fluid from leaking from the capillaries and helps keep the blood pressure normal. This fluid retention may allow the feet and legs to swell (a condition called edema).

Steroids increase blood flow to the kidneys and stimulate red blood cell production. On the other hand, they depress the lymph nodes which produce white blood cells; they also slow the movement of these cells. White blood cells act as garbage men in the body and literally "gobble up" bacteria in an infection, rendering them harmless and disposing of them. Thus, the fact that steroids slow down these cells may aid the spread of infections.

Steroids lead to decreased antibody response. For this reason, they are used in human transplants to help keep the body from rejecting the transplanted organ. This is definitely NOT a desired response in the face of an infection—we need to let the body have all the help it can. Administration of steroids, especially without accompanying antibiotics, may leave the animal susceptible to disease or allow the spread of bacteria which are already present.

Steroids affect muscles by increasing protein breakdown. If used for long periods of time, they may decrease the animal's muscle mass and strength. They also decrease the growth of cells called fibroblasts. These cells form the major part of cartilage and scar tissue and help to heal wounds. By both these methods, steroids may significantly slow growth in young animals. Steroids also interfere with the formation of new bone. Recent studies at Cornell University have pointed to long-term steroid use as causing extensive skeletal damage in growing horses and ponies.

Steroids reduce mucus secretion in the lining of the respiratory system. Mucus helps trap bacteria and viruses that are inhaled and helps keep them from getting to the lungs and causing infection. Less mucus can leave the animal more susceptible to respiratory disease.

Steroids do not actually cure any disease except adrenal insufficiency. Adrenal insufficiency is a lack of production of hormones by the adrenal glands; it is extremely rare in the horse. Steroids may also help specifically in "auto-immune diseases" where the body "becomes allergic" to itself.

In using steroids, we must balance the good effects against the bad. For example, we do not normally use these drugs with broken bones as they retard healing. If, however, the animal is in severe shock, it is better to use them on a short-term basis and save his life; he can't heal if he doesn't survive the initial shock. Cortisones are also valuable with horses suffering from endotoxin shock, such as that occurring in salmonellosis.

Steroids should be used at the site of the problem whenever possible, rather than put into the body as a whole. For instance, injection directly into a joint may cause less long-term damage than giving the whole horse enough to reduce the pain in that particular joint. An ointment may be a much better treatment than an injection of one of these drugs for a skin problem. This usage gives much better results at the site of the problem while reducing the chance of side effects.

Steroids help to relieve symptoms of arthritis and allergies, but do NOT cure these problems. The conditions usually reappear when administration is stopped. In addition, long-term administration of cortisones may lead to destruction of joint cartilage and permanent damage to the joint surfaces, leading to incurable lameness. Poor injection technique into a joint may lead to loss of the animal through infectious arthritis in that joint. If the steroids are accidentally injected into the tissues around the joint, they may induce bone formation in the soft tissues. This progresses over a period of several months and may lead to lameness. To help avoid damage within the joint after a steroid injection, it is of the utmost importance to rest the animal for an adequate period of time after the injection is given. Because they slow down cellular growth, steroids may significantly retard the healing of damaged joints.

Cortisone administration is often accompanied by antibiotics to help prevent the spread of infection. These products are especially valuable when used together to treat pneumonia.

Steroids are used in ointments to help treat allergic and inflammatory skin problems. They may also be used in eye ointments. In this form, they are used on healed corneal ulcers to eliminate the blood vessels which grow out onto the cornea during the healing process. These blood vessels may eventually cause blindness if they are not removed.

IMPORTANT: Ointments containing steroids should NOT be used on eye problems without consulting your veterinarian. Using one of these products on a fresh ulcer, cut, or scrape may result in rapid spread of the lesion and loss of that eye.

Where should you use corticosteroid drugs? They are valuable for animals who are in severe shock and may help to save the animal's life. They are helpful whether the shock is endotoxin shock due to salmonellosis or is shock from blood loss or severe pain because of an injury.

Full doses of corticosteroid drugs should not be given with phenylbutazone, but partial doses of both drugs together may be more beneficial than either given alone. Give an adequate amount of the drug to do the job, as recommended on the label of the product you are using, or as directed by your veterinarian. Harmful effects are most frequently seen with smaller amounts given over long periods of time; this type of treatment should be avoided.

NOTE: Other than using this type drug to treat shock, steroids should only be given on the advice of your veterinarian.

NOTE: There are some conditions in which steroids should NOT be used. They should not be given to horses with kidney disease, rickets, or osteoporosis (weakening of the bone). They should not be given to animals with infections that are not controlled by antibiotics, nor to those with surgical or slow-healing wounds or broken bones. They should not be given to horses under four years of age because they may severely retard bone growth.

They should not be used with septic arthritis (arthritis with infection in the joint, such as joint ill in foals). They are of little or no value in chronic lameness with extensive bony changes, such as ringbone.

Administration of cortisones to horses in the last third of pregnancy may cause abortion or premature labor. This may be followed by foaling problems, death of the foal, retained placenta metritis, or all of these. Steroids should not be used in horses with viral diseases or tuberculosis. They should not be given to animals who are being shown or raced, as they are illegal and may show up in blood or urine tests.

Steroids are frequently sold in combination with penicillin/streptomycin products. The combined products should not be used where you DO need a steroid, as they are not generally in high enough concentration in these combinations to do any real good. Using both the penicillin/streptomycin and the steroid separately allows you to use adequate, therapeutic dosages of each. Using one of these combination drugs where the steroid portion is NOT needed may lead to complications as listed above.

ANABOLIC STEROIDS

Anabolic steroids are drugs which are produced in the body to allow the young animal to grow normally. Synthetic versions of the same thing have been thought to make young horses grow larger and faster for show or racing purposes. They have also been thought to stimulate the animal's appetite and make him put on more muscle faster than he would otherwise—a lot like fattening a beef for slaughter. Recent work at Colorado State University found no difference in height and weight gain between animals treated with these drugs and animals not given any. Trade names of a couple of these drugs are Equipoise (E.R. Squibb & Sons, Inc., Princeton, NJ 08540), and Deca-Durabolin (Organon Pharmaceuticals, West Orange, NJ).

The major problem with these wonder drugs is their side effects, most of which are reproductive in nature. Fillies may become masculinized. Abnormal sexual behavior is also seen. The animals may mount other mares and act aggressively toward them. They rarely come into heat. If they do, the heat is brief and infertile. (57)

Stud colts are also affected reproductively. They have low sperm counts, lowered sperm quality, and smaller than normal testicles. In some cases, they may become completely infertile. Sexual activity was not enhanced by these drugs in the controlled studies.

This author can see no reason to use these drugs, especially if you even remotely may wish to breed the horse later in his or her life, since well-controlled studies have shown them to be ineffective for the purpose of stimulating growth.

SULFA DRUGS

Sulfas were the first class of drugs able to attack and retard the growth of bacteria. This effect allowed the body to overcome the bacteria and survive the infection. Sulfa drugs were developed around the turn of the century and came into widespread use shortly afterward, saving the lives of many people. Sulfas were extensively used on animals until antibiotics were discovered and put into common usage. Sulfa drugs are still occasionally used, either as injections (which must be given intravenously because the solution is irritating) or in eye and other ointments. They are also used in the form of a sulfa-urea solution which is very effective for removing debris from the surface of old, contaminated wounds (see Wound Medications).

ANTIBIOTICS

Antibiotics are a class of drugs extracted from cultures of certain soil and airborne molds. Their mode of action varies from one type to another. Some, like penicillin, actually kill the bacteria, while others merely slow them down so that the body's defenses can attack and kill them more readily.

Here are two important rules for antibiotic treatment:

RULE #1: ALWAYS GIVE AN ADEQUATE DOSAGE OF WHATEVER DRUG YOU ARE USING. Using less than this amount only gets rid of part of the bacteria, allowing the infection to continue, and is likely to leave the rest of the bacteria in better shape than ever, possibly even resistant to the drug. You may end up having to switch to another drug to get the desired effect, which costs both extra time and money, and leaves the possibility that the bacteria may gain enough resistance to overwhelm the animal and kill him. ALWAYS use the recommended amount of antibiotics. If you aren't getting the result you think you should, check with your veterinarian about a possible change to another antibiotic or a change in dosage. And, be aware that the dosages currently labeled on some penicillin products may be too low to be effective (see Penicillin, below).

RULE #2: ANYTHING WORTH TREATING IS WORTH TREATING FOR AT LEAST THREE DAYS. If you give only one or two injections, there is a good chance that the harmful bacteria haven't been killed off, and the ones which survive the treatment may have become resistant to the drug. Then you really DO have a problem. So, if you feel that you only need a day or two of treatment, don't bother to give antibiotics at all. The animal will get well without them. Then, you don't help build up resistant bacteria which will cause problems later. Often, it is necessary to treat for two or three days BEYOND the time when the animal appears well. This allows the drug to finish getting rid of the bacteria. Follow your veterinarian's advice on how long to treat.

One of the first questions to ask is if the animal really NEEDS antibiotics. If a virus is causing the problem and there are no complications from accompanying bacteria, using an antibiotic will do no good, and may do harm.

The next question is WHICH antibiotic to use. Some are more effective than others for a given infection. This even varies from one area of the country to another. Often, a drug which is effective against one type of bacteria in one area will be ineffective against it elsewhere. It is usually best to rely on your veterinarian's advice on antibiotic selection. Do not just pour penicillin or another antibiotic into an animal on a random basis and expect good results.

Do not give two antibiotics at the same time unless instructed to do so by your veterinarian. Some combinations of antibiotics—penicillin and streptomycin is one—give better results when used together than either one used alone. Other antibiotics have differing modes of

action, and can actually cancel each other out, leaving the animal in worse shape than if he had no medication at all. An example of this is the use of penicillin and tetracycline together. Do not mix antibiotics with other medication unless you have veterinary advice to do so. The other medication may neutralize the antibiotic, again resulting in no action. As with any medication, give antibiotics only by the route recommended by your veterinarian or the product label.

If no improvement is seen after 48 hours of treatment, consult your veterinarian. He may wish to change the dosage you are using, or switch to a different drug.

PENICILLIN

Penicillin was the first antibiotic discovered. Its discovery triggered research which is still discovering new compounds useful to both man and animals. It kept many people alive in World War II who would have otherwise died of infections. While penicillin is far from new, it is by no means outdated. It remains perhaps the most commonly used antibiotic for treatment of infection in both humans and animals. It is relatively inexpensive as compared to some of the newer, more exotic antibiotics.

Penicillin is generally very safe, and does not cause problems even when given at many times the normal dosage rate; however, allergic reactions may be seen. Epinephrine (adrenalin) should be handy whenever you give an injection of this drug to an animal, so that it can be given if anaphylactic shock occurs. The fact that you have given penicillin numerous times to the same animal is no indication that he will not have a reaction the next time you give it. Thankfully, these reactions are very rare. This author has seen reactions in calves with a certain brand of penicillin (no longer produced), but has never seen one in a horse. However, keeping the epinephrine bottle handy is cheap insurance against the loss of an animal.

Penicillin is used in horses in several forms. The one most commonly used is in combination with another antibiotic, dihydrostreptomycin. Penicillin/streptomycin combination, as it's usually called, is used in most instances where penicillin treatment is required. The two drugs attack different types of bacteria, complementing each other to give far more benefit than either one alone.

Recent work has shown that dosage rates of 40,000 IU (International Units) per kilogram of body weight should be given. This is approximately 60 ml (cc) of most commercial penicillin/streptomycin preparations in a 1000 lb (450 kg) horse. Figure the dosage at 18,000 units per lb of body weight if you are dealing with a different-sized horse. This quantity is necessary to give an effective blood level for 24 hours. Most dosages of penicillin which have been used only give a usable blood level for 8 to 12 hours. There is no need to calculate a dosage for the streptomycin part of the drug—just for the penicillin. (58)

This drug combination can be used for up to five to

seven days. After that, the streptomycin portion can cause damage to the animal's inner ear, resulting in disturbances in balance and hearing. For this reason, when animals need a longer course of therapy, we usually switch them to procaine penicillin without the streptomycin. Treatment with this drug can be continued for months, if necessary, without harmful effects. One client had a mare with a distemper abscess in her abdomen. The horse looked much better after a week's treatment with pen/strep, but became worse when it was stopped. He ended up treating her with procaine penicillin for over a month—every day! When he stopped, she was completely cured had no more problems.

Procaine penicillin, whether by itself or in combination with dihydrostreptomycin, gives a good blood level of antibiotic for only about 12 hours. For this reason, it is best to split the total daily dosage and give half in the morning and half in the evening. Give the two doses as close to 12 hours apart as you can. Procaine penicillin is not soluble and for this reason, should never be given intravenously as it may cause massive pulmonary embolism and death.

Procaine penicillin should not be used where horses will be subjected to urine or blood testing for drug levels. The procaine will show up, and is illegal. The test cannot distinguish between procaine from the penicillin and procaine used to block a lame joint. Procaine may show up in a horses' urine as much as two weeks after it has been given. (59) This product should be avoided before horse shows and events, such as trail rides, in states like California where horses are checked for drug levels. Use a form of penicillin which does not contain procaine, on the instructions of your veterinarian.

Long-acting penicillins (benzathine penicillins) are often touted for once-every-few-days treatment of whatever ails your beast. Research has found that these do keep a small steady flow of penicillin into the bloodstream; however, they never reach a high enough level to be therapeutic. This results in a situation much like when you give too little in the first place. Anything worth treating is worth treating with a daily injection; if it's not worth a daily injection, it didn't need to be treated in the first place.

IMPORTANT NOTE: Most antibiotics have withdrawal times—periods of time which must be allowed to pass after treatment before the animal is slaughtered for food. Depending on the product, these may vary from a week to two months. If you treat your horse with antibiotics, remember that it may be some time before you can eat him! Actually, since most of us don't eat horses, this warning applies more to a feeder steer you may be raising for freezer beef. The same antibiotics can often be used on both horses and cattle.

TETRACYCLINES

Tetracyclines are another major class of antibiotic drugs. They are mostly given intravenously, although they may occasionally be given as capsules to young foals. They are also used as mixtures in drinking water to treat large numbers of animals or those too wild to treat in any other way.

Some tetracyclines are given intramuscularly to cattle, but they cause severe tissue reaction and damage. Local anesthetics have been added to the solutions to reduce the pain, but this does nothing to lessen the muscle destruction. For this reason, it is not a good idea to use these products intramuscularly in the horse.

Tetracyclines are a useful class of antibiotics having a different spectrum of action than penicillin. They are often used in cases where penicillin administration does not get any response. Penicillin and tetracyclines have modes of action that cancel each other out, resulting in no effect at all. For this reason, they should not be given at the same time. If you are going to change, discontinue the one and begin the other.

CHLORAMPHENICOL

Chloramphenicol is a potent antibiotic which can cure many bacterial problems that are resistant to the more common antibiotics. It can have some side effects if administered for long periods of time, so should only be given under veterinary direction. It is also incorporated into some of the most effective eye ointments in use. Its high cost keeps it from being commonly used, except in foals and extremely valuable horses.

Recent data from the Bureau of Veterinary Medicine has suggested that two human deaths have occurred from contact with veterinary chloramphenicol, as well as a severe anemia which may later become leukemia. While these complications are extremely rare, it is a good idea to use care when handling chloramphenicol products to avoid ingesting them or getting them on your skin.

OTHER ANTIBIOTICS

Drugs such as gentamycin and other specialized antibiotics are used for uterine infusions, flushing draining tracts, and other localized applications. Nitrofurazone is commonly used in antibiotic dressings. Liquid nitrofurazone is also used for uterine infusions and flushing wounds. Neomycin is an antibiotic used mostly in oral solution or pills for foals with diarrhea, or to help prevent digestive problems in foals who are fed milk replacers. Other antibiotics are used only in eye ointments due to their high cost.

OXYTOCIN

Oxytocin is a hormone produced by the pituitary gland (a small gland at the base of the brain). It also occurs as a component of "purified oxytocic principle," a hormone preparation which has much the same action. When given to an animal in labor, oxytocin helps to change uncoordinated, weak uterine contractions into strong, rhythmic ones. Because foaling problems in the mare are usually due to too much straining rather than too little, it is rarely used in this manner for mares. This is different from its usage for the cow or dog, for instance, where this drug is often used to help the mother give birth.

Oxytocin's most common use in the mare is for the animal who has little or no milk. It can stimulate milk production if it is given shortly after the foal is born, within the first few days. When given at this time, it also helps to contract the uterus; this helps to expel any membranes or infected materials which are present. It is often given to mares with retained membranes.

Because this drug can stimulate severe uterine contractions, it may cause colic in the mare if given in improper dosage. For this reason, it is best used on the prescription of your veterinarian.

EPINEPHRINE

Also called adrenalin, this drug is secreted in the body by the adrenal gland (a small gland near the kidney). It primarily affects the heart, blood vessels, blood flow, and circulation. It is used to treat anaphylactic shock which may follow injection of vaccines or antibiotics. It should be part of your medicine chest if you EVER give injections or vaccinations.

For use in anaphylactic shock, the dosage is approximately 4 to 8 ml for a horse (of a 1:1000 solution). Check the bottle and make sure of the specific dosage for the particular product you have—BEFORE you need it. When you have to have it, there may not be time to read the label (see Anaphylactic Shock).

DISINFECTANTS AND ANTISEPTICS

Disinfectants are substances which are used to kill organisms (mainly viruses and bacteria) that can cause disease. Antiseptics are usually weaker substances or solutions that can be used on living tissue. The difference is more one of degree than of different chemicals. Some drugs which are antiseptic in small amounts can kill bacteria and sterilize inanimate objects in higher concentrations. Tamed iodine solutions are an example of this action.

Povidone-iodine (often called "tamed iodine") is more mild than tincture of iodine. Betadine (Purdue Frederick Co., Norwalk, CT 06856) is one of the better-known brand names of this disinfectant. Tincture of iodine can burn tissues and causes staining of many materials, invariably including clothing and skin (your skin as well as

the horse's). The tamed iodine products usually do not stain. They are mild enough to be used on the tissues without irritation and are often used where a gentle cleansing action is desired.

Fresh granulating (healing) surfaces may be washed with a mild solution of tamed iodine. Mix enough iodine into the water to make it the color of weak tea. This "weak tea" can then be gently wiped onto the wound with a gauze sponge. This solution can also be used to disinfect buckets, brushes, and other inanimate objects.

Carbolic acid (one of the ingredients of "Lysol" disinfectant, Lehn and Fink Products Div. of Sterling Drug Co., Montvale, NJ 07645) is an old disinfectant. In fact, it was the first antiseptic discovered, used by Joseph Lister to prevent infection in women who were having babies. It can be irritating to tissues, especially in stronger concentrations. Because it has been replaced by disinfectants which are more effective and less damaging, it is no longer used on injuries.

Chlorhexidine (Nolvasan, Fort Dodge, Fort Dodge, IA 50501) is a modern disinfectant which is both effective and nonirritating. It is pleasant to use, and one of my favorites. It can be used to wash mares and stallions before breeding without irritating the sensitive genital area. It is also used in a soothing wound ointment. Mixed with water according to the directions, it is one of the few products available which is capable of killing viruses, making it an ideal disinfectant (along with other sanitation measures) when upper respiratory viruses are going around. A gallon of this compound, while not inexpensive, will last the average horseman for several years. You might be able to purchase a pint or quart of it from your veterinarian.

Benzalkonium chloride is the long chemical name of another good disinfectant, one commonly marketed under the trade name "Roccal" (Roccal-D, Winthrop Veterinary Division of Sterling Drug, Inc., New York, NY 10016). It has a strong coloring agent in it, and is said to be effective as long as there is any green color in the water. Many veterinarians use it mixed to a light green as a substitute for alcohol before giving injections, as well as for cleansing their hands between handling different horses. It is a good disinfectant for barns and equipment. It is often available from your veterinarian.

Hydrogen peroxide is a solution favored by some for cleansing wounds. This author does not like it and never uses it. My feeling is that it opens up the tissues with its bubbling action, forcing at least as many bacteria deep into the tissues as it removes. It may be dangerous if used in a deep cavity or large wound with a small opening at the skin. In these cases, the pressure buildup may cause even more damage. This is a matter of personal preference— some veterinarians like the product and use it routinely.

Alcohol is usually purchased in the drugstore as "rubbing alcohol." It makes an excellent skin disinfectant, and should be well saturated into the hair. Rubbing it in with a sopping wet cotton ball is usually the easiest way. Be liberal, and soak an area several inches larger than you think you might need for an injection. This gives some leeway for you to miss the exact site when you stick the animal and still hit an alcohol-soaked area. Alcohol products should not be used in open wounds because they are irritating, causing both pain and tissue damage.

Chloride of lime is an old-time disinfectant that is still in use for cleaning contaminated barns and premises. For instance, it can be used when you have a horse die of salmonellosis after he has had diarrhea all over the barn for several days. If your barn has a dirt floor, remove all bedding and the top four to six inches of dirt before attempting any disinfection of the stall.

Mix a solution of 6 ounces of chloride of lime per gallon of water. This can be used to treat the floor of the stall and the walls, as well as treating the contaminated soil before you dispose of it so that it does not present a danger to other animals or birds. This solution should be sprayed on with enough force to penetrate all cracks in the stall, and used on feeders and anything else in the stall.

IMPORTANT NOTE: Because this mixture is both irritating and corrosive, proper protective clothing and eye protection should be worn, and it should be kept off surfaces which it might damage, such as aluminum. Also, remove all animals from the vicinity you plan to disinfect. For more information on this method of disinfection, contact your county agricultural agent or library.

Lime can usually be purchased at a feed store. Powdered lime is occasionally used in moderate amounts to disinfect stalls or corrals by merely sprinkling it on the ground. Used in excess, it may dry the animals' skin and hooves and cause them to crack.

Hexacholorophene is included in many soaps and mild cleansing compounds. This helps to make the soap more antibacterial. Probably the best-known soap containing this disinfectant is pHisoHex (Winthrop Laboratories, New York, NY 10016). This is a good product for cleansing the skin, and is often used as a presurgical scrub. It is good to use on a clipped area before the application of DMSO; it must, of course, be completely rinsed off with liberal applications of water or the DMSO may carry it deep into the tissues under the skin.

Hexacholorphene received some bad press about causing problems in monkeys several years ago. Unfortunately, no one mentioned that after carefully reading the experiment, it was found that the young primates were nearly MARINATED in the drug in its pure and concentrated form. This gave them the equivalent of many lifetimes of usage for occasional washing purposes. Don't hesitate to use the drug as a scrubbing and cleansing agent. You may need a prescription from your veterinarian or physician to purchase it. The same product without the hexacholorophene is called pHisoDerm and is available over-the-counter at your drugstore. It is a good cleansing soap, but has little or no disinfectant action. A few people are allergic to products containing hexachlorophene and will break out in a red, itching rash after using them. If you are one of these, either wear rubber gloves while using it or switch to a different type of cleansing product, such as an iodine scrub.

INSECT REPELLENTS

Numerous insect repellent products are on the market. This brief discussion cannot begin to cover all the main ingredients, much less name all the individual products. Instead of trying to discuss them all, general types will be considered to help you choose the one which is right for you, your area, and your animal.

Begin choosing by considering how you are going to apply the product. Many fine pressurized aerosol sprays are available in cans. They tend to be high in price compared to sprays which come in plastic squirt bottles (much like household window cleaner). There are concentrates which you can mix with water and apply with the same type of plastic sprayer. Before you settle on one of these, the big question is: will YOUR horse tolerate a spray can or bottle? Many animals will, but a whole lot of them won't. It doesn't matter how good the product is if you can't get within twenty feet of your horse with it.

Some sprays are available which say that they only have to be applied every three days. These are mainly products containing encapsulated pyrethrins, which are supposed to release the product over a period of several days. These may perhaps be adequate if you have a minimal insect problem. One of my clients tested a long-acting product in an extremely bad mosquito area; it barely lasted 24 hours. You are not supposed to reapply the stuff for three days. You have to either overdose the animal with it, or use another product meanwhile two days out of three. If you are going to use one of these products, buy a small container and see if it will work in your area with your animals and your insect problem before committing yourself to the giant, lasts-forever size.

While we're on the subject of sprays, there are still other products which can be applied with a garden-type sprayer. These are useful if you have a large group of horses, or even just a few of them and not enough time to apply a product to the individual animals. If you are using a garden sprayer (other than a brand-new one), begin by carefully cleaning it out with several rinsings of hot, soapy water followed by a lot of clear water to remove the soap. This will help prevent irritation (or poisoning) by previously used chemicals that may remain in the cannister. Be sure to thoroughly rinse out the spray nozzle and hose while you are at it. If a garden sprayer is the route you take, the safest course is to buy a new one and use it only for your horse.

If you have a horse who absolutely cannot be approached with a sprayer, then you have to try the next possibility—a wipe-on product. These often have an oily base and are applied with a mitt or rag. You can apply one of these, then keep the application rag in a large, wide-mouthed plastic jar with a tightly-fitted lid. This will keep you from having to get a new rag each day (and saturating it anew with a large amount of the expensive product).

One advantage of oily insect repellents is that they tend to remain in the hair for a period of time. After rubbing one of them thoroughly into the hair for several days according to directions, you can then occasionally miss a day and still have some protection. The disadvantage is that, being oily, they tend to collect dirt and dust. This makes the animal look less than shiny. In areas with sandy soil, it holds some of the sand which dulls the coat even more and creates more work to clean the horse before putting a saddle on him.

Some horse owners are hanging insecticide eartags meant for cattle on their horses. These are usually tied into the mane with a piece of stout string, or hung around the neck with a large loop of baling twine, much like a dog collar. Be sure that whatever you use to attach them will break if the animal gets caught on a post or tree limb. These tags help to keep flies away from the animal's head or neck area. Unfortunately, they do little to help the rest of the horse.

A halter-like apparatus is on the market to help keep flies away from the horse's face. The manufacturer calls it a horse "collar" in deference to governmental regulations. It is a plastic saturated with an insecticide much like that used in flea collars for dogs. This apparatus has a band which goes around the animal's throatlatch, a browband, and several strips which hang down toward the eyes. It looks like these may help with flies that plague the animal's head. It may be worth a try if you have this problem.

Whatever product you use, it is important to patch test it when you are using it on a new horse in your herd—or using a new insecticide on the old horse (see Patch Test)!

Some insect repellents (and many of the tags) contain compounds called organic phosphates. These may interfere with certain tranquilizers or anesthetics. If you know that your animal is going to have surgery, you should discontinue the use of these products a week to ten days before surgery is scheduled. If you are using one of these products or tags and your animal requires un-scheduled sedation or anesthesia, please, please mention to your veterinarian that you have been using this type of insect repellent or tag.

Insect repellent ointments are available which can be placed directly into open wounds. These make a world of difference to animals with sores during the insect season. They are also useful for animals with large numbers of insects in their ears. The animals become extremely sensitive and headshy from the bloody sores made by the gnats or small flies.

One to two treatments have been adequate to cure several of these horses. As soon as you can stop the insects from irritating the ears, the sores heal. Once the skin is healed, the animal is not bothered nearly as much by the bugs. To treat the animal's ears, take a large gob of the ointment on the end of your thumb. Cuddle your hand around the horse's ear, with the thumb inside. Then, wipe it firmly upward to spread the salve along the inside of the ear. Expect your horse to object to the treatment since his ears hurt! However, it's the only way to get the job done and the ears healed.

These ointments are also good for other open sores, as they can be placed directly in them (but NOT, of course, on wounds which are to be sutured).

LINIMENTS AND LOTIONS

Liniments and lotions are mixtures which are painted or rubbed onto the horses's legs. They are supposed to help stimulate circulation and make the animal less lame. Many of them do cause reddening in the skin, but that's not where the lameness is occurring! No matter how much you redden and irritate the skin, it's not going to do much for the underlying tissues.

What DOES do some good is the massaging and rubbing. These can help circulation deep in the tissues, as well as helping to remove the soreness. Remember how good it feels to get a back rub when you have overworked or are tense? Massage does the same for the horse's legs. Go ahead and put liniment on the animal if you like, but remember that it's probably the massage that is helping him. He would probably show the same amount of improvement WITH the massage and WITHOUT the liniment. I have tried liniment on my own legs. My impression was that it made the skin irritated enough that I really wasn't feeling the sore muscles inside—much like putting a twitch on a horse's nose.

WOUND MEDICATIONS

Numerous products have been used through the years on cuts and other injuries in the horse. Many (thank heavens!) have been discarded. Some of these old cures did actual harm, while others did no harm, but didn't do any good, either. Among those that have fallen out of favor (at least with most people) are sulfur, bacon grease, and turpentine. Many of the animals who have healed when treated with these items would have healed in the same amount of time and with the same degree (or less) of scarring if nothing had been used.

Still other old treatments, such as putting dry lime into the wound, usually left more scarring than would have been present if the animal had never been treated. When you get right down to it, these are the main criteria for a good and effective wound medication; it should help the animal to heal faster than without it, it should minimize the formation of proud flesh and scar tissue, and it should, above all, cause no harm. Let's discuss some of the common wound medications used today and where and when to use them.

Nitrofurazone dressing. This is a yellow wound dressing containing the antibiotic nitrofurazone. It comes under many brand names, made by many different companies. Perhaps the oldest and best known is Furacin Dressing (Norden, Lincoln, NE 68501). This ointment can be used on nearly any wound. It is water-soluble. For this reason, it is recommended by some veterinarians when you want a wound sutured and cannot get it to the veterinarian right away. My own preference is just to have wounds kept clean and covered if it looks like I'll be treating the wound within about 6 hours or less. Some veterinarians like to have wounds packed with nitrofurazone dressing. Check with your veterinarian for his preference on this.

Nitrofurazone dressing can be used on any wound, nearly anywhere on the body. For head scrapes and small cuts, it can be used without a bandage. It is often used on cuts and rope burns on the lower leg, under a bandage. It is a good product to put on a wound that is dry and crusty when you find it. It helps to soften the scabs so that you can easily remove them, as well as helping to kill bacteria and remove the infected material from under the scabs.

Nitrofurazone also comes as a yellow aerosol spray. Perhaps the best known brand is Topazone (Norden, Lincoln, NE 68501). This is a good product to use on shallow scrapes and wire scratches. It is also good to use (lightly) on a suture line. Because it does not dissolve, it is not good for use on the surface of an open wound (other than a small scrape or scratch) or in a cavity. It definitely should NOT be used on wounds which are to be sutured. Nitrofurazone dressing is a softening and moistening product; Topazone and other similar products are very drying and should be used where you want to dry a wound rather than soften it.

Tri-dye. This is a combination of several dyes which kill bacteria; acriflavine, methyl or gentian violet, and brilliant green are often used. It is commonly called purple lotion, blue lotion, and similar names because of its bright bluish color. It is usually in an alcohol base and, as a result, is a very drying product. It is perhaps the best product to use when you wish to dry a wound. It is not good for use above the animal's knees, except on fine scrapes (like shallow barbed-wire scratches) on an animal's chest or sides. It is good for small cuts at the knee or below (injuries too small to be sutured). Tri-dye is also good for scrapes on the head. It should NOT be used under a bandage.

Tri-dye comes in aerosol cans or dauber bottles. The aerosol cans are convenient and handy. If your horse does not tolerate a spray can, you will find the dauber bottle much better. Either way is fine. Perhaps there is a bit more soaking action with the dauber as it puts more dye onto

the wound and allows it to penetrate material on the surface more efficiently.

Scarlet oil. Scarlet oil is a combination of a dye, a number of aromatic compounds, and alcohol. It is a softening agent, and is excellent for deep wounds in the fleshy parts of the upper body, such as gaping cuts into heavily muscled areas. It is good for cleaning out wounds which are severely infected. In addition to its antiseptic action, scarlet oil helps to promote the formation of granulation tissue which will heal the defect. It does not tend to stimulate the growth of excessive proud flesh, nor does it retard growth at the skin edges. It is most often used for wounds ABOVE the knee or hock area.

If a wound is scabbed and filthy when found, it is often good to begin by applying nitrofurazone dressing daily for four or five days to help soften the scabs and allow their removal. After this period, swab the wound daily with scarlet oil. Before swabbing, gently remove any scabs that you can from both the surface of the wound and its edges. Then, use a cotton swab to apply the scarlet oil if the wound is shallow. If it is deeper, it may be necessary to use longer cotton swabs which may be purchased at the drugstore. Or, you can use a pair of forceps or hemostats to grasp a gauze sponge. Saturate it with the scarlet oil and smear it onto the surface. Scarlet oil is also available in aerosol cans. Aerosol application is not recommended—the physical action of swabbing the wound is very important to cleaning pus and debris off the surface of the granulating area. If you spray the scarlet oil on the area, it merely treats the scabs rather than treating the wound. Remember, scabs don't heal—but, the wound surface does!

Petroleum jelly. Vaseline (Cheseborough-Ponds, Inc., Greenwich, CT 06830) is one common brand name. Quite often, petroleum jelly can be bought as a generic product in many drugstores. This product can be used by itself when softening is needed, as on a mare with a chapped udder. It is safe if the foal licks it from the mare and eats it. It is also the basis for many types of "patent medicines." These often contain carbolic acid (phenol), as well as other drugs. Corona Ointment (Corona Products Co., Atlanta, GA 30301) is an example of one of these mixtures. They are good for softening small wounds and helping them to heal, but may NOT be safe if a foal could possibly lick them. Some of these products should NOT be used under bandages. Be sure to follow label directions.

Strong Tincture of Iodine. Tincture of iodine (7%) is a mixture of iodine in alcohol. It is called "strong" or "veterinary" iodine to distinguish it from the human product, a much weaker mixture. Iodine is useful for helping to clean and stimulate granulation in small wounds, such as punctures. It is also good for punctures and sole abscesses on the foot, as well as for cleansing abscesses elsewhere on the body.

Strong tincture of iodine will STAIN, and stain badly.

Be sure to keep it off clothes that you value, as well as furniture, floors, and counters. If you get it on your hands, you will have brown stains for a week or so until the outer, stained layer of the skin wears off. If you get it on either hands or clothing, it may sometimes be removed if flushed immediately with alcohol. Otherwise, just be careful where you put it—and where you set the bottle. And don't break a bottle of it or you'll have a real mess!

Sulfa drugs are sometimes used as wound medication. These antibacterials may be combined with urea. The urea helps to dissolve and remove any pus or debris in the area. The urea concentration in a wound product should generally be less than 12 to 15%. In higher concentrations, it may irritate the wound and slow its healing. Sulfa-urea is usually used as an oily solution which is swabbed onto the area being treated. It is a good product for cleaning out an old, dirty, infected wound. One product of this type is called Sulfasol No. 2 (Fort Dodge, IA 50501).

Enzymes. Enzymes are used much as are the sulfa-urea products, to clean out wounds which are filthy and infected. They help to liquefy pus and other garbage and facilitate their removal from the wound. One enzyme-antibiotic combination which is used in this manner is Kymar Ointment (Tech America, Elwood, KS 66024). Enzymes are best used on the advice of your veterinarian.

COLIC MIXTURES

From time to time, products appear on the market which are supposed to treat any and all colics. These can be dangerous for two reasons; first, they may lull the horse owner into hoping that the product will cure his horse, causing him to delay getting an accurate diagnosis and treatment until it is too late. Secondly, there is absolutely no way that one product can treat all kinds of colic. Veterinarians use totally different medication to treat gaseous colic with an overactive, cramping gut than is given to an animal with an impaction and inactive digestive tract.

Some products, such as Canadian "Bells," contain drugs which can permanently stop the horse's intestinal action, leading to death from what may originally have been a minor colic. When dealing with a colic, there is no substitute for immediate and accurate diagnosis and appropriate treatment. Forget the patent medicine and leave the diagnosis and treatment of colic to your veterinarian.

ANTIDIARRHEALS

Foals with diarrhea have very little reserve of fluids (much like small babies). A small loss of fluid can rapidly lead to dehydration and weakness. If the foal begins a diarrhea when you cannot get your veterinarian, treat it with Kaopectate or Pepto-Bismol or any similar human antidiarrheal product which you have on hand. Give two to three tablespoons four to five times a day. Or, give a dosage appropriate to an adult human; this dosage is usually about right for a foal. Kaopectate (Upjohn, Kalamazoo, MI 49001) is available in gallons from veterinary suppliers if you need large quantities of it.

If the product is working and the foal gets better, you probably don't need to consult your veterinarian. If it does not, he should be called to examine the foal and prescribe specific medication. If you have continuing problems with foal diarrhea on your premises, get your veterinarian to give you some extra liquid or pills. No particular antibiotic antidiarrheal product will be recommended here because different drugs work better in different parts of the country and on different farms. Leave the selection of an appropriate product to your local veterinarian. Careful disinfection of stalls and corrals where foals have had diarrhea, or foaling out mares on clear pastures can go a long way toward preventing diarrhea.

COUGH MIXTURES

Cough products are sold as either powders or syrups. Their formulas are generally based on expectorants. Expectorants are drugs which help the respiratory tract to secrete more fluid, lessening the irritation and helping the animal to stop coughing. It also loosens secretions which are in the lungs and bronchi so that the animal can cough them up and get rid of them. Antihistamines may be included to help counteract the role of allergies in producing the cough. Powerful cough-suppressing drugs may be added to some of these products.

Since some animals (such as those with heaves) are kept on cough powders for prolonged periods of time (months or even years), it is best to use the LEAST powerful drug which will do the job. Some powders are available which are made of herbs and minerals. If one of these works for you, stay with it. If not, move up to a product containing expectorants. If this doesn't work, go to one with antihistamines. If that doesn't work, get your veterinarian to prescribe a more powerful medication.

Cough mixtures are also useful for horses with upper respiratory diseases. They help to relieve the animal's coughing (much as we use cough syrup when we have colds). This helps to keep the problem from becoming either heaves or a chronic pneumonia. Don't be afraid to use a cough preparation for a month or so with an upper respiratory problem. It's better to treat a little longer than is necessary than to stop too soon and have the animal go into chronic problems because of it.

TRANQUILIZERS

Tranquilizers are drugs which are used to dull or sedate an animal, adjusting his attitude so that he can be worked with. Some nasty mares, for example, are tranquilized before breeding to avoid injury to the stallion (or to the mare herself). These drugs reduce anxiety, but do not directly reduce pain. They are NOT anesthetics and should NOT be used as substitutes for anesthetics. They may, however, dull the animal's senses enough that your veterinarian can then inject a local anesthetic around the wound so that it can be cleaned and sutured without pain to the animal.

Tranquilizers should not be used indiscriminately. Animals who are given tranquilizers may occasionally have reactions in which they become completely crazed and irrational rather than sedated. Horses who react in this manner may severely injure themselves and people around them. In addition, tranquilizers may lower an animal's blood pressure enough to cause problems with an animal who has lost a large amount of blood from a wound or is in shock from another reason. The loss of blood pressure may be enough to cause the animal's death.

Tranquilizers also reduce an animal's coordination. Animals who must be trailered after being tranquilized may fall down and be unable to get up again. If you must haul a tranquilized horse, drive as carefully as possible and hope he doesn't fall. Animals who are ridden after being tranquilized may stumble and fall with the rider, causing a definite hazard.

Tranquilizers may sometimes be used to catch animals who cannot otherwise be corralled. Tranquilizers are available in powdered form which can be fed with a small amount of grain. Mix a little molasses or pancake syrup with the grain and medication to keep it together so that the animal does not just eat the grain and leave the tranquilizer on the bottom of the feed pan. A tranquilized animal may be uncoordinated and yet still have a fear of being handled. This may cause the horse to struggle and fight even though it is uncoordinated, with the disadvantage that it may fall in its struggles.

Recently one of my clients captured a wild mare this way. She was uncoordinated enough to fall down, at which time they jumped on her head and put a halter on, with a lariat on each side. As they maneuvered her toward a trailer, the mare continued to fight, falling several times. One of the falls was right on her head. The horse dropped dead about an hour later, having apparently broken a small blood vessel in the brain.

Regardless of whether a tranquilizer is administered intravenously, intramuscularly, or in the feed, it takes some time to take effect. If the animal is continuously fought or stimulated in this period, it may never take effect. After a tranquilizer is given, take off the animal's halter, turn him completely loose in a familiar pen or stall, and go away for the required period of time. This has much better effect than if the owner stands holding the lead shank and talking to the horse, moving him around. Most tranquilizers which are given intravenously take about 10 to 20 minutes to take effect, those given in the muscle take 20 to 45 minutes, and those given in the feed take around one to two hours.

If you need to use a tranquilizer, ask your veterinarian to recommend one which he feels will be safe for you. An example of this would be a stallion owner breeding a nasty mare who must be tranquilized each time she is bred. It's a problem to have to call the vet every time you breed her (especially if she's a problem breeder.) Be aware that you might get into problems with overdosage or other reactions. Think twice (or more) before tranquilizing a horse that you do not own!

ANESTHETICS

Anesthetics are drugs which are given to horses to put them completely "out." They are used to put the animal's brain to sleep enough that he will not feel a painful surgical procedure, such as castration. Most anesthetics are given as injections. The majority of these are administered intravenously, although a few are given intramuscularly. With an injectable anesthetic, the drug is put into the body, and the animal does not wake up until his organs clear it from his brain and bloodstream (except for a very few drugs which have injectable products to reverse them).

At university hospitals and large clinics, inhalation (gas) anesthetic may be used after a small dosage of an injectable product to get the animal relaxed enough that a tube may be passed into his trachea. Gas anesthetics are the safest of all, especially when administered by a veterinarian or his trained assistant. They have the advantage that when the procedure is over, the animal is disconnected and wakes up rapidly.

Needless to say, gas anesthesia is usually also expensive. The products themselves are costly, the machines to administer them to something the size of a horse cost thousands of dollars, and highly trained help must be available to use them.

Animals vary in their susceptibility to various anesthetics, especially the injectable ones. Some animals can take as much as four to six times what another animal of the same weight and temperament can handle. One of my clients has a stallion who is laid flat on the ground for 20 minutes by a dosage of a particular drug that is half enough to hold most similar horses still for five minutes (standing). Because of the hazards associated with these products, their usage is best left to your veterinarian.

Any time a horse is anesthetized, there is some danger. The amount of hazard varies with the animal's health and condition and his individual reaction to the drug. Some drugs depress heart function enough to cause an animal to go into shock, especially if he is already on the edge of it. Others depress respiratory function, causing the animal to stop breathing. And it's tough to give artificial respiration to any equine larger than a foal; cardiac massage is impossible! While these side effects do not by any means occur every time an animal is anesthetized, nonetheless, they do occur and may be a cause of death. Most veterinarians do not like to anesthetize a horse unless it is absolutely necessary. When they do, they use the least harmful drug which will do the job, and the least amount possible.

PRODUCTS FOR IMMUNIZATION

A number of products are used to immunize equines against various diseases. Vaccines protect them against viral respiratory diseases such as influenza and rhinopneumonitis, as well as against sleeping sickness. Toxoids protect them against toxic products produced by the bacteria which cause tetanus, thus preventing the disease. Bacterins may be used against the bacteria which cause distemper (when these are commercially available). Specific types of products and immunization programs are discussed with each disease.

It is important to remember that immunization is not a substitute for sound management practices, such as limiting horse movement from place to place, isolation of newly arrived animals, and proper sanitation.

HOME CURES AND HERBAL REMEDIES

Numerous home cures are floating around the horse world, and almost every older horseman has his favorite collection. A few of them actually work. Many times, however, the animal heals IN SPITE of the cure rather than BECAUSE of it. Horsemen have been known to douse wounds with axle grease, lard, sulfur, lime, and sheep dip, among other things. Let's, for the most part, forget 1830 and move into the age of antibiotics and cures which specifically attack the problem at hand. Forget the advice of your neighbor who touts one of these "folk remedies" and give your veterinarian a call. Give him a chance to fix the problem before you've made it incurable, or have allowed the lesion to double or triple in size so that you have a major problem instead of the minor one you had in the beginning.

In the process of preparing this book, this author read many books on all aspects of veterinary medicine and horsemanship. Many of the texts showed old-time remedies which were used in the past when we didn't have any other way of doing things. One of the "modern" books,

which shall remain nameless, detailed herbal cures for everything that ails your horse. A few of these cures had a sound scientific basis; the great majority were sheer wishful thinking.

Among those which may be harmful to the animal is fasting, which was prescribed for many ailments. In general, the sick animal needs food, not starvation. Exceptions to this are horses with colic and founder. They do not need any further food for 6 to 12 hours after they have begun to have problems; then, they may be started back to half their roughage ration. Adding grain back to the diet should be done 18 to 36 hours after the start of the episode.

Another cure which could possibly be harmful is the application of used motor oil to keep flies and insects off the horse. Most horse owners cannot imagine marinating their horse in oil with lead from the gasoline and all the other additives which are put into the product. There is a very real possibility of serious harm to your horse if you follow such advice.

The use of garlic or tobacco as a horse wormer is another practice which is worse than useless. Not only does it not work, but it gives a false sense of security in thinking that you have adequately removed worms from your horse's system. These "remedies" are usually preceded by a couple of days' fast, and a large dosage of some sort of laxative. Why use such a "cure" when we have modern wormers that are 95 to 100% effective against worms? If you were a horse, how would you prefer to be wormed—with a wormer that requires no fast and actually works, or one that requires fasting, laxative, and is of dubious value?

This same nameless book also lists new spring grass as helping to remove worms from the animal's system. The only way this could be even remotely true is by its laxative effect. The same publication lists turpentine as a wormer for one particular type of worms. Now, how is that more "natural" than a modern worming medication? And, it cannot be a fraction as effective, if it works at all. It's your horse so I'll let you decide if you want to rely on "folk remedies" or take advantage of modern technology. The acid test for any remedy that you use for your horse should be, "Would I want that done to or used on me?"

Incidentally, a few of the herbal cures do actually work and have some medical basis. The only problem is that the average horse owner does not have the pharmacological background to tell them from the ones that don't work, or are actually harmful. An example of a natural substance which works is the sauerkraut poultice used elsewhere in this book. The cabbage acts as a drawing agent, while the acetic acid and enzymes in the juice act to clean the wound. This is a case where there is a logical reason for the cure to work. My objection is to the ones which don't work, or are actually harmful. There is nothing sacred about "natural" products. Remember, strychnine is a "natural" product (it comes from a plant!).

Chapter 12

BANDAGES AND BANDAGING

Bandaging Materials
Bandaging Techniques
  Foot Bandages
  Leg Bandages
Emergency Bandages
Robert Jones Bandage
Poultices

Bandages are often needed to cover wounds, especially on the legs and feet. They help to keep dirt and manure out of the wound or injury. With open cuts, they may be used to help keep the edges together, allowing faster and more efficient healing. Pressure bandages help to control excessive growth of proud flesh. Bandages also keep insects off wounds and keep the horse from chewing or rubbing the injured area.

CAUTION: Pressure bandages MUST NOT be used in an area where infection is present. In this situation, the bandage may force bacteria and their toxic products deeper into the tissues. Use a bandage only to cover the area until the infection is controlled by antibiotics.

Let's begin by discussing types of bandaging material and the pros and cons of each, and then move on to talk about how to bandage different areas of the horse's body.

BANDAGING MATERIALS

Gauze sponges are small, folded pads of gauze. They can be used to clean discharges from the surface of wounds to get them ready for bandaging. Sponges may then be dipped into dressings, such as nitrofurazone ointment, and placed directly on the wound. Sponges are also useful because of their bulk, to provide pressure on wounds which are bleeding badly; they also help control bleeding because of their absorbency. The easiest way to buy them is in sterile packages of 100. A convenient size is 2 × 2 inches. Larger sponges do not fit into smaller wounds as well. If you are treating a large wound for a long

period of time, you may find 3 × 3 inch or even 4 × 4 inch sponges better. These can be purchased from your veterinarian or from a hospital or veterinary supply company.

Nonstick pads, such as Telfa Pads (Curity, Colgate-Palmolive Co., NY, NY, 10022), are handy for applying medication to wounds and for placing on an injured surface before bandaging. They are also good to put over suture lines before the area is wrapped (use them here without any medication on them). They keep the discharges from the wound from sticking to the bandage. For this reason, they are preferable to gauze sponges in many situations.

Roll gauze is often used as padding over the sponges or Telfa Pads and under the outer bandaging material. It provides extra padding and slight pressure, especially if an elastic gauze such as Kling (Johnson & Johnson Products, Inc., New Brunswick, NJ 08903) is used. On the other hand, the gauze keeps some of the outer bandaging material from coming into contact with the hair. Thus, the outer bandage is not as securely anchored as it otherwise would be and may have more tendency to roll or slip. Using gauze is a matter of personal preference and habit. Most owners will find that their bandages stay in place better if gauze is not used.

Regular (nonstretch) gauze is not elastic. If it is left in place for more than a day, it may cut into the skin, especially if swelling occurs in the limb. It may cause circulation problems with subsequent loss of skin or development of gangrene. If you are using gauze under a pressure bandage, it should be the "Kling" type as mentioned above. The same problems may occur with regular adhesive tape as with nonstretch gauze. For this reason, elastic tapes are preferred for most injuries, and are well worth the extra money they cost.

Roll cotton or thick quilted pads are used in Robert Jones bandages, or for shipping boots (see Robert Jones bandage). Roll cotton may also be used for padding under bandages for sole punctures or abscesses. Disposable diapers may also be used as bandaging pads.

Elastic bandages (often called "Ace" bandages) are used by many horsemen. They are difficult to put on at the right tension. It seems like they're either too tight and cut off circulation, or they're too loose and they slide down, roll at the edges, or bunch up. They're not good to use on animals. The animal can't tell you that the bandages don't fit or are uncomfortable. While some people use them frequently, my preference is for other elastic products which give pressure without the rolling or tightness problems that these bandages can cause.

Vetrap (3M Animal Care Products, St. Paul, MN 55144) is a stretchy, selfadhesive bandage material. It puts gentle pressure on the injured area, and goes onto the leg well without bunching or creating excessive pressure. It does not stick to the hair and cause the animal any discomfort when it is removed—it sticks only to itself. It works well on many horses, but may not stay in place on very active animals.

It is often helpful to take a wrap of regular 1-inch white adhesive tape at the top and bottom of a Vetrap bandage, as well as sticking a few inches of it over the end of the bandage to keep it from coming loose. If taken off carefully and loosely rolled as you are doing so, Vetrap can occasionally be used a second time if it is not contaminated by manure or wound discharges. These bandages are good in hot climates as they do not seem to deteriorate, whereas adhesive tape vulcanizes into a hopeless lump instead of a roll and the elastic tapes stick to themselves so well that they cannot be pulled apart.

Elastic adhesive tapes—one brand name is Elastikon (Johnson & Johnson)—are useful for the nervous or active horse who moves around enough to loosen other bandages and have them slide or roll out of place. These products also work well for bandaging over joints where much movement occurs. They are much like an "Ace" bandage, but with adhesive on the back similar to regular adhesive tape. As mentioned above, the rolls of tape don't survive well in a vehicle or horse trailer which becomes very hot, as they stick to themselves (meanwhile, becoming nearly worthless for sticking to anything else). For use in cooler climates and times other than summer, they are superb. Place gauze sponges or Telfa pads over the wound itself, and then stick the rest of the bandage directly to the animal's hair so that it will not roll or slide. One of these bandages is often easier to remove by cutting vertically down the side opposite the wound with bandage scissors. Rip it off quickly, rather than trying to unwind it, layer by sticky layer.

Plain old white adhesive tape is occasionally used for horse bandages. It has the advantage of being relatively inexpensive when compared to the elastic bandaging materials. Some white adhesive tape is waterproof. This is occasionally useful for hoof bandages. Do not use the waterproof tape higher up on the leg because it tends to make the area "sweat." A couple of strips of adhesive tape can be placed over the end of an elastic bandage or wrap

to help keep the end from coming loose and unraveling. A strip can also be used at the top and bottom of a bandage to keep dirt from working down into it. As mentioned previously, it should not be used for wrapping legs where swelling may occur.

Duct tape (the kind used by auto mechanics and furnace repairmen) is handy for temporary use to hold silicon caulking in place under a hoof pad until it is dry. It should be removed in three or four hours. It is sometimes helpful when you have a horse who is chewing his bandages off. Place a couple of wraps of it around the top of the bandage. Its slick surface makes it more difficult for the horse to grab the bandage with his teeth. A wrap or two may also be used around the bottom, if needed. Do NOT cover the whole bandage with duct tape, as it will cause sweating—even worse than waterproof adhesive tape—and retard healing.

And, while we are on the subject of horses who chew their bandages, there are several preparations which can help stop this problem. Try putting a light coating of petroleum jelly over the bandage and sprinkling it liberally with powdered cayenne pepper—the hottest you can find! Tabasco sauce will stop some animals when shaken onto the bandage. Be careful that you don't use so much that it soaks through the bandage. It is strong enough to act as a blistering agent and really create a mess. Variton Creme (Schering Corp., Kenilworth, NJ 07033) is a foul-flavored ointment which will keep some animals from chewing when it is applied in a thin coating to the outside of the bandage. Bitter apple flavoring will repel some horses. If none of these solutions work, it may be necessary to put on a head cradle or put the horse on an overhead trolley wire, or muzzle him to keep him from chewing.

Cheesecloth is useful for making a loose shroud to help keep insects off wounds on the upper body which cannot otherwise be bandaged. Clean, old bedsheets can also be used for this purpose. These coverings must be changed periodically when they become soiled so that flies do not start to infest them and so that they are not holding pus and discharges against the wound.

Splints and casts are used to immobilize legs to allow fractures to heal by preventing movement between the bones. They are also used for wire cuts, especially those in the heel and pastern area, as well as on the coronary band. Prevention of movement allows more rapid healing than would otherwise occur. Less scar tissue will form when the skin is not allowed to pull apart every time the horse takes a step. Casts can be used to support injured or severed tendons to help their healing. They may also reduce swelling and inflammation in the injured area.

Various materials are used to make splints and casts—among them are plaster of paris, fiberglass, balsa wood, and aluminum tubing. Casts constructed of different materials are used in different ways to repair fractures, crooked legs in young foals, and similar problems. It is beyond the scope of this book to discuss all their methods of contruction and usage. More information can be found in Adams' "Lameness in Horses," or can be obtained from your local veterinarian. Putting on a good cast—one which does not result in pressure sores or other problems—is a real art. Leave it to your veterinarian.

Whatever bandaging material you choose, don't get it any wider than four inches. Some people wrestle with six-inch wide tape, but it never seems to lie flat around knees and is nearly impossible to wrap around feet. In fact, my choice for bandaging feet is two-inch wide Elastikon, or a similar product. Store any adhesive-backed products in a cool place. If you need to keep bandages in your vehicle or horse trailer in hot climates, Vetrap is the hands-down choice.

BANDAGING TECHNIQUES

FOOT BANDAGES

Feet are bandaged for a number of reasons. Most common are puncture wounds, wire cuts, rope burns, or other injuries. If there is an open wound or cut, decide what medication you are going to use on it. Nitrofurazone ointment is a common choice. Spread a thick coating over the appropriate area on a gauze sponge or Telfa pad—like jelly on a sandwich. You can smear it on with a clean finger, or use a tongue depressor or kitchen knife. Make it a half inch or so larger than the wound you're putting it on—it isn't always easy to get the pad centered on the wound.

If the horse is nervous or broncy, cut a piece of tape eight to ten inches longer than the pad is wide. Stick it firmly across the back of the pad, leaving an equal amount sticking out on each side. The piece of tape should be planned to go sideways around the leg rather than up and down. This whole outfit can be quickly stuck onto the horse's leg. Let him relax and get accustomed to having something around the wound. Then, go ahead and finish bandaging him.

If you are covering a puncture wound in the sole, it will be necessary to pack the sole with absorbent material. Gauze sponges or pads of sheet cotton are often used. In an emergency, clean paper towels or cloth could be used, or even disposable diapers (baby side to the foot).

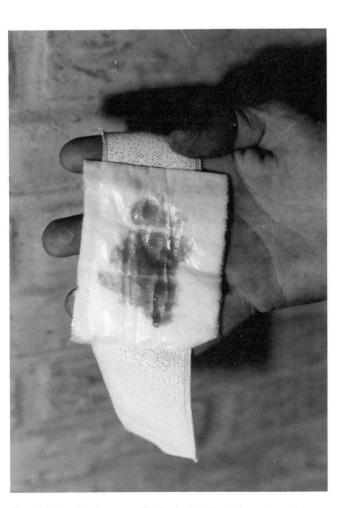

Bandaging the horse—Telfa pad with ointment and tape.

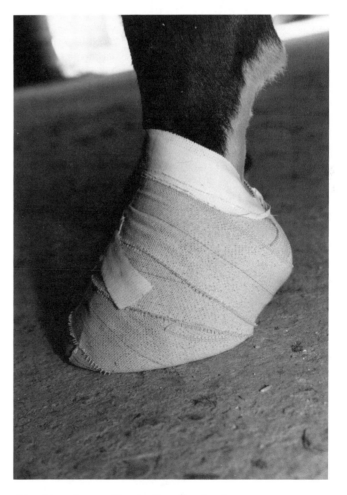

Hoof bandage with elastic adhesive tape.

Wrap over the pad with your choice of bandaging materials. My first choice is an adhesive-backed elastic tape (such as Elastikon). My second choice is Vetrap. Third is plain white adhesive tape. Wrapping feet is one of the few places where white adhesive tape is useful. Whatever product you use, it is extremely important to get it down UNDER the bulb of the heel. This keeps the bandage from creeping upward, which it invariably does if not anchored by the bulb of the heel. It does not hurt to wrap a third or half way across the bottom of the foot, even if the bandage is meant for the pastern area. Of course, if you are putting on the bandage because of a puncture in the hoof, it will go all the way across the bottom of the foot.

If you are using an elastic tape or Vetrap, put a strip or two of white adhesive tape across the end of the bandage to keep it from pulling loose and unraveling. If the animal chews at the bandage, handle the situation as mentioned previously.

LEG BANDAGES

Most of the principles of bandaging legs are the same as those for feet, and the Telfa pad/ointment usage is the same. The main problem is that the animal's movement and the shape of the leg (larger at the top and smaller at the bottom) contribute to the bandage sliding down if it is not carefully applied. If the bandage is too tight, circulation may be affected, resulting in swelling below it. In many cases, it is easier to put a snug bandage all the way down to the hoof than to fight with getting the tension just right higher up. It's quite permissible and often advisable!

Animals with severely injured legs, or injuries (such as bowed tendons or fractures) which are going to take a long time to heal should have the opposite leg wrapped to give it support. This helps keep the tendons from being stretched and dropping the fetlock. Otherwise, you might heal one leg and find that the other one has dropped beyond recovery! A simple supporting bandage of one of the elastic materials can be used. It may be applied right on the leg, or put on over quilted pads or roll cotton (as a Robert Jones bandage). It should be snug enough to give the tendons some support, or you can use knit wraps as are used on racehorses. These are washable and reusable. Like other bandages, these should be changed at least every three days to prevent skin problems from developing underneath, and to allow you to treat them if they occur.

A sprinkling of boric acid powder rubbed into the hair will help prevent skin problems under the bandage when you are going to have the horse bandaged for a long time. This is useful with any bandage placed over unbroken skin. It's the equine equivalent of powdering your feet before you put on your socks. This powder can be purchased at most drugstores.

EMERGENCY BANDAGES

When you have a horse injured out in the middle of nowhere, it's time to improvise protection for his wound. If you have bandaging materials handy, that's a step in the right direction. Pack a fresh bleeding wound with sterile gauze sponges and then wrap snugly—preferably with an elastic tape or Vetrap if you have either one. If not, the gauze may be held in place with anything else that you have—duct tape, strapping tape, or a chunk of bedsheet or shirttail. If you have no sponges, sanitary napkins or disposable diapers can be placed over a bleeding wound before wrapping with tape.

One of the most original emergency repairs was done by a client who was about forty miles into a National Forest on a dirt road. His horse was severely cut from halfway up the neck down into the armpit area. The wound varied from three to six inches deep, and was hanging open. The owner wrapped electrical tape all the way around the animal's neck in great loops from top to bottom. The tape put enough pressure on the area to prevent the wound from gaping, and kept it quite clean and moist—enough to allow it to be sutured when he

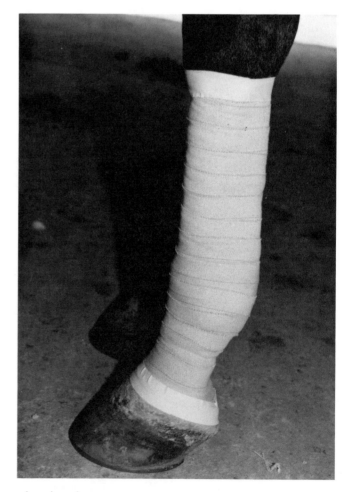

Leg bandage.

arrived at the clinic. The horse made an uneventful recovery.

The foxhunters' practice of wearing a stock tie was traditionally meant to provide a bandage in case his horse (or he) were injured. The cowboy's scarf often served the same purpose. If you are on a pack trip or trail ride into rough country, carrying a couple of rolls of Vetrap and a few gauze sponges is cheap (and lightweight) insurance. Incidentally, either Vetrap or Elastikon is handy to carry when you are backpacking or hiking, and will allow wrapping a sprained ankle and then putting a boot or shoe on afterwards. If you're back a ways and have to walk out, don't bother to take off the boot—just wrap over the whole thing to put on pressure and to help keep the swelling down. Either of these products is durable enough to go quite a few miles if necessary.

ROBERT JONES BANDAGE

This is the bandage equivalent of a cast—basically, a soft cast. It can be used to help support and immobilize problems, such as bowed tendons. It can also be used with large foam pads or bed pillows to stabilize a broken leg if nothing else is available. It can be used to support the limb opposite an injured one. As with any pressure bandage, it should not be used in an area where infection is present.

Begin to build the bandage by putting soft material next to the leg. For bowed tendons, for instance, start by wrapping the leg with two to three layers of thick roll cotton, going continuously around the leg until it is built up about an inch thick. Begin the bandage just below the knee, and extend it down to the foot for lower leg injuries, or higher for upper-leg problems. Wrap elastic gauze around the cotton to hold it in place. Next, using Elastikon, put strips of it vertically on the front and back of the leg and on the inside and outside. Use two to three thicknesses of the tape. These "splints" help to stiffen the bandage. Now wrap Elastikon around the gauze and vertical strips, pulling it more snugly than you would if you were putting it on the leg by itself. When you come to the bottom of the cast, you can either stop or can continue down the fetlock area and around the heel, as described for bandaging feet. If you do not wrap down around the fetlock, it will be necessary to keep a close eye on the leg for swelling below the bandage.

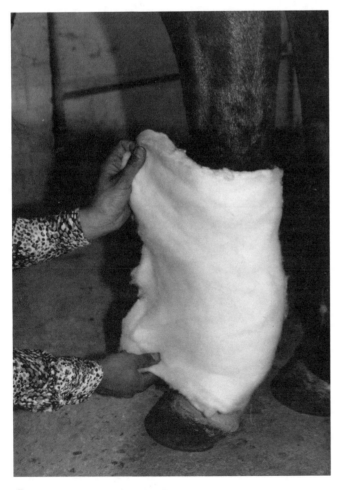

Putting cotton on leg for Robert Jones bandage.

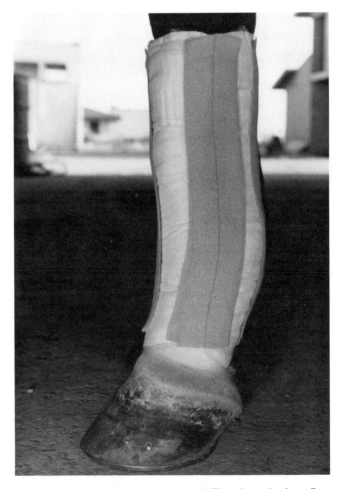

Cotton is covered with gauze and Elastikon "splints."

For bowed tendons, the bandage may be placed over a drawing poultice, such as Gelocast (Biersdorf, Norwalk, CT 06856). The poultice is placed on the leg, then covered with a plastic wrap. The rest of the bandage is applied as described. If the pressure is carefully regulated to avoid swelling below, it can be used just over the cannon area.

A similar bandage may be made with foam rubber, blankets, or even bed pillows to splint a broken leg when nothing else is available. Place the soft material over the leg. Five or six inches is none too thick. Then, wrap firmly over it with any tape or bandaging material which you have; gauze, adhesive, electrical, or duct tape, or even strips of sheet or rags. The object is to make a big, soft, but very thick, bandage.

POULTICES

Poultices are drawing packs which are used under a bandage to help remove fluid or swelling from an area. Mixtures of clays may be used as well as a paste containing epsom salts. Other materials, such as bread, charcoal, and linseed meal. have been used for poultices. Many

herbal and plant mixtures are also used. One of my favorites for heel problems is sauerkraut (see Scratches). Some poultices can be applied only to unbroken skin and are not suitable to use on open wounds. Others can be used on infected or open wounds. Poultices are especially good for use on puncture wounds. Be sure the poultice you choose is suitable for the use you intend. Some poultice materials are available already saturated into gauze and ready to roll onto the animal's skin (Gelocast, above).

The poultice material is applied to the skin or to gauze or other material according to its directions. It is then covered with a sheet of plastic or a plastic bag. A pressure bandage is then placed over the plastic. Packs such as these should be changed every one to two days. Leaving them any longer may result in skin infection. Anyway, after one to two days, the drawing effect of the poultice material has been exhausted and you are no longer getting any benefit from it. A fresh application will again give good results.

If you are going to rebandage a leg which has had a poultice on it, it is a good idea to rinse the leg with warm water to remove any remains of the old material before applying a new one—whether you are using a plain bandage or replacing the poultice. Either dry the leg carefully or allow it to air-dry if you are replacing the poultice with a regular bandage.

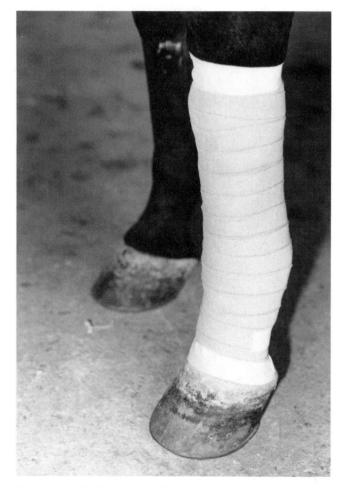

Completed Robert Jones bandage.

Chapter 13

INJURIES AND THEIR TREATMENT

How They Occur
Tetanus
Abrasions
Scratches
Puncture Wounds
    Bullet Wounds
Cuts
    To Sew or Not to Sew
    Treating Fresh Cuts
    Complications in Sutured Wounds
Skin Grafts
Treatment of Open Wounds
    Complications in Open Wounds
    Proud Flesh
Closed Wounds and Other Assorted Swellings
Bones
Fractures
    First Aid for Fractures
    Fracture Repair
Amputation
Osteomyelitis
Avascular Necrosis
Arthritis

HOW THEY OCCUR

Almost every owner who has had a horse for any length of time has had the animal become injured in one way or another. In spite of the fact that they are so large and strong, horses tend to hurt themselves. Or maybe it is BECAUSE of their size and strength that they are easily injured. Like humans, some are accident-prone. Other animals may not be very intelligent, or they may not see very well. Whatever the cause, they can be a constant source of expense and grief to the owner. Often, the least expensive and happiest way out is to trade one of these in for a good animal who is not accident-prone.

Other horses develop habits, such as pawing, which make them liable to injury. A horse who paws with his front feet may not cause any problem—until he does it near a barbed-wire fence. A good example is a mare owned for nearly five years by one of my neighbors. At least once a year, this animal would stick a front foot through the fence and try to saw it off on the barbed wire. As she usually did this at night and some distance from the house, the owner never discovered her until morning after the damage was already done. It didn't help that she was slow to heal and nasty to treat. Vices, such as kicking the barn or other horses, may lead to a continuing series of injuries and expenses.

Other animals are bullies. They may not get injured, but will cause problems by running other animals through fences, or kicking or biting them. The fact that the horses's primary defense is to run from whatever frightens or threatens him also contributes to injury. A horse will often run blindly from a real or imagined danger, in the process blundering blindly into a fence, wall, tree, or ravine—anything! Loud thunderstorms or explosions in an area may be followed by a rash of injured horses as the animals try to get away from whatever they imagine is out to get them.

Animals separated from others with whom they are familiar will often show the same reaction, crashing through fences. One of my clients had a yearling who had never been away from the group of mares she had been with since birth. The client put the animal in a barn and prepared to load it into a trailer to be hauled to another ranch. The horse panicked and escaped during the loading process. In her frenzy to return to her friends, the filly went over or through three barbed wire fences. The result? Cuts on three of her four legs and a slash across the bridge of her nose which stretched from one jawbone to the other. The animal was so crazed that she had to be completely anesthetized before she could be sutured. Horses also seem likely to bump into fences, walls, etc. When a horse gets snagged on a piece of metal or a nail sticking out, horsehide tears like paper.

This section will begin with a discussion of my philosophies of wound treatment in enough detail so that you can determine the best treatment for a given wound. I want you to be able to determine when you should treat the animal yourself and when you should call a veterinarian. After all, that's what this book is all about. Before we begin the discussion of how to treat injuries, let's consider tetanus—which may be a complication with even a minor wound.

TETANUS

This disease is serious and may even be fatal in the horse. It is caused by a type of bacteria which are normally found in the horse's intestine. They are passed in the manure, so they are present in barnyards and other areas where horses have been. The bacteria may persist for long periods of time after horses have been in an area—perhaps as long as hundreds of years. The tetanus organism grows only in the absence of air. Conditions especially favorable for it to grow occur when the horse punctures his foot by stepping on a nail or impales himself on a branch. It can also occur from gunshot wounds or being "quicked" when he is shod. It rarely occurs in surface or clean wounds, but is enough of a danger to revaccinate the animal when any cut or puncture occurs, no matter how shallow.

IMPORTANT NOTE: Tetanus can be a problem in humans from the same sort of punctures and wounds that cause it in the horse. It is especially important for people who work around horses to keep their tetanus immunizations current. Have you had one recently? Check with your physician for his recommendation on frequency.

SIGNS

The incubation period for tetanus varies from several days to nearly four months. By the time the horse has developed tetanus, the injury through which the bacteria have entered may be completely healed. The first sign is usually stiffness involving muscles of the jaw and hindlimbs. Rarely, the muscles in the area of the injury may also be stiff. After 24 hours, the signs become more noticeable and begin to spread throughout the body. The animal will become hypersensitive, and may go into intermittent spasms. He is usually conscious. Muscle spasms of the head cause problems with picking up food and chewing. The tail and ears may be rigid. The legs are usually extended stiffly, so that the animal looks like a sawhorse, with his neck straight and head upward or even bent back toward his withers. The animal cannot pick feed up off the ground, and is usually unable to chew.

The third eyelid may show prominently over the inside corner of the eye. The horse may have an anxious facial expression. The nostrils are usually flared. The animal may have a stiff-legged gait, moving with difficulty, if at all. The horse may show constipation and other signs of colic. Because of this, an early case of tetanus may be confused with a simple colic until further signs develop. He may retain urine. Sweating is common, and the breathing and heart rates are more rapid than normal. The temperature will be elevated, sometimes to as much as 108 degrees F (42.2 C). This usually occurs late in the course of the disease, when terminal brain damage has occurred.

TREATMENT

If the disease is caught early, large amounts of tetanus antitoxin (50,000 to 200,000 units or more) may or may not be of value in helping the animal to recover, but it is worth the attempt. Your veterinarian will probably treat the horse with antibiotics, usually either penicillin or tetracyclines. He may also administer tranquilizers or muscle relaxants to help relieve the severe muscle spasms.

IMPORTANT NOTE: Horses who have been given tetanus antitoxin may develop a serum-sickness type of liver problem 4 to 10 weeks after it is given. The horse should be watched. If any unusual symptoms develop within this time period, they should be promptly reported to your veterinarian. For this reason, tetanus antitoxin should not be used indiscriminately.

As with many other diseases, nursing is of the utmost importance to the animal's recovery. A horse with tetanus should be confined in a quiet, dark barn with plenty of bedding. Feed and water should be placed high enough that the animal can reach them without having to lower his head. Soft foods, such as alfalfa meal, should be fed. If the horse will not eat, it may be necessary for your veterinarian to feed him via stomach tube. If the animal tries to collapse, it may be necessary to support him in a sling.

Approximately 80% of the horses affected with tetanus die, and those who recover take 3 to 6 weeks of careful (and expensive) treatment and nursing before they recover.

PREVENTION

Tetanus is easily prevented. It is avoided by vaccinating the animal against it with a product called tetanus toxoid. Yes, it is confusing! In general, we prevent the disease with "toxoid," and treat it with "antitoxin." If you are giving it to a young horse or to one who has not been immunized previously, he will initially need two injections, two to four weeks apart, depending on the vaccine that you are using (follow label directions on the timing). The first injection is usually given at 3 to 4 months of age, with the second dose two weeks later. Give a third dose six to nine months after that. Then, he needs an annual booster each year for the rest of his life, in addition to a booster if he suffers a cut or puncture wound. This vaccine is often included in a four-in-one injection with sleeping sickness and influenza vaccines. Considering that horses often die from tetanus, it's cheap insurance against this possibility. Tetanus toxoid stimulates the animal to produce his own immunity (called an active immunity).

If the horse has not previously been immunized against tetanus, tetanus toxoid may not be effective if he has been infected with the disease. It takes 10 to 14 days for response to occur with the first dose of the vaccine. Subsequent doses, if given on a yearly basis, give a good immunity. Boosters administered when injury occurs are effective in less time, and allow tetanus toxoid to be used by itself (without accompanying it with antitoxin).

A horse who has never had any tetanus toxoid is usually given a product called tetanus antitoxin as a part of wound treatment. Instead of stimulating the animal to produce his own immune antibodies, this merely puts some into his body, giving him instant protection against the disease. 1500 units of tetanus antitoxin are usually considered protective. When more is given, it does not necessarily give greater protection—it just lasts longer. (60) Tetanus antitoxin is also given to foals of mothers who either are not immunized, or where the mare has lost her colostrum. It is often given to orphan foals on the presumption that they didn't get any colostrum. When given at a few days of age, the immunity will generally last three to four months, at which time the toxoid can be given to begin active immunity. (61)

Adult horses who have never been immunized for tetanus may be given 1500 units of tetanus antitoxin, and a normal dose of tetanus toxoid at the same time. These products should NOT be mixed or given with the same syringe since they will neutralize each other nor should they be given at the same site. In the adult horse, the protection from tetanus antitoxin is usually considered to last about three weeks. By this time, the body will be starting to produce its own immunity from the toxoid given at the same time. (60)

Mares should have a booster dose of tetanus toxoid four to eight weeks before they foal. This gives the animal a durable immunity to protect her if she is injured or torn during foaling. It also boosts the antibodies against tetanus which are in the colostrum; these help to give the foal a good immunity for the first few months of his life. This is considered to be much more effective than giving antitoxin to the newborn foal. (62)

ABRASIONS

Abrasions are scrapes in which the hair is removed and the surface of the skin is badly irritated or abraded. Yellowish serum usually oozes from the wound, and there may be a small amount of bleeding. These wounds occur in a number of ways. One of the most common is due to the animal falling on pavement or gravel. Gravel may be ground into the wound. Remember how you skinned your knees when you were a kid and fell off your roller skates or skateboard onto the sidewalk?

Shallow bites which do not break the skin fall into this category. They often look like burns, or at least what clients imagine burns to look like. Veterinarians are occasionally called by someone who has just turned a horse into a community pasture and frantically reports that "my horse has burns all over his body—someone did something to him." Well, something happened, but not quite what the owner thought. In actuality, the horse has been bitten and chewed by one or more of the other horses in the process of establishing the pecking order.

Hair may be scraped from the horse's shins while the animal is being loaded or unloaded from a horse trailer. Rope burns are a more severe type of abrasion. Because of their similarity to burns, their treatment is discussed in the burn section.

Abrasions rarely bleed. They must feel to the animal much as it does when we burn our hands on a hot skillet— very sensitive and uncomfortable—because they seem to bother the animal more than would be expected for the amount of injury involved. They also heal slowly.

TREATMENT

In general, my wound treatment philosophy tends toward trying to get a wound back to a normal balance with the rest of the body. In other words, if it is hard and dry, soften it; if it is weeping and moist, dry it up. If is is moist and you are treating it accordingly and it changes to dry, change your medication to reflect this shift in the animal's condition. What medications do you use to accomplish these things?

If you are trying to dry up the wound, one of my favorite products is purple lotion. This is a mixture of dyes which kill bacteria which could cause infection in the wound, in a drying, healing base. These products are usually liquid. Before you apply the medication to the horse, wipe the surface with a clean piece of gauze or a paper towel. If there are scabs around the edge, pick them off gently with a fingernail or pair of forceps.

When your animal has a wound that is already dry and you are trying to soften it, any soothing ointment WITHOUT a corticosteroid in it is good. One of the simplest and most common is petroleum jelly. Fancier versions of petroleum jelly include preparations such as Corona ointment. Nitrofurazone dressing is a soothing antibiotic ointment which should be in every horseman's first aid kit. It is good for routine use and excellent if the wound shows any signs of becoming infected, such as drainage of pus. If scabs are hard and dry, you may not be able to remove them before treatment. Just paste on some nitrofurazone dressing and let it soften the scabs.

Then, the NEXT time you treat it, clean off the scabs before putting on the ointment.

Once a day is often enough for treating scrapes. Abrasions do not need to be bandaged as they generally heal better if left uncovered. The exception to this rule is for the horse who chews at the wound. If his scrape is on a leg and is being treated with an ointment, it may be bandaged. Otherwise, it should be treated with the antibiotic dressing or purple lotion, and then sprayed with an aerosol anti-chew product made to be put on wounds. Or, you can put a light coating of petroleum jelly on the hair AROUND the wound and shake a liberal coating of cayenne pepper (from the grocery store spice rack) on it. Do not get the pepper on the wound itself. Some animals may need a neck cradle or sidestick to keep them from chewing their wounds. Most ointments and creams may be used under a bandage, but wounds treated with purple lotion should be left uncovered.

SCRATCHES

These wounds are long, thin gouges into the upper layers of the hide, but NOT through it. They will be red and may bleed considerably, but they should not gap open. You will not be able to see the underlying muscles. If you do see muscles, it's not a scratch. This type of wound is commonly caused by the horse rubbing against barbed wire, but not hard enough to cause serious cuts. They may also be caused by running through brush or dense trees. On rare occasions, they are due to mountain lion attack where the animal was not able to cling to the horse hard enough to cause deeper damage.

Shallow scratches are not a serious problem and require only minimal treatment. While they will usually heal without complications if not treated, it is a good idea to paint them with purple lotion to help prevent infection and to speed healing. Spray a light coating of insect repellent over the area to keep flies and other insects from bothering the animal. One treatment is usually sufficient, and these injuries can then be ignored so long as they do not become infected. The animal should still be treated for tetanus, as with any wound which breaks the skin.

PUNCTURE WOUNDS

Puncture wounds result from a variety of causes. The animal may run into a tree branch or fence rail and drive a splinter of wood deep into his body. Or, he may break a corral pole and have the jagged end go deep into his tissues. They also occur when an animal panics and tries to jump a fence or lunges when tied to a low post and gets his leg over it. Splinters may lodge well up into the armpit or groin area. The object may come out cleanly, leaving

only a small hole. Or, chunks may be left in the wound and prevent healing until they are removed. These wounds are sufficient cause to call your veterinarian.

Puncture wounds in the foot occur when the horse steps on a nail, a piece of wire, or something like a sharp piece of glass. These wounds may be so small as to nearly invisible upon casual inspection. (see Punctures, Hoof).

Pitchfork wounds are occasionally seen from a malicious assault on a horse. On the other hand, they may be seen where an owner defended himself against an unexpected attack by a vicious animal. Punctures also may be caused by horn gores or bites.

In the most severe cases, puncture wounds may invade joint cavities, tendon sheaths, or even the chest or abdominal cavity. Animals having even the smallest puncture into a joint cavity or tendon should be treated immediately by a veterinarian to prevent complications which may permanently cripple the horse. Injuries which penetrate the chest cavity, abdomen, or eye are equally urgent.

The small entry hole seals over quite easily or allows only minimal drainage of infected and dead material from

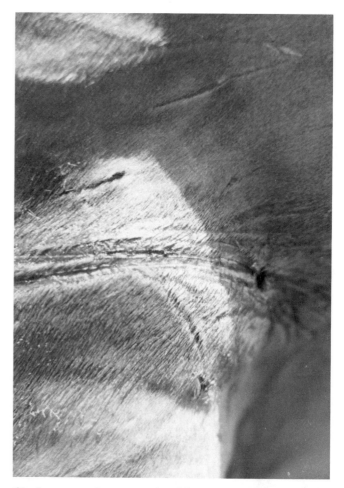

Shallow scratches on a shoulder—no stitches needed.

within. This tiny opening tends to keep air out of the wound, allowing bacteria to grow which prefer airless places—especially the types of bacteria which cause tetanus or other serious clostridial infections. Puncture wounds should always be treated as serious problems because of their tendency to become complicated by serious, life-threatening infections. In general, your veterinarian should be consulted for all but the simplest of punctures.

IMPORTANT NOTE: Antitetanus treatment is even more important with punctures than with the average wire cut or other wound. It should be among the first things you do for a horse with a puncture wound.

BULLET WOUNDS

Bullets cause a puncture-type of wound. A small entry hole from a gunshot wound may camouflage severe damage to the internal structures. An example of this is a horse who was shot in the rump by a stray bullet during hunting season. The entry hole was only about ¼-inch in diameter, but probing into it revealed shredded muscles and severe damage extending about 6 inches deep. The owners couldn't figure why the animal was severely lame and unwilling to move from such a small wound. The hidden damage was sufficient to make him more than just a little bit sore—and took about five weeks to heal!

If your veterinarian determines that the injury was caused by a gunshot, he will probably not remove the bullet unless it is obvious and convenient, or unless it is clearly causing problems because of its location. Don't think that there is something wrong with your veterinarian if he does not rush to take it out. That old line in the movies about "having to remove the bullet immediately" was true in the black powder days. Those bullets were large and slow. They caused large amounts of tissue damage and carried a lot of dirt, hair, and other debris into the wound.

Modern high-velocity bullets are more likely to cause damage because they shatter or mushroom as they hit, shredding and destroying large amounts of muscle and other tissue. They tend to carry in fewer contaminants and can be left in place. Pieces of lead which are left as shrapnel in the wound are unlikely to cause future problems, especially if they are located in a large muscle mass. The body will wall them off with fibrous tissue and they will be no further problem. Sometimes, but not often, fragments will work their way to the surface and be noticed as a hard lump just under the skin. This takes months or years to occur.

The real trouble with bullet wounds is caused by the tissue which is damaged or killed by the traveling slug. Damage can occur at a distance of several inches outward in all directions from the path of the bullet, creating a large tubular area of severely injured tissues and blood vessels. (63) Because the entry hole is small, there is no place for this material to go as it dies and is ready to be expelled from the body. Also, the closed, warm location and dead, often liquefied tissue provide ideal conditions for bacterial growth.

For this reason, it is EXTREMELY important that the wound be kept open. In the previous example of the horse shot in the rump, the small entry hole was enlarged by making an X-shaped incision about 1 inch on each side to help keep the hole open. Another problem in this case was that the large cavity inside was located below the level of the opening in the skin which kept the dying and dead material from draining out. The owners were instructed to swab out the cavity with long cotton swabs and strong (7%) tincture of iodine once a day. They were to remove any scab that formed and keep swabbing until the hole was completely healed from the inside. If pockets formed inside, the owners were to push gently through them so that the hole could be felt to get smaller day by day rather than to suddenly be closed.

The horse described above was placed on penicillin/streptomycin injections for a week. At the end of the week, we evaluated his condition and decided to switch him to procaine penicillin for another 5 to 6 days. The animal was also lightly exercised. The owner rode him two to three miles a day at a walk to prevent stiffness and to help loosen the infected material so that it could be swabbed out. The animal required treatment for well over a month, but made a full recovery.

TREATMENT

The seriousness of other punctures depends in large part on which structures are involved and how much damage has been done to them. Healing time may be very long when severe internal damage has been done.

Wounds which may have wood splinters or other foreign bodies in them should be immediately examined by your veterinarian. Probing around in these wounds looking for foreign bodies may cause damage to blood vessels, nerves, or other vital structures and should be left to him. This is also true when a metal object has penetrated the area which may have caused damage to the bone. Call your veterinarian and let him probe the wound, evaluate it, and advise you on treatment.

Large puncture wounds eventually heal, but will require diligent care for a long period of time—often as long as two or three months. The horse owner rarely sees the progress because it is slow, day-by-day, and hidden from view. It will, however, be obvious to your veterinarian as he checks on the animal every week or ten days (oftener if you have a problem and call him).

Deep or large puncture wounds are no fun to treat. Cotton swabs may not be long enough. You may need to buy a special pair of forceps called sponge forceps. You can then grasp a piece of gauze in them and use it to apply medication deep into the wound.

Do not use aerosol medication for these injuries.

They merely spray medication on the surface of the wound. If you physically swab it out, this helps to remove debris and infected material. In my experience, deep treatment results in faster healing with fewer complications (such as pockets of infection which are walled off and left behind to break open later) than does surface treatment with spray products. This is the reason for my recommendation that you swab out wounds. It allows you to both clean and treat them at the same time. Antibiotic solutions, such as crystalline penicillin or liquid nitrofurazone, may be used in place of iodine in some punctures with equally good results. Sulfa-urea solution is occasionally used to clean out a deep, dirty, puncture wound.

Small puncture wounds—say, those less than an inch deep—which do not involve any joints or vital structures (thus not causing any lameness) may be treated by the horseman. Begin by clipping the hair away from the opening. Electric clippers are good for this, or you may use a pair of scissors or a straight razor. Next, wash the area with soap and water, scrubbing the skin carefully. The object is to get the skin clean so that you will not carry dirt or hair into the wound. DON'T forget about tetanus protection for the horse.

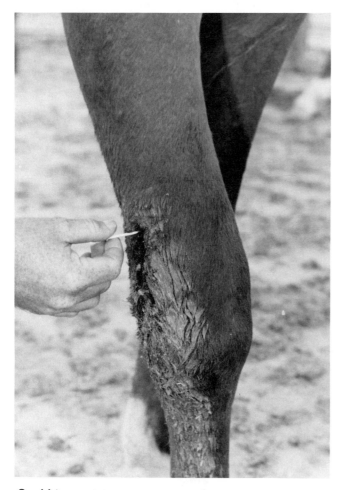

Swabbing out a puncture wound.

Next, saturate a cotton swab with strong (7%) tincture of iodine. Push it gently into the opening and feel around inside the wound. Here, you are trying to clean out any loose debris or infection which may be present. Do not worry about pushing too hard—you are not going to hurt normal areas with moderate pressure. Horses are put together better than that! It may be necessary to twitch the animal or grab a fold of skin above the wound (see Shoulder Roll) in order to take the animal's mind off the pain.

Repeat this treatment daily, removing any scab that forms before you insert the swab. You are using the iodine for two reasons: because it is very effective in killing bacteria or other infectious agents which may establish themselves in the wound; and because it helps scar tissue to form. Scar tissue formation is the method by which the animal heals the wound. Punctures into fleshy areas, such as large muscle masses, or the armpit or groin areas, may also be swabbed with scarlet oil instead of iodine. This acts the same as iodine to prevent infection and help the area to fill with scar tissue.

Puncture wounds in the fleshy parts of the body—especially above the hock or knee, may cause the leg to become enormously swollen with fluid (called edema). This occasionally occurs with wounds in the foot or lower leg. It is due to disturbed blood circulation in the area and also because the animal is not using his leg, thus allowing excess fluid to accumulate in the limb. Edema is easily diagnosed by pushing a finger or thumb firmly into the tissue. Hold it there for five to ten seconds, and then remove it. The imprint of your finger will remain in the tissue for a few minutes. It will be obvious when you feel back over the area with your fingers, and may be visible, too.

A leg with edema can be soaked in a solution of epsom salts (magnesium sulfate) in warm water. Or, it can be wrapped in a gentle elastic bandage to help "wring" the fluid out of it, forcing it back into the blood stream. Be very careful not to get the bandage too tight or you might create more problems than you repair. A bandage for this purpose MUST go clear down to the hoof to avoid swelling below it. The leg can also be wrapped with bandages over a poultice, such as Gelocast. Place a dressing over the wound itself so that the poultice material does not get into it. This poultice will help to remove some of the accumulated fluids. If the original wound is not too serious, it may be possible to exercise the animal which will help to remove some of the edema.

Systemic antibiotic treatment is necessary with any puncture and doubly important when edema is involved. Penicillin or penicillin/streptomycin combination are the drugs most commonly used.

If the puncture is low on the leg or foot, your veterinarian may put a cast or splint on it, or have it wrapped in a heavy, immobilizing bandage to reduce movement and help it to heal.

A horse who has a chronic, draining sinus tract (a nonhealing puncture wound) which does not heal should be checked for the possibility of a foreign object, such as a bone chip or piece of wood, remaining in a puncture wound. These may occur with no apparent previous injury when the horse is out on pasture or the owner was on vacation when the original problem occured. The hole seals over before being noticed.

CUTS

The majority of severe wounds that veterinarians repair are cuts. These occur when horses go through or rub against barbed wire fences. They also occur from cuts on scrap metal and other junk, from trailer accidents, and from falls through cattle guards. Horses occasionally cut themselves on rocks or tear their skin on tree limbs. They think of ways that the horse owner cannot. As one of my clients said of her show horses, "I could raise them in padded stalls and they would find ways to hang themselves."

Walk your pastures, look critically at your corrals, and closely examine your barns and stalls. Try to find anything and everything your horse can step on, rub against, get tangled in, or caught on. Trying to prevent punctures and cuts is better medicine than having to treat the subsequent wounds.

Cuts heal in two ways. If they are clean (uncontaminated), fresh, and small enough or unshredded enough to be readily sutured, they usually heal with relative ease. On the other hand, if the wound is old and contaminated or already infected when you find it or has a lot of tissue missing, healing will probably be by granulation. Sometimes there is a combination of the two types. We often suture a very large wound that is already contaminated, knowing that it is likely to break open, at least in part. The thinking is that whatever we are able to repair by sewing the edges together will be that much less that has to heal by granulation.

And what is granulation? Granulation tissue is the name for the new scar tissue formed by the body to heal a defect. It is made up of new cells which come from the undamaged edges of the wound and migrate in to help fill the void. Other cells grow upward from the depths of the wound. Together, they produce fibers which help knit the defect together. There are plenty of blood vessels in this new tissue, and almost no nerves—at least in the early stages of healing. Granulation is the only way that defects in the body heal. When there is too much granulation tissue, we call the resulting bulge "proud flesh." It's all a matter of degree.

As granulation tissue heals the defect, cells from the skin edge form a new skin surface. When a wound heals without the skin edges being sutured together, this cellular migration is the only way that new skin can form over the defect. Skin cannot grow down into a hollow or up over a hump of granulation tissue. The skin can only grow over a level surface. So, the object of the game when healing reaches this stage is to keep the surface of the granulation tissue level so that the skin may grow out over it and finish healing the defect. We often use fairly strong medications to "dissolve" excess granulation tissue. When using any of these drugs, it is extremely important to protect the skin edges so that delicate cells are not damaged or slowed in their growth. Failure to do this may significantly retard the healing process.

If the defect is small, the new skin may have hair on it. If it is large, the skin in the middle of the wound may be thin and fragile. It can break open if the animal moves the newly healed area (such as the skin over a joint) before it has had time to toughen and become strong. That is why we often advise limited exercise with a wound that appears to be healed. This is especially true of cuts on the back of the feet or the front of the knee or hock.

TO SEW OR NOT TO SEW?

So you've just found your horse with a cut. What do you do now? The first question is whether the cut is fresh or not. A fresh cut will often be bleeding when found. If deeper tissues are exposed, they will be fresh and healthy-looking. They are often light pink or red, depending on whether muscles or the tissues under the skin are showing. If you touch them gently, they will be soft and flexible rather than hard and crusty or stiff. There is no unpleasant odor to a fresh cut.

A cut that has happened 12 hours or more ago will often be dark red or black on the surface. It may have a hard, dry crust. Dirt, leaves, and other material may be embedded in it. If several days have passed since it happened, there may be pus in and around it. At this point, the odor is often quite strong and unpleasant.

Let's begin with discussing treatment of a fresh cut—say, one that is less than six hours old. The first decision to make is whether or not to call a veterinarian. If you can get treatment for it within approximately six hours after it happens, there is a good chance of clean, relatively rapid healing. Any cut which CAN be sutured SHOULD be sutured to give more rapid healing and less scarring. This is especially true of cuts on the lower leg (below the knee or hock). A dozen or so stitches in this area may save two to three months of daily treatment and healing time.

In addition to better healing, there are often some clear-cut economic advantages to suturing a fresh cut. Bandaging the wound and treating it with ointment may look like the "cheap" way in the short haul—until you add up the cost of medication and bandaging material for the duration of healing. In most cases, you could have paid for the suturing job, and NOT have spent the extra time healing it—and also obtained better results at the same time. If you figure the cost of the time you have used in treating the horse, you come out even farther ahead.

Keep the wound clean, and DO NOT put ANYTHING in it unless specifically instructed to do so by your veterinarian. That goes even for washing it out or attempting to clean it (other than picking out obvious sticks, leaves, or large debris). My own preference is to just have the owner keep the wound clean until I arrive and can determine if there is any chance at all that it can be sutured.

It is helpful to discuss first-aid for wounds with your veterinarian before you need him so that you can handle any cuts your horse has according to his guidelines. Putting ointments, creams, fly sprays, or other substances into the wound can result in your veterinarian being unable to suture it, or in its breaking open if he does suture it. One horse owner called me for a sheet metal cut on the side of her horse's foot. She called me promptly after the accident occurred, and I got there within an hour, ready to suture the wound. To my chagrin, I found that her neighbor had "helped" her by putting lime (can you imagine!) into the wound. There was no sense even attempting to suture the cut—the caustic had burned the tissue enough that the stitches would only have pulled out and the surface would slough anyway. We ended up healing this fresh wound as if it were an old one—open, with daily bandage changes. To the owner's credit, her diligent daily treatment healed the problem in about eight weeks. The sad thing was that it would have healed in perhaps three to four weeks if we had been able to suture it as we had planned.

Place something clean over the wound and try to keep it clean until your veterinarian arrives. Sterile gauze sponges are good, if you have them. If not, a clean paper towel or piece of clean rag (such as a piece of old bedsheet) is the next best choice. Place this directly on the wound, if it is on the lower leg. Then, wrap over it with tape, gauze, Vetrap, or more strips of clean fabric if that is all that you have. You are trying to keep the horse from getting dirt and manure into the cut until the veterinarian arrives.

Once you have protected the wound, go call your veterinarian. Make arrangements for him to visit the horse, or for you to trailer the horse to him (if the horse will load into a trailer reasonably well and is not so badly injured that he cannot step into it). If the horse is severely injured, try to tell the veterinarian as much as possible about the extent of his injuries so that you and he can make a decision together as to whether it would be best to have him come to the animal, or whether the animal should be trailered to him.

What do you do while waiting for the vet to arrive? Keep the animal calm. Keep other animals away from him so that they do not chew or push on him. This goes for curious cows, as well as other horses, and for dogs or children who may worry the injured horse. Keep the bandage in place if at all possible. Do not remove it to change it if it becomes soaked with blood. The blood may soak through, but the constant pressure will help the bleeding to stop underneath. It does not matter that the bandage is bloodsoaked when the vet arrives. Keep the animal standing if possible. Do not deliberately move him around, but keep him calm and quiet. Keeping him still also helps keep a leg wound cleaner.

Most veterinarians would appreciate having a bucket of clean, warm water when they arrive, especially if you are in cold country. You should have a bucket available for this purpose. It need not be fancy: a pickle bucket from the local hamburger joint will cost fifty cents to a dollar at the most (if they don't just give them away). Washed and kept clean for this purpose, it will be greatly appreciated by most veterinarians.

How do you decide which cuts need to be sutured and which do not? Fresh cuts that are more than an inch long are almost always worth a try at suturing. Even if it appears that there is a large gaping hole with flesh or skin missing, sometimes your veterinarian can still repair it. Sutured cuts may still break open and have to be healed as if they were old wounds when discovered. But, it's usually worth trying. There is nothing to lose (except money) by suturing the cut, and much to gain if it works. If it does not work, even a half-healed cut will fill in more rapidly than one which is gaping open.

Older cuts may occasionally be successfully sutured if you are willing to go to the expense of trying. One of my clients had a mare who cut herself above the eye, about 2 inches long and an inch deep. It was gaping open about ¾ inch, and had occurred several days earlier. It was explained to the owner that we could heal it as an open wound, but that we might gain a lot by trying to suture it. A thin layer of tissue was carefully cut from the entire inside surface of the wound. Then, a thin strip was trimmed from each of the skin edges and they were sutured together. When the horse was examined several weeks later, the hole had healed completely, without breaking open and without scarring. How well this after-the-fact treatment works depends on how large the cut is, and how much damage has been done inside it. A clean slice will be much easier to repair as an old injury than will one that is shredded, with muscle tags and pockets everywhere. One that has a good, clean, granulating surface will be more likely to heal than one which is infected and covered with pus.

TREATING FRESH CUTS

How does your veterinarian go about treating the wire cut or similar injury? He will usually begin by cleaning the wound. Most veterinarians prefer to remove all hair around the edges, either with electric clippers, scissors, or a straight razor, for a distance of about half an inch. Removing the hair makes the area easier to clean and prevents hair from being trapped in the suture line. It also keeps it from holding any pus or drainage that may come from the wound during the healing process. In addition, if he wishes to have you put any medication on the suture line, it will not make a mess in the remaining hair. Removing the hair also makes the sutures easier to find when it is time to remove them. Hair which is left around the edges of a wound may also cause enough irritation to result in the formation of excessive amounts of granulation tissue. This proud flesh retards wound healing and may make the problem much worse than it would otherwise have been.

After clipping or shaving around the wound, most veterinarians wash the wound using saline solution with an extremely mild disinfectant (such as a "tamed" iodine). Your veterinarian may also use a gentle soap. There is little effort made to "kill" infection if the wound is to be sutured because any disinfectant which would kill bacteria would also cause tissue damage. The subsequent liquefaction of this dead tissue would then cause the wound to break open. Better to treat infection with injections of antibiotics from within, via the bloodstream. But, more about that later.

The veterinarian will control any bleeding which is occurring, either by tying off the vessels with a special, absorbable suture (usually catgut) or by twisting them off with a fine pair of forceps (called hemostats).

The next procedure is usually to anesthetize the wound edges. This is also called "blocking," as in "blocking the pain." A local anesthetic (one which acts in the area where it is used rather than on the animal's brain) is injected under the skin edges to deaden the area so that it can be sewed without hurting the horse. This is similar to the "novocaine" your dentist uses when he fills or pulls a tooth. Before he blocks the animal, however, the vet may give a tranquilizer or other sedative if the animal is not cooperative (or is not likely to stay that way). Or, he may tie up a leg or otherwise restrain the horse so that he (and you) are not injured by the animal. He may use a twitch to take the animal's mind off the needles being stuck under the wound edges. A twitch may be used by itself (if the

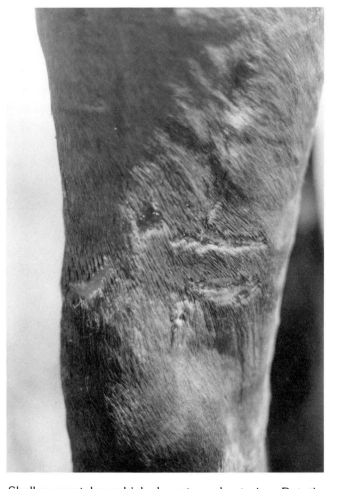

Shallow scratches which do not need suturing. But, the small, gaping cut at the left of the photo should be sutured. Either a purple lotion product or an aerosol nitrofurazone spray is good for the scratches.

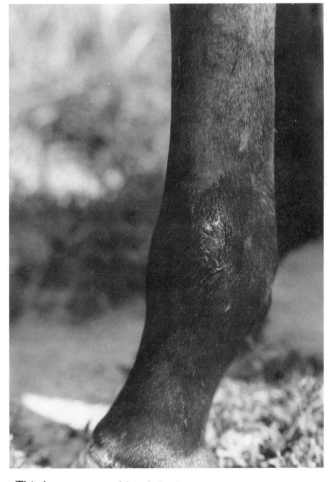

This horse scraped his fetlock in a horse trailer. There is not enough skin left to suture. This wound should be kept under a pressure wrap with nitrofurazone dressing until healed.

animal is likely to allow blocking with it), or in addition to a tranquilizer or other sedative.

After blocking, the veterinarian will then proceed to trim out any pieces of tissue which are dead or unlikely to live. This includes dangling bits of muscle and shredded pieces of tendons, nerves, or blood vessels. Pieces of skin which have been left without blood supply will also be removed if they are extremely narrow and long. If they are more triangular, such as a V-shaped wound with the small point facing upward, he may go ahead and suture the cut, with the knowledge that the decreased blood supply will perhaps cause part or all the flap to die. In the interim, it acts as an attached skin-bandage for the granulation tissue underneath, and that is, in itself, a valuable function. Antibiotics, such as penicillin/streptomycin or nitrofurazone, may be placed in the wound to help prevent (or control) infection.

If the wound is several hours old or if the skin edges have dried because of wind or severe cold or heat, he will probably "freshen" the edges. This means that he will trim a thin strip of skin from each side of the cut. This provides fresh, clean edges with a good blood supply which can be sutured together with a better chance of healing than if they were not treated in this manner. He may also snip a very thin layer of tissue from the surface of the muscles and/or the backside of the skin. This is very often done when the animal has gotten a lot of dirt, hay, or other debris into the wound. Or it may be done if the surface has begun to dry. This is done for the same reason as trimming the skin edges—to provide a fresh, new surface ready to attach itself to the corresponding surface on the other side of the wound.

If there is damage to the underlying muscles which leaves them gaping apart, your veterinarian may stitch them together with heavy, absorbable suture called "gut." This is short for "catgut," a suture which is made not from

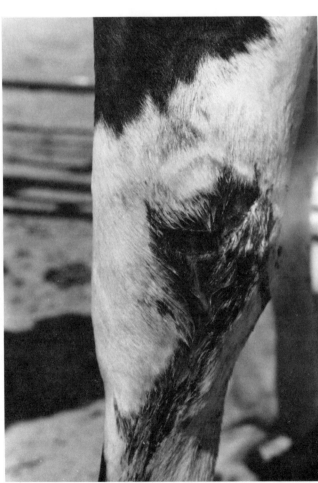

This fresh, deep cut on the outside of the horse's knee should definitely be sutured.

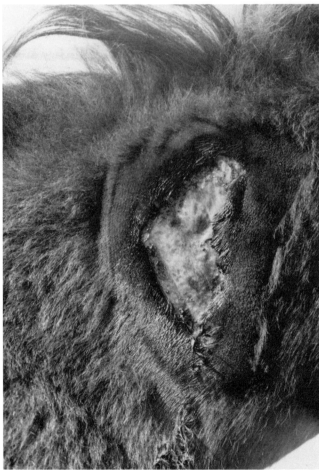

This gaping wire cut on a yearling's neck was discovered the day after it occurred. It was too old and infected to be sutured. The edges were clipped and it was swabbed daily with scarlet oil. The wound healed with only a small, wrinkled scar, completely covered with hair. Don't give up on one of these!

cats, but from thin strips of sheep intestine. There are also synthetic suture materials available that are absorbable. What he is doing is trying to place the muscles together in relation to each other so that they will grow together as they were previously. He is also closing up what we call "dead space." If a hollow is left deep in a wound, the body will fill it with blood and serum. These pockets of fluid have a much greater chance of becoming infected than does normal tissue. Because muscle tissue is very fragile (ever try to sew a steak?) and has little holding power, the stitches must be large and far back from the cut surface of the muscle. These sutures are meant to dissolve within a week or two after healing is well underway.

If nonabsorbable sutures are buried, they are often poorly tolerated by the body, and will eventually form an abscess (called a "stitch abscess"), or will work their way to the surface of the skin and out—usually after a long period of irritation. For this reason, sutures, such as nylon and its various relatives and stainless steel, are buried deep in the body, but ONLY under special circumstances.

Finally, your veterinarian will sew the skin together, using one of the NONABSORBABLE sutures just mentioned, such as stainless steel, nylon, or other synthetic material. The type of suture pattern that he uses depends on personal preference and the location of the cut on the animal's body. There are several suture patterns which are stronger than others for special applications. Most of the time, veterinarians fall into the habit of using one or two favorite patterns.

The stitches will usually be placed well back from the skin edges to allow them a bigger "bite," thus giving greater holding power and more resistance to tearing out through the skin. In general, the bigger the cut, the farther back from the edges we put the stitches, to give more support.

With very large cuts, several large stitches, called

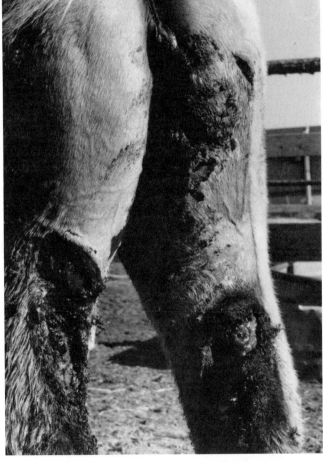

This filly was savagely attacked by dogs, and had bites all over her body. Discovered about eight hours later, the wounds were fly blown and infected. The one to the right of the vulva was about four inches deep. The edges were clipped and the wounds were cleansed with a tamed iodine solution, then swabbed daily with scarlet oil.

This is the same filly a month later. She is nearly healed and has very little scarring. The wounds are becoming covered with hair. She is functionally normal, despite the fact that several major tendons in the hock area had been completely exposed. Careful daily treatment can heal many seemingly incurable injuries.

"stay" sutures, may be placed far back from the edge of the wound—often an inch or more from the cut edge. The purpose of these stitches is to give added support and help hold the tissues together. These stitches may be anchored over buttons, chunks of leather, or pieces of rubber tubing to spread the tension over an even greater area and help keep the stitches from pulling through. The more pressure there is on the stitches along the line of the cut itself, the more chance there is of them tearing out and leaving the wound gaping open. The stay sutures help to avoid this.

It is important to adequately immobilize the injured area to allow healing. If the cut edge is pulled every time the animal takes a step (as it will be in areas like the back of the pastern and the front of the knee), it will tend to tear open. Often, splints or casts are used to immobilize the leg. These must not interfere with circulation in the area.

The general health of the patient affects the rate of tissue repair. Animals with tumors, infections, or other diseases heal more slowly than normal animals. Deficiencies of protein and vitamins retard tissue repair. Sutures should be left in longer in old horses and those who are in poor health.

If the wound is going to have an obvious pocket of infection, your veterinarian may put in a rubber drain tube which will allow any discharges to drain out of the area. Or, he may suture the upper part of the area and leave an opening toward the bottom for drainage. Some very large wounds with severe tissue damage may need to be flushed with a mild antiseptic or antibiotic solution daily until they heal. Or, they may be swabbed with scarlet oil or strong tincture of iodine.

Wounds which are partially healed but have a large granulating surface (especially those that occur in an area which cannot easily be covered with a pressure bandage) may require additional protection to heal well. In these cases, skin grafts or a specially prepared pigskin may be used to cover the area. These coverings help to relieve pain and speed healing. These are often used with large cuts on the front of the hock.

Now that he is finished stitching, the veterinarian may put a wound dressing on the suture line. It is not strictly necessary, so don't criticize him if he doesn't use it. My favorite for this is powdered, aerosol nitrofurazone (an antibiotic). Topazone powder (Norden, Lincoln, NE 68501) is one of the best known of these products; it is also available under other brand names. Use a light dusting, please—not a thick, yellow crust of it. This product is not water-soluble. This means that it will not draw fluid out of the suture line and make a weeping, moist mess over the stitches. It also will help to keep the stitch line dry for a few hours, which can help to prevent infection from getting in through the sutures until the skin has a bit of time to seal.

If it is fly season, shield the suture line with a piece of paper or your hand and spray the areas above and below the cut (or to the sides of it, as the case may be) with insect repellent. This will help keep insects from settling on the wound and bringing infection. It will also keep them from annoying the animal. You can also use a wipe-on insect repellent. Do NOT get it directly on the incision, but wipe it within a quarter inch of each side of the cut. If you are in a screwworm area, ask your veterinarian for a product to spray directly on the wound to help prevent the possibility of screwworm infestation.

Wounds on the rear of the fetlock and pastern areas, as well as in the coronary band area, may have a cast placed over the sutured area. This keeps the wounded area from moving. Movement is perhaps the most common cause of wounds breaking open. The cast or splint helps prevent it. A plaster or fiberglass cast may be used. A window may be cut in the cast for treatment of the injured area, or the whole cast may be removed in one to two weeks to check the wound. It may then be reapplied for a further period if necessary. Wounds in the coronary band which are not adequately immobilized may have each edge of the area heal separately. They will then stay that way indefinitely rather than healing together across the wound. For this reason, casts are commonly used when the coronary band is cut.

If a cut has penetrated a joint capsule (or if you even THINK it may be into a joint or tendon sheath), it is VERY important that you consult your veterinarian. He can recommend treatment which may save the animal for further use. Delaying treatment may result in infection in the joint, with subsequent loss of the use of that joint (which may result in loss of the use of the horse).

While he's handy, ask your veterinarian about aftercare. We usually have the owner remove stitches from the wound in 10 days to two weeks, depending on the nature of the injury. Ask your veterinarian when he wants them to be removed. He may have a reason for wanting them taken out sooner than usual—or left in longer. It helps if you have watched how he put them in and which pattern he used so you can have an idea of how to remove them. If you are not sure, ask him where they should be cut.

The most common suture used is called a simple interrupted pattern. This is simply a loop in one side of the cut (from the top down) and out the other (from the bottom up). It is then tied with an overhand knot (or several of them, depending on the suture). Several knots in each stitch are used to keep it from coming untied, either because of pressure from the stiffness of the suture material, or because the animal is chewing or licking the stitch line.

Stitches are removed by pulling up on one side of the loose end, and then cutting close to the knot on one side or the other. Do NOT cut the knot away from the loop underneath by cutting both sides of the stitch under the knot. This would result in a loop of suture being left under the animal's skin. The skin may grow together over it, which would then form an abscess and work out later.

You can use stitch scissors which have a small notch near the end of the blade, with a small, thin end that slips easily under the stitch. Or, you can use manicure scissors. It may be necessary to twitch the animal before removing the stitches. Try to take one or two out first to see if you can do the procedure without having to twitch the horse. If necessary, it is more kind to twitch the animal or grab a roll of his skin to take his mind off the area than it is to fight him to get the job done.

Other aftercare questions may include whether the animal should have exercise or rest and whether the area should be bandaged or unbandaged. If it is to be bandaged, ask if the bandage should be elastic to put on a gentle pressure, or if it is only to be a covering to keep the area clean. In general, we use elastic bandages (also called pressure bandages) on cuts on the leg and foot to help control the growth of proud flesh.

Upper leg and body or neck cuts are often left uncovered. This is done because they are nearly impossible to bandage, and also because they seem to heal well without pressure. Proud flesh is much more likely to form on the lower legs than on the body or neck.

How often does the bandage need to be changed? Most are changed every day or every two days. They should also be changed when they become wet or soiled. Otherwise, spoilage and severe infection may occur under the damp bandage. If it is rainy or snowy, or if the corral is wet and the horse tends to lie down, it is worth confining him to a clean, dry stall if he must be bandaged.

Find out if your veterinarian wants you to put any medication on the stitch line. Also, determine whether the animal is to have any antibiotic treatment. My own preference is for a minimum of three days of penicillin/streptomycin combination injections for most horses with fresh injuries (see Antibiotics). When the cut is infected, or when there has been severe shredding of the muscles, your veterinarian may wish to treat the animal for as long as five days to two weeks. Follow his recommendation. If there is any question about the amount or kind of treatment, ask him! In my opinion, there are no stupid questions unless they go unasked and you never learn the answer.

COMPLICATIONS IN SUTURED WOUNDS

After you have seen a few injuries and watched them heal, whether on your own animal or a neighbor's, you will have a better idea of how normal wound healing should appear. Healing is different in sutured wounds than in wounds which are left open. Let's begin with wounds which have been sutured.

Swelling often occurs in sutured wounds because the drainage of small blood vessels and lymphatic channels has been disturbed. If the sutured cut is in the lower leg, it is often best to keep it bandaged for at least the first five or six days to help prevent fluid accumulation. The bandage helps keep the wound from literally popping open from the pressure of the swelling, which may occur if bandaging is not done. The leg should be snugly bandaged all the way down to the hoof even if the injury has occurred higher in the leg, to prevent it from swelling below the bandage.

If infection occurs, the area under the stitch line may swell and become hot and tight. The edges of the sutured area may become purplish or reddened. If you leave the stitches as they are, chances are good that the pressure will kill much of the skin edge due to tension on the sutures. This skin will die and slough, and you end up dealing with the whole thing as an open wound.

When you see this infection beginning to occur, it is far better to remove two or three stitches. If the wound is vertical, pull them out of the lower end of the cut. This will allow pus and infected material to drain from the wound. It will also allow you to swab the wound out and keep it clean. If the wound is more horizontal, remove two or three stitches from the lower end, if there is one; if not, take them out at the point where the swelling is most prominent.

If, when you remove the stitches, there is no drainage, take the tip of a small pair of forceps or other blunt object and push it gently into the area of the cut line where you have removed the stitches, moving it back and forth to find a weakened area. There is nearly always a weak spot somewhere along the line where an opening can easily be made. If the swelling is very tight, be sure to stand to one side—the pressure within will often cause pus and fluid to shoot quite some distance from the opening. After you have established drainage, swab out the cavity under the suture line with scarlet oil. Use cotton swabs or a pair of forceps of a length appropriate to the depth of the cavity. This will need to be done once daily until the wound is healed. This whole procedure is similar to handling a puncture wound.

Do not be afraid to push moderately hard on the swabs—you will not undo anything that is already healed. If a scab forms, it is important that you pick it off and then resume swabbing as you have been. Otherwise, the debris and pus that is trapped inside the wound will provide a fertile breeding ground for bacterial growth. The pocket will then fill with pus and you will get to go through the cycle all over again. Diligent daily treatment will heal the hole much more rapidly than trying to "be nice" to the animal and letting it scab over. If the wound totally opens up, it should be treated as an open wound.

SKIN GRAFTS

Skin grafts are often useful for covering large, nonhealing wounds. They are occasionally used within three or four days after the injury has occurred. More commonly, they are used after a bed of granulation tissue has formed. They are often used in areas, such as the front of the hock, where large, hairless scars will be harmful to the animal's movement, and where healing is otherwise prolonged. Nearly 90% of grafts will "take" and cover the wound. They usually become covered with hair, thus also giving a cosmetically suitable result. Splints or casts may be used in conjunction with the graft to keep the injured area from moving and allow it to heal.

TREATMENT OF OPEN WOUNDS

We have already covered the treatment of scratches and small abrasions. Often larger wounds must be treated as what we call "open wounds," either because they are too large and jagged to be sutured, or because too large a piece of tissue is missing to be able to suture the area. Wounds which are more than six to eight hours old when they are discovered are also usually treated as open wounds. "Open" is in contrast to "closed" where the skin is sutured to completely cover the wound. Some wounds may be partially sutured but will be handled as open wounds since the skin doesn't completely cover the underlying tissues.

The edges of these wounds should be shaved or clipped as with wounds which are going to be sutured. They should also be cleaned in the same manner.

Open wounds in large, fleshy areas, such as the forearm and thigh as well on the heavily muscled parts of the body, should be treated with scarlet oil (or another product as recommended by your veterinarian). The wound should be wiped daily with gauze sponges or other clean material to remove pus and debris which is on the surface. If there are scabs around the edges or on the surface of the wound, they should be removed. Otherwise, you are only treating the scabs. If the scabs are hard and dried, do not damage the tissue by removing them. Merely cover the area with your scarlet oil, or apply nitrofurazone dressing or other similar, softening product. Let it work until the following day, when the scabs should be softened enough to remove. Then remove them and continue treating as before.

Wounds below the knee and hock do not heal well when treated with scarlet oil (it is best used on the fleshy or muscular areas). For these, you must first decide whether you are going to bandage or not. They will usually heal faster and with less proud flesh if they are bandaged. Use nitrofurazone ointment under the bandage. Keep moderate pressure on the area with elastic tape or other similar dressing. This helps to keep the skin edges together and prevent the growth of proud flesh.

Lower leg wounds which are so small or shallow as to not need to be bandaged should be treated with a drying medication which retards the formation of granulation tissue. One of the purple lotions is ideal.

COMPLICATIONS IN OPEN WOUNDS

Here we will discuss complications that may occur with wounds which are being treated as open wounds from the start. This will also include wounds which have been sutured and have broken open or have been opened because of infection within.

Foreign objects left in a wound may keep them from healing. There are times when you have treated a wound for what seems like forever, and it still hasn't healed. You are able to swab into it as deeply as you could when you started. First, determine how long you really have been treating it. It seems like forever when you have to go out and treat the animal every day. It's not a bad idea to jot down on your calendar when the wound occurs so you will know how long you really have been at it. If it has been two weeks or more without noticeable improvement, consult your veterinarian. He will need to look at the wound to determine what should be done next.

Here is an example of a wound which contained a foreign body. One of my clients swabbed a wound under her horse's jaw for nearly a month. Not only was it not getting better, it was developing some heavy, hard scar tissue around the opening. My examination found an animal with a hole going up into the muscles between the lower jaw bones at the base of the tongue. My first move was to take a small pair of forceps and probe into the hole to see how deep it was. There was a grating sensation on the end of the forceps. I began grasping with them and soon pulled a rusty scrap of baling wire about three inches long from the hole. Another couple of weeks of swabbing with iodine healed the animal completely. This draining tract would have been a continuing problem had not the foreign body been removed.

Another example is a horse who crashed into a corral pole and shattered it while being chased by another horse. The mare had a wound deep into her left shoulder. The owner called me to examine the wound several days after it had occurred. My probing removed half a handful of large fragments of wood. The animal was sent home with instructions for the owner to swab it out with iodine daily. The client was warned that there was a possibility that there were still some fragments left in the wound, but since I wasn't sure, I did not want to carve up the horse's shoulder at this point just on that chance. She was told that if it did not heal within a reasonable length of time, we might have to recheck it. About two and a half weeks later she called, saying that it had reached a certain point in healing and then stopped making progress. We anesthetized the animal. With the mare lying down, the wound was reexamined, probing some 5 to 6 inches into it. Another half-dozen small fragments of wood were pulled from the hole. Sent home again, the animal made an uneventful recovery.

Another type of foreign body which may be in a wound is the bone chip. These may occur over bony areas, such as the face or hip bone. They may also happen when the horse hits his cannon bone, as with a jumper hitting a solid jump, or a horse crashing into a steel edge while being loaded into a horse trailer. They should be suspected whenever a wound does not heal and shows a chronic, draining tract or opening. Surgical removal is the only cure for bone chips.

Infection may occur in wounds. It shows up as pus draining from a puncture wound or from a sutured wound which has broken open or been deliberately opened for drainage. On an open-surfaced wound, it looks like a thin greenish or yellowish coating across the surface, and often has a foul odor. Clean it carefully from the wound, using gauze or paper towels. If the wound is sutured, it may be necessary to remove a few sutures in order to establish adequate drainage and allow the pus which has formed in the area to drain out. After drainage has been established, the lesion will be treated as an open wound by swabbing it out daily with scarlet oil or strong tincture of iodine.

If you have given the animal an initial course of penicillin/streptomycin at the time the wound occurred it is unnecessary to restart it just because the surface of the wound is infected. The surface of granulation tissue is almost as effectively sealed off from the rest of the body as if it were on another animal. Merely cleaning and treating the surface of the wound is quite sufficient.

However, cleaning the wound before putting on medication IS of paramount importance. If you do not remove the pus, scabs, or other debris as carefully as possible before putting on medication, you are not treating the wound. You are merely treating the scabs or pus. Neither of these items get well, whereas the wound will heal if you get the medication down to its surface.

Cellulitis and gangrene are two serious complications which are occasionally seen. In these infections, the bacteria do not stay on the surface of the wound, but invade deep into the tissues underneath. The area will be hot, painful, and often swollen. It may show a reddish or purplish discoloration. The animal shows signs of feeling ill: fever, depression, and loss of appetite. Discharge from the wound may become thin and tinged with a little blood. The animal should be started on penicillin/streptomycin combination immediately, at a dosage which is adequate for the size of the animal.

If the animal does not show improvement within 24 hours, or gets worse, consult your veterinarian immediately. Treat with the pen/strep for a minimum of three days, and as long as 5 to 7 days or more if needed. Be sure not to stop until the animal is back to normal, and has remained that way (normal temperature, less pain, swelling gone, color of wound area back to normal) for at least 48 hours. This is a case where it is imperative to give sufficient antibiotics for a long enough time to kill off the organisms which are invading the tissues. If you stop too soon, the infection may come back with a vengeance, and

may then contain bacteria which are resistant to the antibiotic. The result of inadequate treatment when a drug-resistant organism invades the body may be a dead horse.

Gas may form in the tissues in cases of gangrene or cellulitis because it is produced by bacteria which have invaded the wound. Or, it may occur because the animal pumps air into the tissues as he moves. This is frequently seen with punctures in the armpit area. If the gas is due to bacterial infection, it is a very unfavorable sign and your veterinarian should be consulted at once. This is especially important if the animal is running a temperature, is depressed, or otherwise doesn't look well, or is becoming noticeably worse. If the air is physically being pumped into the area, it will eventually be taken up by the body if infection does not occur. Confine the animal as much as possible to limit the amount of air that is pumped into the tissues by movement. If enough gas is taken in or produced, it may separate the skin from the underlying tissues and cause it to die. This is a very unfavorable development.

Continuing damage is often done to the wound by a horse who either chews at it or rubs it in an attempt to relieve itching. If at all possible, a wound should be immobilized to aid healing. Cuts in the lower leg are often covered with casts or other solid bandages to prevent the animal from injuring them as well as to prevent flexing which retards healing.

Dead tissue in or around the wound occurs when areas are left without adequate circulation. It is common in triangular tears or cuts, the tips of which point upward. The blood supply to the tip of the flap is severed and the area dries up and dies. The dead area should be removed. It will be dry and hard, without nerve supply, and can be cut off with a sharp knife or scissors. Begin by whittling off a small portion and remove more if needed. It's easy to take more off and impossible to add it back if you take too much! It may be necessary to twitch the animal before working on the area. This is not because the animal can feel you cutting on the area—he usually can't. But, he may object to pulling or pressure on the normal tissues to which the dead area is attached. The twitch helps to take his mind off this feeling.

Muscles which are left hanging in an open wound often die and slough. They often liquefy and become part of the drainage which oozes from the wound. If they do not slough, it may be necessary to cut the hard, dried portion free.

Dirty bandages are another source of dead tissue in the area of a wound. Wet, filthy bandages are an ideal place for bacteria to grow, causing infection in the wound and retarding healing. Most bandages should be changed at least every three days; they may have to be changed more frequently if the wound is fresh and there is still some bleeding, or if it is infected and draining badly. Clean bandages should be used to avoid contamination of the tissues with more bacteria than are already present. Antibiotic dressings or mild antiseptics are often used to prevent infection, especially when the wound is bandaged.

Inadequate drainage may cause complications and severely retard wound healing. If the dead and dying tissue materials cannot get out of the lesion, they form an ideal medium for bacterial growth. This will result in serious infection. Extremely large wounds should be examined by a veterinarian. He may wish to install a special rubber drain tube in the area.

Insect infestation of wounds may occur in the warm months. Wounds which are not properly treated easily become "fly blown." This term refers to the presence of flies and their larvae in and around the wound. Flies can lay great masses of eggs in an open wound. These appear as small yellowish or whitish granules. So many may be present as to amount to a mass several inches in diameter. These hatch into larvae which feed on the dead tissue and infected material within the wound. At this point, wriggling larvae may be seen crawling on the surface (and often deep into crevices) of a wound. These eat only the dead material.

Fly larvae can be controlled by several methods. If only a few are present, careful removal with a cotton swab or forceps may be followed by treatment with a wound dressing, such as scarlet oil. This will keep the flies from laying eggs in the area and solves the problem. In some cases, it may be necessary to spray the area with an insecticide specifically made for use in open wounds. Small cuts may be coated with a wound dressing containing an insecticide.

Do NOT apply ANY wound dressing or insecticide if you think there is a possibility that the wound will be sutured. Cover it to keep the flies out. You can also apply insecticide AROUND but not IN the wound itself. Keep it a half inch or so back from the edges to avoid contamination. In some cases, when the wound is not to be sutured, or if screwworms are present in the area, it may be necessary to use insecticides directly ON the wound itself. Use a product recommended by your veterinarian.

The fly problem is worse in some of the southern and southwestern states where screwworms are present. These flies lay eggs which hatch into larvae who eat living tissues. Thus, a small scrape or cut may become a large, open, festering, life-threatening sore. In these states, proper treatment of wounds is essential to prevent severe damage or even death of the affected animal. Use a wound medication which is recommended for screwworm control. Daily application must be religiously followed to prevent screwworm problems. In most states, screwworms must be reported to the State or Federal Veterinarian so that control measures may be taken.

Another method of fly control in wounds is to use a net or cover over the area. For a shoulder wound, for instance, a cover can be made of an old bedsheet or piece of cheesecloth. These allow air to get to the wound to help its healing, while helping to keep flies out of the area.

Caustic wound medications and irritating antiseptics may cause far more harm than good. They can kill tissue and may significantly slow the healing process. Medications such as lime and alum destroy tissues and slow the healing process, while others such as lard and turpentine do no good at all. Caustic powders will remove excess granulation tissue ("proud flesh"), but may result in excessive scar tissue formation in deeper layers, giving a harder and larger scar than would have resulted otherwise. Surgical removal or treatment with corticosteroid ointments under a pressure bandage are much better, resulting in less scarring and faster healing.

Poor nutrition may retard healing; animals who are lacking in either quality or quantity of feed may heal more slowly than those given proper nutrition. Animals who are not receiving enough feed do not have the reserves to maintain their bodies and heal a wound at the same time. Others who receive enough feed but of poor quality may lack vitamins and minerals or other nutrients which are essential to the healing process. Horses who are heavily loaded with worms or have dental problems may also heal poorly.

PROUD FLESH

As mentioned previously, granulation tissue is the stuff which fills in cut areas and heals wounds. When so much of it is produced that it bulges out above the area of the surrounding tissues and keeps the skin edges from healing together, it is called "proud flesh." It must be brought back to level so that the skin edges can grow back together over it and complete healing of the wound. With wounds on the lower leg, this is best accomplished by pressure bandages which keep a gentle but steady compression on the wound and help prevent the formation of proud flesh.

If proud flesh occurs despite pressure bandages, corticosteroid ointments are among the best products for its removal. If infection is present, the ointment should also contain an antibiotic. With severe infection, it may be necessary to treat the animal with antibiotic ointment (such as nitrofurazone ointment) alone for a few days until the infection is under control. Then, use the corticosteroid ointment on all areas of the wound which are ABOVE the level of the surrounding skin. Protect the skin edges with nitrofurazone dressing or a similar product, coating it carefully over about a quarter-inch of the skin, as well as about ¼ inch onto the granulated area. If this is not done, the corticosteroid ointment will retard the healing of the skin area as much as it does the growth of the proud flesh.

Also use the nitrofurazone to cover any areas of the wound which are BELOW the level of the surrounding skin so that their growth is not retarded by the corticosteroid ointment. A gauze sponge or nonstick pad is then applied over the wound and a light pressure bandage placed over it to hold it in place, as well as to retard the growth of the proud flesh by its pressure and by keeping the wound clean.

Materials, such as caustic powders, have been used in the past on areas of proud flesh. They are less used now because it has been found that they remove the surface of the granulation tissue, while at the same time irritating the underlying areas so that they grow back more rapidly than they otherwise would. This results in heavy scar tissue and often a much larger blemish than would have otherwise occurred. These materials may also, in some cases, result in a wound which does not heal.

If a large amount of granulation tissue is present, it should be surgically removed by your veterinarian. Animals often bleed extensively after this surgery because of the large number of blood vessels in granulation tissue. This is normal and is usually controlled by a gentle pressure bandage. This may need to be changed daily for several days until a new granulating surface forms.

Proud flesh is uncommon in the large muscled parts of the body, such as the buttock, neck, and shoulder. Large defects in these areas are rapidly filled with granulation tissue, which normally seems to know better when to stop growing than it does on the legs (where under some circumstances, it may grow indefinitely). These muscled areas often heal without surface scarring. In most cases, sizeable defects (say, 6 inches in diameter and 3 inches deep) fill in and become covered with hair. Occasionally, some shrinkage occurs after the healing is completed, resulting in a dimpled or wrinkled area being present after the deeper scar tissue finishes contracting.

CLOSED WOUNDS AND OTHER ASSORTED SWELLINGS

Closed wounds include what we call a bruise. The overlying skin is not broken, but a varying degree of damage has been done to the underlying blood vessels and tissues. Smaller bruised areas may have only ruptured a few small blood vessels. These show little swelling. In horses with light-colored skin, a blue or purplish discoloration may be seen. Small bruises heal quickly and rarely cause problems.

Larger bruises may end up with a large pocket of blood in the tissues or under the skin. This forms a clot, which may heal in one of two ways. The clot may contract and squeeze out the serum, leaving a pocket filled with clear yellowish fluid, called a seroma. Or, it may contract and shrink, forming a sunken, shrunken scar. The latter frequently occur in the large muscles of the rump and shoulder. Perhaps the most common cause of blood clots (called hematomas) in these areas is a kick by another horse. They may also occur from the horse hitting his chest muscles against a feeder or other hard object. When the horse is kicked in the neck, one of the muscles is often

torn apart, resulting in a permanent dimple or blemish which will remain for the rest of the animal's life.

If you are present when the injury occurs or shortly afterwards, it is often helpful to apply cold packs or ice, along with as much pressure as possible, to help stop the bleeding. Applying DMSO (Diamond Laboratories, Inc., Des Moines, IA 50317) twice daily for three or four days often helps to reduce the swelling of hematomas or seromas.

In some cases, surgical drainage of hematomas may be helpful. However, drainage may result in continuation of the bleeding or serum production. Many veterinarians get better results by not draining them, relying instead on the pressure produced by the fluid to stop further bleeding or serum production.

When drainage is performed, the opening should be made at the lowest point of the swelling, and religiously kept open until it has healed from the inside. It should be swabbed daily with strong tincture of iodine.

Occasionally, bacteria may be brought into the area by the bloodstream. A pus-filled pocket, called an abscess, may occur. These are often recognized because the skin over them is hot, in addition to being swollen and thin to the touch. If not treated, they may break and drain on their own, running a yellow or blood-tinged pus.

How do you tell which one of these you have? The easy way is to tap it with a needle. Begin by clipping all the hair from the area, or shaving it off with a razor or scissors. Scrub the area carefully with a disinfectant soap, such as pHisohex, and rinse well with water. As you are scrubbing, you can palpate the area to tell whether there is a soft point in the area or not. If there is, the needle will be placed at the softest area. After scrubbing, place it at the most prominent part of the swelling. Now, flood the area with alcohol or other disinfectant. Allow this to dry.

Use a sterile 18 gauge or 19 gauge thinwall needle, 1-½ inches long. Take it firmly in hand and pop it into the swelling, moving it around under the skin, if necessary, to allow a bit of the fluid content to drain. If there is blood, then you have a hematoma. If the fluid is thin and yellow, the lump is a seroma. There is, in most cases, no further treatment for either of these. If you open the area and drain it, it will continue to either bleed or ooze serum, thus continuing the problem. So, these are usually best left to themselves to heal, taking care to see that the lump does not develop into an abscess. The reason it is necessary to take so much care with the tap is that if you are not both careful and clean, you may introduce infection into what was initially a sterile condition, thus turning it into an abscess which is harder to treat and more likely to result in complications.

If you get pus (which may be creamy yellow, greenish, or tinged with blood), it is necessary to drain the abscess. Drain it carefully with a sharp knife blade, making a large enough opening so that the pus will drain out and so that you can swab inside to clean it out. Do not try to be "kind" by making a tiny incision, as this only makes it more difficult to swab out the area and keep it clean. In most cases, an inch-long straight or x-shaped incision is about the right size.

In some cases, this incision is best made over the high point of the lump, especially if it is getting soft (we call this "coming to a point"). In other cases, it is best to drain the pocket toward its lower edge so that the pus will drain out more easily. In either case, it is important to keep the hole open by removing any scab which forms and to swab out the lesion daily with a cotton swab and strong (7%) tincture of iodine so that it can heal from the inside out. If the abscess if very large, the animal should be treated with penicillin/streptomycin combination for a minimum of three days. For small abscesses, careful local cleaning to keep it open and drained will be sufficient.

Occasionally, animals are seen with extremely severe bruising under the skin. The injury has not broken the skin, but there is so much damage to the underlying tissues that the skin later sloughs along with the dead, damaged tissues underneath. These situations are usually seen with heavy blows and similar injuries. One of my clients had this occur to his mare's leg just below the hock. She had rolled down a mountain on an elk hunting trip and was apparently normal after the accident, except for a few minor bruises and scrapes. About four days later, one hindleg swelled tremendously until she was unable to walk. The mare was treated with antibiotics for the infection. Drugs were used to remove the edema, helping her to use the leg (thus further promoting circulation and removing swelling from it). Several days later, the skin ruptured, leaving an open wound which had to be treated by swabbing for another six weeks.

All that can be done for an animal with this kind of problem is to clean out any dead tissue that is visible and to trim the edges of the wound if the skin has died. The wound should be cleaned daily. If in the lower leg, strong tincture of iodine is usually best; if in muscular areas, scarlet oil is often the drug of choice. Check with your veterinarian. In some cases, he may recommend an antibiotic ointment be spread on the surface to minimize infection.

BONES

Mature bone consists of bone cells surrounded by a mineral matrix. If the bone is fractured, some of the cells divide and form a framework on which new bony material is deposited, resulting in healing.

In the embryo, bones are first formed from cartilage, especially the long bones. This material gradually becomes calcified and is replaced by bony tissue. The bone continues to grow in length from growth centers near the end, called epiphyses or epiphyseal cartilages. It can grow in length as long as these cartilages continue to grow.

When the cartilage has all turned to bone, the bone cannot get any longer and the animal will not get any taller. This closure occurs at different times in different bones.

The date of epiphyseal closure is widely used to determine the relative maturity of racehorse prospects, and the likelihood of injury if the animal is put into hard training. He is much more liable to be injured when the area is still cartilage than after it has become bone. X-rays are taken to make this determination. Diseases, such as rickets and epiphysitis, affect the area of the epiphysis and may cause permanent damage if the causes are not remedied quickly.

FRACTURES

Fractures are breaks in the continuity of the bone. Many different terms are applied to them, depending on the severity of the break and its complications. A simple fracture is one in which the skin over the fracture site is unbroken. A compound fracture is one in which the skin is torn or punctured over the fracture site. This may be caused by a broken bone end puncturing the skin from the inside out or it may be caused by an object, such as a piece of metal or a bullet, entering from the outside and causing the fracture. Compound fractures are often a severe problem in horses because their tissues become infected so easily. A fracture in which the bone ends are exposed through a wound and left untreated for more than about six hours will probably require heroic treatment and long-term antibiotic therapy to save the animal, if it can be saved at all.

A comminuted fracture is one which numerous small fragments are formed because the bone is splintered or crushed. An epiphyseal fracture is one which occurs at the epiphyseal plate. Epiphyseal fractures occur mainly in young animals, as do greenstick fractures, in which one side of the bone is broken or splintered while the other side is only bent.

If the broken ends of a fractured bone are brought together and kept from moving, normal healing will usually take place. The ends must be matched as closely as possible to their normal location. If the center of one side is matched with the outer area of the other side, healing will not occur or will be extremely delayed.

At the time of the fracture, bleeding occurs from blood vessels which are torn around the fracture area. A blood clot will form. This clot is invaded by connective tissue cells which form granulation tissue and bring in new blood capillaries. The cells from the surface of the bone divide and form a large amount of bony material called a callus. This callus bridges the gap at the ends of the broken bone, completely covering it. It forms an effective splint which usually prevents movement between the bone ends, and can often be felt as a large, bony knot at the fracture site. The callus gradually becomes calcified, changing into true bone. This bony area is then naturally remodeled into a typical bone shaft with a marrow cavity and supporting outer wall. Slight misalignments will be corrected over a period of time, as the bone cells remove bone from where it is not needed and strengthen that which is in the proper place. The bone cells respond to structural stress within the bone. The result is that the bone will be strongest along the lines of greatest stress when strength and rigidity are most required.

Nonunion fractures occur when there is too much movement between the two fragments, or when the bone ends are separated by too great a distance for normal healing to occur between them. These fractures are held together by a fibrous callus which does not turn to bone as it normally would. It leaves the area weak and wobbly and often requires surgery ("rebreaking") to realign and stabilize the bone ends so that proper healing may occur. Recent studies have used electrical stimulation across the nonhealing area to help stimulate bone growth. Good results have been reported for this technique. It is inexcusable in this age of x-rays and fracture repairs to blister or fire a sore animal only to find later that the problem was a fracture. These treatments may cause a nonunion as well as stimulating excessive growth of useless, nonhealing, new bone which may cause problems by growing around important blood vessels or nerves. (64)

The most rapid healing of fractures occurs in younger animals. A fracture which may take five or six months to heal in an older animal may heal firmly in a month in a foal.

Fractures were at one time considered to be "the end" of a horse, and many horses were shot because of them. Modern methods of stabilization and splinting allow us to repair many fractures which were previously unrepairable. Modern antibiotics contribute to preventing infection. Before you shoot the horse, get a veterinary opinion as to whether he is salvageable. Obviously, if the animal is a gelding and is worth killer price only, is old and has a miserable disposition, and you are sixty miles into the wilderness, a well-placed bullet may be the only reasonable cure. But if you value the animal or would consider salvaging it for breeding purposes, get it examined before you shoot.

If at all possible, take the animal to a veterinarian who works primarily with horses, or to a university hospital. These people will usually have access to the latest techniques and equipment for stabilizing the animal's fracture and giving him the best possible chance of survival. It is extremely important to stabilize the animal's leg (if that is where the break has occurred) so that a simple fracture does not become compounded, or a compound fracture does not become worse. Otherwise, an animal with a repairable fracture may have it become so badly damaged in transit that it is no longer fixable. Your veterinarian will splint or cast the leg, he may put pins or screws into it, or he may wire it together, depending on the type of fracture.

The aftercare is up to you. The animal should have a nutritious, but not excessively rich, diet. It is important to keep the horse's weight down to normal to reduce the load on the fractured leg. An overweight horse may need to be put on a reducing diet. Be sure such a diet is well balanced and contains all essential nutrients.

The horse should have either exercise or rest as prescribed. If the veterinarian says to rest him in a stall, that DOES NOT mean to take him out for walks or put him on the walker. It DOES mean that he wants the animal to stay as still as possible for the healing period. It is important that casts or splints be kept clean and dry to avoid skin problems under them. Allowing a cast to get wet may cause enough of a skin problem, with resulting severe infection, that the animal may have to be put down because of the complications. Don't let this happen. However, accidents do occur and a cast or splint may get wet. If it does, call your veterinarian as soon as possible. He may elect to replace it because of the danger of skin infection.

A horse with a fractured leg (or any serious leg injury) may try to keep all weight off that leg, putting the entire burden on the opposite leg. This can lead to a breakdown of the uninjured leg. What happens is that the tendons are stretched so far that they can never come back to their normal length. When the injured leg is healed, the animal may still have to be euthanized because the fetlock on the uninjured leg is touching the ground and the tendons will not tighten up enough to bring it back to a normal position. For this reason, a horse with an injured leg who is bearing most of his weight on the opposite leg should have it wrapped in a snug, supportive wrap. Race track type bandages are sufficient if the animal only needs support for a week or so. Animals who are going to be incapacitated for a longer period of time may have to have a Robert Jones type bandage, or even a splint or cast applied to protect the good leg.

FIRST AID FOR FRACTURES

Emergency treatment for the horse with a fractured limb is aimed at keeping the problem from getting any worse. If, for instance, you can keep a simple fracture from becoming compounded as the animal moves, his chances of recovery are greatly improved. Stabilizing the leg also helps to relieve the animal's pain and the anxiety that occurs because he cannot control the limb. It will help prevent further damage to the bone ends and the soft tissues that surround them.

Injuries of the lower leg (to just above the fetlock joint) can be splinted with relative ease. A light layer of sheet cotton or gauze padding should be put on the leg. It should not be more than about ⅛-inch thick. If too much padding is used, it will compress as the leg moves, allowing the splint to loosen and permitting excessive movement of the bone ends. It is often necessary to straighten the leg and splint it with the toe pointed downward; alignment in the normal position is usually difficult to maintain with an emergency splint. A light layer of strong splinting material, such as lightweight wood, metal stripping, or strips of plastic pipe, can then be placed down the front of the leg, from the knee to the hoof. If casting plaster is available, it can then be applied over the splint to hold it in this alignment. Fractures of the hindleg are immobilized in the same manner.

Fractures of the middle part of the front leg, from the middle of the cannon bone to above the knee, will need a splint to help hold the entire leg straight. It should extend from the elbow to the ground. A splint which is too short will not adequately stabilize the leg. A Robert Jones bandage, put on in many layers, is a good method for immobilization. A layer of sheet cotton or similar padding is put on the leg. It is then wrapped snugly with elastic gauze or tape. Several layers are built up in this manner. Each layer should be thin enough so that it will not shift or compact. After a number of layers are built up, rigid splints should be put in place on the sides and back of the limb.

A stiff, lightweight material, such as wood or plastic, can be used for splints. Excessively strong material is not necessary. Use regular adhesive tape over the splint material rather than the elastic kind so that it does not expand and allow the splints to slip. Apply the tape as tightly as possible.

Fractures higher in the leg can be stabilized with the same type of Robert Jones bandage, but with splints that extend upward along the side of the chest or hip.

When the animal is transported, every effort should be made to keep the horse from walking. Foals should be carried, if at all possible. If the animal has a fracture in the front leg, it is good to haul him facing backward if possible so that when braking occurs, his weight will be borne by the hindlegs. By the same token, the animal with a fractured rear limb should be hauled facing forward.

Confine the horse in the trailer as much as possible so that he can lean on the surrounding supports to keep his balance. If the animal is allowed to move freely in an open trailer, he may do severe damage to the injured leg while attempting to keep his balance. Cross-tie the animal's head. Although a horse should not be allowed to load up on feed if surgery may be necessary, a small amount of hay will help to keep the animal calm and busy while he is transported. (65)

FRACTURE REPAIR

Many fractures which once required euthanasia of the horse are now repairable. Fractured jaws, for example, may be repaired with stainless steel plates screwed firmly to the bone. Broken legs are repaired by numerous methods, including splints, pins, plates, and wiring. A professor of surgery at the Western College of Veterinary Medicine in Saskatchewan, for instance, feels that there is no apparent upper weight limit for fracture repairs below the knee or hock. (66) In other words, the size of the horse

is not a significant factor in deciding whether or not to attempt repair of a fracture below the hock or knee. If you are in doubt, stabilize the animal until you can get a veterinary opinion (or a second opinion) on the break.

AMPUTATION

Amputation has occasionally been done in the horse, and the animal has been fitted with an artificial leg. Equine amputees suffer from the same problems as do humans: raw stumps, infection, and pain. These problems are compounded immensely because of the animal's size and weight. When a human has a problem requiring amputation, we fix it and keep him alive. I am sure that most human amputees would agree that they are glad to be alive, even without their limb or limbs. On the other hand, the horse is an animal kept for use—for what he can do or produce. I cannot imagine keeping an horse who required an amputation. It would be much kinder to put the animal to sleep than to make him suffer the pain that is present because of his size and sensitivity. Amputation, by the way, works very well in smaller animals, such as dogs and cats, where the animal is not so large and heavy.

OSTEOMYELITIS

Osteomyelitis is an inflammation of the bone and the medullary (marrow) cavity. The term osteitis is occasionally used. It has a slightly different meaning, but the difference is not important for our usage. The inflammatory reaction which occurs in osteomyelitis usually also involves infection.

The infection of osteomyelitis most commonly occurs following a compound fracture where the bone ends have penetrated the skin and were exposed to dirt and bacterial contamination. Osteomyelitis is always a very serious infection. Older horses do not often recover from it. Treatment seems to be more successful in younger horses.

Osteomyelitis may also occur in a fracture where a small chip is separated from the main part of the bone and left without a blood supply of its own. The fragment dies and infection is carried into it through the bloodstream.

A similar avascular (bloodless) necrosis may occur in a fracture fragment when a horse is kicked on one of the cannon bones. An abscess develops in the outer layer of the bone. The chip acts as a foreign body and must be removed before healing will take place. Osteomyelitis may occur in the carpal bones following surgery, especially if the surgery has been done to remove excess bony growth. Infection shows up two or three weeks after the incision has apparently healed cleanly and without complications. As with the previous example, the infection apparently arrives at the weakened area through the bloodstream. Osteomyelitis may also occur with the fracture of a splint bone, where a portion of the bone is left without a blood supply.

SIGNS

Osteomyelitis is often first seen as a draining wound which does not heal. If this occurs with a compound fracture, it will be noticed that the bone is not healing at a normal rate. The bone callus which holds the break together may be very late in forming or may not form at all. This may also occur when a piece of bone is isolated from its blood supply in a fracture with multiple fragments. The wound will continue to drain as long as the dead piece of bone is present.

The wound may heal and then break open repeatedly. Osteomyelitis or a foreign body should be suspected any time this occurs.

TREATMENT

If a compound fracture is present, the wound must be cleaned thoroughly. This, like any other fracture, is a job for your veterinarian. He will completely clean the wound with a very gentle disinfectant. Strong disinfectants would only kill normal tissue and add it to the dead material that must be removed. He will then place a cast or splint on the break, or immobilize it by some other means.

It may be necessary to cut a "window" in the cast to allow access to the wound for cleaning and treatment. The wound may be treated with disinfectants, antibiotics, enzymes, or a combination of these medications. It is necessary to stimulate granulation tissue to cover the bone. It is extremely important—with a window cast—to keep pressure on the portion of the wound exposed through the window to keep proud flesh (excess granulation tissue) from bulging out through the cast. If a dead piece of bone is present, as in a fracture with multiple fragments, it may be necessary to remove it. This is also true of a single chip on a large bone. A pressure bandage will be needed for a couple of weeks after surgery to keep granulation tissue from getting out of control. The animal will be kept on systemic antibiotics, such as penicillin, for a prolonged period of time—generally not less than a week, and often as long as three to four weeks.

AVASCULAR NECROSIS

This problem goes by several other names, including aseptic necrosis, osteochondritis and ischemic bone necrosis. Necrosis means "death," and avascular means "without blood." Thus, the term refers to a situation where portions of the bone die without infection. Avascular necrosis is most commonly seen in young horses while their bones are in the growing stages. All cases seem to involve joint surfaces. This necrosis may involve carpal or tarsal bones, the femur, the shoulder blade (in the shoulder joint), and the lower end of the cannon bone.

The disease apparently begins with loss of blood supply to a small area of the bone just under the joint cartilage. The area of bone left without blood dies, and the minerals are removed from the area, leaving an area of lessened density. It is not known what interrupts the blood supply, but it has been theorized that the cause is a blood clot in a small blood vessel in the epiphysis (growth plate) from which the bone grows.

As the disease progresses, the dead area of bone and the cartilage attached to it may gradually separate from the adjacent bone and cartilage and become a loose body. Injury due to overwork or other hard usage may help to cause the necrosis. In a severe case of the disease, the joint cartilage may be completely destroyed.

The horse may show vague signs of lameness. Pain in the joint is one of the most important signs. Your veterinarian may identify the area of pain by using selective nerve blocks. The joint will usually show obvious swelling. X-rays show the dead spot very graphically, much like a hole in Swiss cheese. Several x-ray views may be necessary to show the lesion and to precisely pinpoint its location.

Based, in part, on experience with similar problems in humans and dogs, conservative treatment seems to be the best approach. Surgery is usually unnecessary, especially if the cartilage over the lesion is still intact. The joint should be protected as much as possible from weight bearing. The avascular bone will, one hopes, remain in place and its blood supply will return to normal within three to seven months.

If a portion of the bone separates, the condition is called osteochondritis dissecans. The outcome of these cases is generally unfavorable, no matter what treatment is attempted. The condition usually occurs in the carpal or tarsal joint and may result in permanent deformity of the bone. Surgical removal of the loose bone is occasionally attempted if the value of the horse warrants it. Large chips may be reattached with a bone screw.

Complete stall rest is usually indicated, as is an examination of the animal's diet to make sure that it is adequate and contains an adequate mineral balance without excesses of any kind. The animal's weight should be kept normal or a little on the thin side to reduce damage to the bone and joint surfaces.

ARTHRITIS

"Arthritis" refers to inflammation within a joint. Early in the process, changes may be minimal. Later, it may be accompanied by degeneration of the joint cartilage, a decreased amount of lubricating synovial fluid, and the development of bony spurs, such as those which occur with ringbone around a joint. Another name which is commonly used for this process is "degenerative joint disease," often abbreviated "DJD."

As with the same disease in humans, many treatments have been used for arthritis in the horse. Corticosteroids have been injected into the joint. In my opinion, this treatment is a lot like putting a "band-aid" on a broken leg. It helps the problem temporarily, but does not in any way fix it. If steroid injections into the joint are used, it is of the utmost importance to give the animal adequate rest afterward. Do not just inject him and then work him if you wish to keep him usable for the long haul. The injection

may relieve the pain enough that the animal becomes overly active and permanently damages the joint.

Many authorities feel that rest is the best treatment for most kinds of arthritis. This allows the inflammation to subside and the body to heal itself. New treatments for this disease are being tried daily, but to date, none has proven to be the cure-all everyone would like to see.

How much rest is necessary? It depends on the type of arthritis and its location. It may be necessary to give the bones time to fuse, or for the bony spurs to stop active growth. This may vary from a month or so to six to eight months. Your veterinarian can give you a better idea of how much is needed after he looks at x-rays of the affected joint.

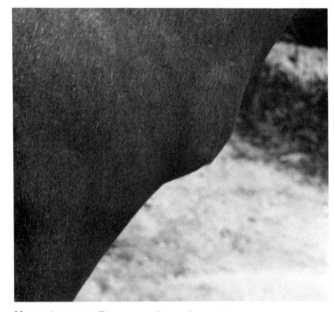

Mysterious swelling on a horse's neck.

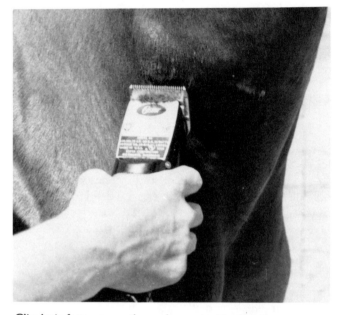

Clip hair from area, then cleanse with disinfectant.

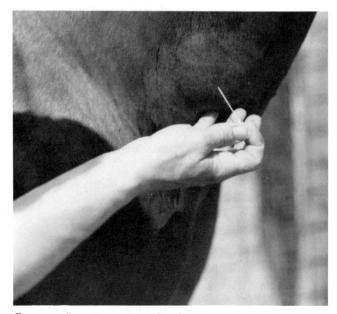

Pop needle into center of soft part.

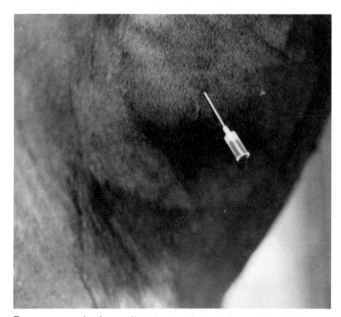

Drop on end of needle shows this to be a blood clot.

Chapter 14

RESPIRATORY PROBLEMS

Roaring
Nosebleed (Epistaxis)
Pulmonary Hemorrhage
Distemper (Strangles)
Respiratory Tract Problems
Upper Respiratory Tract Infections
Pneumonia
Pleuritis or Pleurisy
Thumps
Heaves (Emphysema)
Summer Pasture-Associated Obstructive Pulmonary Disease

ROARING

Also called laryngeal hemiplegia, "roaring" refers to a paralysis of the muscles of the larynx (voice box). The muscles on one side are partially or completely paralyzed. The left side is most frequently affected, although occasionally the right side or both are involved. This paralysis allows the vocal cords to flap loosely into the airway, causing a noise when the horse breathes in. It is seen in racehorses, and is most common in Thoroughbreds and light horses. It is rarely seen in draft horses. Some animals have a higher-pitched roar and are called whistlers. It is felt that whistlers are better able to do hard work than roarers. It is important to remember that not all horses who breathe noisily are roarers; other conditions, while less common, can cause noise as the animal is worked.

The immediate cause of roaring is degeneration of one or both of the recurrent laryngeal nerves, resulting in partial or complete paralysis of the muscles which pull outward on a cartilage beside the vocal cord. The normal tension of the muscles keeps the cartilages from rotating outward when the horse breathes in. This reduces the size of the laryngeal opening, resulting in the noise when the horse breathes in. Paralysis occurs on the left side in over 90% of the cases.

Some authorities have theorized that the degeneration of the nerve is related in some way to irritation produced by the pulsations of the aorta, where the left recurrent laryngeal nerve passes around it. Overextension of the head may possibly cause the problem. It may also be due to infections, such as distemper or pneumonia, or other debilitating diseases. Lead poisoning or certain plant toxicities have been proposed as causes. If an irritating substance has been injected near the recurrent laryngeal nerve, paralysis may occur. If due to an injection, it may be temporary, with the animal recovering in two to four months, or it may be permanent.

A recent study has shown that roaring is hereditary, caused by an autosomal recessive gene. Roarers frequently have offspring who roar. These offspring may not show signs of the disease until they are 3 to 4 years old or older and have been put to hard work. However, offspring of roarers who don't roar carry the gene for the problem. For this reason, roarers should be eliminated from a breeding program. (67)

The most striking sign is a roaring or whistling sound when the horse breathes in. In mild cases, the sound may only be heard after strenuous exercise. When checking the animal for roaring, work him until he just shows signs of respiratory distress; the object is to test his wind, not to wear him out. In worse cases, the noise may be heard after light exercise, or even with the animal at rest. The roaring will usually become more quiet about 10 minutes after exercise is stopped. Animals with these problems are unfit for racing or work. They tire quickly. Horses in the early stages of the problem may have a characteristic grunt when frightened or struck a sharp blow over the ribs. This grunt is said to be a prolonged and deep noise. Some horses with the condition may have trouble breathing when eating grain or when the head is pulled to the side.

An instrument called a laryngoscope is often used to determine if a horse has paralyzed vocal cords. It utilizes fiber optics to allow the veterinarian to see the actual condition and action of the vocal cords.

Occasionally, horses can have abnormalities of the soft palate which lead to difficulty in breathing and a roaring noise. These are usually diagnosed on laryngoscopic examination. These problems may not be significantly improved by surgery.

Roaring rarely cures itself. Generally, the vocal folds are removed by an operation equivalent to debarking a dog. This surgery restores about 30% of the horses to usefulness. (68) In cases which do not respond to removal of the vocal folds, the cartilages may be surgically tied outward, holding the vocal cords out of the way. This type of surgery is felt by some authors to be the more effective of the two.

NOSEBLEED (EPISTAXIS)

Injury is a common cause of nosebleed in horses. Passage of a stomach tube may occasionally result in a nosebleed, even if done carefully. It usually occurs when the horse tosses his head, either as the veterinarian tries to pass the stomach tube or, more commonly, as he is pulling it out. Careful restraint of the horse during passage of the stomach tube will help to prevent nosebleed. It will occur anyway in some animals—this may be due to delicate nasal membranes. If your horse gets a nosebleed when your veterinarian tubes him for routine worming, try the other side of the nose the next time the horse needs to be tubed. If the horse bleeds on the second try, then feed- or paste-worm him from that time on. It still may be necessary to stomach tube the animal if he has colic or other problem requiring veterinary treatment. In that case, go ahead and tube the animal. A horse who has a nosebleed caused by being tubed will generally stop bleeding soon after he is released and allowed to calm down. In unusual cases, the bleeding may last as much as 30 to 45 minutes without serious blood loss.

Nosebleeds may, on rare occasion, occur with nasal tumors or nasal polyps. This is a consideration in an older animal—usually over 15 years or so. Your veterinarian may encounter one of these tumors while attempting to pass a stomach tube. Sometimes, a tumor or obstruction will be found in the nasal passage on one side, while the tube may be passed clearly and freely down the other side. If this occurs, be sure to make a note in your horse's records of this problem and which side has it so that it can be avoided in the future. Some of these obstructions may be due to hereditary malformations in the nasal passages or to previous injury or fractures of the facial bones.

Horses occasionally get nosebleeds from stumbling and falling, and bumping their heads or noses. Horses subjected to a sudden stop in a horse trailer may hit their heads on the front wall or feeder. A client called me to examine a horse who had fallen out of a stock rack on a pickup. To the owner, the horse looked like he was dying. He did look like a disaster at first glance. Careful examina-tion, however, revealed that he only had a severe nose-bleed, a few scrapes, and a whole lot of bruises—nothing that a little time wouldn't cure.

Nosebleeds may occur with a sinus infection. In these, the blood is usually mixed with pus. Poisoning may be caused by a horse eating moldy sweet clover. This destroys one of the factors in the blood which causes it to clot, and may cause the animal to bleed for no apparent reason. (69)

TREATMENT

Begin by removing the cause of the nosebleed if it is obvious. If, for instance, the animal has been restrained for tube worming and is upset, release him into a corral or arena—an area where he is confined, but has a bit of room to walk around. Do not turn one of these out into his pasture until you are sure the bleeding is stopped. Allow-ing him to be on his own and unrestrained will let the horse relax; this in turn drops the blood pressure, thus reducing the volume of the bleeding.

If a veterinarian is present and the bleeding does not stop after the animal is relaxed and allowed to calm down, he may choose to administer drugs that will help to stop the bleeding. In practice, this author has not seen a nose-bleed that did not stop by itself if given the chance. Per-haps an exception to this could occur with an animal on sweet clover hay whose blood isn't clotting normally. One of these animals might need an injection of vitamin K to help its clotting mechanism; severely affected animals may need blood transfusions to save them. The preven-tion for this type of nosebleed is to avoid feeding sweet clover hay, especially before surgery or any other pro-cedure which might inadvertently or deliberately cause bleeding.

PULMONARY HEMORRHAGE

Bleeding from the lungs is common in horses who are worked hard. It is frequently seen in Thoroughbred racehorses and is also seen in Standardbreds. It also occurs in Quarter Horses and horses used in other events requiring heavy exertion, such as steeplechasers, jump-ers, and event horses.

Many of these animals will have bleeding in the lungs and never show any signs of blood coming from the nose. Others will have varying amounts of bleeding from one or both nostrils.

Bleeding on the racetrack is usually brought on by exercise. Blood may pool in the lower part of the lungs, and not drain out until the horse returns to his stall and lowers his head. About 95% of bleeding in racehorses is said to be from the lungs. Blood from the lungs is NOT necessarily frothy, and is NOT always coughed up. Less than 10% of horses with bleeding into the lungs will bleed from the nose. (70)

Look for bleeding into the lungs with horses who experience sudden, unexplained fatigue during a race. The animal may choke when pulled up by the rider or may tire toward the end of the race. He may be excessively winded after stopping and have an anxious, startled expression. He may bleed without coughing at all. The animal may swallow repeatedly, which may be the only sign of the problem.

TREATMENT

If you feel that your horse is bleeding from the lungs, get a veterinarian immediately. If severe blood loss occurs, treatment for shock may be necessary and, in some cases, a blood transfusion may also be required. Some veterinarians feel that an animal with bleeding from the lungs should be walked very slowly and that they may bleed to death if left standing. Horses with massive bleeding into the lungs usually die when the bleeding is due to the rupture of a major blood vessel. Treatment may do little or no good.

After a race, some horses will continue to bleed into the lungs for several days or weeks. These horses may be dull and listless and have a poor appetite. A blood examination usually shows the animal to have an anemia.

Little can be done to prevent bleeding in the lungs. A diuretic called furosemide is often given before a race to help prevent bleeding. Estrogen injections may also be helpful. The amount of blood that may be visible does not necessarily indicate how serious the problem is, as some horses may become severely ill or even die, without showing any bleeding from the nose. The animal who survives the acute part of the problem should have an extended rest period so that the lungs have a chance to heal.

DISTEMPER (STRANGLES)

Also called strangles, this is a bacterial disease caused by a type of bacteria called Streptococcus equi. It has no relationship to dog distemper (which is caused by a virus) or cat distemper (which is caused by a virus totally different from that of dog distemper). Equine distemper is most commonly seen in young animals, but may occur in horses of any age who have not been previously infected. Infection passes from one animal to another in pus from the abscesses which form in lymph nodes around the head, or via the pus which may be discharged from the animal's nose. The bacterium is quite resistant and may survive for months in barns or on objects, such as halters.

The incubation period for equine distemper is usually three to six days. However, horses who are exposed to it may not all come down with it at the same time.

One of my clients had distemper in a herd on pasture which went on among this group of horses for over three months. One horse would come down with it, and just about be healed, when the next one would get sick, and so on—through six animals. Only two horses did not get it. Both were old mares who could have reasonably been expected to have had the disease earlier in their lives and to be immune to it.

SIGNS

Often the first sign that an owner notices is that the horse does not eat or drink. The temperature may go as high at 106 degrees F (41 degrees C). Swelling of the lymph nodes under and behind the jaw will usually develop within a couple of days. Drainage from the nose often looks like pus—thick and greenish or yellowish. The animal may not wish to swallow and may stand with his neck extended. Abscesses may also occur in lymph nodes inside the back of the mouth. These contribute to the discomfort and to problems in swallowing. Abscesses in the throat which are very large may cause the horse to have trouble breathing, giving the disease one of its common names, "strangles." When the abscesses finally break and drain, relief usually follows rapidly. The animal feels better immediately and will show more interest in life. The appearance of abscesses is almost a foolproof sign of distemper. Once you have one case of the disease in a herd, it is a warning to be on the lookout for more of them.

The disease lasts about two weeks in an individual. Like the viral upper respiratory diseases, distemper is rarely fatal. Fatalities usually occur in young or very old animals or in those with another illness which weakens them. When death does occur, it is usually due to central nervous system involvement or internal abscesses. Most horses recover without permanent damage.

Animals with an inadequate immune response may develop a form of distemper commonly called "bastard strangles." This will only affect an individual animal—it is not a herd problem. Also, treatment of the animal with antibiotics, especially when used before the abscesses break, may force the bacteria into the animal's internal organs, creating a case of bastard strangles. This then necessitates very long-term antibiotic therapy—in some cases, procaine penicillin must be given for up to a month.

TREATMENT

Penicillin is often the drug of choice for a chronic case of distemper. In routine cases, most veterinarians do not use any antibiotics at all for fear of causing a case of bastard strangles. Antibiotics may be needed if the abscesses break but the animal is not showing signs of recovery, is still very ill, and not starting to eat. If you do start antibiotic treatment, it must be continued until the temperature returns to normal and has remained there for several days.

The horse should have complete rest and nursing as described under viral respiratory diseases. Hot packs may help the abscesses come to a head. They may then be drained at the soft point. This is usually a job for a veterinarian. You would hate to cut a major blood vessel or nerve while draining an abscess! However, in the absence of a veterinarian, you can make an incision right at the point of the abscess when the skin over it is stretched tightly and the point of it feels soft and ready to burst. Use a very sharp blade (disposable scalpels are best) and make a puncture at the very point of the swelling, about ½ inch long. As soon as you make the puncture, the pus will begin to pour. Let it pour out until it is finished draining.

Now, enlarge the incision to about 1 inch long, depending on the location of the abscess. It is also a good idea to make two cuts at right angles to the original cut, making the opening into an "X" shape. This helps to keep it open and draining. Making a small hole is not a kindness—it tends to close and causes problems. Do not hesitate to cut a good-sized hole! It will heal over, and a lot more readily if it is larger instead of small. Amazingly enough, there is rarely a scar over the abscess area. It will take some time, but nearly all abscess areas heal back to completely normal and hair over. So, don't worry about a large hole in the jaw of your show horse—it WILL heal, even if it looks as if it never would.

After the abscesses break or are drained, the cavities should be swabbed out with strong (7%) tincture of iodine. Using three or four of the long cotton swabs together helps make the job a little more efficient and less unpleasant. You may also want to cover your hand with a plastic bag or disposable glove to prevent both the pus and the iodine from running down it. The disposable plastic obstetrical sleeves that your veterinarian uses for pregnancy testing are ideal for this use—you may be able to buy some from him or from an artificial inseminator or livestock supply house. Saturate the swabs in the iodine and work them around inside the opening of the abscess to clean out the pus and debris.

Make sure the hole stays open. If it scabs over, do not assume that it is healing O.K. It should heal gradually from the inside out like other open wounds. You should be able to get the swabs in a little less each day. You should not be able to get them in an inch and a half one day and not get them in at all the next. The object is to help the hole heal from the inside out. If you allow it to scab over before the infection inside is all cleaned out, it will only break open and drain again, prolonging the course of the disease. So, pick off the scab and keep swabbing!

Occasionally, the swollen lymph nodes will put enough pressure on the animal's air passages to make breathing difficult or impossible. Your veterinarian should be called immediately. It may be necessary for him to perform a tracheotomy to make it possible for the animal to breathe. In some cases, he may insert a metal tracheotomy tube into the animal's neck to keep the incision open until the swelling goes down enough for the animal to breathe by himself.

PREVENTION

Killed vaccines (called bacterins) are intermittently available for prevention of distemper. Many veterinarians do not use these products any more because of some adverse side effects. In the past, some of the available bacterins have caused a disease called purpura hemorrhagica. Many veterinarians decided that they were losing more horses to the purpura than they ever did to distemper. It also caused other side effects, such as swelling and hardening of tissues where the injection was given.

If the bacterin is used, most veterinarians feel that it must be started when the foal is about two months old and continued religiously. Using this bacterin in older horses sometimes causes purpura; this may have something to do with the animal's previously having been exposed to the bacteria which cause the disease. Bacterins for immunization against distemper should ONLY be used on the advice of your veterinarian.

RESPIRATORY TRACT PROBLEMS

Respiratory tract problems may be caused by several agents. Bacteria and viruses are common causes. The bacteria which cause lymph node abscesses and nasal drainage often invade the lungs, where they may cause pneumonia. Viruses which cause upper respiratory tract infections may also have complications involving the lungs. Allergic reactions to dust or molds on feed may cause emphysema (heaves).

When discussing a cough or respiratory problem with your veterinarian, the history of the condition is very important. When did it start and how long has it been going on? Is only one horse in a group affected, or do several have common signs? Have the horses been together for a period of time, or have some been brought in recently—or taken out to go to a show or rodeo? When does the animal cough—while eating, while being worked, or after the workout is ended? Some horses will cough only when in their stalls, showing that the problem is due to dust, lack of ventilation, or dirty, poor quality bedding. If you can answer these questions for your veterinarian, he will have a much better chance of determining what the problem is with your horse, and of fixing it. Also, be sure to tell him whether the horse had been previously treated, what medication was used, and what the results were. This will help to avoid going through the same process again if it did not work the first time.

Be aware when you are dealing with any respiratory problem that treatment may be long and sometimes expensive, even for a simple virus problem. The animal may need a prolonged period of recuperation before he can be used again if permanent damage to his lungs is to be avoided. Also, be aware that some respiratory problems, such as heaves, are unrepairable. Once the damage is done, the animal can never be returned to his original condition. Treatment from that point consists of management to keep the problem from getting any worse and to make the animal as usable as possible within the limitations of the damage that has already been done. Now, let's discuss some specific respiratory problems.

UPPER RESPIRATORY TRACT INFECTIONS

At least ten viruses are associated with upper respiratory tract infections in the horse. Several of these cause groups of clinical signs distinct enough to be recognized as separate diseases, such as influenza, rhinopneumonitis, and viral arteritis. These, along with the rest of the viruses involved and the bacteria which may follow them into the weakened animal make up a group of miseries which resemble the common cold in man. The resemblance is in appearance only, as "colds" do not occur in the horse.

There are two kinds of writers about equine medicine: the lumpers and the splitters. The splitters will define everything down to a gnat's eyelash and bore you to death with unnecessary detail. The lumpers will work in generalities. Rather than boring you with absolute differences among these diseases, this author will lump them together because the treatment is generally the same. Your veterinarian may be able to distinguish among them on a clinical basis, especially if a large group of animals is involved. Or, he may have to send serum samples to a laboratory which will take several weeks to make a diagnosis. The difference is academic; by the time the laboratory decides which disease your horses have, the animals have either gotten better or died.

You can (and should) vaccinate all horses, especially pregnant mares, against rhinopneumonitis; do the same with influenza. The rest of the diseases are, like the common cold in man, something we cannot do anything about, so the exact name of the virus that caused it, in my opinion, doesn't matter. And like the common cold, they rarely cause death unless the animal is very young, very old, or weakened by an existing disease problem or malnutrition. Viral arteritis apparently gives a lifelong immunity to animals who recover. There is no vaccine against it. The only prevention is good sanitation and isolation measures for new horses to reduce the likelihood that infection will be brought to your premises.

Contagious respiratory diseases are more common in young horses, especially those who, like children in the first grade, are away from home for the first time. They get together and pass the viruses back and forth at racetracks, training facilities, shows, and similar events. Crowding and stress both bring on the diseases and help to spread them once they are established.

SIGNS

The incubation periods for the upper respiratory diseases vary from 1 to 10 days. Fever is a constant sign, ranging from 102 degrees to as much as 107.5 degrees F (39 to 42 degrees C). The animal will usually have a nasal discharge; this will probably be thin and clear early in the course of the disease. It may later change to thick and purulent (pus-like) if, as usually happens, bacteria invade the weakened tissues. Tears and/or pus may run from the eyes. The eyelids may be swollen and the animal may be sensitive to light.

There is usually a cough. It may be dry and hacking, but is more commonly moist. Mucus may be heard rattling in the trachea as the animal coughs to get rid of it. The cough often persists for several weeks after all other signs are gone. Breathing may be labored. The horse is usually lethargic and depressed and may have little or no appetite. Rapid weight loss may occur because the horse is neither eating nor drinking. The horse may also have a diarrhea. Occasionally, the diarrhea shows up several days after all the respiratory signs have passed. The virus causing that syndrome seems to be particularly common around racetracks. Muscular soreness or stiffness or central nervous system disturbances (dopiness or unusual attitudes) are occasionally seen.

ABORTIONS

Equine viral rhinopneumonitis may cause mares to abort as long as 1 to 4 months after infection. Also, the infection in the mare may be so mild that it occurs without the owner ever noticing that she has the disease. For this reason, it was some years before the veterinarians in Kentucky connected respiratory infections of young horses in the spring and summer with mares who aborted in the fall and winter or had foals born weak, dying within a couple of days.

Mares with "rhino" commonly abort between the 8th and 11th months of pregnancy. The foal is usually fresh (not decomposed) and looks normal. The mare usually aborts suddenly without any warning signs. She will promptly expel all placental membranes and breed back normally.

Equine viral arteritis may cause abortion in as many as 80% of the mares infected with it. With this disease, the mare usually aborts shortly after a bout with a respiratory infection. This may help your veterinarian to specifically diagnose this problem. Abortions are rarely seen with influenza.

DIAGNOSIS

Positive diagnosis of these diseases is often purely academic, and may involve lengthy laboratory serological analysis. It is easier to give a definite diagnosis if several horses are involved than if there is only one affected. In some cases, your veterinarian may be able to tell you which disease is present, but don't be angry or feel that he's incompetent if he can't—it's tough! If the problem is caused by one of the diseases you can vaccinate for, it's often too late to immunize after the animals have been exposed, although some veterinarians will vaccinate along with treating the disease. In some cases, prompt immunization may keep a few of the horses from getting the disease.

TREATMENT

Medication, as with the common human cold, is rarely indicated. The animals get over the problem in two weeks if you treat them and 14 days if you don't. Good nursing and absolute rest are of the utmost importance in treatment. The animal should be confined in a comfortable building with no exercise at all. Keep the animal warm, dry, and as comfortable as possible. Blanket if necessary, but try not to overheat him. If the weather is good, it may help the horse's attitude to be allowed out in the sun for a bit. Wiping the discharge from the horse's eyes or nose will help him to be more comfortable. Putting Vicks (Vicks Health Care Div., Richardson-Vicks, Inc., Wilton, CT 06897) or Mentholatum (The Mentholatum Co., Buffalo, NY 14213) in the nostrils may help the animal to breathe more easily. A cough syrup or powder may be given if needed.

Many veterinarians do not use antipyretics (drugs to bring down the temperature) unless it is exceptionally high (say, over 104 degrees F (40 degrees C)). If the animal's temperature persists at or above this level, your veterinarian should be consulted. It may be necessary for him to administer medication to reduce the horse's fever so that the animal will feel better and start eating again. Up to the point that the high temperature itself may be damaging, fever is one of the body's mechanisms to help deal with the invading viruses and should be allowed to run its course.

Continued use of these drugs may mask a rise in the animal's temperature, and remove the most valuable indicator that we have as to whether the animal is getting better or worse. These drugs may allow the animal to slide into a pneumonia while temporarily looking much better. We could miss the pneumonia by not having the rise in temperature to indicate its presence.

Some horse owners routinely administer corticosteroids to animals with respiratory disease. These drugs suppress immunity and may significantly slow the animal's recovery. They may also lead to invasion by resistant bacteria, while doing nothing to affect the virus which is causing the disease. For these reasons, it is not a good practice to use steroids with these diseases.

Antibiotics should not be routinely given because of the same problem of invasion by resistant bacteria. They are rarely indicated in equine respiratory disease and should be given only on the advice of your veterinarian. Antibiotics are not usually given unless there are definite signs of an accompanying bacterial infection.

If the animal stops eating for more than two days, your veterinarian should definitely be called. The horse may go into what is called a negative nitrogen balance and may not start eating again without medical assistance. He can go without eating for a couple of days, but beyond that, may need an appetite stimulant and possibly intravenous fluids and amino acids to help get him going again. The horse should absolutely NOT be exercised in any way, shape, or form during the course of the disease.

Recent studies recommend a minimum of a two-week convalescent period AFTER the last symptoms have vanished. Horses who have had severe lung problems may need a longer period to recuperate—in some cases, up to six months. Adequate convalescence is important in preventing chronic bronchitis or emphysema (heaves). This means freedom from exercise and work of any kind. It does NOT mean putting the horse on the hot walker to "keep him in shape"! Failure to completely rest the horse often contributes to having the disease last longer and be more severe than it would otherwise be.

Rest also helps prevent the disease from developing into pneumonia, sinusitis, guttural pouch infection, or other nasty sequel. Most veterinarians have treated these animals and had the owner say that they "had to" ride him in the roping Saturday, or the barrel race at the State Fair, or some other pressing commitment. And we've been called back many times to treat the animal for sinusitis, heaves, or other unpleasant aftereffects of using the animal while he was sick. The point cannot be overemphasized that by trying to use your horse for that one important event when he has an upper respiratory disease, you may be jeopardizing the rest of his useful lifetime. I might also add that other competitors won't appreciate your bringing an infected horse to the event and exposing theirs. In addition, laws prevent interstate shipment of sick animals or those exposed to contagious disease. If you move a sick horse across state lines, you could possibly be subject to legal action.

No drugs any veterinarian can give will make the problem magically go away. Like a human cold, it simply takes time. If you love and value your horse, give him that time. When you start the horse back to work, do so very gradually.

PREVENTION

Two of the upper respiratory diseases are preventable. Vaccines are available for equine viral rhinopheumonitis and influenza.

Two vaccines are commonly used in the United States at this time for "rhino." Pneumabort-K (Fort Dodge Laboratories, Fort Dodge, IA 50501) is a killed vaccine. Rhinomune (Norden Laboratories, Lincoln, NE 68501) is what is referred to as a modified-live virus vaccine. The virus is not killed, but is weakened enough to cause immunity without causing the disease.

Foals should be vaccinated for rhinopneumonitis at three months of age and again a month later. They should be revaccinated around weaning time and yearly thereafter. Nonpregnant mares should be vaccinated before breeding. For young animals and nonpregnant mares, either a killed or a live product may be used. Mares who are pregnant should be vaccinated at 5, 7, and 9 months of pregnancy. My preference for pregnant mares is to use a killed vaccine. The cost of these vaccines is slight when compared with the loss of the foal and the cost of keeping a mare for a year without getting a foal from her.

Many veterinarians alternate between Pneumabort-K and Rhinomune for vaccination of horses other than pregnant mares, feeling that this gives a better overall immunization against the disease.

Reliable vaccine is available for influenza. It should be given to foals about two months of age and again a month later, with a booster when they are weaned, as with rhinopneumonitis. A yearly booster can then be used. Animals who may be frequently exposed (rodeo animals, racehorses, etc.) should have boosters every six months. Many owners routinely give boosters to these horses in midApril and again in October. Others feel that in a racetrack situation, killed influenza vaccines should be given every 2 to 4 months. These animals should be revaccinated within a month prior to going into a high-exposure situation (e.g., racetrack or sales). It has been suggested that immunization of foals prior to 6 months of age is not always effective. (71)

Horses do not get a lasting immunity with any vaccine, so they need to be revaccinated every year after an initial series of two vaccinations about a month apart. Horses with an unknown vaccination history should have two injections a month apart and then a yearly or semiyearly booster, as needed. Animals who are over five years old seem to have some degree of natural resistance to these diseases, but not enough to give reliable protection when the disease sweeps through your stable or neighborhood.

IMPORTANT NOTE: Some horses will become ill or sore if worked after influenza vaccine is administered. Plan to allow a MINIMUM of 48 hours rest after giving this vaccine. Because stiffness or local reaction may occur,

don't give the vaccine immediately before you need the animal for a show or race. These reactions are rare, but can occur. A "catch-22?" Sort of. Your horse may be exposed at an event, yet you forgot to vaccinate him far enough in advance to allow the rest for a couple of days. What to do? If you think the chance of exposure is high, don't take him to the event. He probably wouldn't do well anyway if he's stiff and sore from the vaccination.

Horses who are vaccinated may occasionally get the disease against which they were vaccinated. However, they usually get it much less severely than if they were not vaccinated.

Sanitation and hygiene help to prevent these diseases and their spread. However, do not think that you are home free because you live in the middle of nowhere. One of my Wyoming ranch clients who lived about 35 miles from the nearest town and who had no fence-line horse contact with other ranches lost one year's entire foal crop to rhinopneumonitis. Mare after mare aborted late in pregnancy or had a live, weak foal that died within three days. That was a black spring without any income for this Arabian breeder. It was never determined where the problem came from; it most likely was brought home by one of the mares that they sent to outside stallions to be bred. No signs of previous respiratory infection were seen on the ranch.

With that gloomy note, I will recommend that you provide protection by vaccinating all young animals as soon as they are old enough. Keep up the immunity in older animals. Isolate all animals returning from shows, outside breeding, or the racetrack. Keep them separate and preferably downwind from the other animals. It is a good idea to feed them after you have fed the other animals, and to wash your hands after leaving the quarantine area and before handling any of the "clean" animals. Rubber boots which you can disinfect might not be a bad idea, either. Separate tack should be used on these quarantined horses, especially halters and bridles which are easily contaminated by nasal discharges.

If your animals have fence-line contact with other horses and they are nosing each other regularly, quarantine will probably not accomplish much.

Isolate any mare who aborts to prevent her spreading an infectious agent (if that is indeed the cause of the abortion) to other mares. Clean up any membranes and drainage as well as the aborted foal and dispose of them by deep burial or burning so that dogs, birds, or other scavengers do not eat the carcass and thus perhaps spread the disease. If you have outside mares arriving for breeding, it is well worthwhile quarantining them, the stallion(s), and your own mares which are being bred separately from any mares already in foal. A three-week quarantine should be adequate to show most contagious diseases if they are present.

What about those respiratory diseases for which we

have no vaccine? There are two schools of thought. One says that we should keep the horse isolated from any other horse who coughs, sneezes, or looks cross-eyed. The other says to go ahead and expose him to the problems, let him get over them, develop an immunity, and go from there. This author is in agreement with the second approach. Protect foals and young horses from contagious respiratory problems as much as possible. Because they may not yet be equipped to deal with these diseases, the danger of permanent damage or death is too great.

When they are coming two-year olds, haul them to shows or other events with the rest of your horses. Let them drink out of every common trough and get all the common diseases. Do all this, of course, AFTER they have had all their immunizations against the diseases for which we have vaccines. It can be an inconvenience to deal with a sick two-year old when traveling. Do this in good weather so that rain or snow do not complicate the procedure. In this way, the young horses get over many of the common minor infections and develop some immunity to them, thus avoiding a lot of trouble when you need the animal later in his life for serious showing, performance, or use. Otherwise, Murphy's Law invariably strikes; the animal will get sick when taken to the most important show of the season or to the National Finals in whatever you do with him, even if he's a five-year-old at the time!

PNEUMONIA

Pneumonia, like diarrhea, is uncommon in the horse, but often severe or life-threatening when it does occur. Pneumonia is most commonly a disease of young horses, aged horses, and debilitated animals. In foals and young horses, it is an acute problem. In aged or debilitated horses, it is usually chronic and progressive. Any of the upper respiratory viral diseases can lead to pneumonia. A horse with the sniffles bears watching because of this possibility.

A viral respiratory infection such as influenza or rhinopneumonitis may predispose the animal to pneumonia. Bacterial diseases, such as distemper (strangles), may lead to pneumonia, as can parasitism. Several bacteria specifically cause pneumonia in foals. These can cause large numbers of foals to die or be permanently incapacitated on infected farms. Foals often get pneumonia after they are weakened by scours, navel ill, or joint ill. Overcrowding, poor sanitation, and contaminated feed or water, as well as stress due to weaning or rough handling, may bring on this condition in foals.

Hauling the horse for long distances in an open trailer or truck may start pneumonia. Dusty corrals or stalls may bring it on. Malnutrition weakens the animal and makes him more susceptible to pneumonia. Smoke inhalation, as following a stable fire, often leads to pneumonia, as can the inhalation of irritant chemicals.

When animals are stomach-tubed for worming or some other procedure, putting the drug into the lungs instead of the stomach almost surely will result in pneumonia. This is why I do not recommend that the horse owner attempt to stomach tube his own horse; this procedure is best left to a veterinarian. Aspiration (another name for inhalation) pneumonia may also follow an attempt to drench the horse with mineral oil. He cannot taste the clear, flavorless liquid, and is as likely to inhale it as to swallow it. This kind of foreign, unremovable material in the lungs nearly always results in a severe pneumonia and subsequent death of the animal. Inhalation pneumonia may also occur when a horse who is choked inhales saliva or feedstuffs.

SIGNS

By the time pneumonia develops, the problem which initially caused it may be gone. There may be a clear nasal discharge for a few days to a week before the pneumonia starts without any other unfavorable signs. In foals, a navel or joint infection may be noticed. The horse may have had a recent case of distemper. The horse will have a poor appetite and little energy. He may appear dull or dopey.

Affected animals will have an elevated temperature. It will be at least 102 degrees F (39 degrees C). Some cases will go as high as 104 to 105 degrees F (40 to 40.5 degrees C). These horses usually will sweat profusely. The horse often quits eating, but may still drink a little water. It will be depressed. The pulse rate may be a little above normal. An occasional cough may be heard. The breathing will be more rapid than normal and may be shallow and labored.

Horses with acute pneumonia which goes untreated rarely live more than 96 hours. The prognosis is favorable if treated early. If treatment is delayed or is inadequate, as many as half of the affected horses either die or turn into chronic cases. Chronic cases may require long-term treatment. Emphysema (heaves) often occurs in these animals after they recover from the acute pneumonia.

TREATMENT

Acute pneumonia is an emergency, one in which you should call your veterinarian IMMEDIATELY. Prompt antibiotic and supportive treatment may result in saving an animal who would otherwise be lost. Some antibiotics work better in some geographic areas than others. Your veterinarian will be able to advise you in this matter. If you follow your veterinarian's instructions to the letter and the horse does not improve, be sure to consult with him again. He may then wish to change to another drug.

If you do not have access to a veterinarian, give the animal penicillin/streptomycin mixture, at the rate of 18,000 units of penicillin per pound, intramuscularly. The animal should be treated for an absolute minimum of 7 days, and often as much as 10 days or more. Penicillin is definitely not a cure-all for pneumonia. Indeed, in some areas, other drugs may be immensely more effective. However, it is one of the safest to give until you can get specific veterinary advice on the infection. Be sure not to stop antibiotic treatment as soon as you see improvement because the organisms causing the pneumonia may not be well enough controlled to allow the animal to overcome them. They may then come back with a vengeance and overwhelm the animal with fatal consequences.

As with many serious diseases, nursing and care can make the difference between saving the animal and losing it. A horse with pneumonia should have draft-free quarters. Clean the stall frequently to avoid irritation by ammonia fumes from the animal's urine. Adequate ventilation will help to keep the air fresh and avoid this problem. Do not have the stall so closed that it becomes damp and stuffy. This is more harmful than having a bit of a breeze going through. Good, deep, clean bedding will allow the animal to lie down and relax if he wishes. Blanket the animal during the fever stage and, if the weather is cold, keep him blanketed throughout the disease, if needed.

Clean, palatable feed will help tempt the animal to eat. The horse should have water available at all times. If the animal shows dehydration, your veterinarian may wish to give fluids intravenously. Keeping the horse as close as possible to a normal fluid balance is of the utmost importance in helping to ensure his survival. Favorable signs are: temperature returning to normal, increased alertness, improved appetite, and renewed interest in life. The animal should be rested for a minimum of three to four weeks after apparent recovery from the disease to help avoid relapse, or undesirable aftereffects, such as bronchitis or emphysema (heaves).

PLEURITIS OR PLEURISY

Pleuritis and pleurisy refer to an inflammation of the lining of the chest cavity, called the pleura. You are unlikely to diagnose this condition yourself; these terms are mentioned so that you will know what your veterinarian means if he uses them. He may use these terms in reference to sounds that he hears through a stethoscope. He will hear characteristicly squeaky sounds caused by a lack of normal lubrication between the lining of the chest cavity and the surface of the lungs.

In horses, pleuritis is usually secondary to a respiratory infection or pneumonia. If you could open the chest of a living animal affected with pleuritis, you would find, usually, excess fluid which had been produced in response to the original problem. There would be threads of fibrin; this is the part of the blood which helps to hold a blood clot together. These fibrin threads may, if not treated with care (or if you're unlucky) form adhesions which could bond the outer surface of the lung to the inner side of the chest cavity.

Pleuritis causes severe pain, so the animal may breathe very shallowly and uncomfortably. Horses with pleuritis are often reluctant to move or lie down and, initially, may look as if they have colic. The condition often accompanies pneumonia or other respiratory disease. When pleuritis occurs by itself, it is usually due to an injury such as puncture of the chest cavity caused by a broken rib.

The significance of pleuritis is that if the inflammatory process is allowed to continue with subsequent adhesion formation, the animal may suffer permanent damage and a lessened usefulness. If pleuritis occurs, it is doubly important to heed your veterinarian's instructions and not to exercise or use the animal for a minimum of three to four weeks after all symptoms of the original problem have disappeared. In most cases, pleuritis is just one more indication that the problem your horse has is serious.

THUMPS

"Thumps" refers to a condition involving spasms of the diaphragm. It occurs simultaneously with the horse's heartbeat and is thought to be due to an irritation of the nerve which enervates the diaphragm. You can confirm the presence of thumps by putting one hand on the animal's flank and the other over his heart area, or by listening to his heart with a stethoscope and holding a hand on his flank at the same time.

A horse with thumps will have heavy, labored breathing with such a pounding in the flanks that it appears as if the heart were beating there. The muscular contractions may jerk heavily enough to shake the whole animal.

Thumps are caused by severe exertion, especially in a horse that is not in good physical condition. Thumps are not so important in themselves; they are a sign that the animal is in serious physical distress and should be rested and receive veterinary attention immediately. Many horses will recover from thumps by themselves after they have been rested, but a horse who is stressed sufficiently to cause thumps should be checked for other problems which may occur along with them.

This problem is often seen on trail rides with unconditioned animals—the equine equivalent of the "weekend athlete." On endurance rides, it may be seen after the horses have gone a number of miles. Some horses may have thumps once and never have them again. More commonly, horses who tend to get the thumps will do so again. For this reason, a horse who has had the thumps should be watched more closely than usual when he is worked hard at a later time. He should be conditioned gradually and carefully before being put to hard use. His pulse recovery rates should be carefully monitored to be sure that he is getting into condition. He should have a thorough physical examination to be sure that he is capable of doing the work being asked of him.

HEAVES (EMPHYSEMA)

Heaves is also called chronic pulmonary emphysema, chronic alveolar emphysema, chronic obstructive pulmonary disease (COPD), and broken wind. It is characterized by an expiratory distress; that is, when the horse attempts to breathe out, he is unable to fully empty his lungs. This results in extra effort trying to do so, a heaving motion of the abdomen from which the disease gets its name. Animals who have this disease may have a continuous cough. The cough is a deep, dry, hacking one that seems to come from the bottom of the horse's feet. There is rarely a nasal discharge, and the animal (at least early in the course of the disease) will otherwise look and feel normal. These horses may make a wheezing noise when they breathe, particularly on breathing out.

Both the coughing and wheezing often get worse as the disease progresses. The horse may lack stamina and become thin. A horse with an advanced case of heaves may be almost impossible to keep at a normal weight.

CAUSES

Heaves is usually started by an allergy to something that the horse is inhaling which causes a chronic cough. This cough leads to a chronic bronchitis and then to the lung damage which causes the difficulty with breathing that occurs later in the disease. It is commonly caused by dusty or moldy hay. This problem seems especially bad with alfalfa hay, perhaps because it is more difficult to put up good alfalfa hay than good grass hay (if baled too wet, it molds easily). Or, if it is stored in stacks without shelter, molding may occur when it is rained on after baling. Dusty pens or stalls may initiate the coughing. Dusty straw or other poor quality material used for bedding may start the horse coughing.

Some researchers feel that heaves may be more frequently seen when horses are kept in close contact with chickens, as when chickens use horse stalls for roosting areas, or old chicken coops are used for housing horses. Just because you do not now have chickens may not mean anything if you have an old barn—it could have been used to house them even 20 or 30 years ago and still have material from them in the dust. The condition is felt to be an allergy to chicken dander or the dust that they cause. Thus, it is perhaps a combination of an allergic reaction and irritation from the dust itself. Virus or bacterial infections of the respiratory tract may start the cough that starts the heaves. Extreme exertion, especially if the animal already has a respiratory disease, may lead to this problem.

Whatever the initiating cause, the horse begins coughing. This, in time, causes a chronic bronchitis, which, in a vicious circle, helps to keep the horse coughing. After he has coughed for a period of time, the small air sacs in the lungs, called alveoli, begin to rupture. Their walls break down, leaving less area for absorbing oxygen, leaving the lungs much less efficient. As they break down, relatively large air pockets form in the lungs. These pockets are the cause of the difficulty on expiration and account for the wheezing. Heaves is not a contagious disease, but may be seen in whole groups of horses who are exposed to the same environmental causes. Speaking of causes, smoking is thought to contribute to the development of emphysema in humans, although we don't call it heaves.

SIGNS

When the horse takes a breath, he will often hurry as if gasping for air. His nostrils may be flared. Early in the disease, there may be a slight nasal discharge. The horse has to make an extra effort to try to push the last of the used air out of his lungs in preparation for taking another breath. This produces what we call an "expiratory lift." If you watch one of these horses closely, you first see him breathe out. After he has finished a breath (before he inhales the next one), he will make an extra push upward with his abdominal muscles. These belly muscles are used to help expel the air from the animal's lungs. After a period of time, this continued effort thickens these muscles into a ridge along the lower side of the abdomen. This ridge is called a "heave line." In a severe case, this muscular ridge may be extremely thick and prominent. The ribs may be permanently rolled forward, giving the appearance of an enlarged chest cavity.

The horse with advanced heaves falls into a breathing rhythm: gulp a breath of air (quickly); breathe out (slowly); and push (and often wheeze or grunt at the same time). While a nasal discharge is rare in an early case of the heaves, a small, constant amount is commonly seen in advanced cases. The cough is still observed, but may get weaker and less deep at the disease advances. It may be worse after feeding the grain ration.

Heaves is usually a progressive disease. It is very similar to smoker's cough in humans. If a person smokes enough for long enough, he may develop chronic emphysema, with loss of strength, wheezing, shortness of breath, and a continued cough even if he has stopped smoking. This is due to the chronic bronchitis which he has developed. Horses go along the same course: they start coughing, get bronchitis going, and then continue to cough. The disease may appear to be worse at some times of the year than others. It is often worst in hot, dry weather and will be more severe when the horse's surroundings are dusty.

Early cases of heaves may be difficult to diagnose, even for your veterinarian, because they look much like other respiratory diseases. Heaves is a good bet if you have several horses and only one is affected, especially if the affected animal is an older one—say, 10 years or older. It is also a likely diagnosis if you have been feeding dusty or moldy hay, if the weather has been exceptionally hot or dry, or if you are keeping your horse with chickens or in an area where they have been. Heaves is also probable if the horse has coughed for a week or more with little or no nasal discharge and is otherwise feeling bright and well.

Horses with heaves usually have a normal temperature. In an advanced case, your veterinarian will be able to hear a characteristic sound through the stethoscope. It really can't be described in words so that you could know it when you heard it. But, once you hear it, there's no mistaking it. This sound and/or the heave line give a positive diagnosis of heaves. The wheezing noise is also very characteristic. When you buy a horse, take him out and work him hard enough to sweat him and get him to breathing hard. If you hear any wheezing, you should have the animal checked by a veterinarian to see what is causing the noise before you buy him.

Lungworm infection in the horse looks exactly like heaves. Tests used for cattle lungworms do not detect the worms in the horse, so it can be very difficult to determine whether this problem is present. These worms are not considered common.

Animals who are excessively fat and/or have large hay or grass bellies may make sounds similar to heaves or roaring when they are worked. This type of animal should either be examined by a veterinarian with a stethoscope or rechecked when he has slimmed down to a normal size and weight and is in better physical condition. Wheezing may be entirely due to the fact that the animal is overweight and out of shape. A horse who is ridden with his head pulled hard into his chest and his neck arched may wheeze or whistle. This noise is easily distinguished because it goes away as soon as the animal's head and neck are allowed to move freely.

TREATMENT

How do you cure heaves? The answer is that you don't, no more than a smoker with emphysema can undo the damage which has already occurred. This is not to say that nothing can be done for the animal, or that they are not usable. The only thing that can be done, however, is to manage the disease so that it does not get any worse. If the horse has a mild case, you may keep it at the same stage of development for a prolonged period of time. One of my mares had a mild case when I purchased her at seven years of age; the condition was kept static so that she had not gotten any worse by the time she was sold at 14. The mare was used hard during this period. Animals with a mild case, given careful management, can lead useful, productive lives. While you should not normally purchase an animal with heaves (even though I did), except perhaps as a breeding animal, there is no reason why you should not treat and continue to use an animal that you already own.

The very best treatment is to get the animal out on a good, clean pasture. My mare, for instance, never coughed when out on pasture. When brought into the corral and fed hay, she could go about four days before the cough started. Then, it would persist the entire time she was fed hay. Many horses with heaves lead long, useful lives if they are kept on pasture all the time.

If the animal is just starting a case of heaves, dampen the hay when you feed it—with a nozzle on a garden hose or with a watering can. Better yet, put the hay in a hay net and completely immerse it in a tub for five to ten minutes until it is soaked. Soak it until it's dripping wet, throughout. Most horses do not like wet hay, but given a bit of time, they get used to it. It is necessary to clean out any leftover feed at the next feeding, since the wet hay is more prone to mold or spoil than dry hay. If the grain is dusty, dampen it lightly, too. A lightly molasses-treated grain isn't dusty, but be careful not to let your horse get fat if you use it.

If this does not control the cough, the next step is to feed one of the anticough products which are available. You may be able to get one from your feed store or veterinarian. If it looks as if your horse is going to be on them for a long period of time, try them all. In general, the syrups are more powerful, but cannot usually be used for long periods of time. They are also much more expensive than powders. The powders give less cough control, but may be enough after you get the cough slowed down with a syrup. Powders are generally less expensive than syrups and some of them can be fed indefinitely. Read the label for recommendations regarding length of feeding, or consult your veterinarian for this information. Some animals, if they are being kept in and fed hay, will have to have one of these preparations every day in order to not cough and to be usable. If damp hay plus cough powder does not give enough control for the confined horse, you may need to feed alfalfa cubes or a complete pelleted feed (see Feeds). Some people recommend that hay cubes also be soaked before feeding, as with hay.

Chronic lung infections may be a component of some respiratory problems diagnosed as heaves. Some veterinarians start horses who are diagnosed as having heaves, on a course of antibiotics. Penicillin/streptomycin is one antibiotic which is commonly recommended. It should be given for 5 to 7 days (see Penicillin). Cough suppressants should be given at the same time.

If you have a horse with both heaves and laminitis (founder), you have a problem. The horse will go lame if you put him out on green pasture; he will cough if you keep him in and feed him hay. The best solution for this situation is to keep him in and feed hay cubes or a pelleted feed (or trade him in on a new model).

As with most diseases, the best cure is not to develop the problem in the first place. The best prevention is to keep the horse on pasture rather than keeping him in and feeding him hay. If you must confine the horse, keep him in dust-free surroundings. Feed good quality, mold-free and dust-free hay. If the hay shows any signs of dust or mold, dampen it before you feed it so that the mold does not fluff up into the horse's nose as he eats. If you are unable to obtain quality legume hay, feed grass hay instead. If the grass hay is not up to par nutritionally, supplement it with grain and a vitamin/mineral mixture if necessary, rather than feeding a nutritionally better but dusty or moldy alfalfa hay.

If you have a horse who is out of condition, start him to work gradually. Do not force him to work hard until he is back into condition. Do not make a horse work for any reason if he is coughing. Allow adequate recovery time after upper respiratory diseases, such as influenza and rhinopneumonitis. Waiting two weeks after he has STOPPED coughing is none too much; three to four weeks is even better. These measures help to prevent the chronic cough and bronchitis that can later become heaves.

SUMMER PASTURE-ASSOCIATED OBSTRUCTIVE PULMONARY DISEASE

A problem which looks exactly like heaves has been seen in Louisiana, Florida, Georgia, and Mississippi. The big difference is that it occurs in the summer when the animals are on pasture. It has been called "summer pasture-associated obstructive pulmonary disease" (SOPD). While the exact cause is not known, it is currently thought to be due to certain compounds in lush feeds which act to constrict the bronchial passages. The constriction may be caused by an allergic reaction, or the compounds may act directly on the passages to produce the constriction.

Many animals affected with this problem will become normal within a week to ten days after being removed from the offending pasture. Treatment consists of removing the animal from the pasture and treating with drugs to help reduce the cough and to decrease any allergic reaction, much as for heaves.

Chapter 15

THE DIGESTIVE SYSTEM

Normal Teeth
Examining the Horse's Mouth
Ageing the Horse
Signs of Tooth Problems
Congenital Mouth Defects
Other Dental Problems
  Retained Caps
  Retained Incisors
  Retained Temporary Premolars
  Wave Mouth
  Smooth Mouth
Mouth Injuries and Fractures
Miscellaneous Mouth Problems
Lampas
Choke
Vomiting
Colic
  Chronic Colic
  Sand Colic
Diarrhea
  Foal Diarrhea (Scours)
  Protozoal Diarrhea
  Mycotic Diarrhea
  Virus Diarrhea
  Diarrhea Caused by Water
  Diarrhea Due to Other Causes
Colitis-X (Salmonellosis)

NORMAL TEETH

The horse has two sets of teeth. The baby teeth, often called "milk teeth," begin to erupt during the first week of life. Some of these teeth are in use as long as 4–1/2 years. The permanent, adult teeth begin to come into the jaw in the molar area first, at 10 to 12 months of age. The last ones are in place around 5 years of age. Unlike human teeth, equine teeth are not susceptible to decay. However, they can suffer breakage and other damage.

The teeth in the front of the mouth are called incisors. These do the heavy work of grazing. Then, there is a space, called the "bars." This is where the bit rests. In most mares, this space is about four inches long before the rear (cheek) teeth begin. Stallions and geldings have a small stub of a canine tooth on each side, usually in both the upper and lower jaws. This tooth is located in the middle of the bars.

The first permanent upper premolar is commonly called the "wolf tooth." It is a small stub of a tooth that your horse may or may not have. This tooth is the remnant of what in prehistoric times was another full-sized molar; it is gradually disappearing in the evolution of the horse, much as our wisdom teeth are doing. It occurs just ahead of the main section of strong rear grinding teeth (the molars and premolars). A wolf tooth is usually just a nubbin. It may, however, cause the horse considerable discomfort if it is bumped by a bit. If your horse is tossing his head when you put a bit on him, look for this tooth. If it is present, consult with your veterinarian regarding its removal. This is a common cause of head-tossing on the racetrack. Trainers invariably have these teeth removed, thus effectively removing the problem.

The remaining cheek teeth are divided between premolars and molars. They do the serious grinding, getting the horse's roughage and grain ready for swallowing.

All the permanent teeth of the horse (except the canines) are continuously erupting. They start as long teeth, extending four or more inches into the upper and lower jaw bones. As the surfaces are worn off, the teeth are pushed upward by slow growth of bone under them, keeping a constant tooth level.

When a tooth is lost or removed, the tooth from the opposite jaw will grow into the space, becoming very much longer than the others. This process can greatly hamper chewing. Animals with this condition may become very thin. Once a tooth is discovered to be without its opposite, plans should be made to trim the tooth once or twice a year. If it is done frequently, your veterinarian may be able to remove the growth rather simply with a dental float. If you let it go, the animal may have to be sedated, and the extra tooth clipped off with a large pair of molar cutters.

Another peculiarity of equine teeth is that the upper and lower rows are not directly opposite each other. The upper teeth are spaced slightly farther apart than the lower ones. This allows a side-to-side grinding, shearing motion. Careful chewing is important to a beast who eats roughage but does not get a second chance to chew it. This is compared to the cow who at her leisure regurgitates her food and rechews it in the form of a cud.

This grinding action causes the pattern of wear which makes horses' teeth form points and hooks, parts of the teeth that are not evenly worn down. If the sharp spur is on the front of the first upper premolar, it is called a hook. If it is along the side of the teeth (the outer side of the upper teeth or the inner side of the lower teeth), it is called a point (or, more usually, "points"). These sharp protrusions may cut the animal's cheek or tongue, causing raw and painful sores. This will cause the animal considerable discomfort when he is eating and may also cause it to throw its head when a bit is used. The term "hooks" is also used to refer to a sharp angle on the back of the upper corner incisor. These hooks help, at certain stages, to indicate the animal's age, but do not generally cause problems.

If allowed to grow to great length, the points may make the animal unable to grind efficiently, and often accounts for an older horse being thin. Any horse above about seven years of age should have his teeth checked once a year and floated if necessary. Floating is done by your veterinarian with an instrument that looks like a chunk of wood rasp on a long handle. Or, it may be a chip of metal with tungsten carbide flakes applied to one surface. He will grind off the sharp points and hooks. He will NOT grind the surface of the teeth flat. The chewing surface is not meant to be flat. It is meant to be at an angle. If you grind it flat, the animal would be nearly unable to chew!!

A horse older than about 14 should definitely be checked every year. Regular attention to the teeth will do more to help an older animal than almost anything else that you can do for him. This is especially important if the animal is out on pasture and expected to scrounge his own feed throughout the winter. Check all your horses' teeth before autumn and have them floated, if necessary,

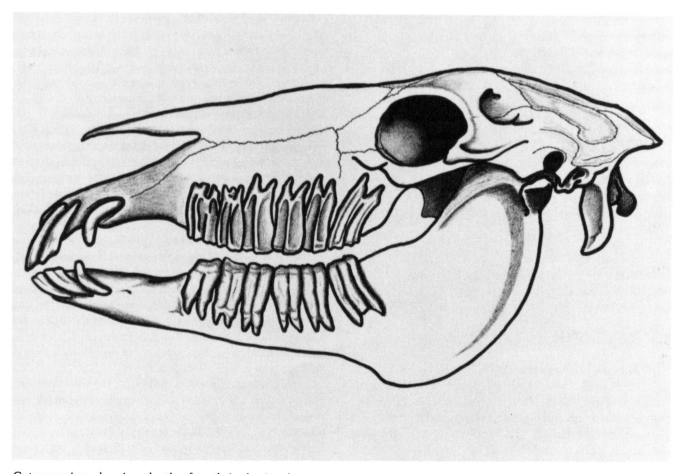

Cutaway view showing depth of teeth in the jaw bones.

to help insure that they will come through the winter in good condition.

When buying a horse, examine his teeth. Look for the animal's age, as well as the general condition of the teeth. Check for the proper angle of the cutting surfaces. Also look for abnormalities, such as parrot mouth, or shear or wave mouth (in which the grinding surfaces of the rear teeth, instead of being level from front to back, dip up and down like an ocean wave). Wave mouth is both abnormal and inefficient. It is also nearly impossible to correct. An animal with a severe case of wave mouth may need to be fed special feed.

Special feed may also be needed by very old horses. The teeth continue to wear and when their length is used up, the stubs fall out. This occurs between 25 and 30 years of age. This will leave sizeable gaps in the grinding surface and severely reduce the efficiency of the animal's chewing. He will need to be fed the best quality feed. Try feeding a very fine-stemmed, leafy alfalfa hay. If this is not available, the most efficient solution may be to go to a complete, pelleted feed. It is usually best to get it in the largest pellets available, but try all the sizes you can get and buy the one that the animal seems best able to handle. With a

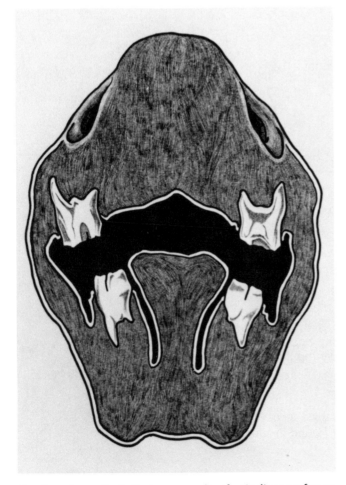

Section through skull shows angle of grinding surfaces.

bit of extra care, the elderly horse may continue to give years of companionship and pleasure.

EXAMINING THE HORSE'S MOUTH

Begin examining the horse's dental equipment by looking at him from the outside. Are there any draining tracts or sores on the face? Lumps on the jaw bone— upper or lower? Run your fingers along the outside of the face where the upper teeth overlap the lower ones. Both hooks and points may often be felt in this manner. Smell his breath. Does he have bad breath or any rotten or infected odors? Is there any drainage from the mouth or nostrils? Now proceed to examine the inside of his mouth.

Most horses do not like to have their mouths opened or handled. But because the horse's teeth are so important to his health and well-being, it is important that the animal allow them to be examined. Training is best started when the foal is only a few days old and is being halter broken and otherwise trained. While you are working with him, teach him to allow you to put your fingers in his mouth and let you open his mouth and hold it gently open. Work with him easily so as not to frighten or hurt him and he will soon accept this handling as normal. Then, do it once or twice a month from then on to keep him in training for it. In addition to making it easier for you or the veterinarian to handle him and check his teeth, there is the added bonus in that the horse usually accepts the bit more easily when his education reaches that point.

For a full dental examination, the animal should be positioned so that he is facing a bright light, or a strong flashlight should be available. Facing the animal toward the sunlight is usually adequate for examination outdoors. The mouth should be rinsed with a dose syringe and lukewarm water to clean out any hay or grain. This allows problems to be more easily seen. If the animal shows any pain when his mouth is rinsed, make a note of this so that you can tell your veterinarian. Dental examinations are enough trouble that they are worth doing right the first time.

If you are dealing with an older horse whose mouth must be examined, you do not have the advantage of gradual training. He may already have bad habits. Try to restrain him as little as possible and handle him as gently as you can. Work slowly and carefully. Make sure that the halter you put on an animal for a dental examination has plenty of room in the noseband area. It is impossible for the animal to cooperate with you and open his mouth if the halter is clamping it tightly shut.

If the horse protests too strongly about being examined, it may be necessary to tranquilize or otherwise sedate him. It is often useful to put the animal into crossties or a good set of stocks. There is a very real danger to the person checking the teeth that the horse may strike him with a front foot. Indeed, these blows can be fatal.

AGEING THE HORSE

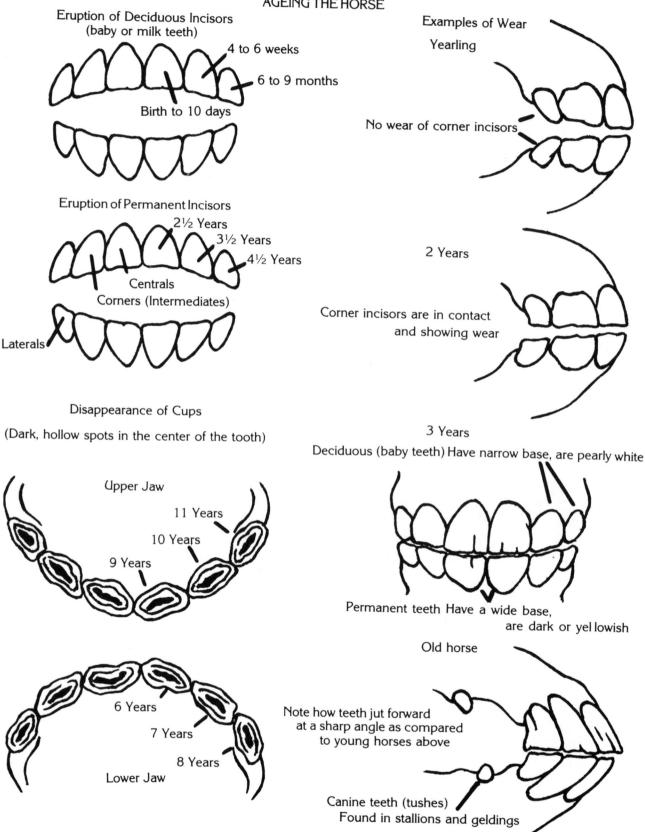

Eruption of Deciduous Incisors (baby or milk teeth)

4 to 6 weeks

6 to 9 months

Birth to 10 days

Examples of Wear

Yearling

No wear of corner incisors

Eruption of Permanent Incisors

2½ Years

3½ Years

4½ Years

Centrals

Corners (Intermediates)

Laterals

2 Years

Corner incisors are in contact and showing wear

Disappearance of Cups

(Dark, hollow spots in the center of the tooth)

3 Years

Deciduous (baby teeth) Have narrow base, are pearly white

Upper Jaw

11 Years

10 Years

9 Years

Permanent teeth Have a wide base, are dark or yellowish

6 Years

7 Years

8 Years

Lower Jaw

Old horse

Note how teeth jut forward at a sharp angle as compared to young horses above

Canine teeth (tushes) Found in stallions and geldings

Change of Shape of Lower Incisor Surfaces with Age

Galvayne's Groove

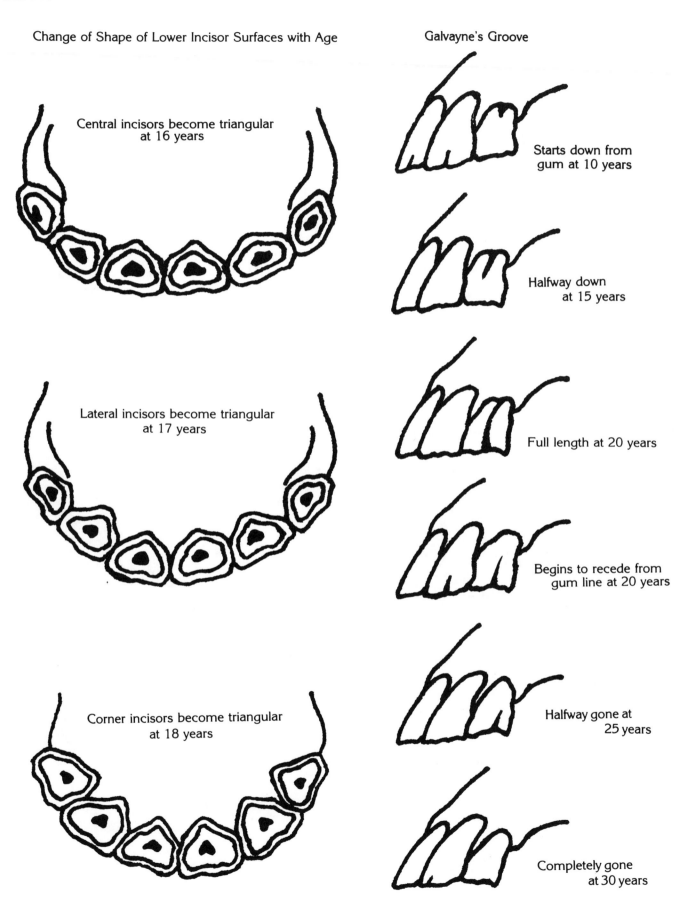

Central incisors become triangular
at 16 years

Lateral incisors become triangular
at 17 years

Corner incisors become triangular
at 18 years

Starts down from
gum at 10 years

Halfway down
at 15 years

Full length at 20 years

Begins to recede from
gum line at 20 years

Halfway gone at
25 years

Completely gone
at 30 years

Even a normally well-mannered horse may object to having his mouth opened and his teeth examined. So, take precautions to guard against being hurt. If you have no good way to restrain the horse, take a horse blanket (preferably a heavy quilted one with a closed neck), and put it over the animal's head. Allow the main part of the blanket to dangle in front of the horse's forelegs like an apron. This will give considerable protection against being struck. Some horses will stand for a dental examination if a twitch or lip chain is applied; for others, this only makes them fight harder. Use as little restraint as possible, but use enough to be safe.

Begin to open the animal's mouth by working your fingers into the corner of his mouth. Some people like to wear leather gloves because it allows them to grip the tongue more easily and there is less likelihood of its slipping from their grasp. Begin by putting your fingers in through the space between the front and back teeth. In mares this is especially easy because there is no canine tooth. In geldings and stallions, a sharp canine tooth is present in this interdental space, and it is necessary to work around it to avoid being gouged.

Gently grasp the horse's tongue and pull it out of the side of his mouth. If you are pulling it out of the left side of the horse's mouth, you can then step around to the front of the horse (still holding the tongue out the left side). From this position, you can examine the front teeth and the rear teeth on the right side. When you have finished checking these teeth, step to the horse's right side. Keep your grasp on his tongue, but do not pull excessively hard. Switch the tongue so that it is now pulled out the right side of his mouth. This will allow you to examine the rear teeth on the left side. You are looking for hooks or points and other abnormalities, such as uneven wear surfaces, broken or missing teeth, or teeth that are abnormally long.

Some people like to use a speculum, which is a device to hold the animal's mouth open. There are several kinds on the market, ranging from a simple wedge with a handle on it to full lever-action gadgets that strap on the horse's head and mechanically prop his mouth open. These are not good for two reasons. It seems that the horses fight more when one is used, and they are big, heavy pieces of metal which become dangerous projectiles if a strap should break or they otherwise come loose as the animal swings his head. This can result in injury to the examiner or his assistant.

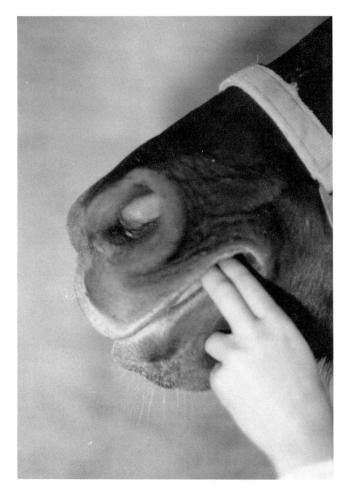

Opening the horse's mouth.

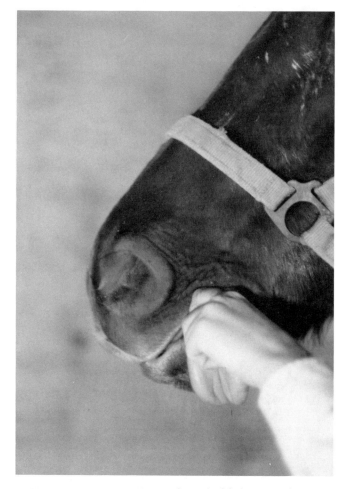

Pulling the tongue to one side to hold the mouth open.

If abnormalities are seen, contact your veterinarian for treatment. Points and hooks are removed with a float (dental rasp). X-rays may be necessary to help determine how badly a tooth is damaged or whether there are problems with the underlying jaw bone. Trimming excessively long teeth or removing broken teeth are major surgical procedures and often require that the animal be totally anesthetized.

SIGNS OF TOOTH PROBLEMS

One of the most common signs of dental problems in the horse is called "quidding." The horse spits out balls of roughage or hay as he eats, dropping these half-chewed green wads around the feeder and on the ground. The horse may accumulate a wad of food in his cheek between it and the cheek teeth. He may also dribble grain from his mouth, spraying large amounts of it around as he chews. If you have a grain dribbler, have his teeth checked. If you find that they are normal, then the dribbling is probably just a habit with that individual animal. Others will drool saliva.

Some animals with tooth pain will appear to eat more slowly and carefully than normal. Others will eat their hay, but leave grain. Animals with tender teeth occasionally refuse to eat and may also refuse to drink cold water. They may show pain when the mouth is rinsed with cold water. A horse with a toothache may suddenly stop chewing, throw his head to one side and slightly open his mouth, acting as if a sharp object had punctured the mouth. When held to the side, the affected side is often held upward. A horse with a sore tooth may pull to one side while being ridden with a bit in his mouth. If you do not find anything on examination, the animal should be checked further by your veterinarian to determine which tooth is affected and what should be done about it.

CONGENITAL MOUTH DEFECTS

1) Cleft Palate
This is a congenital abnormality that is occasionally seen in foals. In a small number of cases, the defect is definitely hereditary. (72) In other cases, there is some evidence that intake of some toxic agent by the pregnant mare, or some virus infections during pregnancy may cause it. Other causes include exposure to radiation and vitamin or hormone deficiencies.

Milk is noticed to drip from the foal's nostrils when he attempts to nurse. The foal may get aspiration pneumonia from inhaling milk. If you open the mouth and examine the palate (roof of the mouth), the defect will be seen. Cleft lips may occur along with the cleft palate and may cause difficulty in suckling. In extremely valuable animals, surgical correction is often attempted. This is usually more successful if done before the foal is six to eight weeks old. The ethics of this are questionable when hereditary problems are involved due to the possibility of the animal passing the defect on to its offspring.

2) Parrot Mouth and Undershot Jaw
Animals with these conditions have front teeth which do not meet as they should but overlap. In parrot mouth, the upper teeth lap over the lower ones, like a parrot's beak. With undershot jaw, the lower teeth protrude past the upper ones, jutting out sharply.

Either problem keeps the animal from grazing efficiently. When such an animal is put on pasture, it may stay extremely thin and be malnourished. These are hereditary defects. Animals with parrot mouth or undershot jaw should not be used as breeding animals. Ideally, they should be castrated or spayed so there is no temptation to use them for breeding.

There are no cures for these congenital conditions. All that can be done is to manage the animal as well as possible. Keeping the animal in a stall or corral and feeding him nutritious feed will usually allow him to live a perfectly normal life. Indeed, it is probable no one will know that he has the problem without looking at his teeth as long as the animal is not expected to scrounge for himself in pasture.

If you are buying an animal who is definitely going to be kept in a stall all of his life and not used as a breeding animal, the fact that he has a parrot mouth may be totally irrelevant. What is, in fact, an unsoundness for a breeding animal or animal who is to be kept on a pasture is no more than an inconvenience for a performance horse who is valued for what he can do and is never out of a stall. Be warned, however, that the condition may reduce the resale value of the animal. Like a dent in the fender of a car, it is less than perfect; it's up to you to decide if you want a "dented fender" or not!

The teeth on a parrot-mouthed horse should be checked from time to time, as the lower teeth may become long enough to bruise the upper jaw. If this occurs, call your veterinarian to have the teeth trimmed to a normal length.

OTHER DENTAL PROBLEMS

Mechanical irritation and infections due to grass awns or other plant material may be seen. These are discussed elsewhere (see Poisonous Plants).

RETAINED CAPS

This is the name given to the condition that occurs when the baby teeth in the cheek area are not shed when they should be. The temporary tooth sits on top of the permanent tooth and prevents it from erupting from the gum as it should. Or, the cap may stay firmly attached to the top of the tooth so that it grows upward with the permanent tooth. The retained cap may fit so closely that a line of separation cannot be felt. You may be able to move the cap if it is loose. Once you are sure that the problem is a cap, it can often be popped loose with a screwdriver. This works best on upper teeth. A pair of pliers will work better if the tooth is a lower one.

Once you have removed the cap, examine it to see that it is not broken. If it shows signs of breakage, this means that you have left part of the tooth in the jaw. This may cause the animal considerable pain and may also cause the permanent tooth to grow crooked. If this occurs, call your veterinarian to sedate the animal and remove the offending piece of tooth. Also, call the veterinarian if the animal needs to be tranquilized to do the job, or if you are unsure of what to do. These problems usually occur in animals under the age of five, but may rarely be noted in older horses. Removing these teeth if they fail to pop out by themselves will help to insure that the permanent teeth can grow in normally. No training time will be lost due to teeth interfering with the bit, or pain when the animal is chewing.

RETAINED INCISORS

These are retained caps which occur on the front teeth (the incisors). These teeth may remain firmly embedded in the jaw, with the permanent teeth attempting to grow in behind them. If they are not removed, they may cause the permanent teeth to grow crooked, and cause severe problems with the bite as these teeth become solidly set. Indeed, you can cause an animal to have a sort of parrot mouth by inattention to this problem.

If you check the animal and the permanent teeth are well grown in, with the deciduous teeth still present behind them, try gently to move the baby tooth. If you cannot remove it easily, this is generally a job for your veterinarian. He will sedate the animal and then use a special instrument called an elevator to loosen the tooth and prepare it for removal. This instrument helps him to undermine the tooth to make sure that he gets the whole root. This is why you do not just want to pull on this sort of tooth with a pair of pliers (nope, it's no place for a string on a doorknob!). Occasionally, the veterinarian will have to make a slit in the gum and remove the fragments that remain. You can see from this that removing caps on the incisors is not usually a do-it-yourself procedure!

RETAINED TEMPORARY PREMOLARS

This problem occurs with the first few of the cheek teeth (called premolars). It is similar to the retained caps, as above. It most commonly seen in animals 2–1/2 to 3 years old, but may occasionally be seen in older animals. It most commonly affects the first lower premolar (the first of the cheek teeth). The failure of this cap to fall off can be

seen by a bony enlargement on the lower surface of the jaw. This is especially prominent in Arabians and finely-boned animals of other breeds who have less mass of jawbone to hide the problem. This lump can also be caused by a root-canal-type infection or a cavity, but these are uncommon, especially in this age group. In the absence of other signs of discomfort or pain, the lump should be considered to be caused by a retained cap and treated accordingly.

Treatment is as mentioned above for retained caps. The cap can usually be removed with the horse standing and twitched. Occasionally, the cap does not come off easily. In this case, call your veterinarian as he may need to sedate the animal, or even lay him down. He will possibly need to make an incision and loosen the tooth with a root elevator as described above.

Retained caps in any location usually occur in pairs. If you find one, look on the opposite side of the mouth for another. If they are left in place, they may cause abnormal growth of the permanent teeth. The permanent tooth becomes impacted, much as do our wisdom teeth. The permanent tooth may then need to be removed.

Serious horse dentistry is a job for your veterinarian.

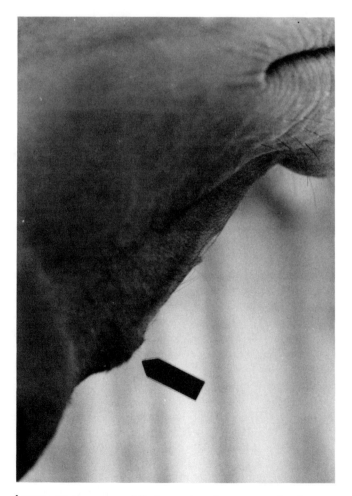

Lump on two-year-old's lower jaw from a retained cap.

He will sedate the animal or may anesthetize the horse totally. If the tooth is in the upper jaw, he may trephine (a fancy name for cutting or chipping) a hole in the skull. He will then take a mallet and punch and remove the offending tooth. It's tough to use finesse when you're dealing with something as large and as well attached as a horse's tooth. If the tooth is in the lower jaw, he will chip the bone away from the base of the tooth and proceed in the same manner.

If you have a tooth removed from a horse, remember that the tooth opposite it will no longer be ground off properly. The animal will need to have the tooth floated or clipped once or twice yearly for the rest of his life. And that's definitely one of those things that's easier to maintain than to let go and try to fix later.

WAVE MOUTH

This condition results from uneven wear on the grinding surfaces of the molars and premolars. The surface, instead of being level from front to rear, undulates like an ocean wave. Mild cases may be helped somewhat by floating. Severe cases may have so uneven a surface that one set of teeth is totally worn down, and the other protrudes enough to gash the gum. This may cause severe pain and infection. These animals may be helped a bit by cutting off the offending teeth so they do not cut the opposite jaw. When wave mouth is this severe, it seems to recur even if the teeth are floated and clipped back to nearly normal. It seems to be somewhat like trying to balance a tire with a bump on it: it works for a while, and then gets back out of balance again.

SMOOTH MOUTH

This is usually found in old animals, but occasionally occurs in young horses. The grinding surfaces of the teeth have become flattened because of severe wear or because they are congenitally defective. The animal may be thin and often is more prone to colic. It can be caused by improper floating in which the person doing it removed too much material, thus creating the problem. The teeth should NEVER be ground level from side to side when they are floated.

An animal with a smooth mouth will need to be fed chopped roughage and soft mashes, or a complete pelleted feed. If it is a younger animal, this diet may give the teeth a chance to reestablish their proper angle and rough cutting surfaces.

The term "smooth mouth" is also used to refer to horses over 11 to 12 years of age. The small central hollows in the permanent teeth, called "cups," have worn off the surface of the upper and lower incisors. The animal's age can no longer be told with great accuracy. Old-time horse traders used to grind new hollows into these teeth and darken them to make the horse appear younger than he was. The shape of the teeth differentiates them from those of a young horse because the incisors become more triangular as the animal ages.

MOUTH INJURIES AND FRACTURES

Injuries and fractures of the mouth are most commonly due to accidents. Horse trailer accidents can cause this sort of injury, as can an animal being thrown from a stock rack on a pickup. Being kicked by another horse occasionally causes damage to the mouth. This often occurs when a stallion is breeding a mare who is not properly restrained (or is being pasture bred). Mouth injury can also be caused by the horse falling and landing on his mouth, or running into a fence or wall.

Any time that a horse is injured around the head, it is worth opening his mouth and checking to see that he does not have any jaw fractures or cracked teeth. Part his lips and examine the teeth and gums. Look for cracks on the teeth. Push on the teeth to see if any are loosened and look for any misalignment of teeth or jaw.

Large bluish or purple bruises on the gums may be a clue that a fracture is present. See if you can wiggle any part of the jaw bone. If you can, get the animal to a veterinarian as soon as possible. Broken jaws can often be wired back together or pinned, saving the animal. Also, after such an injury, make sure the animal continues eating. Refusal to eat should warn you to call your veterinarian and possibly have the animal sedated and examined very thoroughly. If any teeth are broken, you should also call your veterinarian, even if it appears that it is broken off deeply into the gums. Part of the root may be left in the jaw, and will cause infection and complications if not removed.

MISCELLANEOUS MOUTH PROBLEMS

Other mouth problems are seen, but they are rare. An older horse may develop a tumor or tumors in the mouth. Some older horses who have lost one or more teeth (especially the front ones) will have the roof of the mouth grow forward and downward, forming a bulging pad which looks much like a tumor. Have this sort of problem checked so that it can be treated if it turns out to be a tumor.

Horses do get infections resembling cavities in humans, but these are infrequent. These are usually noticed by their foul smell. Indeed, any foul smell coming from the mouth should alert you to check the horse carefully and call your vet if you cannot determine a cause for it. Reluctance of the horse to eat is another clue that further attention is needed. The development of lumps or knots on the jawbone or any area of the upper jaw near the teeth is also a clue to examine the animal further.

LAMPAS

The hard palate ends in a ridge just behind the upper incisors. Some old-timers decided this was a swelling due to "bad blood," and called it "lampas" or "lampers." They insist that this ridge is a disease and "cure" it by scraping or scarifying it with a sharp knife. This ridge of mucous membrane is NORMAL, and it is normal for it to be filled with blood when the animal is eating. At that time, it may even project below the level of the teeth. The same swelling may occur when the horse is cutting teeth, or if he has gotten foxtails or other grass awns into the roof of his mouth or around his teeth. If the grass awns are causing the problem, removing them will cure it. If not, nothing is to be gained by cauterizing, cutting, or otherwise injuring the membrane which is not diseased in the first place.

CHOKE

Horses most commonly choke on dry grain which they have eaten too rapidly. The grain is not well chewed or mixed with enough saliva. It gets part way down the esophagus and stops. The animal continues to eat, packing more grain on top of that he has already eaten. This is complicated by the fact that the lower part of the esophagus is very thick and narrow, making it relatively easy for dry or lumpy food to catch there. The same thing may happen if bran is fed dry. It should be dampened when fed to avoid this problem, unless well mixed with other grain.

Occasionally, horses will choke on hay, potatoes, or other root crops, or on an ear of corn or an apple. Wheat or oat chaff may also cause choke. Dry, pelleted feeds may cause choke, especially if the horse gulps them rapidly. If the animal is startled by a human or dog when feeding on one of these feeds, choke may occur. If left to themselves, these animals very rarely attempt to swallow an object until it is sufficiently chewed. Lawn clippings used as feed may cause a choke because they are fine and short-chopped, and the horse does not chew and mix them with adequate saliva. The saliva provides lubrication for the food as it travels down the esophagus.

Choke may be secondary to existing damage to the esophagus from previous injury or inflammation, or from a constriction which gives the grain or other material a place to catch.

SIGNS

Symptoms of choke vary somewhat with the location. If the choke is high in the esophagus, the animal will be in great distress; he will usually have rapid respiration and frequent cough, together with excessive salivation, sweating, trembling, or stamping the forefeet. The abdomen may become distended with gas. Often, the object causing the choke may be felt by running the hand down the upper part of the neck.

If the choke is located lower in the esophagus, it is still often possible to palpate it along the animal's neck. Here, the signs are not usually so severe. The animal will occasionally draw himself up, arch his neck, and act as if he wished to vomit. He may swallow repeatedly. He may make chewing movements. Here, too, the abdomen may be filled with gas.

If the choke is located in the chest, the symptoms are still less severe. Feed and water may run from the mouth after the animal has taken a few swallows. There may be some symptoms of distress, with coughing and occasional attempts to vomit. Again, the abdomen may appear to be full of gas.

Sometimes choking horses will groan. The facial expression may appear anxious and the eyes may be bloodshot. In any choke, food and saliva may be regurgitated through the nostrils. The animal may paw or stamp his feet and get up and down, generally showing signs of distress. Within a short period of time, the animal may calm down and relax. If the choke occurs in a nursing foal, milk may run from the nostrils.

If the problem goes on for more than a day or so, there is great danger that pressure from the blockage will cause the death of the lining of the esophagus. If this occurs, the animal may have scarring and constriction in that area even after the choke is relieved. He will be more susceptible to choke for the rest of his life because of the narrowing of the passageway. If the animal inhales any of the material which has come back up into the throat, inhalation pneumonia may result.

TREATMENT

Cases of choke occasionally clear up by themselves in horses as the obstruction is softened by saliva. Make sure the animal has water available, but do not give him any food or allow him to graze. If the choke has not cleared within a few minutes, call your veterinarian. He will probably treat it with relaxants and sedatives. If the choke is due to grain, he may pass a stomach tube down the horse and flush the grain out. If the choke persists, surgery may, in rare cases, be necessary. Surgery is very likely to leave a stricture (small, inflexible area) that will make the horse more likely to choke again in the future.

The signs of choke may mimic those of rabies. For this reason, it is important NOT to put your hand into the animal's mouth or down his throat unless the cause of the choke is obvious, such as a horse in an orchard who has swallowed an apple. When a choke is promptly relieved without complications, the prognosis is good.

Horses who have had choke should not be fed pellets, as they may easily cause an obstruction in the esophagus. Allowing the animal to graze, free-choice, on grass, is perhaps the best permanent management for a horse who is prone to choke. Animals who are greedy eaters should have large rocks put in their feeders to slow them down as they eat. Making the animal graze for a living will accomplish the same thing.

VOMITING

Vomiting is difficult for the horse for several reasons. One is that the stomach is small and does not lie on the floor of the abdominal cavity so that when the abdomen is forcibly contracted, it does not press upon it directly as it does in many other animals. In addition, there is a loose fold of mucous membrane at the point where the esophagus enters the stomach; this forms a sort of one-way valve which does not hinder the passage of food into the stomach, but does interfere with exit of food back into the esophagus.

Vomiting may occur when the stomach is severely distended with food or gas. When it is stretched tightly, it may eradicate the valve-like fold. More pressure can be put on the stomach as the abdominal muscles contract. The distension must be extreme to permit vomiting. At this point, the extreme pressure frequently leads to rupture of the stomach walls. This has given the impression that vomiting cannot occur in the horse without rupture of the stomach. This is not entirely true, as it is possible for the animal to vomit and be normal afterwards. Often, however, the pressure is so great that the animal vomits and rupture of the stomach occurs at the same time, leading to peritonitis (infection of the lining of the abdomen) and death within 12 to 24 hours. After the stomach has ruptured, the animal will usually show considerable relief and appear to feel much better, temporarily. After rupture of the stomach has occurred, the animal can no longer vomit.

COLIC

Colic is a general term for any pain in the abdomen. While it most commonly arises from disturbances in the digestive tract, the term is also used to describe pain that is caused by problems in the urinary tract, uterus, liver, or other organs. Peritonitis may cause signs of colic, as abdominal tumors can do. Animals with tying-up (azoturia) problems may appear to have colic. Colic may occur because of certain infectious diseases or poisonings. These are rare.

Colic in the digestive tract may be caused by spasms or by gas. It may also be caused by twists and torsions of the intestines themselves. Adhesions within the abdomen may cause constriction of the intestine, or may be the site of a torsion or similar problem. Obstruction of the blood supply to the intestine will cause colic. Animals with diarrhea will often show colic. Severe intestinal irritation, as caused by colitis-X, will often cause signs of colic to appear. Constipation (or impaction) may also appear as colic.

Prompt diagnosis and treatment of colic may prevent a simple colic, such as one caused by excess gas in the intestine, from becoming a more severe one (such as a torsion), resulting in loss of the animal. Delay may cause the problem to go from a $50 or $100 call to the loss of an animal worth thousands of dollars. In all too many cases, the owner tries to save money by waiting, hoping a bellyache will go away, or walks the animal until he is too exhausted to be saved. DON'T WAIT TO CALL FOR VETERINARY ASSISTANCE!

According to Rhulen Insurance Agency, their most common reason for horse death or euthanasia was colic. This was the largest SINGLE cause of horse loss, causing 33.5% of the claims paid by the agency. The second place cause of horse death was miscellaneous sickness, at 15.3%. (73)

CAUSES

Probably no other set of symptoms can be caused by so many different things. The basic reason for colic is the horse's internal anatomy. His stomach is very small, so feed passes through it essentially undigested. The small intestine is very long; his large colon is enormous. There are several points in the digestive tract where food must move uphill. The fact that we keep the horse in confined quarters and feed him abnormal feeds on an artificial schedule contributes to the occurrence of colic. The horse is an animal which, through the ages, has become accustomed to eating small amounts of roughage, day and night, on his own schedule.

The immediate causes of colic are many and varied. With the exception of sand colic, colic is, in general, caused by stress of one sort or another. One of the most common causes of colic is parasitism. The worms disturb the circulation to the intestines, causing signs of colic. Or, blood clots or pieces of dead worm may break off and go down the bloodstream to other parts of the intestine where they cause blockage of blood vessels, with loss of circulation to the area. If this area is large enough, a portion of the intestine may die; this will appear as a colic. In young horses, large numbers of ascarids may form a physical blockage in the intestine and cause an obstructive colic.

Overfeeding the horse (or accidental entry into a storage area) may cause colic. This may also occur when the horse receives two meals because of lack of communication between the persons feeding him. A horse who is undernourished for a period of time may be more susceptible to digestive upsets. A normal quantity of a feed to which the horse has not been gradually accustomed may also cause colic.

A feeding schedule so irregular that the animal is extremely hungry when fed and then wolfs down his food may result in a colic, usually within a few hours after feeding. Feeding a horse immediately after work, especially without adequately cooling him out, may bring on colic. Exercising the horse right after he has eaten, particularly without warming him up slowly, may also cause colic. Changes from hay to pasture, or even from pasture to hay, are sure causes of problems for some animals.

In many cases, feed quality is even more important than feed quantity or schedule. Feed which is moldy or soured may cause colic. Sudden changes from mediocre feed to good feed, or from feed of lesser nutritional value, such as grass hay, to hay which is quite rich, such as alfalfa hay, can cause problems.

Grain which has been finely ground may pack together into a sort of dough in the digestive tract, leading to an impaction. If ground grain must be fed, it should be well mixed with very coarsely chopped hay (see the Feeds section for a further discussion of feedstuffs which may cause colic). Cribbers who swallow air may get colic from that practice. Problems with the teeth in which the horse does not adequately chew his feed may cause colic.

Weather changes are often felt to cause colic in horses where nothing else has changed. Colics tend to occur in batches, often accompanied by cattle with bloat. Veterinarians often see three or four cases of colic and/or bloat in one day, and then none of either of these problems for several weeks. The only common factor which can be found was an impending weather change.

Foreign bodies, such as stones, or built-up concretions of plant material which occasionally occur in the equine intestine, may cause colic. Ingesting sand by eating off the ground or eating roughage which has been flooded may cause a sand colic.

Certain poisonings cause signs of colic. Most common among these is mold poisoning from eating moldy hay, grain, or bedding. Phosphorus and arsenic poisoning are among those which exhibit signs of colic.

Twisting of various sections of the intestine may cause severe colic. These problems have various names, depending on which portion of the intestine is twisted, and which way the twist goes. Portions of intestine may also flip through tears in the mesentery (the thin membrane which supports the intestines) and then become twisted or caught. This is also called a strangulation. The intestine may crawl into the inguinal ring in a stallion or gelding and go through the same process, with the blood supply being cut off due to the twisting and pinching of the gut. This is usually called an incarceration. One portion of the intestine may telescope into another; this problem is called intussusception and is more common in foals than in older horses. It usually occurs during or after a bout with diarrhea (scours). Torsion and volvulus are names given to other twists within the digestive tract.

SIGNS

Restlessness and abnormal behavior are generally the first symptoms noticed with a colic; some horses may show a definite personality change. Many animals will show a lack of appetite, and may be dopey or lethargic. The temperature may range from normal to 101 degrees F (38.3 degrees C). The pulse may be normal and the respiration rate may be normal to slightly elevated.

Other early signs of colic are: kicking at the belly with a hindfoot; alternately cocking and resting one or both hind legs; pawing the ground with one or both forefeet; looking around at the flank; yawning; raising the upper lip in a curl (a smile-sort of action, called fleering or flehmen); grinding their teeth; and stamping the feet impatiently or even in a vicious manner.

The animal may stand stretched as though attempting to urinate. This action gives rise to many calls for "a horse with kidney problems," when that is not the problem at all. He may switch his tail, or pump it jerkily up and down. Laziness and a stumbling gait may be noted. The horse may have feed, but not wish to eat. He may groan or sigh. Any or all of these signs may come and go according to the discomfort of the moment.

As the animal begins to feel worse, he may lie down for a short time, and will often pull his legs up to his abdomen. He may then get up and lie down again within a very few minutes. As the pain becomes stronger, the animal may lie on his side and stretch his legs, then pull them back up to his belly and roll back up to his chest. He may get up from this position, or lie back onto his side and stretch again.

From this point, it is only a small step to rolling and thrashing on the ground. This is one of the classic signs of colic. The roll of a horse with colic differs from a normal roll. It is more of a thrashing than a calm, happy roll. The horse may roll from side to side, or may lie on his back in an attempt to ease the abdominal pain.

Careful observation, and knowing what IS a normal roll for your horse will help to differentiate between normal rolling and colic rolling. When lying down, the horse may be so bunched up that his shoes will injure his elbows. Animals who are in severe pain may throw themselves to the ground with considerable violence.

The animal may grunt loudly at times. During the periods when the pain is severe, the horse may sweat profusely. Some animals will move constantly in a circle or show other signs of hyperactivity. Others may be lethargic. In any case, a marked personality change is usually evident.

Continued gas production within the digestive tract will cause increased pressure on the diaphragm. The horse may take short, rapid, panting breaths. The horse's temperature may rise at this point to 101 to 103 degrees F (38.3 to 39.4 C). The respiratory rate will rise to 20 to 40 breaths per minute and the pulse may reach 60 beats per minute. Animals who have a spasm in the intestinal tract may show severe pain, but be passing feces normally because the gut beyond the spasm is still functioning normally. Others may pass no feces at all or have diarrhea.

In a really severe case of colic, the animal may be impossible to keep on his feet. He may throw himself violently to the ground, thrash around, and jump to his feet again. Periods of obviously intense pain may alternate with periods of nearly complete relief, during which the animal may be calm and quiet and even possibly interested in food or water. During these periods, the animal may appear depressed, standing sleepily or dazed, with his head down and eyes closed. He may lean his head against a feeder or wall. The horse may grind his teeth. He may, if loose, walk into walls or fences, and can injure himself in his aimless travels. The horse may stretch as though attempting to urinate or pass a bowel movement. He may strain and moan without results, although he may pass gas.

The horse may look as if he is attempting to vomit, but without any results. During attempts to vomit, the animal may show labored breathing, an upturned upper lip, and contraction of the flank. He will move his throat and draw his nose in toward his chest, causing high arching of the neck. If he does vomit, this is one of the most unfavorable signs possible. It is frequently followed by rupture of the stomach and death of the animal. Vomitus will run out the nose. The pulse rate is elevated, usually 70 to 80 or more beats per minute. The respiratory rate rises to 60 breaths per minute or higher. The temperature may be much higher than normal; the higher it is, the more unfavorable the prognosis.

The mucous membranes of the mouth and eyes may be unusually colored. They may be pale and lighter than normal, or they may be a dark, muddy color. They might, in severe cases, be flaming red. Other than appearing abnormal, there is no set pattern to this shade and color. The vessels may stand out prominently. The membranes of the mouth may be extremely dry. Normally, when a thumb is pressed firmly into the membranes of the upper gum, the white spot that is left should fill rapidly. With a severe colic, the capillary refill time, as this test is called, is three seconds or more.

Know what is normal with regard to your horse's temperature, pulse rate, and capillary fill time. A list of these readings plus a description of the symptoms your horse is showing will help your veterinarian determine how serious the colic is. This will allow him to give you instructions as to what to do until he gets there. It will also help him to determine whether the problem is very serious; if he cannot get there shortly in one of these cases, he may recommend that you call another veterinarian.

History can be very important in helping your veterinarian to determine the cause, and therefore to be more sure of the necessary treatment for a colic. Jot down on your list any items that you think may have caused the problem. When did you first notice symptoms? Has the horse had any diarrhea or constipation? Are there any other abnormal characteristics of the feces? Have you changed feed? What kind of feed did the animal have at his last meal before the colic occurred? When was he last fed and watered? Was he worked shortly before or after this feeding or watering? Has he had a regular supply of drinking water?

Has he suffered from any other disease lately? Recent infection with diseases such as distemper may leave the animal with internal abscesses which will cause a colic. If a mare, is she pregnant? Is the animal on a regular worming program? When was he last wormed, and with what product? Be sure to tell your veterinarian if you have administered any medication to the horse. This may make a great deal of difference in what drugs he uses to treat the animal.

Your veterinarian will use a combination of the history which you give him, the clinical signs he observes, and perhaps some examinations and tests to tell him how to treat the colic. He may do a rectal examination, an abdominal tap (also called a paracentesis), or other tests to help him make a diagnosis. Do not allow a well-meaning friend or neighbor to examine your horse rectally. If they accidentally puncture the rectum, there is a good chance that the ensuing infection will result in the animal's death. An untrained person who is not experienced in rectal examinations is quite unlikely to be able to tell anything of value, anyway.

TREATMENT

A colic which was minor in the beginning may be converted to a serious one if the animal is not treated promptly, or is allowed to roll without control. Colic can quickly turn into a severe abdominal crisis. If you already have a torsion or other serious problem, delay can make the difference between a live, repaired horse and a dead horse. Waiting five or six hours can make it impossible for your veterinarian to save the horse. Prompt diagnosis of the type of colic that your horse has, and treatment of it, along with pain control, are vital to saving the horse's life.

Now that I've frightened you badly about colic, how do you handle a case of it? Let's say you have just found your horse with signs of a mild colic. He is looking uncomfortable, but not rolling. Begin by taking the animal's temperature. It should not be over about 101 degrees F (38.5 C). Also count his pulse rate—preferably BEFORE you begin to walk him. Look at his membranes and see what their color is. Press your thumb into the gum, making a bleached white spot. After you pull it away, count how many seconds it takes to come back to its normal color to determine the capillary refill time. List all the symptoms you are seeing so that you can describe them to your veterinarian when you call him. It is a good idea to write them down so that you do not forget any. Keep cool. Your calm attitude and clear mental state during this emergency may well be the salvation of your horse.

Begin by walking the horse for about 15 minutes.

Then, turn the horse loose in a pen or corral if he is acting more comfortable. Observe the animal and see what he does. If he lies down, this is O.K.—IF—AND ONLY IF—the animal will lie quietly. If he wants to thrash or roll, get him up and continue to walk him. If he stays quiet and calm and you are seeing fewer symptoms, just keep an eye on him.

Do not give the horse any hay or grain and take away any edible bedding, such as straw. Make sure that he has adequate bedding of shavings or something inedible in case he wishes to lie down. Be sure he has plenty of water. If the symptoms go away, either feed the horse half his hay and no grain, or nothing at all at the next meal.

And what if the animal is thrashing severely and bashing his head against the ground? Call your veterinarian IMMEDIATELY, after jotting down the heart rate, temperature, and other signs as mentioned above. When obtaining this information, BE CAREFUL. A horse with severe colic doesn't care who or what may get in the way of his head or feet. If you cannot get your regular veterinarian, you may have to call any veterinarian whom you can get within a reasonable length of time.

Get the animal to his feet if possible and walk him. It may be necessary for one or two persons to help steady the animal if he is staggering or trying to drop. It may also be necessary to use a whip to keep the animal moving. If you absolutely cannot keep the animal on his feet, try to keep him from rolling or thrashing. Hold him in a folded-up position if at all possible. If he is banging his head on the ground, pad it by slipping old pieces of blanket, jackets, or other soft material under the halter.

If the weather is bad—either very hot, very cold or very wet—try to get the animal into shelter, even if it is only a shed or garage. Blanket him if he is cold. If you take him into a place like a garage, don't turn him loose, but have someone hold the halter so that he does not blunder into things, or take the place apart by rolling and thrashing his hooves into objects.

Walking a colicky horse is, in my opinion, an act which can be severely overdone. If a short bit of walking will not relax the animal and fix the problem, hiking him around the block all night will probably not cure it. If the animal is bad enough to be walked for more than an hour, it is a severe enough problem that you should get immediate treatment for your horse by a veterinarian. If you have a severe colic case which ends up needing surgery, how good a candidate will your animal be if you have walked him 6 or 8 (or as some owners have done, 24) hours? He will be tired and weak and may not live through the surgery as a result. It is my firm opinion that you should not add exhaustion to his problems. Also, when the animal is walked to the point of exhaustion, his nervous system automatically shuts down because he is tired, compounding the problem in the digestive tract. You may have literally walked him to death.

If there is a university veterinary hospital or good veterinary clinic within a reasonable distance, your best bet may be to haul the horse there, particularly if you cannot get a veterinarian to come out right away. If this type of facility is not near, by all means have the veterinarian come out to examine the animal. This avoids having to haul an already upset, ill animal, and avoids the chance that he may thrash around and harm himself in the trailer. Even if you have a colic which is extremely severe, it is probably worthwhile to have a veterinarian visit your premises, give the horse sedatives and painkillers, and then haul him to a clinic if it is determined that surgery is necessary. If you have to haul the animal, try to use a stock trailer or large horse trailer with removable dividers so that the animal may lie down if necessary.

Do NOT use a product called "Canadian Bells." If given to a horse with colic, it may shut down the intestinal motion which is needed to help expel a blockage and may make a colic very much worse. Some other "patent medicine" type colic mixtures may contain atropine. This is a drug which slows down or stops intestinal action and it relieves the pain quite rapidly. Atropine is DANGEROUS because, sometimes, intestinal movement does not start again and, meanwhile, the bacteria inside the gut continue producing gas. This excess gas production may lead to severe distension of the intestine. This, in turn, may push on the intestinal walls so much that the blood supply is reduced and causes serious, permanent (or even fatal) damage. Enemas, by the way, are all but useless in the adult horse. All they do is increase the discomfort and straining for an animal who is already miserable.

When your veterinarian arrives, what principles does he use in treating the animal? For constipation or impaction-type colics, or with gaseous (tympanic) colics, his first action will usually be to administer some sort of laxative. The same treatment will be used if the animal has overeaten on grain or other substances, as well in some poisonings and several other types of colic. He may stomach tube the animal and administer a gallon or more of mineral oil. In most cases, the fact that the animal passes some of the oil through his digestive tract (as evidenced by oil on the hind end and tail some hours later) means that the animal does not have a blockage. On rare occasion, the oil can pass around a blockage without moving it or breaking it down.

For some colics, your veterinarian may use a water-soluble laxative in powder form which is mixed with water and administered by stomach tube. He will probably add an antibiotic solution to kill some of the gas-forming bacteria which are helping to cause the animal's discomfort. This medication also helps to reduce the number of bacteria available to invade weakened tissues if there is any damage to the intestinal lining. He may also add a surface-tension-reducing agent. This agent acts to help break down gas bubbles which may be trapped among the food material (causing pressure and pain) and aids in their dispersal. Some veterinarians, in certain cases, also add activated charcoal or a similar product to help absorb toxins.

He will also usually administer some sort of pain-relieving drug. Phenylbutazone or one of its synthetic analogs, such as Banamine (Schering Corp., Kenilworth, NJ 07033) may be given. He may, on occasion, wish to give both. Dipyrone is a drug related to aspirin which may be used to bring down the temperature if there is one, and also to give pain relief. He may use a laxative-type injection if he feels the problem is an impaction. If, on the other hand, he feels that the colic is due to spasms in the digestive tract, he will give a smooth-muscle relaxant which helps to calm the muscle cramps and allow the intestines to resume their normal push-pull-squeeze onward motion.

If the horse does not respond to routine treatment, or if the veterinarian feels that the horse has a serious problem such as a twisted intestine, he may recommend exploratory surgery. This procedure is also called an exploratory laparotomy. A sterile surgical facility should be available for the operation. There should be enough personnel to do the surgery, as well as experienced persons and adequate equipment to provide safe anesthesia. If a section of intestine is twisted, or has a thrombus (blood clot) blocking its blood supply, it may be dead and gangrenous. In this case, the section of intestine is removed, and the gut is then "anastomosed." This means that the cut ends are put back together and sutured or stapled to make the gut whole again. Special feeding is often necessary for several weeks after surgery so that the surgical site has time to heal. This aftercare is of the utmost importance.

What do you do if you are in the middle of nowhere camping or hunting with your horse as many do in the western states, and he colics? It's not a bad idea to know about the other people in the area. On a recent elk hunting trip, several hunters consulted me, and I didn't even have any horses in my camp. They had found out that I am a veterinarian and came to me when something went wrong. So, check around! Help may not be as far away as you think. If you can't find help fairly quickly, walk the horse. If you are near a trailhead or road—say, within a couple of hours from it, it would be a good idea to walk him in the direction of the outside. He may die before you get there, but chances are that he won't. You may be able to get him out to civilization and get help. Or, the walk may, if you are lucky, shake things back to normal and alleviate his pain.

And what if you are absolutely in the middle of nowhere? If you plan to be that far from civilization, you should be carrying a first-aid kit for the horse. It should include phenylbutazone tablets. Give these according to your veterinarian's instructions or the label directions, at the first sign of colic. Bear in mind that they may mask the signs of his getting worse. But, on the other hand, the drug may give the animal enough pain relief that he will relax and get well. Walk him for a half-hour to an hour, and then allow him to rest if he will.

Another drug worth carrying into the back country is called Jenotone (Burroughs Wellcome Co., Kansas City, MO 64141). It is an anti-spasmodic, and helps to return intestinal action to normal, and to stop cramping. Many times, an injection of this drug, with or without phenylbutazone to accompany it, is enough to relax a colicky horse and allow his digestive tract to return to normal. It can be given intramuscularly, which is an advantage to the horse owner.

Veterinarians occasionally use tranquilizers to sedate and relieve a colicky animal. Bear in mind that tranquilizers are NOT painkillers. Also, they lower the animal's blood pressure, which may be harmful in some cases of colic. You have to weigh this risk against the possible relaxation and its benefits to the animal. Most veterinarians only use tranquilizers on an animal who is so out of his mind with pain that he is trying to throw himself on the ground, and on whom other painkillers are not working rapidly enough. In these cases, we administer enough tranquilizer to dull the animal's mind and keep him from hurting himself. Most of us do NOT use it as a regular treatment. You should not risk administering drugs if you can get veterinary attention for your animal, as they may not be appropriate for the type of colic which he has. The above measures are NOT recommended as routine treatment, but as EMERGENCY measures ONLY!

PROGNOSIS

If the pulse rate is not over 60, the temperature not elevated, and the animal's symptoms are relieved by simple treatment, chances are very good that he will come out of the colic without any serious aftereffects. These make up, by far, the bulk of colic cases. A pulse over 80 is an unfavorable sign, although some animals whose heart rate has risen this high may survive. There is often a poor prognosis for animals whose symptoms are not relieved within a few hours after treatment. Colics which last more than 24 hours frequently have unfavorable outcomes. An abdominal tap which shows blood is also an unfavorable sign.

Overall fatalities due to colic run around 10% of the affected animals. Colics due to the various intestinal torsions or twists are nearly 100% fatal if not treated. If the veterinarian diagnoses a torsion or other twist-type problem, do not delay if you are going to have surgery done. If you wait for another six or eight hours before making the decision to operate, you have significantly reduced the horse's chances of survival. Decide to operate while you (and the veterinarian) still have a chance to save the animal.

Vomiting is a very unfavorable sign, as it almost invariably accompanies rupture of the stomach. Vomitus will run from the horse's nose. Sudden relief from severe pain is not necessarily favorable. When the animal's stomach ruptures, he will, in many cases, appear to be much more comfortable and will show less signs of pain than he had previously. The animal will subsequently die from peritonitis and shock due to release of stomach contents and bacteria into the abdomen.

Continuing, severe pain may indicate a poor prognosis. Animals who are going to get well usually show relief following treatment. If the mucous membranes have a continuing muddy color or are a very bright red, this also gives an unfavorable prognosis. Bluish or yellowish coloration of the membranes may also be unfavorable.

So your veterinarian has treated the horse. What do you look for now? Keep an eye on the animal's general attitude. He should be alert, and within a short period of time (say, an hour after treatment) should show relief from the symptoms that alerted you to the colic in the first place. He should look relaxed and comfortable rather than anxious and pained. The pulse rate should stay normal (or drop back to normal if it had been elevated). The temperature should be normal. There should be no further sweating (if outside temperatures are not elevated). The horse should begin to pass normal bowel movements without straining or apparent pain. If any previous signs of colic return, consult with your veterinarian immediately.

CHRONIC COLIC

Some horses will show a touch of colic (or worse) on a regular basis. These attacks may come several times a year; sometimes, as with an extremely valuable Arabian mare owned by one of my clients, every six to eight weeks, without fail. These attacks may not be serious in themselves. The danger is that you might not be home when one starts, and the animal may roll and twist an intestine or cause other serious harm due to the pain. Chronic colic is a definite unsoundness.

If you do not make an attempt to control the attacks, you may ultimately lose the horse. Begin by checking the feeding program. Cut down on grain even at the risk of having an animal that is a bit thin. If you are feeding alfalfa hay, it is worth changing to a good-quality grass hay, if you can get it. This will sometimes make a difference.

Feeding bran regularly is beneficial to many of these animals. You may give as much as three to four cups twice daily, mixed with a bit of grain. Make sure that your worming program is up to par. It may even need to be better than usual. For the Arabian mare mentioned above, the only factor that consistently controlled the colic was regular worming—every SIX weeks, with a different product each time.

Moderate, regular exercise will help passage of food through the digestive tract and add to the animal's well-being. It also helps the circulatory system to be more efficient. This may make a difference if there is a circulatory problem in the animal's intestines. Another of my

clients has a stallion whose tendency to colic is controlled by bran, exercise, and the utmost care with his feed. He seems to need to be fed on a very strict schedule; being an hour or two late frequently brings on an attack even when he is being fed the same feed as he has had for months. He also seems to need a carefully controlled quantity. Feeding him more than he is accustomed to may precipitate an attack.

The client who has the stallion with chronic colic has been instructed to always keep a gallon of mineral oil on hand. She either buys four one-quart bottles from the drugstore or will occasionally purchase it by the gallon at the feed store. That way, if she calls another veterinarian and he is out of mineral oil when he arrives, she has it available for him to administer. She realizes that UNDER NO CIRCUMSTANCES should she ever attempt to give this drug by mouth, as the horse could inhale it, with fatal results.

SAND COLIC

Sand colic is generally a chronic colic and is caused by the horse eating sand with his food. This is common when the pasture is overgrazed and the animal is eating forage close to the ground. This often happens in sandhill areas, such as parts of Nebraska. Or, the animal may be fed from the ground, taking in sand with his hay as he tries to pick up leaves and stems. If starved, the horse may eat dirt, sand, or other material. He may also take in sand with pasture forage which has been flooded and has sand clinging to it. Another way to get sand and dirt is by drinking from a waterway that is muddy; the dirt will be suspended in the water and taken with every mouthful the animal drinks.

By the time the animal has ingested enough sand or dirt to cause problems, he is probably carrying somewhere between 30 and 80 pounds of it in his digestive tract. The horse often becomes thin and suffers chronic colic. The bouts may become increasingly severe, with each lasting longer than the one before. Occasionally, sand may be found if the feces are examined closely. This does not occur in all cases.

Sand colic may be very difficult to diagnose. If your horse colics and you think sand may be the cause, ask your veterinarian about it when he examines the animal. Occasionally, he will be able to feel the mass of sand on rectal examination.

Treatment of sand colics usually involves repeated treatments with some sort of laxative. Feeding bran regularly may also help to flush out the sand. Whatever treatment is used, it will be a long-term procedure. Be warned in advance that even after all your effort, the case may not turn out well if so much sand is present that it has settled in parts of the intestine. It may lie there against the membrane on the inside of the gut and cause it to die because of weight and pressure.

DIARRHEA

Diarrhea in adult horses is uncommon—and often serious. It frequently occurs in foals, and may result in their deaths if not promptly treated. Sometimes when we do everything possible, they still die. Foal diarrheas are usually due to bacterial infections. Animals between one and three years of age seem to be susceptible to protozoal diarrhea. Animals who have received prolonged antibiotic treatment (say, more than five or six days) may be susceptible to diarrheas caused by mold growth because all of the normal intestinal bacteria have been killed by the antibiotics.

Contagious diarrhea due to a virus is often seen at racetracks. It is important to differentiate this disease early in its course from colitis-X which may also be seen in this stressful situation. If the problem is colitis-X, starting treatment promptly may mean the difference between life and death to the horse. Usually, only one horse (or at most a small percentage of horses) will be affected with colitis-X, while virus diarrhea may involve many animals. The virus diarrhea is a mild problem usually only lasting for a day or two, unless there are other complications. In some outbreaks, the animals come down with diarrhea a few days after an upper respiratory disease has occurred, suggesting that the two problems are linked. Either they are caused by the same virus, or the respiratory virus weakens the animal enough that the diarrhea virus can invade the gut. In either case, contagious diarrhea is more annoying than serious. Let's begin by discussing diarrhea in foals.

FOAL DIARRHEA (SCOURS)

Diarrhea in foals (also called scours) is frequently due to a bacterial infection, although some diarrhea in foals is probably caused by viruses. The animal is generally weakened by other factors. He may have been weak and chilled by bad weather right after he was born. He may have been born into a dirty environment, picking up the infection from filth around him or from surroundings contaminated by sick calves, lambs, or pigs now or at some time in the past. Or, there may have been another foal with scours in the same stall previously. Foals who are fed milk replacers or cows' milk are much more likely to develop scours than are those who are nursing a mare. The problem may also be seen with a mare who is a good milker and a foal who is greedy.

The foal may show scours when the mare comes into heat. This is called "foal heat diarrhea." It has been thought by some to be due to the foal licking vaginal secretions from the mare while she is in heat. However, foals who are raised on bottles may show a similar type of diarrhea at the same time period, when not exposed to a mare. The diarrhea lasts approximately two to five days, about the duration of the mare's foal heat. Foal heat diarrhea rarely shows complications and there is NO

TEMPERATURE RISE. Reducing the amount of feed given mares who are nursing foals at this time may help reduce the effects of this problem.

SIGNS

Foal diarrhea may be preceded by mild signs of colic. The bowel movements may vary from thin and sticky (but not normally formed) to thin and watery. They may be yellowish, orange, dark, greenish, or white. Fresh, bright red blood is a sign that you have a serious problem, as may be a black color. The temperature usually is not elevated early in the disease.

When the diarrhea begins, just keep an eye on the foal. Make sure that he is feeling well and frisky and looking bright. If he does not show any further signs of illness, antibiotics or other medications are usually not given.

If the temperature begins to rise and stay up (over 102 degrees F (39 degrees C), or the foal looks droopy or weak, the problem may be getting serious. Blood in the diarrhea can also be an unfavorable sign. Depression or lack of appetite (often first noticed because the mare's udder is tight and painful) can also be signs of a serious problem. If any of these symptoms are noticed, contact your veterinarian immediately so that he can examine the foal and treat it as necessary.

Foals, like human babies, are small and have limited reserves of fluids and energy. They dehydrate and become ill very quickly with scours. Diarrhea in foals may be a sign of a generalized infection within the body (called a septicemia), or an infectious gastroenteritis. With either of these problems, the temperature will rise. The foal usually stops eating and may appear colicky. He may be depressed and lethargic. The membranes may be reddened. As the diarrhea progresses, the foal will dehydrate rapidly. The feces are often very fluid and have a foul odor.

TREATMENT

Good nursing is important to treating any case of diarrhea in the foal. Medications to protect the intestinal lining are commonly given. These mixtures may also contain antibiotics. They may have drugs to slow down the violent, painful cramping motion of the intestines. They may also contain drugs to slow fermentation and gas production in the digestive tract. If there is a significant temperature rise or other signs of generalized infection, your veterinarian may recommend giving systemic antibiotics. He may take a sample of the feces to send to a laboratory to find out exactly which antibiotics will kill the bacteria causing the diarrhea.

If you don't have any medication specifically for diarrhea, give Kaopectate (Upjohn, Kalamazoo, MI

49001) or Pepto-Bismol (Norwich Pharmaceuticals, Norwich, NY 13815) until you are able to get more specific drugs and veterinary care. Give about two ounces (1/4 cup or 60 ml) four times a day, or about as much as you would give an adult human. Lift the foal's head only slightly above level as you give the liquid. Holding it too high can cause the foal to inhale the liquid, resulting in inhalation pneumonia. Place the medication in the foal's mouth from the side. A handy way to measure and give the medicine is with a clean syringe. 45 ml. are equal to an ounce. Fill the syringe with the required amount of medication and place it in the corner of the foal's mouth like a miniature dose syringe.

It is important that the foal have warm, dry, well-ventilated surroundings, preferably with clean, deep bedding. This is especially vital when the weather outside is wet, cold, or snowy. All the medication in the world will not save the foal if he is wet and shivering from exposure.

The foal's hind end may become "scalded" by the feces which get onto the tail and hair. Cleanse the area carefully and gently with warm water, and pat dry with paper towels or a clean cloth. Then, cover the area with petroleum jelly or mineral oil. This procedure should be repeated daily. It is best to not use any soap on the already irritated skin.

If the foal has diarrhea because the mare is milking too heavily, he may be muzzled for part of the day to keep him from overeating. The mare can be milked out to help reduce the amount available to the foal. This type of overeating may occur if the mare and foal are separated for some time, and he is hungry and greedy when they are reunited. It can also happen when the mare reaches her peak milk production, which usually occurs sometime during the first month of lactation.

Sudden dietary changes, as from milk to milk replacer or vice versa, may cause diarrhea. The presence of sugar or products, such as Karo syrup, in a formula may cause problems with a very young foal, because of his inability to digest the sugar. If diarrhea occurs, reduce or eliminate sugars in the diet until it is under control.

Some foals may have diarrhea because of infestation with worms, such as Strongyloides westerii and Parascaris equorum (strongyles and ascarids). A fecal exam should be run to rule this out, especially if these worms are known to cause problems on an infected premises.

Foals may have diarrhea because they have been treated with antibiotics, especially if these are given orally. Some drugs are more prone than others to kill off the foal's intestinal bacteria—the critters which help him to digest his food! If antibiotics have been administered, it may be necessary to give the foal buttermilk or yogurt to help reestablish his digestive bacteria. Or, you can give him fresh feces from a healthy adult horse, mixed with water and given as a drench. Given a choice, start with the yogurt. If you go the "fresh feces" route, be sure the donor horse is healthy.

PROTOZOAL DIARRHEA

Diarrhea caused by protozoans such as Trichomonas or Giardia may occur in horses of any age. The problem usually shows up as a long-term, chronic diarrhea. Recent antibiotic treatment may have killed off a sufficient number of normal intestinal bacteria to allow overgrowth of the protozoans. Animals who are kept in dirty stalls with poor sanitation may be especially susceptible to these infections. Under some conditions, this diarrhea may be contagious and affect more than one animal. Animals affected with chronic, long-term, protozoal diarrhea rarely die from it, but may be poor and thin.

Chronic cases of this protozoal problem show a frequent diarrhea. It may be present all the time, or it may be intermittent. The animal usually has a good appetite and appears to feel well and look well other than having diarrhea. His temperature is normal. However, young animals who have this problem for a long time may become stunted and appear malnourished or parasitized. Longstanding, chronic cases may show laminitis, slight anemia, and generally look poor.

You may suspect this disease, but are unlikely to confirm it by yourself. Consult your veterinarian for any horse with chronic diarrhea. Diagnosis of protozoal diarrhea is often made only by microscopic examination of fresh fluid from the diarrheic material. A veterinarian will usually do this procedure by setting up his microscope at the stable so that he can examine the material when it is as fresh as possible.

There are several new drugs available which can cure protozoal diarrhea, but are not available to the public. They may have toxic side effects, and are not drugs to be used lightly.

MYCOTIC DIARRHEA

Mycotic diarrhea is a chronic disease most commonly seen in foals and young horses. It usually occurs after treatment with oral antibiotics. It may also occur in the presence of a severe load of worms. A mold called Aspergillus may be cultured from the feces by the use of special techniques.

Antibiotics will not heal this problem—it should be suspected in an animal which has previously been treated with antibiotics and which still has a severe diarrhea. A special antifungal drug will be necessary. Your veterinarian will need to get this one for you. Try to prevent reinfection by cleaning and disinfecting the stall or corral. As this fungus can be carried in hay, changing the feed may be helpful.

VIRUS DIARRHEA

Diarrhea may be seen with some of the upper respiratory virus diseases. Virus diarrhea problems may also occur in stables or racetracks, unaccompanied by respiratory problems. Viral diarrheas are usually acute conditions in which the animal generally feels well or is only slightly depressed. They usually clear up by themselves. Cut the animal's feed down, and give Pepto-Bismol (Norwich Pharmaceuticals, Norwich, NY 13815) if you do not have any other medication handy. Give about 1 cup (250 ml) two to three times a day to an adult horse. Make sure that clean, fresh water is available at all times. Watch to see that the animal's temperature remains normal. Keep an eye on his membranes to see that his color remains normal and that he is not developing a more serious problem, such as colitis-X.

DIARRHEA CAUSED BY WATER

In some areas of the country, water contains minerals which may cause diarrhea. If you have several animals with chronic diarrhea and you have eliminated other causes of diarrhea, have the water checked. Your health department can do this, or people there can tell you where you can get it done. One of my clients had two horses with chronic diarrhea caused by well water. The neighbor's well (about 150 feet away) did not cause his horses any problems. So, don't assume that since no one in the neighborhood is having problems, that it could not be your water. It may be worth hauling water for a couple of weeks to see if that clears up the problem. Water with a high alkali content or large amount of magnesium sulfate (epsom salt) will cause diarrhea.

DIARRHEA DUE TO OTHER CAUSES

Diarrhea may be seen with sudden changes in feed. This often occurs when the horse is switched from a grass hay to alfalfa. Alfalfa is a good, nutritious feed, but may be too much for the animal if he is suddenly switched to it from a less rich feed. Make the change over four to seven days. Gradually increase the amount of alfalfa hay fed and reduce the amount of grass hay as you make the conversion. Changing types of grain may lead to the same kind of problems. Grain changes should also be made gradually.

Diarrhea can occur when horses are fed large amounts of grain. Often, all that is necessary to cure the problem is to decrease the amount of grain. In other cases, feeding a larger amount of grass hay along with the animal's grain will result in improvement.

Horses who have diseases associated with the large intestine, such as chronic salmonellosis, may be unable to digest fiber in a normal manner and may show chronic weight loss. These animals may do better on a high grain diet. While this does not cure diarrhea that may be present, it does allow them to extract a greater amount of usable nutrients from the higher-quality feedstuffs. Thus, they may show improved body condition even though the original disease remains.

COLITIS-X (SALMONELLOSIS)

Also known as colitis, this disease is presumed to be due to endotoxin production, probably by the type of bacteria called Salmonella. The disease is also called salmonellosis. Several other species of bacteria are thought to produce or contribute to the problem. The disease is acute and strikes with little or no warning. It will often strike only one horse in a group; on rare occasions, it may infect several animals (up to 20% of a group of horses). It occurs in all parts of the United States on a sporadic basis, with no regard to age of animal, or time of year.

The only common history among animals affected with colitis-X is recent stress or upper respiratory disease. Some animals had been shipped long distances (especially in hot weather) or were deprived of food. Others had recently had surgery or been under general anesthesia or had major medical problems. Even these factors are not present in some animals. Many horses have no history of prior illness or stress. Sometimes, no causative factor is ever determined. There is some feeling that an excess of protein and lack of cellulose may initiate the disease in some animals. (74)

Colitis-X can affect horses of any age. It may rapidly cause death in foals. The affected animals need not be run down or otherwise ill. They may appear perfectly normal up to the onset of signs. Colitis appears suddenly with depression and weakness. The animal may lie down and be unable to rise. His heart rate may be very rapid, up to 100 beats per minute.

The horse may show colic or moderate abdominal pain. The temperature may rise, but usually does so only briefly, in the very early stages. By the time you notice that the animal is ill, the temperature may be back to normal or even subnormal. The animal's gums may appear reddish or muddy-colored. The membranes of the eye may be a flaming red and the small blood vessels on the eye may stand out prominently.

Death can occur from colitis-X in as little as three hours, with signs of severe shock and nothing more. If the horse lives one to two days, he will usually show a profuse diarrhea. It will appear to be normal manure diluted with copious amounts of water. In some animals, the diarrhea may be bloody. It often has an especially fetid odor. The fluid loss leads to a severe dehydration, which adds to the shock which is already present. Call your veterinarian IMMEDIATELY if you suspect a case of colitis. Time is of the essence in treating it. Colitis must be treated immediately and aggressively. Many horses with colitis die in less than 24 hours.

The prognosis with colitis is always very poor. Without treatment, only a handful of affected animals will survive. Even with prompt, intensive treatment, many horses still die. Your veterinarian will treat the animal with large volumes of intravenous fluids to try to counteract the massive shock that is a major feature of this disease. It is not uncommon to administer more than 7 gallons (28 liters) of fluids intravenously within a 24 hour period. Antibiotics and other supportive medications will also be given.

Nursing is of the utmost importance in the treatment of colitis-X. The animal should be put in a warm, dry place, and blanketed if necessary. He should be offered water frequently if he wishes to drink. Your veterinarian may wish to stomach tube him to give extra water and electrolytes. This helps to replace the enormous amounts of fluid that the animal is losing.

The animal should be attended 24 hours a day, if at all possible. If you are near a veterinary school, you may wish to take your horse there. These are perhaps the ideal places to take a colitis case, as the large number of staff members assures that your animal will be treated as well as he possibly can be. Be warned that colitis can be very expensive to treat because of the large amounts of medication needed, and the time and labor necessary to care for the animal.

Because we don't know what causes colitis, it is hard to prevent. About all that can be said is to avoid stress, which is the key to preventing so many other ailments. Although the disease is generally of low contagiousness, it is worth taking sanitary precautions when you have a case. Disinfect your boots and wash your hands before going to another barn or onto someone else's property, and before handling or feeding another horse.

All organic material must be carefully removed from the barn before disinfection and destroyed, preferably by burning. Leave the pen or stall vacant for a few weeks to allow sunlight and drying to help kill any infectious bacteria. Then, clean all infected areas with a strong disinfectant solution. Bleach, diluted 1:32 in water, or a 2% formaldehyde solution may be used. (75)

Other animals on the premises should be carefully observed to allow prompt treatment if any of them should come down with colitis-X. It is a good idea to take their temperatures daily for several weeks so that the disease may be detected early. Prompt, aggressive treatment may allow horses to be saved who would otherwise be lost.

Chapter 16

EYE PROBLEMS

Eye Examination
Corneal Injuries
Conjunctivitis
Medicating the Horse's Eye
Eyelid Lacerations
Cataracts
Tumors In and Around The Eye
Occlusion of the Tear Duct
Eyeworms
Periodic Ophthalmia
Spasm of the Eyelids
Blindness
Eye Removal
Other Eye Problems

EYE EXAMINATION

Before you can begin to treat a horse's eye, it must be examined to see what the problem is. Correct diagnosis is of the utmost importance for correct treatment. If the eye is swollen shut so you cannot examine it, leave the job to your veterinarian. It may be necessary for him to sedate the animal and/or to anesthetize the nerves to the eye (with a nerve block) in order to do a thorough examination and make a diagnosis. In some cases, it may be necessary to anesthetize the animal completely in order to check the eye and determine the cause or the problem.

If there is a film or cloudiness associated with the eye, the next task is to determine whether it is on the surface or deep within the globe. Injuries to the cornea and some other problems will cause a whitish or bluish film on the surface of the cornea. Cataracts cause a cloudiness deep within the eye. This appears to be about a half inch behind the cornea and is viewed through the pupil. The horse's pupil is the dark, horizontal oval slit in the center of the eye. If you look closely, you will see dark, rounded bodies along the edge of it. These are normal.

The tissues surrounding the eye must be examined to determine whether or not they are involved in the problem. Are there any cuts or lacerations in the eyelids? Are the eyelids rolling inward or otherwise causing problems? Is the conjunctiva (the white membrane which lines the eyelid) inflamed, oddly colored, or injured?

Animals with sudden blindness should be examined by your veterinarian as soon as possible. This may result from many causes, including injury and disease. Blindness may be due to problems within the eye itself, or it may be due to abnormalities in the nervous pathways to the brain. Problems, such as detachment of the retina (a membrane in the back of the eye which makes vision possible), can be repaired if they are detected promptly and treated before permanent damage has occurred. Occasionally, if you are a long way from a veterinary school or a veterinarian competent to treat eye problems, your veterinarian may call in a human ophthalmologist to consult with him as to what the problem is. Physicians will usually not look at a horse without considerable restraint, especially if they are using some of their expensive instruments which could be damaged if knocked out of their hands by the animal.

At times, it is valuable to examine an animal with a severe, healed eye problem in order to know what to expect in the future. One of my clients was worried about a stallion who had suddenly become blind in one eye due to a cataract. He was concerned that the animal might become blind in the other eye and that the problem might possibly be hereditary (as some kinds of cataracts are). Arrangements were made for the horse to be examined by a veterinary ophthalmologist who was in town for a special seminar. This man's opinion was that the cataract was due to an injury, and that it was neither hereditary nor likely to occur in the other eye. With this information, the client was then able to trace the problem to a period when he had been out of town for several weeks, and the horse had been cared for by someone who did not know enough to call a veterinarian when the animal had injured his eye.

CORNEAL INJURIES

Horses injure their eyes by running into objects, such as tree limbs and fences. They hit their heads on starting gates. They get hit in the eye by horsemen attempting to discipline the animal by hitting the side of his head or neck and missing their target.

Injuries to the cornea (the clear part of the eye) may be superficial scrapes or may be deep cuts. If the injury has just occurred, the obvious sign is severe pain, with the eye being clamped tightly shut.

When the eye is opened, a scrape or scratch may be seen when you look across the cornea. Use a penlight to first look directly into the eye, and then across the cornea from the side. The scrape can be often be seen from the side angle. The wound may only be a small depression, but the pain can be intense. If it is just a small scrape, treat it immediately with an eye ointment containing ONLY antibiotics. Neomycin ointment may be used as can a multiple-antibiotic product, such as neomycin-bacitracin-polymyxin-B ointment. Do NOT use an antibiotic containing any corticosteroid (such as prednisolone), as it can cause enlargement of the lesion and subsequent loss of the eye.

Put the ointment in the horse's eye a MINIMUM of four times a day. This should only be done with smaller scrapes, say, less than ¼ inch in diameter. During the course of the treatment (which should usually not last more than three or four days before the eye is healed), make sure that the lesion is growing smaller instead of larger.

Fluorescein strips should be part of every horseman's first-aid kit. These are small pieces of paper saturated with a fluorescent dye. They are packaged in small, sterile, paper wrappers. When you suspect an eye injury in the horse, open one of these strips. Hold it by the green end, letting the orange end hang free. Moisten the orange end with ONE drop of clean water (no, spitting on it isn't legal!). Put the end of the strip gently in the inner corner of the horse's eye to allow the dye to float into the eye. If you do not have any clean water handy, place the strip in the corner of the eye and allow it to be moistened by tears. Try not to let it touch the cornea, because that may be painful. The dye will be carried over the surface of the cornea when the animal blinks. If there is a spot on the cornea where the green dye sticks, you are seeing either a corneal laceration or an ulcer. A veterinarian should be consulted IMMEDIATELY. If the dye doesn't stick anywhere, you next have to determine whether the animal's problem is an infection or a foreign body in the eye. Bear in mind that infections may be introduced by foreign bodies.

If the animal has suffered a laceration (cut or tear) in the cornea, it is imperative that you call a veterinarian or get the animal to one as soon as possible. Waiting five or six hours before suturing a cut may leave the horse with a blind eye—or no eye at all. Occasionally when the cornea is punctured, it can be saved by a technique called a conjunctival pedicle graft. If your veterinarian cannot do this, consider consulting a human ophthalmologist to see if he will do the surgery. Otherwise, it may be necessary to remove the eye. The graft is only feasible if the structures within the eye are basically sound. If they are damaged or torn, it is useless to attempt this type of repair.

IMPORTANT: If a corneal injury involves a cut rather than a scrape, does not heal within three days, or appears to be getting larger, CALL YOUR VETERINARIAN IMMEDIATELY. Waiting longer to "see if it heals by itself" can lead to loss of the eye. This is because these problems are sometimes difficult to heal in the horse, especially if the animal is rubbing his eye on his knee to scratch it.

Your veterinarian will probably use drugs to reduce the pain in the animal's eye. He will most likely sedate the animal and then sew his eyelids together. This is because it is almost impossible to bandage a horse's eye in any other manner. The sutured eyelids act as a bandage to cover the cornea and allow it to heal. Having them sewn together also removes the irritation which is caused by the lids opening and closing over the injury. This, in turn, reduces the pain and makes the animal much more comfortable. During the period that the horse has his eye sewn

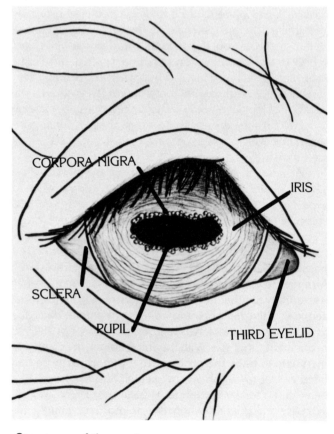

Structures of the equine eye.

shut, he should be kept in a stall or small corral rather than expected to navigate in a larger, brushy pasture. Be sure to talk to the animal when you approach him so that you do not startle him. Approach the horse from his good side so that he can see you.

It may be necessary for you to put eye ointment in the horse's eye several times a day. This treatment is very important and should not be neglected. It helps the eye to heal under the closed lids and helps to prevent infection which might otherwise occur. The animal may be reluctant to allow you to put ointment in the closed eye, as you will be working from his blind side. Talk to him continuously and touch him a lot. Make firm contact with the side of his face before you touch the eye area and work slowly up to the eye. Occasionally, you will encounter a horse who, after all this, will throw his head so high that you cannot treat him. Use a lip chain on these animals (see Lip Chain).

CONJUNCTIVITIS

You have stained the surface of the cornea with fluorescein dye and determined that it is undamaged. And, you have checked carefully to determine that there is no scrap of hay or weed seed caught in the conjunctiva. Yet, you are still faced with reddened membranes and a painful eye.

Conjunctivitis is the name given to an inflammation or infection of the conjunctivae. These are the membranes around the eye and down inside the eyelid. They occasionally become reddened and inflamed. This can be caused by various bacteria, by physical conditions such as dust and dry weather, or by irritation from insects. Some cases are probably caused by various viruses. Conjunctivitis may accompany other diseases (especially upper respiratory viruses).

The membranes around the eye with conjunctivitis are swollen and reddened. They may exude pus which will drain from the corner of the eye and down the face. No signs of corneal damage are seen with fluorescein staining, and no foreign bodies are seen within the eye.

The UNDAMAGED eye with conjunctivitis is the place to use an ophthalmic ointment containing both antibiotics AND a corticosteroid. One of the best known of these products is Neo-Predef (Upjohn, Kalamazoo, MI 49001). Put the ointment in the animal's eye four to five times a day for three days. If the problem has not cleared in two to three days, or if it should become worse, have your veterinarian examine the animal. While you are treating the animal with a corticosteroid ointment, you should stain the eye every other day. If the cornea shows any sign of holding the stain, discontinue the corticosteroid treatment immediately and call your veterinarian.

MEDICATING THE HORSE'S EYE

As mentioned previously, when you go to treat the horse's eye, work your hand gradually up the side of his face, talking to him and petting him. Most people find it easiest to rest the hand containing the ointment tube against the side of the animal's face so that if he moves, the hand will move with him. This helps to avoid bumping the horse in the eye with the ointment tube. Squeeze about a quarter inch of ointment into the horse's eye, preferably onto the cornea just above the lower lid. Then, blink his eye open and closed three or four times with your fingers. The blinking helps to spread the ointment across the surface of the eye.

If the ointment cannot be squeezed into the corner of the horse's eye, it is sometimes possible to put ¼ inch or so of it on a clean finger, and gently smear it onto the conjunctival (inner) surface of the lower lid.

In some cases, eye drops may be prescribed for the horse. It is usually necessary to put drops in more often than you would ointment, because they have a lesser contact time with the cornea. A tuberculin syringe (which holds 1 cc.) may be helpful to squeeze the eye drops into the inner corner of the animal's eye.

Some horses can be extremely difficult to treat because they clamp their eyelids firmly shut when touched. If you cannot get the prescribed ointment or drops into the horse's eye, contact your veterinarian so that he can arrange for another method of treatment, or suture the animal's eyelids shut if the problem is serious enough. Better to call him out an extra time for no reason than to let the problem go untreated and end up with a blind horse!

In some cases, a catheter will be punched through the upper lid of the affected eye and left in place. The other end is passed to the side opposite the injured eye (where the horse is not wary). Medication may be injected with a syringe from that location. At other times, your veterinarian may treat the animal by injecting medication into the membranes under the eyelid.

EYELID LACERATIONS

Eyelid tears and cuts often occur when the horse catches the eyelid on a fence wire or piece of brush. If neglected, these lacerations can lead to an abnormally shaped eye opening. They may support a large growth of granulation tissue ("proud flesh") and cause pus to drain down the side of the face, as well as attracting flies and other insects which make the animal miserable. Call your veterinarian as soon as you discover a cut eyelid. Prompt treatment frequently leads to perfect cosmetic healing. These cuts usually take only a few stitches, but these few can really make a difference in the healing because there is no way to bandage the area.

CATARACTS

A cataract is a cloudiness or series of lines or scars in the lens of the eye. The lens is seen deep inside the eye, through the pupil slit. A slight cloudiness (a sort of ground-glass appearance) is normal in the horse; know what is normal for your animal. Cataracts may be hereditary, or they may occur from trauma or from problems such as periodic ophthalmia.

When cataracts occur in the foal, they are usually present at birth. These should be considered to be hereditary and should eliminate the animal from consideration as breeding stock. They may, on rare occasion, occur because of severe malnutrition in the mare during pregnancy, especially when her diet is deficient in vitamin D. If they encompass the entire lens, they may cause blindness.

Cataracts which occur in the older animal may be small pinpoints, long streaks, or a cloudiness of the whole lens. The animal usually can see around the cataract if it involves only a small part of the lens and may have near-normal vision. If the entire lens is involved, the horse will probably have decreased vision or may be completely blind.

Cataracts are rarely treated in the horse unless the animal is of exceptional value. In these animals, the lens may be surgically removed. This can usually be done at one of the veterinary colleges, or by a veterinarian who specializes in eye surgery. Once cataracts begin, they often become progressively worse. For this reason, they must be considered an unsoundness.

TUMORS IN AND AROUND THE EYE

Several types of tumors can occur in and around the horse's eye. These are not common, but you should be aware of them in regard to certain animals. Gray horses have a susceptibility to a tumor called a malignant melanoma. This neoplasm ("new growth") occurs on skin and may grow at the edges of the eyelids or elsewhere on the face.

White ("albino") horses and those with bald faces, or paint horses with white patches over their eyes, are susceptible to a type of tumor called a squamous cell carcinoma. This is the same problem as "cancer eye" in cattle. This may occur on the edge of the lid or in the corner of the eye. It may also be seen on the third eyelid.

If you see a lump that you suspect to be either of these problems, consult your veterinarian. They may often be treated by prompt removal. Loss of the eye may result if they are neglected. When ignored, these tumors may invade the whole side of a horse's head.

OCCLUSION OF THE TEAR DUCT

Technically called the nasolacrimal duct, the tear duct extends from the inside corner of the eye to the inside of the nose. The lower opening is a small hole which may be seen inside the nostril, on the inner wall. Normally, it drains excess tears from the eyes into the nose (ever notice how your nose runs when you cry?). These ducts may become plugged due to injury or debris. They may fill with pus because of infection.

The first sign is that the horses's tears spill out of his eyelids. He will have a damp or pus-like streak down the side of his face. Flies and other insects are attracted to this moist spot and may severely annoy the animal. The problem can occur in one eye or in both. The membranes of the eye may be reddened because of the insect irritation, but usually will not be as red as they would with an eye infection.

Call your veterinarian for this one. He will use a small tube and sterile saline solution to flush out the duct through its opening into the nostril. Often the pus will exude in a long chain or string and float across the surface of the eyeball. This procedure may need to be repeated daily for several days until pus is no longer flushed from the upper opening.

EYEWORMS

A long thin worm called Thelazia lacrimalis is occasionally found in horses' eyes. These parasites have been reported from Indiana, Kentucky, Tennessee, and Canada. The animal will try to avoid light and will show severe conjunctivitis. He will usually have increased tear production. Severe cases may lead to keratitis (an inflammation of the cornea) and blindness. Most worms can be found on the surface of the conjunctiva. They are often surrounded by a sticky, light brown fluid. They are occasionally found on the surface of the cornea and on the eyelashes, as well as behind the third eyelid and within the tear gland and duct.

Treatment consists of removing the worms. They can usually be picked out with a pair of forceps or tweezers. The eye is then treated with a soothing antibiotic ointment for a few days to speed healing and kill any infection which may be present.

PERIODIC OPHTHALMIA

The cause of periodic ophthalmia is not positively known, but it is thought to be an allergic sensitivity within the eye to infection with certain bacteria. Serologic studies have linked the disease with leptospirosis, a disease spread by cattle in urine and abortion discharges. (76) Often, no cause can be found.

Whatever the cause of periodic ophthalmia, the animal ends up with an inflammation inside the globe of the eye. Early in the disease, the animal will show severe pain in the eye. He may hold it squeezed tightly shut, resisting any efforts to open it. He may be extremely sensitive to light. The eye may drain pus. After two or three days, the cornea will often appear cloudy. The membranes around the eye will be reddened and usually swollen. Pus or other white material may often be seen in the front chamber of the eye (just under the cornea), often by the second or third day of the attack.

The pupil is often narrowed to a fine slit. A heavy red line may be seen around the outer edge of the cornea. The first attack may last as long as a month. The problem may occur in one eye or both in the first attack. It may occur in the opposite eye on the next attack. The disease recurs at intervals, with as long as a year between episodes. As the disease progresses, cataracts usually develop within the eye. These may be partial, or may occupy the complete lens, causing blindness.

Early in its course, this disease looks much like a simple eye infection (conjunctivitis). If you have stained the eye and feel sure that there are no lesions on the cornea and have checked for foreign bodies, treat the animal as for conjunctivitis, using an eye ointment containing a corticosteroid. Keep the animal in a darkened stall.

If the horse is not significantly better by the end of three days, consult your veterinarian to have the animal examined and the diagnosis confirmed. At the present time, there is no specific treatment or prevention for periodic ophthalmia. The best that can be done to manage each individual attack is to try to minimize damage to the eye and make the animal comfortable until remission occurs. As mentioned above, blindness frequently is a sequel to periodic ophthalmia; because of this, periodic ophthalmia is an unsoundness.

SPASM OF THE EYELIDS

Newborn or very young foals may suddenly blink one or both eyes tightly shut. The animal shows evidence of severe pain. What has happened is that the eyelid has rolled inward, and the eyelashes and hair are rubbing the surface of the cornea, causing severe pain. Often all that is necessary to fix the problem is to roll the eyelid gently back to where it belongs. This is best done when the foal is lying down to avoid stressing the newborn by wrestling with him. This can be done several times a day. If this does not fix the problem, or if it recurs, consult your veterinarian. There is a simple surgical procedure which can be done to permanently "uncurl" the eyelids.

BLINDNESS

When a horse becomes suddenly blind in one eye, he may tilt his head peculiarly to one side. With time, the animal adjusts to the handicap and the head is usually held normally. A horse who is blind or has poor vision may balk or shy; these may be mistaken for dispositional problems rather than the true medical problems that they are. He may be overly sensitive to sounds, and move his ears continually.

A type of night blindness is seen in some horses. It is common in Appaloosas, but may occasionally be seen in animals of other breeds. Affected horses may frequently injure themselves in familiar surroundings in darkness. There is no known treatment for this condition. It is considered hereditary and affected animals should be removed from breeding programs. (77)

Waving a hand in front of an animal's eye is not a reliable test for blindness, as he may blink because of the shadow, the movement, or because he feels the movement of the air against his eye. If there is any doubt about whether or not your horse can see or whether an animal you are going to purchase has normal vision, have him examined by your veterinarian (see Blindness in the section on unsoundness for further information).

EYE REMOVAL

Occasionally an eye is so badly injured that it must be removed. An ulcer or cut which has been neglected can become so badly infected that the eye must be taken out. Removal can also be necessary because of tumors. Your veterinarian will sedate the horse before surgery. He may do the operation with the horse standing, or may prefer to have him lying down, depending on the animal and the facilities available. The entire eyeball is usually removed. If a tumor is involved, other structures in the eye socket, such as muscles and fat, will also be taken out. The eyelids are then trimmed along the edges to allow them to grow together after they are sutured shut. After the wound is healed, the animal will learn to cope with having only one eye—a feat which they usually accomplish rather easily and calmly.

OTHER EYE PROBLEMS

A few truly exotic eye ailments are seen in the horse as in any other animal. If you do not find the problem to be one of the common ones, consult your veterinarian for a diagnosis. If he is at a loss as to the problem, ask him to recommend a specialist for you, or take your animal to one of the veterinary schools for examination.

Chapter 17

SKIN PROBLEMS

Allergies
Hives
Photosensitization
Sunburned Udders
Sunburned Noses, Lips, and Eyes
Burns
    Chemical Burns
    Rope Burns
    Lightning Strike
Frostbite
Saddle and Cinch Sores
    White Spots (Saddle Marks)
Pyoderma
Chapped Hocks and Knees
Scratches
Ringworm
Virus Skin Diseases
Warts
Vesicular Stomatitis
External Parasites
    Flies
    Mosquitoes
    Screwworms, Blowflies
    Face Flies
    Lice
    Ticks
        Ear Ticks
    Mange
    Streptothricosis
    Onchocerciasis
    Habronemiasis
    Cattle Grubs
Skin Cancer (and Other Tumors)
Sarcoids
Fistula of the Withers and Poll Evil
Ear Problems
Tail Rubbing (Including Washing the Sheath)

The skin is the largest organ of the body. It has a multitude of functions, including keeping out foreign influences which might hurt the animal and regulation of his temperature. The skin contains large numbers of sensitive nerve endings which makes it an important sense organ. It would seem that when you're dealing with something so large and prominent, it would be a cinch to diagnose problems. Sometimes, with diseases such as warts or ringworm, it IS easy. Other times, despite bacterial cultures or tests as sophisticated as biopsies, we still can't determine the cause of a skin disease which is staring us in the face. So don't think your veterinarian is lacking if he can't come up with a reason for a skin disease. Perhaps it will help to assure you that the great majority of the undiagnosable skin diseases go away with time. Of those we CAN diagnose, most are repairable or controllable. Let's discuss some causes of skin problems.

ALLERGIES

Allergies to substances applied to the skin can cause an animal considerable misery. This problem can result from using insecticides or insect repellents—like the time one of my clients raised four-inch wide welts, an inch high and several feet long across the side of a mare she'd just bought. She was using a repellent that had served her long and faithfully on several other animals. The only difficulty was that this mare was allergic to it! She switched to another product and the bumps went away in five or six days, during which time she was unable to ride her new animal because of the welts in the saddle area.

The way to avoid this situation is to patch test all new animals with any product that you intend to apply to their hides. Test products which are new to your horse in the same manner. Pick a spot that you can remember, in an area that is not critical, such as the side of the neck. Put some of the substance you will be using in a spot about 2 inches square, rubbing it in thoroughly. Use slightly more than you will be using normally, but don't get carried away and marinate the spot with it. Wait two days, observing the spot at least once a day (twice or three times a day is better) to see if there is any swelling or heat. Watch for any bumps that may suggest hives and for weeping or tenderness in the area.

If the animal survives the patch test with flying colors, then you can feel reasonably safe in using the product all over his body. Even so, use it lightly the first couple of times to make sure that when it is used in large amounts all over the body, there will be no reaction. It is a good idea to test grooming sprays, coat conditioners, and other products in this manner.

Horses may show allergic reactions to insect bites. Some will not have any bumps or only very small ones from mosquito bites at the beginning of the insect season, while later in the year they will have large spots and look like they have been through a war. This is thought to be due to the animal's becoming increasingly allergic to the bites as the season wears on. Bee, wasp, or hornet stings may also cause an allergic reaction. The animal may become quite miserable because of the bumps that these cause. In Australia, a disease called Queensland Itch has been shown to be caused by an allergic reaction to the bite of a particular type of sandfly. In severe cases, an injection of a corticosteroid drug may provide some relief.

Then there are the cases of nonspecific bumps that we occasionally see. Animals may be covered with lumps up to about ¾ inch in diameter, often interspersed with many smaller ones. The lumps usually start on the front end of the horse, covering the head, neck, forearms, and withers. In the worst cases, they may spread all over the horse. They do NOT go away in two or three days. Indeed, they often do not go away in two or three months! But the good news is that, finally, they usually do go away.

Current thinking is that the lumps are due to an autoimmune problem in which the animal is allergic to something within himself, much like systemic lupus in humans. Talk about an allergy! The only treatment seems to be large amounts of corticosteroid drugs for long periods of time. If left alone, the lumps are usually is gone by the next summer. Even when one of these lumps is cut out and sent to a laboratory, there is yet to be any good answer as to the cause of the problem.

HIVES

Also called "nettle rash" or "urticaria," hives is an allergy problem. Hives may result when the horse eats plants to which he is allergic. They have been reported in horses who had been grazing clover or buckwheat. Hives may be due to systemic causes because of the absorption of toxins from the digestive tract after constipation or intestinal inflammation. They may also be seen after sudden changes in feed. Horses get hives from eating certain foods much as we do: one author reports a horse who was severely allergic to carrots!

These bumps may also occur after skin contact with certain plants which contain irritating chemicals. The rash that follows contact with stinging nettles (Urtica species) gives this condition one of its names. Well over 100 species of plants can produce some form of allergic reaction in an animal sensitive to them. Walking through plants, such as poison oak, poison sumac, and nettles, may cause hives on some horse's legs. As with humans and poison ivy, not all individuals are susceptible, but the reaction can cause considerable misery to those who are.

Hives may be seen as a mild form of anaphylaxis due to vaccination reaction or after an injection of a foreign (non-equine) protein material. They may be seen after medication with drugs, especially penicillin.

SIGNS

Hives appear suddenly. They are ¼ to 1-½ inches in diameter, and may be raised as much as a half-inch. They are usually worse over the neck and trunk, but may totally cover the body. The lips and eyelids may be swollen in the worst cases. On rare occasions, there may also be swelling of the mouth, vulva, or perianal area. The animal may be obviously uncomfortable and may have little or no appetite. Some (but not all) animals may show severe itching.

Hives may be easily diagnosed because they pit (dent) if you press a finger firmly into them. The pit will remain for a minute or two after you remove your finger. This is especially obvious immediately after they have occurred, and becomes less evident after they have been present for several days. Sudden onset of a bumpy skin disease usually points to either hives or a batch of insect bites (bee or hornet swarms). In either case, treatment is similar.

TREATMENT

Horses tend to recover from hives by themselves, and hives often leave as suddenly as they appeared. Severe cases and those persisting more than two or three days should be examined by a veterinarian. He will usually give drugs, such as antihistamines and corticosteroids.

If you have determined that there is a plant or dietary agent causing the problem, take steps to see that it is removed. Has there been a change in feed? A "change" may be that you bought your feed from a new or different supplier, or even that a new batch of your old feed was made with different ingredients. If there has been no sudden change in the feed and the animal continues to have problems, begin by removing all sweet feed and supplements from the diet. Then, reintroduce feeds one at a time to see if the reaction recurs. If it does, then the feed you introduced just before is probably the culprit.

If insects are the cause, take proper control measures. Bees may attack sweaty horses more readily than dry animals. If beehives are present in the horse pasture, it may be necessary to move them to another location or to remove them entirely to avoid problems. If hornets are the cause, it may be necessary to destroy their nests, if you can locate them. This is best done at night when the insects are inactive and inside the nest. Don't stand right under the nest when you get rid of them! Mosquito repellent may make it possible for the animal to be outside. It may be necessary to keep the horse covered with a sheet or in a screened stable during the worst time of the day.

PHOTOSENSITIZATION

The name of this condition indicates an abnormal sensitivity to light. It is caused by substances in the bloodstream which make the animal react to light by becoming burned. Two main causes are seen in horses: 1) the ingestion of certain poisonous plants which contain sensitizing substances or intake of certain chemicals which have the same effect; and 2) photosensitization due to intake of substances which damage the liver and prevent the elimination of a liver byproduct called phylloerythrin. This byproduct builds up in the bloodstream, causing the horse to become sensitive to light.

Plants which have been said at times to cause photosensitization include alfalfa, red clover (Trifolium pratense), burr clover (Medicago denticulata), and alsike or Swedish clover (Trifolium hybridum). The problem may also be seen in animals who are mostly fed vetch (Vitia sativa). St. Johnswort (also called Goat Weed, Tipton Weed, and Klamath Weed) has been incriminated in causing photosensitization. Like many other poisonous plants, St. Johnswort is usually not eaten by animals if they have a choice of anything else. Buckwheat (Fagopyrum sagittatum) is grown for its grain; when grazed, it will, on occasion, cause photosensitization. Agave lechugilla, found in the Southwest, can produce photosensitization accompanied by liver damage.

SIGNS

If noticed early in the course of photosensitization, the animal may appear restless. The skin becomes reddened, especially in areas which are white, such as blazes and stockings. It is usually worse in thinly haired areas such as the muzzle and bridge of the nose. The reddening is followed by leakage of serum from the capillary beds in the skin. Severe cases may show leakage of yellowish serum through cracks or tears in the swollen, thickened skin. The hair may be thickly matted with the exudate, and bacterial infection or attack by flies may follow.

The horse may peel thin flakes of skin much as we do following a severe sunburn. Large areas of the skin may die and slough if the problem is severe and not treated in time. There may be a foul odor from the dead skin material and exudate. There may be intense itching and the animal may rub, causing trauma to the already weakened skin tissues. Animals rarely die from photosensitization itself, but death may occur in untreated animals from secondary infection, from liver damage caused by the plants in the first place, or from starvation. This is a miserable ailment for a blaze-faced animal with two or three white stockings. It is a disaster for a paint who is half white. White hair means pink skin underneath and less protection from sunlight.

Photosensitization caused by alsike clover may occur only on areas of the animal that have been in contact with the clover, particularly the mouth. This seems to at times occur with a lush, new growth of the plant. The fact that it occurs in the summer with bright, sunny days and nights that are cool with heavy dew has given this condition the name "dew poisoning." Painful sores in and around the mouth have been reported in this condition, causing the horse to quit eating and to become emaciated.

Diarrhea, colic, and other digestive disturbances are sometimes seen with clover poisoning. The horse may show a severe yellow discoloration of the membranes of the eyes (called icterus). This may be followed by sluggishness, lack of appetite, depression, and either unconsciousness or continuous walking around. The urine is usually dark colored. It progresses to unconsciousness and/or paralysis. Alsike clover poisoning is usually fatal unless reversed in its early stages. If photosensitization is the major problem, the animal will usually recover promptly if treated and removed to an alsike-free pasture.

TREATMENT

Remove the horse immediately from the pasture or feed suspected of causing the photosensitization. Place the animal in a closed stable to keep it both in the dark and free from insects. Control insects in the stable by spraying or other control measures. Do not use insect repellents on the animal unless absolutely necessary. They can be very irritating to the raw surfaces of the lesions.

Use a healing ointment on mild cases without severe skin sloughing. Good products include nitrofurazone dressing and zinc oxide ointment. More severe lesions should be cleaned with a mild soap such as pHisohex and patted gently dry with paper towels or clean, soft cloths. Then apply an antibiotic ointment, such as nitrofurazone dressing. Panalog ointment (Upjohn, Kalamazoo, MI 49001) which contains a corticosteroid to help reduce inflammation is also good.

Severe cases may require the administration of systemic corticosteroids to help reduce the inflammation and pain. Injections of antibiotics may be necessary to control infection in the damaged skin.

If at all possible, determine what caused the problem before you turn the horse back out into the pasture. If it is determined to be due to a poisonous plant, make other arrangements for pasturing the horse, or put him in a corral and feed hay. If you put him out on the same pasture, you are likely to go through the same problem all over again. Put the horse back outside during the day gradually so as to slowly reaccustom him to being in the sunlight.

If the area affected by the sunburn is small, you may wish to paint it with purple lotion. This helps to screen out the sunlight. It is not pretty to have a horse with a blue nose and a blue foot or two, but it can allow you to turn the animal out if necessary after he is healed, and avoid the need to gradually reaccustom him to sunlight.

SUNBURNED UDDERS

Sunburned udders are occasionally seen in mares with unpigmented udders, such as Appaloosas, in the northern states where it snows frequently in the spring, interspersed with days of brilliant sunshine. This occurs because sunlight is reflected from the snow up onto the udder. Naturally, this usually happens just about the time mares are ready to foal (the equine version of Murphy's Law!).

The first sign often noticed is that the foal acts hungry or uneasy; he may be down and weak. The mare may not allow him to nurse or moves away or kicks at him. He may even chase her, trying to make her let him have a meal.

Examination shows that the mare's udder is tightly swollen and hard, visibly reddened, and miserable-looking. You may need to have the mare sedated before she will even allow you to work on her. Gently soak her udder with towels which have been dipped in lukewarm water. Milk out as much milk as you can by hand, checking it to see that there is no mastitis or other infection present. By this time, the swelling should be reduced and the udder softened to where the mare will allow the foal to nurse. If not, you may need to milk the mare and bottle-feed the foal until the sunburned areas are a little less tender. In some cases, it may be necessary to administer painkillers to the mare so she will allow the foal to nurse.

Keep the mare and foal in a barn, in a deeply bedded stall, so that she can lie down if she wishes without too much discomfort. Apply a thin layer of petroleum jelly to the udder after you are finished working with the mare. Be wary of putting other ointments or salves on it. Remember that the foal may lick and nuzzle off anything that you put on; be sure whatever you use is edible for his sake.

The mare can usually be turned out when the sunburn is cleared up, if the snow has melted or the weather is cloudy. If the sun/snow combination is still present, you may need to keep the mare confined until better weather conditions prevail. This condition can be the cause of loss of foals in pasture-foaling mares. If this occurs and no one is around, the mare may abandon the foal or kill him as he attempts to nurse her tender udder. In this case, the ultimate cure to the problem is not having mares with white udders.

SUNBURNED NOSES, LIPS, AND EYES

The same sort of sunburn is frequently seen on horses with white on their faces or around their eyes. Horses who have white around their eyelids frequently have burned and peeling spots. These may weep and exude serum, as described under photosensitization. The white of the eye is often more reddened than usual, as are the conjunctival membranes. This causes excess tears to be formed in response to the irritation. They then spill down the side of the face, making dirty tracks as dust collects on the moisture.

Many a bald-faced horse spends the entire summer blinking and weeping and trying to fight off the flies that are attracted to the sores and exudate. Perhaps the simplest solution to the problem is not to own bald-faced or white-faced horses. In lieu of this, paint large circles with purple lotion around each eye (being careful not to get the solution in the eye itself). This has several actions; it protects the skin by acting as a sunscreen, it helps to dry out and heal any sores that may be present and, when placed around the eye, it acts as sunglasses or the charcoal that football players place on their cheeks to help prevent the sunlight reflecting from the white skin into the eye where it can sunburn the conjunctiva. Obviously, this cure is tough to use if the animal is a show horse. It may be necessary to keep one of these horses inside and only allow him to graze outside at night. The same purple lotion may be used on noses and lips that show sunburn.

BURNS

Burns on horses are occasionally seen in the horse after a stable fire or other accidental fire. The superheated air and/or smoke that the animal has inhaled may cause pneumonia. This is one of the more common problems after a fire (see Pneumonia). The animal may suffer burns over a significant part of the body. Burns may also be seen after a lightning strike in an open pasture or from contact with live electric wires.

It is advisable to call a veterinarian to help make a determination if the animal can be saved at all or if he should be put out of his misery. If it is decided that the animal can be saved, you may be looking at months (perhaps as long as 6 to 8 months) of treatment. Treatment will be required at least once a day, and perhaps more frequently.

Consider also whether the animal will be usable if you save him. A gelding who is severely burned across the back may be useless as a riding animal because of the scarring that will inevitably occur. Scarring may not be a problem in a mare who is to be used only for breeding. There is considerable pain and infection involved with a serious burn. Do you wish to put your horse through that, or would it be kinder to put him down? Animals with burns over more than 50% of their body are generally euthanized.

The skin of a burned animal is usually thickened with fluid and may have small blisters and dead spots. Severe burns may have charring of the skin. If large areas of skin are lost, there may be great loss of fluid and protein in the exudate which weeps from these sites. Enough plasma may be lost to put the animal into shock. The burned surfaces are very susceptible to infection and heal slowly. Animals with severe burns may be lethargic and indifferent. They frequently resent handling and are reluctant to move.

TREATMENT

Burns involving less than 15% of the animal's body are treated with relative ease. Systemic antibiotics are usually not needed. Ointments such as nitrofurazone dressing are used. Apply the ointment and cover with a sterile bandage. Clean the wound daily, wiping off any exudate with sterile gauze sponges and reapplying ointment and dressing.

Be careful not to pull off any skin while changing the bandage. If the gauze sticks, try to pull it loose gently. If it does not come loose, cut around the pad and leave it on the wound, rebandaging over it. It will fall off when the scab that forms over the area falls off.

Do not use greasy products, such as petroleum jelly or lard, and do not put loose cotton on the wound, as the fibers will catch on the surface and help hold the exudate. This contributes to the possibility of infection.

Burns involving more than 15% of the body surface will need systemic treatment. This is definitely a time to call your veterinarian. He will consider the condition of the lungs and respiratory system. The pulse, respiration rate, and temperature should be carefully noted.

Oral fluid therapy, begun immediately, may avoid the need for intravenous fluids. The animal may have fluids given through a stomach tube. A solution of one teaspoon of salt and ½ teaspoon of bicarbonate of soda (baking soda) per quart of water can be used. As much as 10% of the animal's body weight may be given the first day, and up to 5% the second day.

Your veterinarian may also give corticosteroids for the stress. The amount used should be reduced and then stopped as soon as they are no longer needed for treating the shock, as this type of medication retards healing severely. Burns heal slowly enough as it is, without anything else to slow them down. Antibiotics such as penicillin/streptomycin should also be given. Electrical burns are treated in the same manner.

Animals with any type of burn may need to be restrained to keep them from lying down and tearing off healing, new skin, and to keep them from chewing bandages or biting or scratching the burned areas. Good nutrition is a necessity for the healing burn patient. The larger the area of damage, the greater the need for a diet high in protein to help replace that lost with the plasma exudate. Ample water is a necessity.

CHEMICAL BURNS

Chemical burns result from accidental or malicious contact with acids, alkaline substances, or other chemicals such as phenol. One of the most commonly encountered substances is battery acid, because of its ready availability.

The basic treatment principles outlined for heat or electrical burns hold for chemical burns. The first step in treatment is to neutralize whatever is causing the problem. If the burn is caused by an alkali, vinegar or lemon juice may be poured over it to neutralize it. Baking soda (sodium bicarbonate) mixed with water is the logical choice for acid burns or for burns caused by unknown chemicals. If the accident just occurred, immediate flushing of the affected area with water alone will help to dilute the substance and to rinse it off the animal.

After neutralizing the substance as well as possible, wash the lesion with pHisohex or other mild soap. Then rinse it with large quantities of a solution of one teaspoon of sodium chloride (table salt) per quart of water. A moist bandage kept damp with the same salt solution may be helpful if kept in place for a few hours.

Petroleum jelly, oils, or ointments should be avoided with chemical burns. Consult your veterinarian for further treatment of these problems.

ROPE BURNS

Rope burns and other friction burns are often treated with antibiotic salves, such as nitrofurazone dressing. As they frequently occur in the pastern area, you may wish to cover the burn with a sterile dressing to keep it clean. If it becomes weepy and moist, change to purple lotion. The basic principle on this type of wound is "If it's dry, soften it, and if it's weeping, dry it up."

A rope burn that has been left untreated for some time will often be covered with dirt, crusts, and exudate which you cannot easily remove. One of the easiest ways to handle this is with a sauerkraut poultice (see Scratches). This will clean it up, after which you can decide to use a softening ointment with a bandage, purple lotion without a bandage, or leave it without further treatment.

LIGHTNING STRIKE

Horses are struck by lightning because of their tendency to stand under trees. Unfortunately, no one has explained to them that it is hazardous to stand under lone trees or small clumps of trees on the top of a hill. They also occasionally lean against wire fences or pipe corrals. In this case, a lightning strike anywhere along the fence line may be carried quite some distance to where the horses are standing.

Another problem is that horses frequently huddle together in a storm. If the lightning is carried down a fence to one of them, it may be conducted through that animal to any others who are touching him, resulting in the death of several animals. Death from lightning usually is instantaneous, resulting from cardiac arrest or respiratory stoppage due to the passage of electrical current through the brain.

In lightning death, the animal or animals may appear to have dropped without a struggle. Lightning is especially suspicious if several animals are found dead around a tree or near a fence shortly after a storm with lightning. Burn marks, splitting of fence posts, or welding of fence wires are definite evidence of a lightning strike.

Singe marks are said to occur in 90% of lightning deaths. These marks often appear as lines on the insides of the legs. If the animal or animals are insured, call a veterinarian immediately for a postmortem (necropsy). Without a prompt examination, your insurance company may refuse to pay the claim.

Occasionally, an animal is unconscious, but may recover completely within several hours. Some of the recovered animals will have nervous signs, such as partial paralysis, incoordination, or depression; these abnormalities may persist for weeks. If lightning burns occur, treat them as for other burns.

FROSTBITE

Frostbite occasionally occurs when horses, especially foals and young animals, are exposed to storms and severe cold. It is worse when the animals are poorly nourished. The ears are most commonly affected, but if the animal is weak and lying down, any part of the skin may be damaged.

Mild frostbite causes the blood vessels in the skin to constrict, leaving the area without blood. After thawing, the area will be hot, swollen, and very painful. When the swelling goes down, the area may remain reddened, itchy, and irritated for some time. The animal will be abnormally sensitive to cold for the rest of his life.

If freezing is more severe, the frostbitten area may be swollen and extremely painful. It will remain cold to the touch and later begin to shrivel. In severe cases, patches of skin die. A line of separation develops between the frostbitten area and the normal tissue. The dying skin develops a dry gangrene and finally drops off, leaving a raw area.

TREATMENT

Small areas of frostbite may be cleaned with a mild antiseptic, such as tamed iodine. Cover the affected area with an antibiotic ointment, such as nitrofurazone dressing. If the frostbite is noticed early, warm the area in a lukewarm water bath (104 to 108 degrees F (40 to 42 C)) for 15 to 20 minutes. Massaging the area gently every day may help stimulate circulation and relieve pain. Severe frostbite should be treated similarly until it becomes obvious that the area is dead. It should then be surgically removed and the area treated as an open wound.

SADDLE SORES AND CINCH SORES

Saddle sores and cinch sores are common in horses who are ridden hard. They are also seen in animals used with ill-fitting saddles so that the tack either rolls or pinches.

Cinch sores are common with dirty tack. Cinches which are allowed to become caked with mud and dirt can quickly rub sores on the animal's tender hide. Cinch sores must be distinguished from girth itch, a type of ringworm. Girth itch will often be seen in a number of horses in the group, while cinch sores may occur in only one or two individuals.

Saddle and cinch sores are more common when the rider sways from side to side or slouches to one side, resulting in a rubbing action or unbalanced load on the animal's back. Both are seen more often in horses who are fat and out of shape. The extra blubber allows the saddle to roll and twist. They may also be seen in horses who are so thin and gaunt as to not have enough flesh to pad the tack.

Saddle sores may be seen on horses who have been on a conditioning program. The horse started out fat, with a saddle that fitted. As the animal becomes trim and gets into shape, the saddle no longer fits his contours. Do not assume that because the saddle fit at one time, it will always fit the same horse, especially if his shape changes radically!

These sores are more common in horses who have little or no withers; it is necessary to cinch the saddle more tightly in an attempt to keep it from rolling or turning. This helps to create the pressure and irritation which cause sores.

Saddle and cinch sores begin with inflammation of the skin tissues. A saddle sore which is not visible yet may often be felt by running the hand over the skin of the back.

Raised, hot, swollen spots are the beginnings of the sores. If the rider continues to use the horse who has one of these lumps, it will be subjected to even more friction and rubbing from the saddle because it is raised.

The hair over the area may be standing up slightly or may be rubbed short. The future site of a sore may either be sweaty—on a back that is otherwise dry—or it may be a dry spot on a wet back. When you see one of these spots, keep an eye on it. Some horses will have a dry spot or wet spot from either too much or too little saddle pressure on a given area from a particular saddle. These conditions may indicate an oncoming saddle sore.

The next step in the development of a saddle sore is for the hair to be worn off, leaving a hairless spot. Blisters, weeping sores, and swollen, bloody areas may follow. If the situation has been going for a long time, it may be called a "saddle gall."

In serious cases, abscesses may develop in the skin and underlying tissues. These can be hot and painful and may break and drain a clear or pinkish to bloody fluid. Severe damage to deeper tissues may result in death of the skin in the area, with eventual sloughing. Chronic saddle sores may have hardened spots under them. After healing occurs, the hair in the area may turn white. The white patches, if soft underneath, will not generally cause any problems in the future.

TREATMENT

Early saddle sores are usually treatable with a minimum of trouble. Prompt treatment may keep them from becoming worse. Early treatment is especially important if you are out in the middle of nowhere on a pack trip or long trail ride. Begin by resting the horse, if at all possible. If the sore is weeping, use a purple lotion product to help dry up the sore. Later, use a soothing ointment, such as nitrofurazone dressing, to soften the area if it becomes dry and crusty. Use nitrofurazone dressing or neomycin ointment or solution on saddle and cinch sores which are infected. If the sores are very large or severely infected, penicillin injections for three to five days may be needed in addition to the local treatment. Dead tissue should be removed surgically by your veterinarian.

If the sore is severe, it will be necessary to stop using the animal until he is healed in order to prevent complications. Less severe sores may be managed by cutting a hole in a thick saddle pad, and then using another pad over it to take all pressure off the area. This must be done with care; in some cases, the animal will just develop another sore area (or enlarge the present one) around the edge of the hole.

The extra-thick, high-quality, hospital acrylic (pile fabric) pads can be used on horses with saddle sores, and the animal can sometimes be healed while still being ridden. Beware of cheap "fake fur" pads. These are little or

no improvement over a plain saddle blanket or pad and will not allow this healing to occur.

The same acrylic material can be made up into a cinch cover to protect the animal. When used over cinch or saddle sores, these materials must be scrupulously clean. Many can be washed in a washer. Run them through one or two extra rinse cycles to be sure that all soap is removed. After they are dry, take one of the wire "doggy combs" and comb the pile until all knots and lumps are gone and it is uniformly smooth.

Cinch sores may be avoided in some animals by cinching the horse in a different location—either farther backward or farther forward. In an emergency, sheepskin covers can be made to cover the cinch or the offending cinch ring.

PREVENTION

Getting a horse into condition gradually so that his skin has a chance to toughen up for use along with his muscles, tendons, and hooves will help prevent some saddle and cinch sores. Keeping the horse at a consistent normal weight also helps. Keep tack clean. Wash blankets frequently, or hang them over a clothesline or fence and curry the worst of the dirt off them, and then beat them until clean if they are not washable. Wash cinches when they become dirty (if they are washable). Leather girths should be cleaned with saddle soap. Be especially careful to remove mud from tack so that it does not irritate the horse the next time you ride him. Badly fitting saddles should be replaced. A saddle which is perfect for a Quarter Horse may be sheer torture for a Thoroughbred, and vice versa.

Check your riding habits. Do you ride lightly and with the horse, or are you a bit overweight and less than totally graceful so that you lurch around in the saddle? Slewing the saddle around can literally wear holes in the horse's hide, as can habits such as slouching one hip to the side, or riding with most of the weight in one stirrup. If you need to do these things to rest yourself, they are going to put a lot of strain on your horse. If you want him to continue to carry you, get off and walk for a bit when you feel the urge to slouch. Give him a break so that he can continue to do a good job for you. This author has examined a couple of horses on competition trail rides who were literally worn through the hide by riders who moved a lot in the saddle. One of these poor animals had such severe sores and was hurting so badly that the officials pulled him out of the ride.

WHITE SPOTS (SADDLE MARKS)

White spots are often found on the withers and backs of horses who have been used. These are caused by wear and tear and mean nothing more than that the animal has been ridden; they are saddle marks. Draft horses may have similar spots from where the collar has worn. White spots may also occur where the animal has been injured, cut, or branded, or had a cinch or saddle sore. They are occasionally seen at the corners of a horse's lips from contact with a bit. Unless accompanied by soreness or other problems, these white spots are NOT a sign of disease. Check saddle marks to make sure there is no scar tissue under them which could cause problems when the horse is ridden hard.

PYODERMA

Pyoderma is similar to acne in humans. It is a bacterial infection which shows up as pustules ("pimples") on the skin. It often occurs in the saddle area or on the neck and shoulders. Rubbing a hand over the animal feels like there are small bumps everywhere. Small yellow drops of serum may be seen on top of the lesions.

Severe cases may spread over the entire body, even possibly causing ulceration. If the disease is widespread, the animal may have an elevated temperature and an anemia. Before you decide that the horse has pyoderma, check VERY carefully for parasites. Animals with lice or ticks may show the same skin lesions and yellowish exudate.

Avoid irritating affected areas. A 10% Clorox solution may be sponged on the bumps, or they may be painted with purple lotion if there are not too many and you don't mind having blue spots on the horse. Consult your veterinarian if the problem gets worse or does not improve.

CHAPPED HOCKS AND KNEES

Old-timers called scaly, weeping sores around the hocks and knees mallenders and sallenders. They were known as mallenders on the front legs and sallenders on the hind legs. Now we call them chapped hocks and knees.

The spots usually start as dry, rough patches with the hair standing up, and progress with swelling and heat. They then develop into weeping, moist sores. These crust over with yellow scabs which easily break off and start over again, often in a seemingly endless procession. Soon they are completely hairless, with cracks or an eroded, hollow spot. They may be crusty and then become fissured and raw. If they continue for a time, the skin may become thickened and rigid. When they are extremely bad, they can make a horse stiff or lame.

One of the most obvious causes of chapped hocks and knees is stable filth. The skin being caked with urine and manure is almost a sure way to start these spots. They are also common in horses who lie down frequently on hard surfaces or inadequate bedding, such as a hard floor or packed ground. It may be seen in horses with knee-deep bedding—when the bedding was tree chips that had

been run through a city shredder—they were very coarse and rough.

Chapping also seems to start when a horse is ridden through mud and the mud is allowed to remain on the hair for a long period of time. Alkali mud seems to be especially bad. The same problem occurs when corrals are muddy. It is also said to be caused by limestone dust or dry sand. Washing the legs with too-strong soaps (or failing to rinse off a milder soap) can also begin the irritation. Having a leg bandaged and allowing the bandage to get wet and not changing it promptly can also start the chapped spots. Thin-skinned horses seem more prone to chapping.

The immediate cure begins by cleaning the legs. They may be washed with a very mild soap; just hosing them off with clean water will often make a world of difference. Gently remove as many of the crusts as possible. The spots may then be softened with any mild ointment—from nitrofurazone or Corona to bag balm to plain old petroleum jelly. The use of fly spray in season will help avoid adding fly insult to the existing injury.

The permanent cure (and future prevention) depends on finding and eliminating the cause. Changing to softer bedding, or providing bedding if there is none, is a start in the right direction. Taking a minute to rinse mud or manure off the animal's legs will often prevent months of treatment that may be necessary to cure the chapping. When treating chapped hocks or knees, don't give up. The problem didn't develop overnight, and it won't be cured overnight.

SCRATCHES

Also called grease heels, grease, cracked heels, or mud fever, this condition is a dermatitis (inflammation of the skin) of the heel and rear side of the pastern area. While it is most common in the hindfeet, it may affect the front ones, or be any combination thereof. It was very common in draft horses, helped by the long hair (called "feathers") on their legs. This long hair held dirt and moisture, and often covered up beginning signs of the scratches, so it was not noticed until quite advanced. The disease is not contagious, but several horses in the same stable may be affected because they are exposed to the same conditions.

Scratches is frequently associated with dirty stables. It can also occur when horses stand in muddy corrals for long periods of time without relief. Horses whose legs are "stocked up" (swollen and tight) for longer periods of time may have scratches. Shoeing the horse at an improper angle—forming a fold of skin on the rear of the foot—may provide enough irritation, friction, and moisture to cause the problem.

Soaps, salt solutions, or irritating liniments may cause enough dermatitis to start a case of scratches. Lime dust from roads or floors and other chemical irritants may do the same. Photosensitization caused by poisonous plants or chemicals may initiate scratches. Contact dermatitis from alsike clover (dew poisoning) or poison ivy can also start scratches. Infection by bacteria and/or fungi usually occurs as the disease progresses. In some cases, it is impossible to determine the original cause of the problem.

Early in scratches, the skin is sensitive and swollen; it may itch severely. As it progresses, the skin may show heat and be reddened. Serum begins to ooze from cracks and sores on the skin. The exudate may be yellowish or grayish and will have a foul odor. Edema (swelling with fluid) may extend up the leg. By the time it has reached this point, the animal is usually lame and shows severe pain in the area. Dead patches of skin may begin to slough, leaving raw, red sores.

If not treated, the problem becomes chronic. Granulation begins; growths commonly called "grapes" may appear. The skin becomes thickened and hard. The foot may be so swollen as to look like an elephant foot. In severe cases, the infection may extend into the frog. It can even undermine the frog and sole.

Begin by removing the cause, if it can be determined. Cases of scratches which are diagnosed early have a good chance of recovery. Clip all hair from the affected area. Remove feathers if the animal has them. If the weather is wet, it is best not clip them off totally, but remove most, and leave a pointed tuft of hair on the back of the fetlock to help drain water off the leg. If you remove all the hair from the fetlock, any water that falls on the animal will run down over the affected area. Wash the skin gently with a mild soap, such as pHisohex. Then pat it dry with paper towels or a soft cloth towel. Remove any loose, dead skin. Apply a mildly antiseptic product, such as calamine lotion (from the drugstore: Caladryl lotion, Parke-Davis Div. of Warner-Lambert, Morris Plains, NJ 07950) or purple lotion, for a few days to help dry the area. Then change to ointments such as zinc oxide to prevent overdrying it.

If the infection extends deep into the heel or into the frog or if severe granulomatous growths are present, call your veterinarian for treatment of the problem. Small granulations may be removed with a pressure bandage, placed over a soothing ointment or a product containing a corticosteroid, such as Panalog (E.R. Squibb & Sons, Inc., Princeton, NJ 08540). Corticosteroid ointments are also useful for cases of scratches where the skin is not broken. A mixture of sulfanilamide powder and mineral oil is said to work well when the animal cannot be removed from wet conditions. The oil would act to keep moisture off the skin, and the antibiotic would help to heal the lesions. (78) Larger growths ("grapes") will require surgical removal, again, a project for your veterinarian.

The basic theory in treating a problem like scratches is to dry it up if it is wet, and to moisturize and soften it if it is dry. Now that I've told you all the fancy cures for the problem, let me tell you about an old-time remedy. It has cured many minor cases of scratches and also seems to work well on rope burns in the heel area.

Get a large can of sauerkraut, a plastic bag (a bread wrapper is O.K.), and some bandaging material—adhesive tape, Vetrap, or Elastikon. Pull the bag up over the affected foot. Pour the entire can of sauerkraut into the bag, putting most of it on the back side of the foot. Wrap the whole thing well with the tape, putting on gentle pressure and wrapping plenty of tape around the bottom of the hoof to help protect the plastic bag there. Leave it unchanged for three days. When you remove it, the skin is usually clean and fresh-looking and the problem is much improved. Treat it with either softening or drying products as needed. In a few cases, sauerkraut treatment for another two or three days may be necessary. The treatment works especially well with those cases that are exuding pus and are generally messy.

RINGWORM

Ringworm is caused by a fungus which attacks the skin and lives in the hair follicles. The organisms cause the hair shaft to become brittle and break. They do their damage, spreading outward from their central starting point. This often gives the bare spot a rounded appearance, from which it gets the name "ringworm." Ringworm which occurs in the cinch area is often called "girth itch." There are several species of organisms which cause the same symptoms. Since the treatment is the same, the exact type of fungus involved is of academic rather than practical importance.

By far the most common mode of spreading is from one infected horse to others. Horses share this disease by rubbing on each other—in the same corral or over the fence. Or, they may get the fungus from saddles, halters, blankets, brushes, or other equipment which has been used on infected animals. In this way, ringworm may spread rapidly throughout a stable. Infection may also come from infected soil or even from contact with humans who have ringworm. It is occasionally transmitted by rats who have ringworm.

The incubation period for ringworm is usually one to four weeks, but may be as little as four days. Dirty, warm, damp stables encourage ringworm infection. Sun and fresh air help to prevent the spread, but do not necessarily kill the infection once it starts on a horse's skin. Thin-skinned horses seem to be especially susceptible. Animals which have been treated excessively with antibiotics may have a lowered resistance to ringworm. Nutritional deficiencies will make the animal more likely to get ringworm.

In the northern states, ringworm may be seen to affect nearly all the animals in a stable or herd in late winter. The hay or pasture is of poor quality and severely lacking in vitamin A by late winter. This weakens the skin's resistance to the fungus and allows it to attack the animals easily. Feeding a vitamin A supplement throughout the winter often significantly reduces the problem; in some cases, it may eliminate it completely. On some ranches, the problem occurs every winter. The fungus spores may remain infectious for over a year, providing a ready reservoir for reinfection each season. Ringworm may also be seen in cattle at the same time on these ranches. The infection may be passed from cow to horse or vice-versa.

SIGNS

Ringworm appears as hairless patches. They may be rounded or irregular in shape. The patches may be scaly, or they may be covered with serum and thick crusts. Hairs may be growing through the crusts. If the scabs are removed, the area underneath may be red and raw and may also contain pus. In some infections, the area may appear blistered or may be covered with small pustules. Spots are often first seen on the head and neck. From there, they may spread until they appear all over the body. Itching is occasionally seen, but most animals show no apparent discomfort.

TREATMENT

Good nutrition helps to get the skin into condition to fight off the fungus. If the diet is lacking in vitamin A, supplementing this product will help considerably in getting rid of the ringworm. The diet should also have adequate protein. If stable management is a problem, the area should be cleaned thoroughly. Getting the animal out into the sunlight will help dry up weeping lesions and aid skin health.

Strong (7%) tincture of iodine should be rubbed into all of the ringworm spots, using a piece of burlap or rough cloth to help remove the scabs and assure that the iodine reaches the skin. Be extremely careful not to drip it into the animal's eyes. Also, don't get it on your clothes; it stains both fabric and hands a deep brown. Another cure which works well for ringworm is household bleach, such as Clorox (The Clorox Co., Oakland, CA 94612), diluted half-and-half with water and dabbed onto the lesions.

You may want to use one of the commercial preparations for ringworm. They are not necessarily any more effective than iodine and are usually more expensive. If the animal is valuable or you wish to show it, it may be worth giving griseofulvin (Fulvicin, Schering Corp., Kenilworth, NJ 07033). This is a specific antiringworm medication. It does not kill the ringworm. It incorporates itself into the new hair, making it resistant to the fungus. Thus, when new hair tries to grow out of the bald spot, it is not weakened and broken off as it had been previously. As a result, the bald spot will fill with new hair. This medication comes in packets of powder or in bolus form. It

appears to be tasteless, as most horses eat it readily when mixed with grain. If you can only get it in boluses, crush these with a hammer and feed the resulting powder mixed with grain.

If the animal has large parts of his body covered with ringworm, treat the bare spots with iodine; the spaces between that still have some hair with Clorox water; and give the animal griseofulvin orally. Even doing all this, there will be no apparent progress until new hair grows in, which may take as long as three to four weeks. Don't expect results immediately.

Ringworm is contagious to humans, so normal sanitary precautions should be taken. Do not touch your skin or hair after handling the animal. Wash your hands after working with him. Wash all blankets, towels, bandages, and other washable materials which have contacted the horse in hot water with detergent, adding chlorine bleach to the wash water. Soak all brushes, combs, halters and lead ropes, etc. in 10% bleach solution for several hours and then rinse well. Soak girth covers and washable cinches in the same solution. It doesn't hurt to set them out in the sun to air out and dry. Sponge saddle and bridle surfaces which have touched the horse with water containing bleach. Use separate tack and brushes for the affected horse(s) to avoid spreading the disease to other animals. Avoid borrowing or loaning tack and grooming tools when ringworm is present in a stable. If you catch ringworm, consult your physician for his recommendations.

VIRUS SKIN DISEASES

Two viruses frequently cause skin problems in the horse. One is vesicular stomatitis, a disease which is endemic to some parts of the country. The other is warts, a common disease of young horses.

WARTS

Also called equine cutaneous papillomatosis, warts is a disease of young horses or animals who have never previously been exposed. It is most commonly seen in horses up to three years of age. The warts are knobby, often cauliflower-looking growths. They may be up to half an inch or larger in diameter. If the warts are small, there are often a great number of them. If only a few are present, they may each be larger in size. They may be seen as high as the eye area, but are more common on the muzzle and lips. Some may also be found in the mouth or on the tongue and gums. Occasionally, warts occur on the legs. It is thought that these are caused by the horse transferring the virus from its muzzle by rubbing it on his legs, or by grooming tools.

The incubation period is about two months, so by the

time one horse shows warts, it is likely that the rest of the horses on the farm have been exposed. This disease is occasionally seen in newborn foals; in these cases, they may occur anywhere on the animal's body.

Warts are a self-limiting disease. It's one of those problems that goes away in about three months if you treat them, and in about 90 days if you don't! They may last anywhere from two to six months. Most veterinarians don't remove any of the warts unless they are causing irritation or are interfering with eating, as they may do if they occur in large masses at the edge of the lips or on the tongue. There is some thought that if the lesions are removed early in the disease, this may stimulate the growth of many more of them than you would otherwise have had. If you feel that the warts need to be removed, call your veterinarian to ask him do the job. Careless removal may cause serious scarring. Cryosurgery (freezing) is sometimes used to remove these growths, and is often more successful than "knife" surgery.

Warts look ugly, but they generally don't cause any serious harm. Once the animal gets over them, he will probably be immune for life. Vaccines used to prevent warts in cattle do not do much good in horses, as the two diseases are caused by different viruses. If warts persist for a long period of time, the affected horse may have a deficient immune system.

Warts are contagious from one horse to another. This author views them much the same as the viral respiratory diseases. Expose the animal to them when he is young and before you start using him. Let him get the disease and get over it. Then, he won't be coming down with it when you are headed for a crucial show or race when he is a two or three-year-old.

If warts are a continuing problem on your farm, it is possible to get a vaccine made from them that is specific for your individual problem. Ask your veterinarian about this. The vaccine has a short shelf life and can only be kept about two months after it is prepared.

Older horses occasionally get bumps and lumps on their skin; these are usually not warts and may be some type of skin cancer or sarcoid. Unless it is obviously a face full of warts (as is seen in the younger animals), the animal should be checked by your veterinarian. If the problem is a tumor or sarcoid, the sooner it is detected, the better chance there is of a permanent cure.

VESICULAR STOMATITIS

This disease is caused by a virus; the same virus also attacks plants, and it is not known whether it goes from plants to animals or from plants to insects to animals, or just what and how. It was seen in horses during the civil war. Vesicular stomatitis is rarely fatal, but can cause the animal considerable misery. It may last one to two weeks, during which the animal will be unusable. A lactating mare

may quit giving milk, leaving the owner with the problem of an "orphan" foal. It is also contagious to sheep, hogs, humans, and cattle, where it can severely reduce milk production in dairies.

One of the most important reasons to be concerned about vesicular stomatitis is that it looks much like some foreign diseases, such as the notorious Foot-and-Mouth Disease, which could wipe out our livestock industry. If you live in an area where vesicular stomatitis is endemic (occurs frequently), you will no doubt be familiar with it. If it is not a common occurrence in your area, and you find your horse with some sort of unexplainable sores on his mouth, it is a good idea to call your veterinarian at once. In an outbreak, from 30% to 90% of the animals may be affected and inapparent infections may occur in the remainder.

SIGNS

The incubation period for vesicular stomatitis is one to five days. Often, the first symptom noticed is that saliva drips liberally from the animal's mouth. The horse may be depressed and usually stops eating—not because he is not hungry but because his mouth hurts too badly to do so. I would guess that the pain is similar to having a lot of cold sores or fever blisters in your mouth. His temperature may be as high as 104 degrees F (40 C); this occurs early in the disease and often lasts for only a few hours.

Sores may be seen on the lips. They look like blisters or may look like scalded or burned spots. They may be pink, red, or even deep purple in color. Some horses do not have any sores on the outside of the mouth, but may have a large sore or sores on the tongue. These may start out as small blisters or dimpled spots early in the disease. Later, areas of the membrane may peel away, leaving large portions of the tongue looking as if they had been boiled. If no other signs are present, the owner often says that "someone has been riding my horse and cut his tongue." Occasionally, sores may be seen at the coronary band. If they are severe enough, the pain may cause the animal to limp.

This disease is seen frequently in the southern and southwestern states. Cases are most frequent in the summer. Approximately 90% occur in August and September, with only rare cases as early as April or as late as November. Cases are seen over a longer season near the Gulf of Mexico than toward the Canadian border. The disease spreads through areas of dense horse population. In a 1945 outbreak in Colorado, the disease spread along streams rather than along main travel routes. A similar spread was seen in the 1982 outbreak in Wyoming as cases moved up the North Platte River some sixty miles from the start of the outbreak near Douglas. Even in Mexico and South America where there is no frost, the disease is not seen on a year-round basis. It is almost totally confined to the rainy season. The incidence and pattern of spread point to its being carried by an insect or biting fly, or perhaps by mosquitoes.

All horses do not get a clinical case of vesicular stomatitis even if exposed in the same corral or by direct contact. One stable had 90 horses when an outbreak occurred. The only animal to became ill was a mare who had recently been moved there, and was extremely upset, running the fences and worrying. It is likely that stress is a significant factor in the development of the disease.

Your veterinarian can send a serum sample to a laboratory to confirm that this is the disease present in your horse. However, if there is an outbreak going in your area, he is likely to already have confirmed that it is vesicular stomatitis. Tests need not be done on each animal.

TREATMENT

As with many viral diseases, there is no specific treatment for vesicular stomatitis. An animal who is having trouble with infection and complications may need treatment with penicillin/streptomycin combination or other antibiotic. Sores on the lips may be bathed with warm water, using a washcloth or paper towel. They may then be patted dry and any soothing ointment, such as petroleum jelly or Corona, may be used to make the animal more comfortable.

Keep the animal well treated with insect repellent for two reasons: it will make the animal much more comfortable not to have insects chewing on his sores, and it will help to prevent his being bitten by insects who would then carry the disease to someone else's horse. Aerosol or water-mix sprays will be less trouble to apply to the animal than wipe-on products.

Good insect control measures around the stable in the face of an outbreak, through use of insect sprays, baits, or electric insect lights, will do more to reduce the spread of this disease than almost any other measure you could take.

Observe careful sanitation with vesicular stomatitis. Handle affected horses as little as possible. Do not use their halters on other horses. Be sure to wash your hands in a disinfectant solution after handling the horse and do not eat, drink, or smoke while around affected animals so that you do not get the disease yourself. Do not touch your face or mouth while handling the animal. The disease is not terribly contagious to humans, but is moderately so. Don't be afraid of it, but DO respect it.

EXTERNAL PARASITES

Horses are attacked by a multitude of flying, stinging, biting insects. These pests can make the animal miserable, as well as transmitting disease from one animal to another. In fact, just a couple of hundred years ago in France, horses with docked tails were charged a lower pasture fee than were horses with full tails. The reason was simple; those animals without tails spent more time chasing insects and less time eating than did the others.

Flies, such as the common housefly and the stable fly (sometimes called the "biting house fly"), can make the animal uncomfortable, as well as spread disease and, not incidentally, cause humans many problems as they invade our dwellings. Other biting flies, such as the horse fly and deer fly, cause discomfort as well as spread some blood-borne diseases, such as swamp fever. Mosquitoes can spread diseases; allergy to their bites may raise large enough welts in the saddle area to make the animal unrideable. Bee stings can inflict the same damage in an animal who is allergic to them. Lice, ticks, and mange mites complete the list of parasites waiting to attack your horse's hide. Let's begin by discussing flies.

FLIES

Stable flies bite the horse, mostly on the legs. If there are many of them, the animal may get no rest during the daylight hours. Horses may run, stamp their feet, or stand in water trying to get away from these pests. They will also crowd together and swat flies for each other. When severely attacked by these pests, the animal may lose as much as 15% of its body weight because it is spending time fighting them rather than eating. The horse's joints may become so swollen and stiff from standing in a creek or pond to avoid the flies that he can scarcely stand. Stable flies have been shown to carry swamp fever.

House flies act as an intermediate host for one of the roundworms that inhabit the horse's stomach, a worm called Habronema. Horses are infected by swallowing infected flies or larvae of the roundworm which escape from these flies. When the worms reach the horse's stomach, they produce nodules in which they complete their development. House flies may also act to spread diseases from one horse to another by physical contact, as they land on one horse and then travel to another.

CONTROL

Both stable flies and house flies have a life cycle of two to three weeks from egg to fly. They breed and lay their eggs in manure and in wet bedding. Manure should be removed from the stall or pen on at least a daily basis. It can usually be stored for up to a week before further disposal without serious fly problems. Then it can be spread thinly on a field to allow the sun to dry and kill the fly eggs and thus prevent their hatching. It could also be composted in a mound so that the heat within will kill the fly eggs and larvae. This method is useful if you don't have a field on which to spread the bedding. Composted animal bedding is a tremendous fertilizer for your garden. If it is composted, you may need to spray the surface of the pile lightly with insecticide in order to help kill flies which are attracted to it.

Sprays help to reduce the number of flies around a stable. Fogging systems are available which spray a fine mist of insecticide into the area at measured intervals. They are said to be very good for fly control. Poisonous baits can be a valuable addition to a fly control program. Be sure to keep the bait containers out of the reach of horses, children, and pets.

The horses themselves may be sprayed with sprays containing pyrethrins. These products leave a residue on the animal's coat which will kill flies for several hours after spraying. For stable flies, it is especially important to spray the legs well. When spraying with any insecticide, avoid contaminating the horse's food, water, or salt block.

HORSE FLIES, DEER FLIES, GREENHEAD FLIES

These flies cause bites which are severely painful to the horse. This is obvious if you've ever seen a horse attacked by a half-dozen inch-long flies at the same time. The animal will buck, run, or roll in an attempt to get away from them. Remember the old folk song about the man who was killed when his horse was bitten by the "bluetailed fly?" These insects may also carry swamp fever and several other diseases from one horse to another.

These flies are most commonly found in swamp areas and along streams. They may also be plentiful in irrigated pastures. They seem to be more common in wet years than in dry years. They lay their eggs on plants near streams and other moist areas. Control in their habitat is not usually possible, as they are strong fliers and may go a mile or more from where they hatch to the horse that they consider to be dinner.

Using repellents (especially those containing pyrethrins for the residual effect) is about the only solution. In very marshy areas, the horse may have to be kept stabled during the day and only turned out at night to graze. A stable sheet will often provide enough protection that the animal can graze in relative comfort. If you are turning the animal out with a sheet on, be sure that it fits well and is fastened securely so that it will stay in place even if the horse rolls. My experience has been that those sheets provided with leg straps that go individually around each hind leg, plus a belly band, stay in place the best. It does not hurt to spray the sheet lightly with repellent to help keep insects from lighting on it and biting through, as some horse flies will do. You may need to experiment with several repellents to find one that works well with flies, as they are not all equally good on all insects.

MOSQUITOES

The principles outlined in this section will include blackflies, buffalo gnats, and sand flies, because their irritation and their control is similar to that of mosquitoes.

Mosquitoes are the primary insect vector for sleeping sickness (equine encephalomyelitis). Animals who are allergic to the bites of these insects may get large welts from them.

Mosquitoes breed and hatch near or in water. If you can trace your problem to a single pond or swampy area, it may be possible to effect permanent control by draining it or filling it. An oil-based insect repellent may be used on driveway puddles which are starting to breed mosquitoes in an extremely wet year. Just a few drops per puddle are enough to kill the larvae (which because of their motion are often called "wigglers"). A well-screened stable will protect horses from mosquitoes, but sand flies will readily pass through because of their extremely small size.

If there are no animals drinking from the pond or source of the infestation, it may be possible to spray the surface with an insecticide. Consider before you do this how many birds, rabbits, and other wildlife you may be killing by doing this. Consider also if your problem is going to continue due to a neighbor's pond supplying insects.

Repellents have some use. It is often necessary to try several in order to find one that works well on mosquitoes; some repellents work well on flies and not on mosquitoes, while others, vice versa. Stable sheets offer good protection against mosquito bites, especially if combined with spraying the horse once or twice a day with an insect repellent on the neck, legs, and belly where the horse is not protected by the sheet. Some fine-skinned, allergic horses may be unusable in the summer without protection from biting insects. One of my mares would come to me to get her sheet put back on if she had been turned loose without it. She seemed to appreciate it and wore it all summer because of her thin skin. Make sure the sheet fits well and is not going to rub sores on the animal because it is too tight.

Nets may be used over the animal's face or ears when gnats are intolerable. Ultraviolet insect killing lights may be useful in reducing mosquito populations in stable areas. In some areas, gnats or mosquitoes may be so numerous that the only solution is to keep the horse inside a screened stable during the period—either day or night—when the pests are most numerous.

SCREWWORMS, BLOWFLIES

Screwworms survive only in living flesh. This makes them a possible problem any time a horse receives an injury which breaks the skin. As small an opening as a tick bite can allow a screwworm infestation to start. Screwworms used to be a common problem throughout the southwestern states, bordering Mexico. Even now, the Federal Government wages war against these dangerous pests.

The female fly lays batches of eggs on the edge of the wound, where they hatch. The larvae invade the wound, feeding and forming pockets in the flesh. Wounds already infested with screwworms seem to be more attractive to the flies, compounding the problem. The infested wounds often bleed and may have a distinctive odor.

Blowflies lay their eggs on dead tissue, such as the rotten tissue in a old, festered, untreated wire cut. They eat damaged tissue, but stop short of invading healthy tissue, in contrast to the screwworm. They do not attack living flesh, but crawl around in the surface debris.

Contact your veterinarian if you think you have a case of true screwworms. The government has made considerable progress in eradicating this pest by releasing large numbers of sterilized flies. It needs to keep track of new cases in order to be able to stop their damage and spread.

The infested wound can be treated with insecticides, such as lindane, ronnel, or coumaphos, to kill blowfly or screwworm larvae. Use these according to your veterinarian's directions. When you are rid of the worm larvae, you can then proceed to treat the wound. The wound should be cleaned as much as possible and prepared for the use of healing products. Good insect control and fly repellent on the animal will help to prevent reinfestation of the wound. Some small, open wounds may best be treated with healing ointments containing insect repellent.

Blowfly numbers may be reduced by removing carcasses, afterbirth, and other materials in which they lay their eggs and breed. Garbage containing meat scraps should be burned thoroughly or buried so as not to provide homes for them. Some types of blowflies also lay eggs in fruit and vegetable wastes, pet droppings, and decaying garbage. Good general sanitation will significantly reduce blowfly numbers.

FACE FLIES

Face flies are common on cattle, and may attack horses who are pastured with cattle. These flies visit the horse's face only for a brief feeding period which makes them difficult to control. Wipe-on or stick-type repellents must be applied to the animal's head daily to keep these flies away. Fly swishes made of many fine strings may be attached to a halter to hang down over the horse's face and remove the flies. Mesh eye covers have been made of nylon netting or fine plastic window screen. These can be fastened to a halter to keep the flies away from the animal's eyes.

LICE

Lice commonly infest horses in the northern states, often in late winter and early spring. The animals are in close contact in corrals or wintering areas. They often stand together for warmth, which helps lice spread from one animal to another. The lice thrive in the animal's thick winter hair. They drop to very low numbers as the animal sheds its winter hair and the weather becomes hotter. Some horses seem to carry lice all the time, and may be responsible for reinfecting a number of other animals the next fall when conditions are again favorable. The horse's skin is often deficient in vitamin A because the forage or hay is leached and this vitamin is not present in adequate amounts for proper skin health. This deficiency helps make the animals susceptible to lice.

There are two kinds of lice which affect horses: sucking lice and biting lice. The biting lice feed on particles of hair and flakes of skin. The sucking lice pierce the skin and feed on blood. They feed often, and each feeding produces a new and irritating puncture wound. Lice are species specific; lice from cattle, chickens, or other animals will not affect horses, nor will horse lice affect other animals, birds, or humans. A horse louse may walk around on you, but he will not usually bite you.

SIGNS

Horses infested with lice often itch badly. They will rub and scratch on corrals. They most often scratch their heads and shoulders, but may rub flanks and rumps as well. They will bite at areas which they can reach. They will also kick and paw or bite each other. They may be grouchy enough to seriously injure themselves or humans handling them. Young horses with large numbers of lice may fail to gain weight as they normally would. They may lose weight and appear stunted. Lice are most commonly found under the jaws, at the base of the tail, on the sides of the neck, and on the flanks. In a severe case, they will be found all over the body.

When you have a horse in winter or spring who is itching and losing hair, begin by checking for ringworm. Horses with ringworm do not usually itch, or will only itch a little. The spots are definitely hairless, but the hair does not appear to have been rubbed out. If you can rule out ringworm, then the next choice is lice. Scrape your fingernails along the skin between the horse's jawbones. Shake the "scurfy" material that you are able to get loose into the palm of your hand or onto a sheet of white paper. Both ticks and lice leave tiny bits of bloody or brown dirt. They may also cause rough spots on the skin. These spots may be like small pimples, with small drops of dried yellow serum on the top. Along with the dandruff-like material and the bloody or yellow spots, you should see some small lice.

Lice are cream-colored or grayish, yellowish, or light brown. They are small, being less than 1/8-inch long. A magnifying glass is often helpful to see these critters. Ticks are dark brown or reddish, and larger—as much as 1/4 to 3/8 inch. If engorged with blood, ticks may be nearly an inch long. Lice are cigar-shaped (much longer than they are wide), while ticks are nearly round.

When an animal who has lice is introduced into a herd, the lice spread rapidly. They are easily passed from one horse to another by direct contact. Lice may also be carried from one horse to another on brushes, blankets, halters, or tack. When conditions are favorable, eggs attached to fallen hair may hatch. Young lice can survive away from a horse for two or three days. Biting lice may live away from horses for as long as 10 days if kept on hair. It is possible for premises to remain infested for 25 to 30 days.

CONTROL

Dust the horse with louse powder or spray with an insecticide spray approved for killing lice. If the weather is extremely cold, do not dampen an already weakened horse. Use one of the dust products until the weather warms up and you can bathe the horse properly. Mix dips according to instructions on the bottle or as recommended by your veterinarian. Apply the dip with a sponge or rag, soaking the horse until he is totally wet. Wear rubber gloves or disposable plastic gloves to apply the mixture so you won't get it on your hands. Be sure to apply it especially well under the horse's jaw, between his hind legs, and under the belly and tail. Do not rinse it off, but allow the insecticide to dry in the animal's hair.

Repeat the procedure in about two weeks; two treatments will be sufficient for most animals. Add another treatment in two weeks if the first two aren't enough. The additional one or two treatments are necessary to kill lice which hatch from eggs not killed by the first treatment. Sprays should also be mixed according to instructions, soaked well into the horse's hair, and allowed to dry. Horses who do not tolerate spraying should be sponged or dipped instead.

The barn should be sprayed to kill any lice that have fallen from the animals. Hair that has been groomed or clipped from infested animals should be gathered and burned. Be careful not to get sprays or the dip mixture into feed or water, or into the animal's eyes, nose or mouth.

TICKS

Several species of ticks attack horses. In the mountain states, ticks can cause serious debilitation by causing severe blood loss and constant irritation through heavy infestation. They are seen in large numbers in late winter to early spring when the horse's resistance is lowest and when horses are crowded together in barns or corrals. Animals who have ticks may also have lice—check carefully for the presence of both problems if you find that you have one or the other.

Tick problems are especially bad in mountain foothills and often seem to run in cycles. Some years there will be many of them and nearly all horses in the area will be affected. Other years, few animals may be infested. In the southern states, the ticks are of a different variety from those found in the western mountains, but cause similar damage and discomfort.

SIGNS

Horses infested with ticks may appear rough-coated and in poor condition. They may rub on fences and on each other due to the irritation caused by the ticks. Horses who have large numbers of ticks may become weak and anemic and may have a poor appetite. In severe cases, paralysis and death may occur.

Female ticks who are feeding may become engorged with blood, becoming nearly an inch long and plainly visible as they bulge out through the hair. Begin the search for ticks at the same place as for lice; between the horse's jaw bones. Scrape the skin with your fingernails and hold a sheet of white paper underneath to catch any ticks (or lice) which may fall off. Ticks may be found anywhere on the body, but are usually most common under the jaw and between the hind legs. The ticks are hard-shelled and usually round in shape with eight legs. They are usually about ¼-inch in diameter and often dark in color; reddish, brown, black, or gray. In contrast, lice are very small and more cigar-shaped.

TREATMENT

Insecticide treatment with the same products used for lice will give good tick control. Sponging the horse with lindane dip until he is soaked will give tick control for two weeks to a month. Sprays and dusts have also been used. Check with your veterinarian for products which are currently available. Infected barns may be treated with toxaphene or other insecticide.

Reinfestation may occur from untreated horses, from ticks left on the premises, and from ticks occurring naturally in the brush in foothills areas. In some cases, it may be necessary to spray corrals or stalls to help prevent ticks who have fallen off from moving back onto the horses. The infestation usually is worse from winter to spring and diminishes later in the season. Controlling the ticks for the winter season may require several treatments, two to four weeks apart, depending on the species of tick involved.

EAR TICKS

Ear ticks are seen in horses in arid and semiarid areas of the United States, primarily in the southwestern states. The larvae of these ticks crawl into the horse's ears and attach themselves to the tender skin inside the ear canal below the hair line. They feed there for one to two weeks. They then molt and continue to feed for as long as 6 to 7 months. When their life cycle is completed, they drop out of the ear to the ground, becoming adults.

SIGNS

Horses with ear ticks rub and scratch their ears in an attempt to rid themselves of the pests. They will shake their heads and swing them from side to side. The animals may be difficult to handle and be nearly impossible to halter or bridle. If you suspect ear ticks, examine the ear thoroughly. If there are only a few ticks, they may be hidden deep in the folds inside the ear or as far down as the eardrum.

It may be necessary to twitch the animal to take his mind off his ears in order to examine them. Debris and ticks may be removed with a cotton swab. Take out only the wax and dirt that you can see—do not probe down deep into the ear canal for two reasons: it is very easy to slip and puncture the ear drum, and excessive poking around tends to pack dirt down onto the ear drum. This makes an even better home for the ticks and makes the horse even more irritated than he was in the first place.

TREATMENT

Low-pressure sprays containing lindane, DDT, or toxaphene applied into the ear canal work well with ear ticks. These materials may prevent reinfestation for as long as a month. A bulb syringe may be used to apply the medication down in the ear. A mixture containing 5 parts lindane, 10 parts xylene, and 85 parts pine oil may be applied into the ear canal. It can be put into a small oil can and a few drops squirted into the animal's ear. Place a small piece of rubber tubing over the end of the spout to avoid injuring the horse's ear. Continuing application over a period of time may be needed to help prevent reinfestation.

MANGE

Mange is also called scab, scabies, and itch. Three types of mange occur in horses. The one usually called scabies is the most harmful and injurious. Foot mange (also called chorioptic mange) primarily infests the horse's feet and legs. In general, mange is an uncommon problem in horses. Hair loss is far more frequently caused by ringworm and the itching caused by lice or ticks.

SIGNS

Often the first sign of mange is that the horse itches intensely. He may rub on any solid object and will often bite at the worst areas. Rubbed or broken hair may be an early sign (in addition to the itching). Soon there are small hairless patches. There may be small bumps. The first signs may be seen on the head, neck, and shoulders. Sometimes, they first may appear at the foretop, base of the mane, and base of the tail. They may also occur in any part of the body thickly covered with hair.

Early in the disease, the spread is of mange slow; later it may be rapid and will result in irregular hairless patches all over the body. Small blisters may form over and around the burrowing mite. The discharge from these blisters forms small scabs and crusts. They may be dry and flaky or moist and weeping, depending on the type of mite

which is causing the mange. The horse rubs constantly, making large, raw (or even bloody) areas. In time, the skin becomes thickened, wrinkled, and dry. Bacterial infection may occur in the weakened tissue.

Foot mange is usually confined to the lower parts of the legs around the fetlock and below. Occasionally, these mites may spread higher on the legs and onto the abdomen. They are, however, more commonly seen on the hindlegs, especially the feet. Horses with foot mange may stomp and rub their legs together. They often try to bite or chew the itching areas. The horse may lick and rub the spots, removing some of the hair and leading to hardening and thickening of the skin.

If you have a horse with hairless spots, first eliminate the possibility of ringworm (the lesions are usually not as raw, and if they itch at all, do not bother the animal so intensely). Check under the jaw with your fingernails and a white sheet of paper to see if there are any lice or ticks causing the problem. If you have tentatively eliminated these causes, it is time to call your veterinarian. Mange is a very contagious disease.

To positively diagnose mange, it is necessary to take a scraping from the skin and look at it under a microscope to see the mites. When scraping for mites, we often have to go down to the live layers of the skin to find the beasts, so don't think that the vet is abusing your animal when he scrapes down until the skin bleeds. That is often a necessary part of the examination. If the skin has become dry and leathery, several scrapings may be necessary for positive identification of the problem.

Mange is controlled with a drug made specifically to kill mites. Standard insecticides, by themselves, usually do not touch mange, so don't bother trying them. The animal must be saturated thoroughly with the proper miticide for effective control. Be careful to keep the product out of the eyes, ears, nose, feed, or water.

Two treatments a couple of weeks apart are usually needed. Occasionally, more treatments may be necessary to control the mites. Treat all affected animals at the same time to prevent their reinfecting each other. As with other contagious skin problems, mange can be spread by contaminated tack, halters, or grooming equipment. Use separate equipment on infected animals until the disease is controlled.

STREPTOTHRICOSIS

Streptothricosis is caused by an organism that is somewhere between a fungus and a type of bacteria. The organism is thought to enter the skin through a cut or abrasion, or through the cracks caused by chapping or excessive moisture on the skin. The disease is most commonly seen in New York and Vermont. It is known in wet, cold areas as "rain scald." The hair pulls out in tufts, leaving raw areas on the skin. There is little itching. It can usually be cured by applying 7% (strong) tincture of iodine daily.

ONCHOCERCIASIS

Onchocerciasis is caused by a fine, thread-like worm. The adult lives in the ligament along the top of the neck, forming small calcified nodules. The larvae live under the skin, where they may cause hair loss and sores. The skin on the face, neck, chest, and the lower midline of the belly becomes scaly, and much of the hair falls out. The disease is seen as a severe problem in Texas, but most horses in the country are affected with at least small lesions, usually on the midline of the belly.

In areas where it is a severe problem, animals are fed diethylcarbamazine (Dizan, Tech-America, Elwood, KS 66024) daily at a rate of 2 mg. per lb., given from March through October. Administration of corticosteroids will help to control the itching until the diethylcarbamazine begins to take effect. The worms are spread from one horse to another by small biting gnats. Insect control plays an important role in helping to prevent spread of the disease.

HABRONEMIASIS

Habronemiasis is also called "summer sores." It is a skin disease which occurs at the site of minor wounds or naturally moist spots on the body, such as near the eyes and sheath. It occurs when Habronema larvae are deposited by various flies. Summer sores are caused by the body's allergic reaction against these larvae.

Summer sores look like masses of proud flesh covered with red or brownish drainage. They may have a greasy appearance, and some may become quite large. Sores at the inner corner of the eye are usually smaller and more granular in texture. Consult your veterinarian for diagnosis and treatment of this problem.

Fly control is important to the control of summer sores, especially on farms or stables which have a continuing problem with them. Wounds or open sores should be promptly treated with wound medication or an insecticidal paste, or should be protected until they can be sutured.

CATTLE GRUBS

Also known as warbles, cattle grubs are members of the Hypoderma species. While they are primarily a parasite of cattle, they occasionally infest horses in the western states. They are a sporadic parasite, occurring on some premises in an area and not on others, and occurring in some years, but not seen other years. They appear as lumps about ¾- to 1–¼ inch in diameter, and are raised about ½- to ¾-inch high. They occur on the neck, chest, and shoulders of the horse, as well as on the back. When

present on the back, they are often seen in the area of the backbone.

In cattle, these grubs mature, create a hole in the skin, and emerge through that opening to drop to the ground and complete their life cycle. In horses, they may form the hole, but are usually unable to emerge through it. The usual cure for grubs in cattle (when there are only one or two of them) is to push on them until they pop out through the hole. When this is attempted in the horse, it usually result in a crushed grub and subsequent infection. Or, if the grub does not form a hole, it may die and form a pocket with a sterile, fluid-secreting lining, or an abscess. When this happens, the lesion is often as much as two to three inches in diameter, but usually no higher than it was before. These pockets also occur when pressure from the saddle crushes and kills the grub inside the skin.

The only cure which is consistently effective is to remove the entire grub and secreting pocket surgically, and suture the area back together. Adequate time must be allowed for healing before the animal is used, especially if the grub is on the back. Occasionally, ranchers will cut a hole in a saddle pad or blanket, finish using the animal for the season, and then have surgery done late in the fall when the animal is no longer needed. This does not make the problem go away, but does sometimes allow the horse to be used until he can be rested long enough for surgery and the healing afterward.

SKIN CANCER (AND OTHER TUMORS)

Cancers, also called tumors or neoplasms (new growths), occur in the horse much as they do in man. They occur when cells become abnormal, but the body does not recognize them as being abnormal. Thus, the immune system does not destroy them and they continue to grow, causing an abnormal lump of tissue. A cancer is a group of cells which no longer respond to limits which are normally imposed by the body, growing wildly and without restraint.

Cells in your body (and every other living animal's body) are being replaced daily. This replacement occurs because some of the cells in the tissue divide to fill the new need. Somehow, the cells know when to stop dividing, so as to just replace themselves. This limitation is what keeps your fingers, feet, indeed all body parts and organs in about the same size and relationship throughout life. Without these limits, your index finger, for instance, might continue to grow until it was the size of your foot. Thank heavens for limits!

When a tumor occurs, the involved cells no longer respond to growth limits. They divide and expand, producing a swelling or "growth." At the same time, depending on the type of tumor, roots are sent down into underlying tissues. How rapidly the cancer grows and how deeply it invades depends on the type of cancer; some grow very slowly and never spread, while others invade deeply and rapidly into the body in addition to spreading to other parts of the body (a process called metastasis or metastasizing). As with human cancers, some cancers in the horse are easily cured, while others are untreatable.

Two particular types of skin cancer are commonly found in horses, and both are related to the animal's color. Squamous cell carcinoma is commonly found in horses, such as paints and Appaloosas, who have pink (unpigmented) skin around the eyes. These tumors begin as a pinkish or reddened raised patch, or as a weeping sore. They may occur on the eyelids, or on the third eyelid (the pink structure in the inside corner of the eye). Less commonly, they may occur elsewhere on the animal's face, as well as on the penis and sheath of stallions or geldings; occasionally, they may be found on other white areas of the animal's skin.

Like "cancer eye" in cattle, squamous cell carcinoma is thought to be at least partially caused by the action of ultraviolet light from the sun acting on the unprotected, unpigmented skin. Additional support for this thinking comes from the fact that these are most commonly seen in the southwest, which has many sunny days, and in high mountain areas, where there is less atmosphere between the sun and the animals to screen out the ultraviolet rays.

Several treatments have been used for squamous cell carcinoma, including surgery, freezing, cauterization, and radiation therapy. The treatment of choice will depend on the type and location of the lesion and how advanced and invasive it is. Prompt treatment is worthwhile, as these tumors tend to invade the underlying tissues if allowed to remain.

This author was unfortunate enough to be called upon to euthanize a horse who had the problem on one eyelid and had not received any treatment at all. Over a period of some eight months, the lesion invaded and destroyed the eye on that side of the face, in addition to severely involving the skin and muscles above and below the socket for a distance of several inches. Do you suspect that your horse might have this problem? Why not call your veterinarian right now?

The second type of skin cancer related to skin color is malignant melanoma. This tumor is most common in gray horses, especially Arabians. It is a black-pigmented tumor. Most of these occur in the perineal region, the underside of the tail, or between the hind legs. They look like a black lump or nodule on the skin.

Unfortunately, this type of tumor tends to metastasize (spread) rapidly, often causing large masses of cancerous growth inside the abdomen. It may also spread to the lungs or other internal organs. Animals with severe involvement usually die or are euthanized for humane reasons.

My own policy is to remove, immediately, any nodular growth on a gray horse and to send it to the laboratory for analysis. Often, by removing them early ("cut wide and cut deep," as the old saying goes), spread may be prevented. If one of these is removed from your horse, it is a warning to observe the animal carefully and frequently for the appearance of more of them. If everything goes right, surgery may remove all of the tumor the first time around.

Other tumors are rarely seen in horses—the numbers are so small and so rare that it is not worth discussing them here. If your horse has a tumor, your veterinarian should be able to give you an estimate of the probability of removing or killing it. These educated guesses can be made on the basis of the slowness or rapidity of growth or the tendency for spread of a given type of tumor cells. These predictions are remarkably consistent with the same type of tumor from one species of animal to another.

As with humans, horse tumors are often removed surgically. Chemotherapy (treatment with chemical agents to kill the tumor) is not usually practical in horses because of their size. Treatment with systemic medication would take huge amounts of very expensive drugs. In some instances, freezing with liquid nitrogen may be used; in others, cauterization (burning) may be used for removal, as may laser surgery.

SARCOIDS

Sarcoids are a common, tumor-like growth which occur on the skin of equines. They are somewhat like a type of tumor called a sarcoma, which accounts for their name "sarcoid," meaning "sarcoma-like." They resemble ordinary granulation tissue in many ways and may occur after a wound has injured the skin, especially in areas around joints where there is constant motion. They can also occur without any history of injury. There is some thinking that they are caused by the same virus that causes warts on cattle. Sarcoids usually begin as a single, isolated growth on the head, leg, chest, shoulder, side of the body, or on the sheath.

At first, the growth may resemble a wart. It then begins to grow more rapidly, often breaking open and showing an ulcerated surface. The raw surface may then become infected with bacteria, resulting in an ugly, weeping, pus-covered sore. More than one of these lesions may be found on the animal's body. Sarcoids may occur in horses, donkeys, and mules of any age.

Surgical removal is often attempted, but the lesions recur with discouraging frequency. This is, in part, due to the fact that these growths invade neighboring tissues, and it is difficult for the surgeon to tell if the sarcoid has been completely removed. Some progress has been made with either freezing or cauterizing them, often with better results than when surgery is used. Occasionally, it seems that surgery actually stimulates enlargement and spread of the sarcoid. Radiation therapy has been used with some success to stop these lesions from recurring.

Regardless of what treatment is used, the sarcoid should be kept as clean as possible. Hair should be clipped away from it every 10 to 14 days. Any pus or drainage should be gently wiped from the surface with a dry gauze sponge, or you may use a gauze sponge moistened in a tamed iodine solution diluted to the color of weak tea. The surface should be protected from flies.

Corticosteroid ointments may be used on the surface, and lesions on the lower leg may be covered by a pressure bandage. Bandages should be changed at least every two or three days, and must be used until skin has COMPLETELY healed over the defect. If you stop bandaging it too soon, the sarcoid may resume growth. Indeed, getting the skin to grow together seems to be a key to permanent healing of these growths. In some cases, skin grafts or pigskin coverings have been used to help heal the skin defect and lead to permanent recovery. Veterinarians sometimes use plastic surgery techniques to move skin over the void left by surgical removal of a sarcoid.

If the lesion has been treated with cryotherapy (frozen), there may be a foul odor when the tissue which has been killed starts to slough from the surface. In some cases, after healing occurs in the area, there may be no pigment left in the skin, leaving a white or odd-colored patch. Sarcoids are the sort of problem which won't usually kill the horse, but lead many to be euthanized because the lesion will not heal, or enlarges to the point where it destroys the animal's usefulness.

FISTULA OF THE WITHERS AND POLL EVIL

Poll evil is an infection on top of the head, at the poll. It occurs in the bursa (a fluid-filled sac) located between and just behind the ears. Fistulous withers involve the bursa on top of the upper processes of the spinal column at the withers. At one time, they were considered to be due to injury at these areas. However, they have been proven to be due to Brucella bacteria, which the horse acquires from cattle or swine, or from other horses infected by the same organism.

A swelling or bulge may be seen on top of the head with poll evil. It may be evenly centered, or may bulge more to one side than the other. Fistulous withers begin with a large rounded swelling on top of the withers. Occasional cases are seen where the whole crest of the neck appears thickened and looks as if it is going to fall over sideways. These seem to be more common in ponies.

The swelling may be hot and tender, or may show no pain at all. Most, however, are painful enough that the horse is reluctant to move his head. The fistula may break and drain by itself if not treated, oozing pus and infected fluid. If it does not open, surgical drainage may be needed.

If the problem has been going for some time, extensive surgery may be necessary. We did surgery on one horse with fistula of the withers in which draining tracts of infection had invaded not only the withers but had eaten down behind the shoulder blades. We anesthetized the animal, and started cutting out the infected material. Following lines of infection that kept going down deeper and deeper, we ended up nearly removing his front leg from his body, and recommending that the horse be euthanized because of the extensive involvement.

Fistula of the withers and poll evil are problems for your veterinarian rather than for home treatment. One of the most important aspects of the disease is that it can be contagious to cattle, other horses, and humans. The Brucella bacteria cause the disease called undulant fever in man. This disease is extremely hard to cure, and may result in a recurrent fever similar to malaria for the rest of your life.

Do not allow the pus from one of these lesions to come into contact with your skin. Animals with these draining sores should not be allowed near streams or other common watering areas which they may contaminate. Your veterinarian may want to take some blood to send to the laboratory to determine for sure that brucellosis is causing the problem before beginning to treat the animal.

The earlier treatment is started, the better the possibility is for curing the disease. Treatment tends to be long-term, and may be expensive. These factors need to be intelligently considered before you place a horse on a treatment program. If the infection has entered the bone, surgery may be necessary to remove the dead bone. The disease may be prevented by not allowing horses to come into contact with cattle who are infected with brucellosis.

EAR PROBLEMS

Horses who are not infested with ear ticks may still have considerable problems with their ears. The ears may be filled with flat white plaques, as well as attacked by insects who cause tremendous irritation. These conditions can be stubborn and difficult to control. Begin by clipping as much hair out of the ears as you can (or as much as the animal will allow). Some animals become extremely headshy when their ears are sore. Then, use one of the healing creams with an insecticide in it. The easiest way to put it in is to take a big lump of it on the end of your thumb. Stabilize the animal's ear with the rest of the hand, and smear the ointment inside the horse's ear as you pull your thumb upward. The animal may need treatment every two or three days for several weeks.

TAIL RUBBING (INCLUDING WASHING THE SHEATH)

Tail rubbing is not a disease as such. It is a common symptom of many other problems. As mentioned above, it can be seen with mange. It can also be seen with lice or other skin problems. In both these instances, other lesions will be seen—there will be hairless patches on other parts of the body.

But what about the horse who is rubbing his tail and there is no obvious reason? In geldings, there may be an accumulation of dirt and grease called smegma in the horse's sheath. There may also be a large accumulation of this material called a "bean" in the small pouch on the end of the penis. Mares may have the same sort of dirt between the halves of the udder and occasionally between the outside of the udder and the inside of the leg. Geldings may be observed when they drop the penis to urinate. Note the crusts and scales of debris, as well as a greasy black material on the penis. If this is present, the animal is definitely in need of washing.

The mare is more easily examined. Look between the halves of the udder for the black, greasy accumulation. Be careful not to tickle the animal, and watch that she doesn't kick your head off. Most mares take this examination rather calmly, but an occasional one will protest violently.

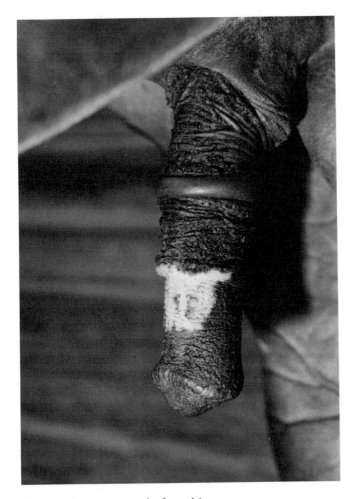

Gelding badly in need of washing.

Infrequently, the tail rubbing may be seen in horses who have pinworms. These worms cause irritation as ruptured female worms (who have crawled from the anus to lay their eggs) irritate the skin under the tail.

Injury to the tail may occur during a ride in a horse trailer. The horse may lean on the butt chain or back door, starting a raw sore which may go unnoticed. An eczema develops which may cause the animal to itch enough to continue to rub his tail. This may also occur with a rope horse who accidentally catches the rope under his tail and gets a rope burn, or on a harness or pack horse who is irritated by a crupper. Once in a while, tail rubbing is seen as a true vice, for which we can't find a cause, and for which there is no cure.

TECHNIQUE

If mange or another skin problem is causing the tail rubbing, it will quit when the rest of the disease is cured. If internal parasites are causing it, it will go away when they are eliminated by worming with the proper medication. Nearly all wormers which eliminate strongyles will also kill pinworms.

If the tail rubbing is caused by filth (smegma or beans), the solution is to wash the animal. Geldings and stallions, if trained carefully and gently, may allow you to wash them without sedation. One of my clients treats the animal with mineral oil several days in advance of when he wants to wash him. He wears a disposable glove and pours a liberal amount of mineral oil on it. He then massages this around thoroughly inside the sheath. When he washes the animal in two or three days, the mineral oil has helped to soften and loosen the greasy debris, and allows it to be removed much more easily (and with less discomfort to the horse). Use lukewarm water and a very mild soap such as pHisohex. You may wish to wear disposable plastic gloves or rubber gloves during this procedure, as the odor from the debris is often unpleasant, and may cling to your hands for quite some time.

Gently pull the animal's penis out and work the grime loose, using liberal amounts of soap. If you are unable to pull the penis out, it may be necessary to have your veterinarian tranquilize the animal. This forces him to relax and drop down to where the washing is easily done. Pieces of cotton batting may be used for scrubbing, but rub very gently. You do not want to start an eczema in this tender spot, and end up with a worse problem than you had in the beginning. Wash the surface thoroughly, as well as up into the sheath, and where the sheath folds toward the belly.

Reach into the pouch above the opening on the end of the penis and pull out any lumps of smegma that are present. Perform the whole procedure with the utmost gentleness to help keep the animal from dreading it in the future. When finished, rinse with liberal amounts of lukewarm water. Be sure that no soap is left on the skin, as it may cause irritation.

Stallions who are not washed during breeding (such as pasture-bred animals) and geldings will usually require washing once a year. Many mares will also need to be washed once a year. It is a good idea, also, to wash a

mare's udder before she is due to foal so that the foal does not end up eating this dirty material.

Tail rubbing due to trailer injury or rope burn should stop when the sore(s) are cured. If you have eliminated all other causes and find that the problem is due to a vice, there may not be a cure for it.

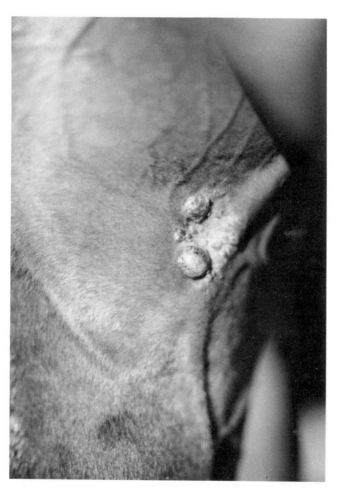

Sarcoid inside a mare's hindleg.

Chapter 18

INTERNAL PARASITES

Problems Caused by Strongyles
Small Strongyles
Strongyloides
Ascarids
Bots
Pinworms
Tapeworms
Types of Wormers
Equine Strongyles and Drug Resistance
  Control Programs for Strongyles
Prevention of Worm Problems
  Worming Methods

A large portion of the following material is excerpted, with permission, from "Drug Resistance and the Control of Equine Strongyles," by Dwight G. Bennett, D.V.M., Ph.D., and was first published in The Compendium on Continuing Education for the Practicing Veterinarian (reg. trademark), Vol. 5, Number 6, June 1983, p. 343–349, who also gave their kind permission.

Horses act as host to many different types of internal parasites. The nematodes or "worms" are the most common of these; these are the ones that cause the most damage, and loss of life. The most important group of worms is known as strongyles, and the infection that they cause is called strongylosis. Both large and small strongyles are usually present in the large intestine. The large migratory strongyles include Strongylus vulgaris and S. edentatus, as well as occasional other species. These worms spend a portion of their life cycle traveling through other parts of the horse's body, especially the lining of the major abdominal blood vessels.

Nonmigratory small strongyles, such as Trichonema, are usually also present. Their parasitic development is confined to the intestinal mucosa (intestinal lining). Heavy infections are most commonly found in young animals, especially those under two to three years of age. Severely infested animals may show a poor growth rate or loss of weight, rough hair coat, and anemia. Less badly infested animals may have reduced food conversion efficiency and less than optimal performance. Although small strongyles are less harmful than large strongyles, infestation with them has been associated with diarrhea, fever, colic, lack of appetite, lack of growth, and blood abnormalities.

Foals may suffer significant anemia from large worm loads. In untreated animals, this anemia will fluctuate with the seasonal worm load. Parasitized animals may grow as much as 30% slower than those kept free of worms.

Drugs used to reduce the worm population in the horse's intestine are called anthelmintics, or wormers. Many different drugs are used for this purpose, and more are being developed at all times. Unfortunately, the worms keep changing (mutating) in response to being attacked by the worming medications. What happens is the worms which are susceptible are killed off by the wormer. Worms who are resistant and who have survived the medication multiply. The next time you worm the horse, the wormer does less good, and the time after that, if you again use the same product or one in the same family, it may do almost no good at all. At first, attempts may be made to explain the failure by saying that the drug was not given at the proper dosage, that the method of administration was not correct, or that other factors caused the failure, such as the animal being ill with some disease at the same time, or that the animal was reinfested immediately after worming. Inevitably, we must quit hauling out these excuses and accept the fact that, in some cases, we have created a population of worms which are resistant to the wormer.

Experiments with worms in sheep have shown that resistant worms were more infestive to sheep, produced more eggs, and had greater development and survival of eggs and free-living larvae. Resistant worms also produced more severe damage in their hosts. It seems that by stimulating the development of resistant worms, we are indeed developing some "super worms."

When a given group of worming drugs is no longer used, the percentage of susceptible worms will increase.

How rapidly this occurs is not yet known. In one study, a thiabendazole-resistant population of small strongyles was selected by treatment every four to six weeks for four years. When medication with this drug was stopped, they reverted to nearly full susceptibility after six months. Other reports are less encouraging. In another experiment, there was no reduction in the level of resistance to cambendazole following passage through 24 generations without exposure to the anthelmintic. Once the worms revert to susceptibility, it seems that reemergence of resistance has been more rapid than normal when the same drug is again used. Therefore, once a population of parasites becomes resistant to a wormer, there is little or no hope of that drug being effective against them in the near future.

One method used to monitor the effectiveness of horse wormers is the fecal egg count. This count measures the number of eggs in a certain amount (usually a gram) of horse manure. However, we can't distinguish resistant worm populations from susceptible populations with this technique. The eggs of small strongyles are for the most part indistinguishable from each other, as well as from the eggs of large strongyles. Also, the number of eggs found in the feces has little or no direct relationship to the number of adult worms present in the large intestine.

If one species of worms is laying great numbers of eggs, this may camouflage the presence of another. Thus, most or all of the worms of one species may be killed by worming medication, while the total number of worms in the body is scarcely changed. Also, some horse wormers may temporarily inhibit egg production, thus reducing the number of eggs appearing in the feces, without reducing the actual numbers of worms.

The numbers of eggs present in the feces may vary from one time of day to another, as worms lay eggs in cycles. Doing a fecal egg count at a time of low egg production could lead to a false impression of low numbers of parasites. Egg counts after treatment may be as high as those before because large numbers of larvae (young worms) which are encysted in the wall of the intestine were not killed by the wormer and have matured and started producing eggs. Experience in cattle has shown that the development of larvae in the intestinal wall may be retarded if there are large numbers of adult worms in the intestine.

Worming may remove large numbers of adults, allowing the previously inhibited larvae to develop into adults and begin producing eggs. Then, the eggs produced by the newly matured parasites may be mistaken for those of resistant worms. Apparent drug resistance may also occur in some individual horses because of diarrhea or impaction changing either the action of the drug or the subsequent egg count. Lack of response to worming due to poor condition, disease, or other causes may be mistaken for drug resistance.

There is also a seasonal variation in the number of strongyle eggs present in the feces. Adult horses show higher numbers of eggs in summer and lower counts in winter.

Several other tests for the amount and type of worms present in the horse's intestine are available. However, they are used mainly for research, as they are extremely expensive. One of these procedures tests the eggs for hatchability when exposed to small amounts of certain wormers.

To date, the only wormers to which strongyles have been shown to become resistant are the benzimidazoles and phenothiazine. Intensive use of other wormers has not resulted in resistance. Phenothiazine-resistant strains have been reported only in North America, but benzimidazole-resistant strongyles have been reported in the United States, Canada, Britain, and Australia. One report details a mild resistance to phenothiazine among large strongyles. All other reports of drug resistance have involved small strongyles only. Only 7 of more than 40 species of small strongyles have been reported to show resistance to benzimidazoles. Only five of these resistant species are common in North America. Strongyles which are resistant to benzimidazoles or phenothiazine are not resistant to either when these drugs are combined with piperazine salts. The intensive use of benzimidazole-piperazine combinations does not seem to lead to resistant parasites. This probably reflects susceptibility to piperazine.

PROBLEMS CAUSED BY STRONGYLES

It is important to understand how parasites damage the horse and what problems might be expected in the wormy horse.

Large strongyles (S. edentatus and S. vulgaris) in their adult stage live in the caecum and colon. They have large mouths equipped with sharp hooks with which they grasp the lining of the gut. A worm grasps a "bite" of the intestinal lining and sucks it into its mouth, eroding a portion of the lining. This enables it to draw nutrition from the horse and is severely irritating to the intestinal mucosa.

The female worm lays eggs which travel through the gut and are passed with the animal's manure. The eggs hatch into larvae; these larvae go through three developmental stages. The third stage is the infective stage. The horse ingests them in the course of grazing or eating from ground contaminated by manure. After the third stage larvae are eaten, they undergo a molt and penetrate the gut wall. They migrate through the body tissues for long periods of time, finally ending up in the lining of the larger arteries, causing extensive damage. After about five months in the arteries, the larvae return to the intestine for further development, becoming adults. (79)

One of the most serious problems of strongylosis is the damage caused to arteries by migrating larvae of

Strongylus vulgaris. Lesions made by these larvae begin with roughened, fibrous tracks on the lining surface of the artery. Small blood clots (thrombi) form where these tracks cross. An inflammation of the artery, called arteritis, follows this damage. Thrombosis (in which blood clots form on the roughened interior surface of the artery) and embolism (in which bits of the previously formed thrombi or portions of worm larvae break off and flow down the inside of the artery) can then occur.

Thrombosis and embolism cause many of the signs of severe colic seen in horses. This is because much of the larval migration occurs in the aorta and the main blood vessels branching from it, especially the anterior mesenteric artery which is one of the major blood vessels to the digestive system.

If clots break off, they flow down the vessels until they lodge at a point beyond which they can no longer travel, thus shutting off the blood flow to the area of intestine distant to that point. If this thrombosis is very near to the intestine, the result may be a small area without blood, which causes a mild and temporary colic. It is later healed by vessels which supply blood from the normal intestine beside the bloodless area. If the shutoff occurs to a larger area, a severe colic may result. If too great an area is left without blood and dies, the animal may die if surgery is not done to remove the necrotic (dead) area of the intestine. Animals with this type of colic can be in severe pain; in their thrashing and rolling, they may complicate the problem by tearing the mesentery and getting part of the intestine caught in the torn area or by twisting an intestine.

Arteriosclerosis and atherosclerosis may occur secondary to the arteritis. The inflammation due to the larval migration reaches deep into the lining of the artery, and may result in the lining being separated from the deeper layers by a space filled with debris and larvae. This produces the atherosclerotic lesion which can result in decreased blood flow to the intestine, and may result in an animal with chronic colic because of an inefficient blood supply.

Aneurysms are frequently found in horses infected with migrating strongyle larvae. They are not found in newborn foals, but may be found in animals as young as 10 to 40 days. (80) These lesions are weakened, thin-walled ballooned areas in the arterial wall and are seen in the aorta and the major vessels leading to the abdominal viscera. They may lead to colic as clots break off the roughened lining, or to infection due to dead worms and worm by-products being released into the blood stream. At worst, they rupture and the animal dies quickly of hemorrhage.

Thrombosis (blood clots) may occur where the aorta splits to go the two hind legs. These clots, and other damage due to larval migration, can cause severe weakness and stumbling because of the reduction in the blood supply to the hind legs. Often, a swaying gait or hindleg incoordination is seen. In some horses, this lameness begins shortly after the animal is exercised. It may be confused with azoturia. The horse gets enough blood to supply the muscles when he is at rest, but the clot prevents the passage of sufficient blood to supply the animal at work. Some horses show lameness when walked. The animal may sweat profusely and show severe pain. One of the most common characteristics of this lameness is the fact that it comes and goes, disappearing with rest and reappearing when the animal is worked or walked again.

Animals who have clots large enough to reduce the blood supply to both hindlegs may be cold to the touch in that area. Surface veins on the affected limb(s) may appear collapsed. This is especially dramatic when one leg is normal and the other has a reduced blood supply due to a clot. Your veterinarian will confirm this problem by his findings on a rectal examination. Treatment is only occasionally successful. If the animal has a large clot or severe damage to the linings of the arteries, worming and other therapy may not work. Severely affected animals are even less likely to be helped by treatment. If the animal can be kept alive and comfortable long enough, other circulatory channels may develop to carry blood to the hind legs, enabling the animal to survive. The chances that he will ever be entirely normal again are very small.

Colic due to worms (called thromboembolic colic) should be suspected whenever an animal has chronic colic. It should also be suspected when colic appears without other discernible cause, especially if it occurs during or shortly after the animal is worked. One of my clients had an extremely valuable Arabian filly who would routinely colic if she were not wormed every six weeks. Another client has a stallion with the same problem.

SMALL STRONGYLES

Small strongyles encompass some 40 different species of parasites. They are often bright red in color and live inside the large intestine. Members of the genus Trichonema penetrate the intestinal mucosa (lining) in their larval stage. Here they form small cysts. The size of the cyst increases as the larval worm grows, until it ruptures to release a young worm, which escapes into the intestine. When the larval worms leave their cysts, a severe inflammatory response may occur in the mucosa (intestinal lining). Other species of small strongyles may cause ulceration and irritation to the lining of the digestive tract. Diarrhea has occasionally been associated with these infestations.

If the horse is receiving plenty of food, he may harbor large numbers of these worms without apparent ill effect. However, the animal would certainly be better off without the damage to his intestinal lining. And, if complications develop, these worms will make him just as dead as any others.

STRONGYLOIDES

Also called intestinal threadworms, these parasites are common in foals. They are the first worm infestation which develops in young foals. They then decrease in numbers until only few, if any, are found in horses over six months old. The infective larvae are passed in the mare's milk for a period of time after foaling, beginning about the fourth day after the foal is born. Many farms routinely worm the mare the day the foal is born to help reduce the numbers of these worms that she will pass on to the foal. Diarrhea is the most common sign of strongyloides infestation in foals. This may be difficult or impossible to distinguish from foal-heat diarrhea, which occurs around the same time.

Therapy for these worms is included when routine worming of foals is begun at eight weeks of age. In areas where this parasite is a special problem, foals may be wormed with a mild, safe wormer, such as thiabendazole, as young as two weeks of age. This should only be done on the advice of your veterinarian. If you treat a foal with severe diarrhea for worms when they are not causing his problem, valuable treatment time may be wasted, possibly resulting in the death of the foal.

ASCARIDS

Parascaris equorum is another roundworm which parasitizes the horse. It is usually 6 to 9 inches in length. It is primarily seen in young foals. Horses quickly develop an immunity to this worm, and they are rarely seen in adult horses. As with the other worms, the eggs (up to 200,000 per day) are laid by the female and passed onto the pasture with the manure, where they become infective. (81)

The horse ingests the embryonated (partially developed) egg. Once in the intestine, it hatches a worm (larva). These larvae migrate through the liver and lungs, where they enter the air spaces. They then travel up the trachea to the mouth. They are swallowed and return to the gut where they remain for the rest of their life cycle.

Many young horses play host to amazingly large numbers of these parasites without apparent ill effects. Other animals may be severely affected by the worms causing perforation of the small intestine and peritonitis; in some horses, this may be fatal. This situation is most often seen in the fall and winter in weanling foals who have accumulated large numbers of ascarids. The damage caused in the lungs by the larval migration may result in pneumonia. They are also thought to be responsible for many otherwise unexplained coughs in young horses. Large balls of these worms in the intestine may cause impaction and subsequent colic.

Ascarids should be suspected whenever you have a young horse (especially in the 3 to 5 month age group)

which fails to thrive on good feed. Often, the animal will have a rough hair coat or will fail to shed his hair when he should. It often has a severe potbelly. These animals should be wormed once a month for three months to remove the ascarids. With some wormers, masses of worms that look like spaghetti may be passed. With other products, the worms are digested before they get to the outside so that none are visible in the manure. Improvement following a good worming program is often quite dramatic.

Because ascarids can persist on an infected premises in large numbers, a rigorous worming program should be kept in effect once these worms are diagnosed. Foals may be treated as early as eight weeks of age and should be treated every two months thereafter. This schedule should be continued until the foals become yearlings. (82)

BOTS

Bots are another of the common horse parasites in the United States. Several species of Gasterophilus are known as bots; the most common is G. intestinalis. Bots are insects; bot flies look much like bees, and may be seen buzzing around the horse, especially around the front legs in the knee area. They lay small, yellow eggs (about $\frac{1}{16}$ inch long) on the hairs. When the horse licks his legs, the larvae hatch and are ingested.

Eventually, the bots (fly larvae) reach the stomach where the they attach themselves to the stomach lining with their biting mouthparts. A portion of the stomach may be solidly lined with attached bots, so that none of the lining is visible between them. Another species of bots has larvae which attach to the terminal part of the intestine just inside the rectum, and may occasionally be seen protruding from this area.

Some horses may have a large number of bot larvae attached to their stomachs without ill effects. On the other hand, these parasites may perforate the stomach wall, producing an ulcer and subsequent peritonitis. Occasionally, they may cause colic. Bots are not diagnosed on fecal examinations used for other parasites unless one of the larvae happens to be present in the sample. Animals who have bot eggs present on their hair can be presumed to be infested with bots.

One of the easiest ways to prevent bot infestation is to remove the eggs from the horse's hair on a daily basis. They may be removed with a commercially-made "bot block" which is a coarse scrubbing material. Or, they may be scraped off with a dull knife blade or picked off with a fingernail.

Some people have advised sponging the horse's legs with warm water to remove bots. This causes the larvae to hatch, where they can still be ingested by the horse if they are not immediately removed. The egg cases are left clinging to the hair and cannot be distinguished from new eggs. For these reasons, sponging is not a satisfactory removal method.

Wormers which kill strongyles do not necessarily also kill bots; often, special products must be used to remove them from the digestive tract. Unless the directions on the horse wormer which you use say that it removes bots, do not feel sure that you have killed them. Among the best wormers for removing them are the organophosphates. A product called trichlorfon (Combot, Haver-Lockhart, Shawnee, KS 66201) is perhaps the best known of these drugs. Conversely, if you have used a wormer which says it is for bots, do not think that you have also wormed the animal for strongyles or ascarids, unless the wormer indicates that it kills both.

Traditionally, we have wormed for bots about a month after the last killing frost in the fall gets rid of all the adult bot flies, assuming that this allows enough time for the worms to migrate to the stomach where they can be killed by the wormer. Recently, it has been found that some of the larvae may take much longer to complete their migration into the digestive system. For this reason, my advice to clients has been to worm their horses for bots at the traditional time in the fall, and again when they worm them in the spring. Twice a year is usually adequate to treat most horses for bots. The twice a year schedule is also necessary in areas of the country where killing frosts are infrequent.

PINWORMS

Pinworms (Oxyuris equi) has no relationship to the pinworms which infect humans. These worms are a parasite which lives in the rectum of the horse. They move to the animal's anus to lay their eggs on the skin. Some may also crawl to the outside, where they may be found as collapsed, dead or dying worms. Pinworm eggs are passed onto the pasture and infection occurs when the horse ingests eggs in which the young worms are sufficiently developed.

These worms do not cause any major damage, but their presence around the anus and under the tail may severely irritate the animal. Fragments of the dead worms may cause intense itching, causing the horse to rub itself on any handy object. The horse may rub all the hair from the head of the tail. In some cases, the entire tail may be rubbed bare, resulting in a "rat-tailed" appearance. A show horse's fine tail may be partially rubbed out. The animal may also scrape or tear its skin and then get an infection in the abraded area.

These worms are more common in younger horses. Routine worming will remove the pinworms and give the animal relief. A similar irritation may occur in stallions or geldings who have dirt in the sheath and on the surface of the penis. Rule filth out as a cause of tail rubbing, as it is more common than pinworms.

TAPEWORMS

Tapeworms are occasionally seen in the horse. They are reported from Illinois, where they have caused a problem called intussusception. This is the telescoping of one piece of intestine into another which can cause a severe colic and, in some cases, may be fatal. The worm involved is called Anaplocephala perfoliata. Some farms may have a majority of their horses affected. The eggs are passed in the feces, but are not well demonstrated by conventional fecal examination methods. Treatment of the affected animals with pyrantel pamoate eliminates the tapeworms. (83)

TYPES OF WORMERS

Wormers may be divided into several groups according to their action and chemical composition. These groups have different modes of action, and thus are less likely to develop cross-resistance. In other words, just because a species of worm is resistant to one type, it is not likely to be resistant to another type (except as noted). The main groups of horse wormers available at the present time include:

1) Phenothiazine. This is one of the oldest available horse wormers. Its exact mode of action is unknown. It is fairly effective against large and small strongyles. However, the dosages necessary to kill the worms are near those which are toxic to the horse. For this reason, it is usually combined with piperazine. The drugs work together, allowing phenothiazine to be effective at half the dosage that is needed when it is used alone. There have been reports of large and small strongyles which were resistant to phenothiazine, but they are not resistant to the two drugs in combination. Cross-resistance between phenothiazine and benzimidazoles and febantel have been reported. Phenothiazine has a reduced efficiency against benzimidazole-resistant worms in sheep, and the same cross-resistance has recently been demonstrated in equine strongyles.

Low levels of phenothiazine have been used where this drug is fed for three weeks of each month in the feed to all horses on a farm. While providing better parasite control than single doses of the drug, this method has fallen out of favor. One reason was the tendency of worms to develop a resistance to phenothiazine. Another is that it was thought to produce hypothryoidism, which impaired the performance of racing animals. With the advent of newer, more effective wormers with fewer side effects, this regimen is no longer used.

2) Piperazines. Piperazines work by changing

transmission of impulses in the worm's nervous system, effectively "drugging" the worms. They then become disoriented and are flushed from the intestine along with the feces. These drugs are as much as 90 to 100% effective against small strongyles, but have poor action against large strongyles. Drug resistance has not been reported with piperazines. Strongyles that are resistant to benzimidazoles and phenothiazine are susceptible to those drugs when combined with piperazines.

3) Benzimidazoles and probenzimidazoles. Benzimidazoles include drugs, such as the old classic thiabendazole, as well as the newer cambendazole, mebendazole, fenbendazole, oxfendazole, and oxibendazole. The probenzimidazole group is represented by febantel. These drugs interfere with carbohydrate metabolism in the worms. Drugs in this group are 90 to 100% effective against large strongyles, and as much as 98 to 100% effective against small strongyles. Small strongyles may develop resistance to these drugs. Once they have developed resistance to the benzimidazoles, they are usually resistant to febantel as well. Reports of this resistance began to occur after the drugs had been used for three to four years. To date, small strongyles which are benzimidazole-resistant have been susceptible to oxibendazole; this may change in the near future. (84)

While all the benzimidazole drugs are effective against adult strongyles in normal dosages, it is only recently that studies have been done to assess their activity against developing larvae. At increased dosage rates (4 to 10 times normal), both fenbendazole and oxfendazole (not yet marketed for use in the horse) have been shown to be highly effective against all stages of small strongyles. They also have some activity against certain stages of developing S. vulgaris and S. edentatus larvae. A similar effect has been achieved by 5 daily doses of fenbendazole at the normal dosage rate.

4) Pyrantel and morantel. These drugs work on the worms' nervous systems, but in a different way than do the piperazines. They are 90 to 100% effective against Strongylus vulgaris and small strongyles. Resistance to these compounds has not been reported. Levamisole (Pitman-Moore, Trenton, NJ 08619), a wormer which is heavily used in cattle, is related in action to these drugs. It is not effective against equine strongyles. A new tube worming product has come on the market which combines levamisole with piperazine to kill strongyles, as well as other worms.

5) Organophosphates. Drugs such as dichlorvos (the stuff in the plastic fly strips which you hang in your house) also act against the worms' nervous systems. This drug is only effective when given orally to the horse. When dichlorvos products are fed, the horse should be hungry. The wormer should be mixed with grain and fed immediately. If allowed to set for a time, an acid reaction is produced, and the animal is unlikely to eat the product. These wormers seem to have a bit of an odor or perhaps an unpleasant flavor, as many horses who are sensitive to foreign substances in their feed will not eat them. One of these products (Combot, Haver-Lockhart, Shawnee, KS 66201) is commonly used as a tube wormer, especially in combination with other drugs. No worm resistance to organophosphates has been reported.

6) Avermectins. This is one of the newest groups of horse wormers. Like some of the other wormers, they attack the worms' nervous systems so that they lose their coordination, become paralyzed, and are expelled. Ivermectin is the first of these drugs available in the United States (under the name Eqvalan, produced by Merck and Co., Inc, Rahway, NJ 07065). It was first offered in an injectable form which has since been removed from the market because a small number of clostridial infections occurred at the injection site, a few of which were fatal to the horses involved. It is currently available in a paste form. Ivermectin is so new that there has not been time for resistance to develop.

EQUINE STRONGYLES AND DRUG RESISTANCE

In the past, we have recommended that horses be wormed every 40 to 60 days, using a different type of anthelmintic every time. However, in light of current understanding of strongyle biology and drug resistance, better recommendations can be made.

In order to design an effective control program, we must consider the time required for development of infective larvae, as well as the survivability of eggs and larvae under different climate conditions. Migration patterns of infective larvae are important, as well as defecation and grazing patterns of horses.

Optimal conditions for development of strongyle larvae are not the same as optimal conditions for their survival. The minimum temperature for hatching strongyle eggs is 45 degrees F (13 C). Freezing inhibits hatching, but does not kill the larvae within the eggs which develop normally and hatch when the temperature increases. Preinfective larvae (first and second stage) are killed by freezing, but eggs and infective third stage larvae are not. During midwinter thaws, when the temperature increases to above 45 degrees F (7 C) and then decreases to freezing within a week to ten days, the larvae that hatched when the temperatures increased will be killed before they can reach the resistant third stage. So, alternate freezing and thawing is more damaging than continuous freezing to strongyle larvae on pastures.

Development from eggs to infective larvae requires as little as 92 hours at 80 degrees F (27 C), but takes 12 days to 7 weeks at 53 degrees F (12 C). Development does not occur at all at less than 53 degrees F. Third-stage larvae survive longer (up to 31 weeks) at winter temperatures than they do at summer temperatures (up to 7 weeks).

Drying of feces inhibits larval development. However, only the first-stage larvae are killed rapidly by desiccation. Second-stage larvae are quite resistant; development will stop when they are dried, but will proceed on to the third stage when they are moistened. Larvae take longer to develop to the infective stage when dried, but seven days of hot, dry weather are required to completely desiccate a compact pile of horse manure. The bottom layer remains moist long enough for infective larvae to develop. Egg hatching was prevented by drying when fecal pellets were broken up and dried rapidly. Third-stage larvae are resistant to drying.

Infective strongyle larvae develop and migrate up foliage in response to moisture. Moist conditions are thus favorable for development and migration of infective larvae, but not necessarily for their survival. A possible reason why infective larvae survive longer under cold or dry conditions than under warm or moist conditions is that they consume their energy stores more rapidly when it is warm and damp.

Almost all strongyle larvae are found within 1 foot (30 cm) of a fecal mass, and 89% are found within 6 inches (15 cm). The proximity of grazing to areas of defecation is therefore important. Adult horses tend to defecate in one part of a pasture and graze in another. Foals are less discriminating and tend to graze in areas where adults defecate and thus are more likely to be exposed to infective larvae. Larvae migrate up grasses in response to small amounts of moisture—as little as $1/10$ inch (2.5 mm) of rainfall. The majority remain within 4 inches (10 cm) of the ground.

The generation time of parasites is also involved in the development of drug resistance. It is defined as the time required for development from the egg to the infective larvae plus the survival time of infective larvae on pasture plus the prepatent period (the length of time between the entry of the larvae into the final host and the time when it can be demonstrated that the parasite is present, such as by eggs in the animal's feces). The development from egg to infective larvae of strongyles requires four days to seven weeks, depending on climatic conditions. Third-stage larvae survive for 7 to 31 weeks, and the prepatent period of the small strongyles varies from 42 to 70 days.

Therefore, the generation time can vary from 18 to 48 weeks. This maximum generation time has been cited as the period during which anthelmintic groups should not be changed to avoid multiple drug resistance. Perhaps the longevity of a single adult parasite in the intestine would be even more valuable in determining this timing.

For example, in the case of S. vulgaris, it is apparent that horses are most likely to become infected during the summer and subsequently have a larger population of arterial larvae three to four months later in the winter.

CONTROL PROGRAMS FOR STRONGYLES

An effective program for strongyle control must prevent the rapid reinfection of horses at certain times of the year while minimizing selection of drug-resistant parasites. Methods for achieving these ends may, at times, be opposed to each other. During the summer months, worming as close as every six weeks may not necessarily result in effective control. At the same time, such frequent treatment greatly increases the probability of selecting resistant parasites. No anthelmintic-resistant strongyles have been detected in horses treated less frequently than 16-week intervals.

One method of reconciling these problems is to treat intensively with anthelmintics at certain times of the year and less intensively or not at all during other times. It is probably an invalid assumption that strongyles develop in horses at an equal rate year round.

It has been suggested that in the northern U.S., horses may pass greater numbers of strongyle eggs during the spring, just prior to the period when climatic conditions are most suitable for development of eggs to infective larvae, than in other seasons. The summer build-up of infective larvae might be prevented by giving horses three spring treatments at monthly intervals, starting just before the grazing of new spring pastures. It has been shown that as few as two treatments in the early spring can provide parasite control for dairy replacement heifers for the entire grazing season. Eggs passed in the fall and winter may survive, either as unhatched eggs or infective larvae, until the following spring, but there is relatively little chance of infection of horses during the winter months, so less frequent treatment during the winter might be possible.

Periodic strongyle egg counts may be used to keep track of whether a given treatment regimen is keeping egg and larval contamination of pastures below a dangerous level and if drug-resistant strongyles are becoming a problem. It should be safe to assume that horses will be protected from serious infection if fecal egg counts are kept below 50 eggs per gram. Less than 70% reduction of egg counts 7 to 14 days after treatment may indicate drug resistance. In this way, the counts are being used not as an absolute gauge of the number of worms present, but to indicate the rising or falling trend of infection within the group of horses.

An approach to determining the frequency of anthelmintic treatment required on a given farm would be to begin with three monthly treatments in the spring, with the exact time of treatment based on climatic factors, followed by monthly fecal egg counts to determine when the next treatments are advisable. So long as counts on ALL horses remain below 50 eggs per gram, no further treatments need be given.

If monthly egg counts rise or fail to decrease, counts should be conducted seven days after the next treatment to check for the possible emergence of drug resistance. After one to two years of treating and checking, it should be possible to determine the timing and frequency of anthelmintic treatment required for control on each farm on an individual basis without having to continue monthly egg counts. Periodic egg counts following treatment would still be advisable to check for drug resistance.

It has been suggested that alternating anthelmintic groups every six to eight weeks might result in multiple drug resistance. The theory is that exposure to more than one group of drugs during the maximum generation time of the small strongyles (approximately 48 weeks) would at least result in more rapid selection of a population resistant to more than one medication if it did not result in a surviving population resistant to every anthelmintic used during that period. Changing anthelmintic groups no more frequently than once every 48 weeks would presumably result in less rapid selection of multiple resistant strains. It has been shown that populations resistant to more than one anthelmintic may be selected simultaneously.

In determining how frequently to alternate anthelmintic groups and which specific one to use, the following should be considered:

1) It is not a valid assumption that all parasites surviving anthelmintic treatment are resistant to the wormer used—a certain small percentage of parasites would probably survive all but the harshest treatments.

2) It is unlikely that a horse will be exposed to strongyle larvae during only one month of the year; so regardless of the program of alternation of anthelmintics, parasites will be exposed to different wormers at different ages. This is because the animal is constantly being reinfected, resulting in worms of different ages in his body at all times.

3) The argument as to whether multiple anthelmintic resistance is likely to emerge more rapidly following frequent versus infrequent alternation of anthelmintic groups is not yet settled; it must be determined with further studies.

4) It is unlikely resistance would develop more rapidly following yearly alternation than following 60-day alternation.

5) Alternating more frequently than once a year helps cancel the weaknesses of certain anthelmintics. For example, pyrantel and the piperazine-phenothiazines are relatively weak against S. edentatus. So, if pyrantel were used for a year without alternating with another group, S. edentatus might start to build up in the herd. If a benzimidazole were used twice during the year, S. edentatus would have less chance to increase.

6) The use of combination anthelmintics, such as a benzimidazole-piperazine combination, seems to delay the selection of resistant strains and to control the resistant population already present.

7) One way to prevent resistance would be to attempt eradication of the parasite population, thus avoiding the escape of survivors that would carry resistant traits. Alternation of unrelated anthelmintics that are 95% effective against small strongyles during 40- to 60-day periods might theoretically accomplish this.

8) All horses joining a resident population should be treated with an anthelmintic and isolated for 72 hours. From this point, treat them along with the resident horses.

9) Daily removal of manure helps to prevent the animals' picking up worms at their infective stages because the parasites do not have time to get that far in their development. Manure may be composted which will kill the worm larvae, if the pile is allowed to heat sufficiently. Or, it may be spread thinly on an unused pasture where drying will help to kill the larvae.

10) Good grazing practices help to limit parasite numbers. Keep the least contaminated pastures for nursing mares and their foals. If you have cattle or sheep, rotating grazing on an annual basis between horses and another species is helpful in preventing parasitism in both.

11) Treat all horses on a farm at the same time to keep worming schedules coordinated and consistent. Use the recommended dosages.

PREVENTION OF WORM PROBLEMS

Prevention of parasite infestation is far better and more efficient than having horses infected with worms and then trying to remove them. All wormers are toxic; the object of the game is to select drugs that are more toxic to the worms than they are to the horse. If it is unnecessary to give wormer to the animal because he has no worms, you are miles ahead of having the worms and attempting to get rid of them. As mentioned previously, bots can be prevented by removing the eggs from the hair. An adult horse with an "average" infection of strongyles may produce about 15 million eggs per day. And that's a lot of contamination to drop on a pasture! (85)

Some research has been done with raising foals who are free from worms. Mares were wormed several times until they were free of worms before the foal was born. Then, they were foaled out in carefully cleaned barns. Manure was removed daily so that none of it laid long enough for the eggs to become embryonated and reach the infective stage. In this manner, the foal had little or no opportunity to pick up worm infestation. Following this sort of procedure shows that it is possible to raise relatively worm-free foals, but that it requires a good deal of attention to cleanliness of every element involved a long while before and a long while (months) after the foal's birth.

IMPORTANT NOTE: Young foals frequently eat their mother's manure, as well as that of other older horses. This practice does NOT give them worms, as the manure they eat is too fresh and has not become infective. They only do this when young, usually between a few days and five months of age. It is thought that this practice evolved so that the foal could get the proper bacteria introduced into his digestive tract to enable him to digest roughage. It may also provide certain vitamins that his body is not yet producing. Manure eating does not indicate mineral deficiencies or illness.

Once a pasture has been grazed by horses, it will carry infective stages of the worms passed by those horses. Parasite loads on pastures may be reduced by several methods. Plowing the pasture at least 10 inches deep and reseeding it should bury worm eggs and larvae deeply enough that they will not survive. Even this drastic treatment may not be completely effective. Of course, it temporarily renders the area unusable for grazing. If the pasture is rested through a hot summer and for the next winter, the number of eggs and larvae will be reduced.

The pasture may be grazed in rotation with other animals, such as sheep or cattle. This system helps because cattle parasites do not affect horses, and horse worms do not bother cattle. When cattle are grazed after horses, they will ingest many of the infective larvae and eggs. Because the cow is different from the horses, the larvae will not develop and will be destroyed. Horses will do the same with cattle worms. In this way, each species will help to reduce worm numbers for the other.

Chemical control of worms on pastures has been attempted, but no economical method has been found so far.

Harrowing is commonly used to help spread the manure to allow it to dry out and kill the worms. This has mixed effects on parasite control. Horses are not inclined to graze near patches of manure and will often ignore lush patches of forage if the manure is not spread. Examination will show that these areas are filled with mounds of horse manure. This selective feeding helps to minimize the animals' chances of picking up infective worm larvae.

Picking up the manure in pastures can avoid all these problems and is perhaps the ideal method of worm control. Removal once or twice a week is adequate to offer good control of worm infestation. This method has been used on some breeding farms with good results. Pasture contamination by infective stages of worms is thus avoided because they take 10 days or more to develop. Fresh manure should not be spread on horse pastures because this will only add to the contamination. Instead, it should be allowed to compost until it heats thoroughly; ideally, even then it should be used on land which is used for crop production, or pastured by other animals. This method is, however, impractical for most of us, unless we have both strong backs and free time, or lots of free or cheap labor. The majority of horse owners will have to be content with controlling worm numbers in their animals by a regular worming program.

Worm production in the mare reaches a peak at the same time as the foal is being born and getting a start in life because of the greater egg production by the worms in spring and summer. This leads to heavy pasture infection and thus to an increased worm burden on the new foals. A worming program to help remove worms from the mare will, in turn, reduce the parasite burden on the foal. The mare may be wormed about a month before foaling. Be sure that you use a product which is compatible with pregnancy. Worm the mare again, using the same wormer about 10 days after the birth of the foal. These two treatments will help to reduce the numbers of worm eggs that are passed in the mare's manure to be picked up by the foal. If you have a problem with strongyloides, the mare should be wormed the day the foal is born.

Horses who are new to a group should be turned out on pasture only after they have received a full dose of the wormer that you are using. One animal who is turned loose without treatment can contaminate a whole pasture and can thereby disrupt a control program which has taken months or years to achieve.

All horses on the premises should be treated when worming is performed. It does little good to intensively treat some animals while leaving others untreated. The unwormed animal can shed large numbers of eggs, quickly reinfecting the others. It is a good idea to keep them in for a couple of days after worming so that any eggs which are shed in the manure do not go to infect other horses. Any transient or board animals should either be kept strictly separate from the treated population, or should be wormed before turning them out with treated animals.

Foals are born free of worms, but begin to pick up infective larvae within the first few days of their lives as they begin to graze. The worms then go through their migration and return to the foal's intestine, where they begin to lay eggs which will, in turn, help to contaminate the pasture. Worm eggs may be seen in the foal's feces between 8 and 11 weeks of age, depending on the type of worm involved. Foals should receive their first worming about 8 weeks of age and again at 12 weeks of age. The next treatment should be given at about 24 weeks of age. Important protection of foals is given by carefully worming their mothers, thus minimizing the amount of worm eggs they will encounter.

It is often worthwhile to have periodic fecal egg counts run at a veterinary clinic or laboratory. These are not as valuable as an index of infection in an individual horse. They are more important in showing trends of worm infestation in the group of animals.

WORMING METHODS

Several methods are used to worm horses. Wormers may be placed in the feed. If you are using one of these products, be sure to read the directions carefully. Some of them tell you to fast the horse for a few hours before giving the wormer. There are several reasons for fasting. Having the horse hungry before the medication is given will make him more inclined to eat the wormer. Some wormers need to be given on an empty stomach so that their action will not be diluted by a large quantity of food.

The wormer should be mixed with clean, fresh, palatable grain—give it with whatever your horse is already eating. If he has not eaten the grain-wormer mix within about 12 hours, he probably is not going to eat it. At this point, the mixture should be discarded in a safe place where other horses or animals, such as dogs, will not get it. Some wormers, such as those containing dichlorvos, actually cause a chemical reaction with the grain after a period of time causing it to become sour and unpleasant. The horse is not inclined to eat it at that point, and its effectiveness may be questionable even if he does consume it. Some animals will not eat wormer in their feed even after days of starvation. Obviously, worming in the feed is only effective if the horse will eat the feed. If not, we must look to other methods.

Paste wormers have become quite popular in the last few years. The wormer is compounded into a paste mixture with the consistency of peanut butter. It is deliberately made tacky so that it sticks to the animal's mouth. These products work well with many animals and are easily given by the horse owner. If you are using a paste wormer, follow the directions on the package. If the package has a calibrated plunger, adjust it to the weight you have estimated your horse to be. Do not use more than the recommended amount. Excessive dosages may be perfectly safe with some drugs, yet toxic with others.

It is especially important to have the animal's mouth empty at the time the paste is placed there. If the horse has any hay or grain in his mouth at the time, he may spit it out, taking the wormer with it and thus wasting it. It is often helpful to either keep the animal off feed for several hours before administration of the wormer to make sure that his mouth is empty, or to wash it out with a dose syringe or garden hose if the horse will tolerate you taking such liberties with his mouth.

Inject the medication into the side of the animal's mouth between the front and back teeth (at the interdental space where the bit rides). Quickly deposit the whole calculated dose as far back as possible on the animal's tongue. Some horses react quite violently to having the paste placed in their mouths. For this reason, you should be standing safely at the animal's side during the procedure, not in front of him. After you have dosed the animal, place a hand on his lower jaw and raise his head for a few seconds. This helps the animal to swallow the wormer, whether he wishes to or not.

Worming via stomach tube is a common and reliable method. Tube worming should be done by your veterinarian because of the danger that the worming compound may be placed in the animal's lungs. This mistake is easily made if you do not know what you are doing. When a stomach tube is passed down the horse's nose, it is far easier to get it into the trachea than into the esophagus; for

this reason, it is not a job for the horse owner. If you attempt it and get the wormer in the animal's lungs, he will probably die of what is called an "inhalation pneumonia" or "foreign body pneumonia."

Why have a veterinarian pass a stomach tube to worm a horse, an often expensive and bothersome process? There are several good reasons. Wormers that no sane horse would ever eat, even in a paste, can be given via the stomach tube. The owner is assured that the animal has gotten his full, correct dose of wormer. And, worming time is a good opportunity for your veterinarian to check over your animal's general health, float his teeth if necessary, and answer any questions that you may have about the animal's health and well-being. We generally tube wormed in the spring and fall (about a month after the first killing frost). That program is now being rethought with the new advances in knowledge about strongyle lifestyles, as noted above.

Whatever worming product is used, the LABEL INSTRUCTIONS SHOULD BE FOLLOWED CAREFULLY AND COMPLETELY. If the manufacturer recommends that feed be withheld before the wormer is administered, this should be done. If the label says that the animal may be fed normally, or SHOULD be fed, this also should be done. Some products are irritating to the horse, and may cause colic if feed is withheld before or after worming. Nonrecommended feeding practices may cause toorapid absorption of the wormer, or may cause it to pass too fast or too slowly through the animal's digestive tract when it is fed, again causing it to be less effective than it should be.

Rarely, a horse may show an allergic reaction to a wormer. Reactions may include hives, anaphylactic shock, and even complete collapse. Get veterinary help IMMEDIATELY! Be sure to note the product which caused the reaction on the horse's records so that it will not be used again.

What happens to the worms after worming the horse depends on the medication which is used. Some products kill the worms so that they are digested before they are passed. When an animal is wormed with one of these products, no worms are seen in the manure. This often leads the horse owner to think that the animal either had no worms or that the wormer was not effective, when neither of these may actually be the case.

Other products make the worms disoriented and dopey so that they lose their grip on the intestinal wall and cannot find their way back to it. These wormers may result in large numbers of live worms being passed in the feces, which may produce fertile eggs before they die. Or, if ascarids are passed without being digested, their bodies may decompose and release large numbers of fertile eggs. These may result in an extra heavy contamination of a small area of the pasture. For this reason, it is often best to worm horses in a stall or small paddock where the manure which is passed after worming may be collected and carefully disposed of to avoid this contamination problem.

A sandwich bag or other plastic sack is a handy container for a fecal sample. Put your hand into the bag like a glove and use the outside of the bag to pick up a sample of manure. One fecal ball is enough. Then, turn the bag inside out over the sample and twist or tie the top shut. The sample which you collect should be fresh. If you cannot take it to the veterinary clinic right away, place it in your refrigerator until you do get there. In general, it should be collected the same day as you deliver it to the laboratory for examination.

Chapter 19

HERNIAS AND CASTRATIONS

Hernias
    Scrotal and Inguinal Hernias
    Umbilical Hernia
    Ventral Hernia
    Diaphragmatic Hernia
Castration
    The Operation
    Complications After Castration
    "Proud-Cut" Geldings
Cryptorchid Stallions
Spaying Mares

HERNIAS

Hernias begin as defects in the abdominal wall. They may first appear as soft swellings without heat or pain, caused when a loop of intestine crawls through the defect and is hanging encased by skin. They generally become larger when the animal is on full feed, and decrease when the bowel is empty. The loop of intestine or other abdominal contents may sometimes be easily returned to the abdominal cavity by gentle pressure. Some of them cannot be pushed back. The gut may fill with feces and be unable to return to the abdomen, causing severe illness. Many hernias are congenital and hereditary, being passed from one generation of animals to the next; a few are acquired through strain or injury.

SCROTAL AND INGUINAL HERNIAS

Some foals have a scrotum which appears enlarged from birth due to the presence of intestinal loops inside it. The scrotum of a six-month old colt may appear as large as that of a grown stallion. This is a congenital problem.

Scrotal or inguinal hernias are occasionally seen in older stallions, but very rarely in mature geldings. The animal may have been exercised hard shortly before the pain began, or just have bred a mare. Acute pain is frequently seen with these hernias.

These hernias are caused by enlargement of the sheath of the testicle combined with a relaxation of the fibrous tissues surrounding the inguinal ring (where the nerves, blood vessels, and reproductive structures pass through the abdominal wall). This allows a piece of intestine to descend into the scrotum. At first, it is intermittent, descending during work and returning to the abdomen when the horse is at rest.

A scrotal hernia may not cause any severe problems for a long period of time. Eventually, however, a loop of intestine becomes filled with feces and is unable to return to the abdominal cavity. This situation is called a strangulation or strangulated hernia. At this point, the animal may not be inclined to move and will appear dull and dopey. He may have little or no appetite, and may have signs of colic resembling those from an impaction elsewhere in the digestive tract. Cases of colic where the horse kicks with his hind feet while standing or lying on his back are said to be especially characteristic of scrotal hernia.

Signs of colic appearing shortly after a stallion has been exercised hard or has bred a mare should cause the owner to suspect an inguinal hernia. If the animal is examined carefully, one testicle may be noticed to be suddenly firm and enlarged. Surgery is the only cure for the problem, and often involves castrating the horse on the involved side.

Gentle pressure on the scrotum may force the piece of intestine back into the abdomen if it has not become too enlarged with feces. If there is any possibility that the problem has existed for some time (say, the horse was out in the pasture and you have not seen him for a few days), do not press on the scrotum. If the gut has been there for some time and has become weakened or dead, it may rupture easily, causing peritonitis and causing the animal's death. The horse might have a chance if you get him to a veterinarian and surgery is performed to relieve the blockage and repair the hernia.

Inguinal hernia is just an incomplete scrotal hernia. Like the latter, it may cause no signs of distress, or it may become strangulated and cause illness or death. These hernias are most commonly seen in stallions, occasionally in geldings, but rarely in mares.

Surgery is the only permanent cure for inguinal or scrotal hernia. If the problem is detected before strangulation occurs, it is a matter of the veterinarian replacing the abdominal contents and then closing the inguinal ring. If the hernia has become strangulated, the procedure may involve removing a section of intestine and suturing the cut ends back together (this procedure is called an anastomosis). Of course, this is more serious than a simple hernia repair.

Many veterinarians recommend castrating the animal at the same time because of the hereditary nature of the problem; this avoids passing it on to more animals who will have to go through the pain (and owners who will have to go through the expense) of the surgery at some time in their lives. And the horses who do receive the surgery are often the lucky ones. A few surely die while out on range, where they become ill and there is no one near to help them.

UMBILICAL HERNIA

Umbilical hernias occur at the attachment of the umbilical cord, or behind or ahead of this area on the midline of the horse's belly. They are caused by defects in the peritoneum. Normally, this is a tough, fibrous sheet of tissue that lines the abdomen. In the foal's development, both sides (right and left halves) must unite at the middle to form an entire, unbroken lining. Where there are defects in this union, omentum or intestine are allowed to descend from the abdominal cavity. They are then contained only by the skin and underlying tissues as the muscles in this area are nearly nonexistent. The size of the hernial pouch depends on the size of the defect in the abdominal wall and how much intestine or other tissue crawls out through it.

Some small umbilical hernias seem to disappear when the animal gets older. It is not so much that it becomes smaller, but that it stays the same size and the animal grows larger around it. Tiny loops of foal intestine which could easily crawl through the opening are replaced by large folds of grown-horse intestine which can no longer do so.

Uncomplicated umbilical hernias can be distinguished from umbilical abscesses or strangulated hernias because the latter two cannot be pushed back into the abdomen when they are squeezed gently. Both abscesses and strangulated hernias may be hot and painful. Either may be accompanied by lack of appetite, ele-

vated body temperature, and signs of abdominal pain. Call your veterinarian for diagnosis and treatment of either of these problems.

Many umbilical hernias need to be surgically corrected. My personal preference is not to do the repair before the animal is about four to six months of age unless the hernia is causing severe problems or becomes strangulated. This gives the animal time to get a good start in life and become strong and sturdy before being subjected to the stresses of anesthesia and surgery. Up to that point, the owners are instructed to check the animal daily, gently pushing the contents of the hernia back into the abdomen. This makes sure that a loop of intestine is not caught in the sack to become strangulated. They are also instructed to keep an eye on the animal for signs of illness or colic, and to let me know right away if these should appear so that the horse can be examined before it becomes seriously ill.

Surgery usually involves completely anesthetizing the animal and turning him on his back. He is then clipped and prepared for surgery. The surgeon opens the skin and reveals the defect. He may then overlap the edges of the

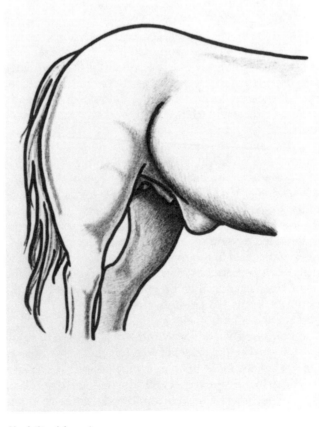

Umbilical hernia.

opening so as to strengthen it or may reinforce it with some synthetic material. Because the surgery involves opening the abdomen, it is best done under sterile conditions to avoid infection. While the defect may be small, the surgery is still a major undertaking because of the horse's susceptibility to infection. If the foal comes down with a respiratory infection prior to surgery, the operation should be delayed until he is completely well.

Over the years, many nonsurgical methods of correction have been tried, including wooden blocks, skewers, clamps, and other devices. While almost any method will work occasionally, many of these are painful to the animal, as well as involving risk of infection. The application of bandages with pads to push the herniated material back into place has also been used, as have blisters and other potions. Surgery is the only sure cure, and is probably, overall, less painful to the horse. The thing that the surgery can do that none of the other methods are able to do is to repair the defect in the peritoneum. If the defect isn't repaired, the hernia is very likely to recur.

VENTRAL HERNIA

This hernia occurs due to rupture of the abdominal wall at a point other than the midline. They are usually due to injury, as from kicks or blows, jumping, pulling, or because the horse has caught himself on some object. They are perhaps most common in pregnant mares. In these animals, they are due to weight of the foal combined with degenerative changes in the abdominal layers. They may also be caused by excessive fluid buildup (edema) adding extra weight to the load borne by the abdominal wall.

This added burden results in rupture of the prepubic tendon. In a pregnant mare, the defect may be so large that the animal appears to have her belly wall hanging down another ten to twelve inches, "overnight." Because of the tremendous weight of the animal's intestines plus the foal, and the fact that the peritoneal layers are generally shredded beyond repair, this problem usually necessitates euthanasia of the mare. If she is near to her foaling date, this is perhaps best done by one clean gunshot to the head. Her belly may then be opened quickly and the foal removed. If it is old enough, it may survive with careful nursing and a lot of luck.

Polypropylene or plastic mesh may be used to repair sizeable abdominal defects in the horse. These implants are not entirely ideal, but may be the only way to close a large gap in the abdominal wall, whether due to hernia or injury. They may be used in some cases to repair mares with ruptured prepubic tendons, if the defect is not too large. They have been used on hernias up to about 3 × 12 inches.

DIAPHRAGMATIC HERNIA

Diaphragmatic hernia is a rare condition in the horse. This is a defect or tear in the diaphragm, the thin sheet of muscle and fibrous tissue that separates the abdominal cavity from the chest cavity. Foals are occasionally born with these hernias. In the older animal, they are usually acquired from an injury, such as being hit by a car, violent exertion, or increased pressure within the abdomen. The abdominal pain is a colic resembling that from other causes, or may be so acute as to be a severe abdominal crisis. This problem is VERY difficult to diagnose. The only cure is to do surgery to repair the tear or defect.

CASTRATION

This is the name given to the surgery which changes a stallion into a gelding and renders him unreproductive by removal of the testicles. It is also (uncommonly) used to refer to spaying mares. The procedure is also referred to as "gelding."

Horses are castrated for several reasons. Removing the testicles eliminates the source of male hormones in the body. This takes away the animal's sex drive, resulting in a horse who acts more like a mare than like a stallion. This allows the gelding, as the resulting animal is called, to be used around mares without undesirable breeding behavior. It also makes the animal much safer to handle and to be around.

A gelding usually has a more consistent disposition and performance than either a stallion who is excited by mares around him or a mare who comes into heat every 21 or so days. Many ranches in the western United States use whole herds of geldings for range work, feeling that they have fewer problems than they would if they had both geldings and mares in their herds. Another very important reason for castration is to keep inferior animals from reproducing; this is important to the improvement of all breeds of animals, not just horses.

As with many other types of surgery, the earlier it is done, the easier it is on the animal. Horses may be castrated at a few weeks of age. There is a problem with this procedure at such an early age. The resulting gelding often has thin, poorly developed front quarters, neck, and head. For this reason, most people wait until the animal is at least a year of age; for heavily muscled breeds such as the Quarter Horse, two years is perhaps even better.

The difference between doing the surgery at one year and at two years of age is somewhat a matter of personal preference. It is also very much a matter of facilities, as many stables will not board a stud colt over a year or so of age. When the animal begins to act like a stallion, they no longer want him on their premises. This may force the owner to do the surgery in order to have a place to keep the animal. Veterinarians often get a batch of stud colts to castrate in the spring of their two-year old year. As the animals begin to come to sexual maturity, they try to cross fences to get to mares that they can smell, often severely injuring themselves in the process. At this point, the owner will often suddenly decide that he doesn't have the facilities to keep the animal, doesn't want his horse ruined for life by cutting some vital muscle or tendon in a fence, and that he does not want the animal for breeding purposes. Veterinary bills for repairing the horse may be getting expensive. It is not uncommon to suture wire cuts and castrate the horse under the same session of anesthetic.

Many ranchers castrate their own colts. This is generally a rough-and-ready rodeo, with the animals roped and tied down and some cowboy wielding a sharp knife. My opinion is that this is a rather barbaric way to do a major operation on an animal as sensitive as a horse. For that reason, this book does not include a description of how to castrate your own horse. It is worth the price to most owners to have the surgery done under anesthesia to lessen the animal's suffering. If you have a large number of horses to castrate and would like to do them in a manner that is easier on them than the bust 'em and cut 'em method, it is often possible to arrange with a veterinarian to join your crew and anesthetize the animals while you do the brute labor. Or, he may give you a herd rate for the surgery. A final word on this point—the shock resulting from the excitement combined with the pain of the surgery can kill a horse. That makes a veterinary bill look small in comparison.

THE OPERATION

The horse should be in good health when the surgery is done. He should not be recently recovered from any serious disease, especially distemper. Be sure to tell your veterinarian if the animal has been on sweet clover pasture or has been fed sweet clover hay, as these feeds may make the animal more prone to bleeding. The horse should not have been recently wormed, especially not with organophosphate wormers; some of these make the animal more susceptible to some of the anesthetics that are used and may cause serious complications. If at all possible, surgery should be done in spring or fall, either before fly season, or after a frost has killed most of the flies. Most veterinarians do not like to castrate horses during cold, rainy weather. Not only is it miserable work, but it seems to me that horses have more complications if castrated during these periods.

Veterinarians give some sort of anesthetic before starting to castrate the horse. Your veterinarian has developed a routine which works for him. This may range from a small dose of tranquilizer and local anesthetic injected directly into the spermatic cords and nerves as he does surgery with the animal standing, to completely anesthetizing the horse until he is flat on the ground. He

may or may not tie the animal up after it is asleep. He will then make incisions—usually one over each testicle—and remove the testicles. He uses a clamp called an emasculator to crush the cords and blood vessels. This helps to prevent bleeding from the surgery site. After the testicles are removed, many veterinarians open the scrotal sack as far as they possibly can. This is to allow the area to drain well and to help prevent swelling and complications.

AFTERCARE

Some veterinarians administer penicillin after surgery; others do not. This is a matter of personal preference; a single dose probably does more for the owner's peace of mind than it does for the possibility of infection. If your horse has not had a recent booster of tetanus toxoid, the veterinarian may administer either this or tetanus antitoxin, depending on the horse's immunization history. If it is fly season, it will be necessary to spray the surgical area daily with a good fly spray. Don't spray it directly into the wound unless the flies are so bad that this is absolutely necessary. For most animals, spraying the vicinity is good enough.

Aftercare by the owner does more to prevent swelling and infection than anything the veterinarian can do. It is of the utmost importance to give the animal adequate exercise after surgery. This helps the opened area to rub together and drain out blood clots, as well as helping to remove infected material if there is any. It prevents swelling. If left to himself, the new gelding may stay in one place, nursing his sore spots. The worst possible thing that you as an owner can do is to just allow the horse to stand and become swollen. If a significant amount of swelling occurs, your veterinarian may have to reanesthetize the animal and reopen and clean the wound. Some horses who have been allowed to stand will swell up larger than a basketball. Needless to say, they will be in misery. The local swelling is usually accompanied by edema of the hindlegs, often called "stocking" or "stocking up."

How much exercise should you give the animal? My personal policy is to let the animal rest on the day he is castrated. The day after, the owner is to exercise him 30 minutes to an hour. The second day after surgery, an hour is the absolute MINIMUM! Two hours are even better, continuing this amount of work DAILY until the animal is completely healed, which usually takes about two weeks. What kind of work? Spending that amount of time walking—whether leading the animal, ponying him, or on a hot walker—is the least that should be done. Spending some of the time at a trot or a lope is even better.

My advice to clients is that this is the ideal time to break their two-year old colt. The animal is too sore to buck or protest when you start riding him. By the time he is healed, you have him pretty well broken and all those ideas are out of his head. So, get out that saddle and go to work. And if you want to trot or lope him, go to it—it's fine with me and great for him! Owners who have used this method have been well pleased with the results. One of my clients started riding an older, spoiled stallion (who was more than a little bit bronc) two days after his surgery. By the time the animal was healed, he had remembered his good manners and the fellow gave him to his grandchildren, with satisfactory results. It's also easier to spend the required amount of time riding the horse than it is to walk around leading him.

Several other methods of castration have been advocated at various times, including the use of clamps (called "Burdizzos," among other names). These are used to crush the spermatic cord and blood vessels. No incision is made in the scrotum. Some people like the fact that no blood is visible. In my opinion, this is a flimsy reason to use them, considering the complications and infection that frequently follow their use. Think of it: the blood vessels are crushed so that the testicles no longer have a blood supply. They die and must be removed by the body—difficult to do without a blood supply. The end result can be bags of fetid material hanging between your horse's legs. Also, if the cord is not adequately crushed, the animal may still be fertile. Or, the procedure may have to be repeated, resulting in still further pain and distress to the animal. Castration is one of the times when a good, large, open wound is the kindest cut of all.

Do NOT assume that since your colt has been castrated, it is safe to turn him in with mares who are in heat. While sperm cells are no longer produced by the testicles, live semen may remain in some of the glands of the reproductive system for several weeks. Thus, the colt may be fertile enough to get a mare pregnant—usually the one you DIDN'T want bred. If it is important that the horse not be fertile, a semen sample should be checked by your veterinarian before he is allowed out with mares. Otherwise, assume an absolute MINIMUM of ten days for all fertile sperm to die. Two to three weeks are even better if you can allow that much time.

Also, it takes a period of time for the hormones to leave the animal's body. He may exhibit stallion-like behavior for a varying period of time, depending on how rapidly these are removed from the bloodstream. This usually requires a few days to a few weeks, depending on the individual. It also depends on how old the animal was when castrated. An older stallion may retain sexual behavior for a longer period of time than a younger animal would who was not fixed in this behavior pattern.

COMPLICATIONS AFTER CASTRATION

BLEEDING

Bleeding often occurs from the edges of the cut on the scrotum; it may also occur from a small artery in the spermatic cord. The horse may appear to bleed quite heavily, especially in warm weather. Untying the animal, if he has been restrained, and allowing him to relax will help reduce his blood pressure (which has been raised by the excitement and handling). This in itself helps the bleeding to stop. It rarely lasts more than 15 minutes. A small amount of dripping (a drop to a few drops at a time) beyond this time is not a problem. If the animal appears to be bleeding heavily more than an hour after surgery, consult your veterinarian and have him recheck the animal to make sure there are no problems or complications.

SWELLING

Swelling of the scrotal area may occur after castration, as well as swelling of the animal's penis, sheath, and hind legs. The animal may be reluctant to move; when forced to do so, he may move stiffly with a straddling gait. He may have an elevated temperature and little or no appetite. These complications can be almost entirely prevented by adequate exercise after castration to help keep the circulation moving in the area and to remove infected material. If exercise is neglected, the animal's scrotum may swell as large as a basketball, interfering with circulation to his hindlegs so that they swell, too.

If severe swelling occurs, call your veterinarian AT ONCE so that he may reopen the area, clean it out, and get it to draining adequately. He may wish to put the animal on antibiotics for a period of time. If he does use antibiotics, be sure to give the prescribed amount of medication for the correct length of time. Failure to do so may lengthen the animal's recovery time or result in his dying from infection. To reiterate a point made previously, this problem can largely be prevented by adequate exercise after the surgery. If you have an animal swollen like this, it is probably your own fault. By trying to be "kind" to him, you have caused him a considerable amount of extra pain and discomfort and possibly endangered his life.

"PROUD-CUT" GELDINGS

"Proud-cut" is the term given to geldings who still exhibit a stallion-like behavior. This may range from merely snorting at and teasing mares in heat to full-blown mounting behavior, including (rarely) development of an erection. While the animal may mount, he usually does not enter the mare. Old-timers attribute this to the veterinarian (or other person who castrated the horse) failing to remove the epididymis, a portion of the reproductive tract which wraps around the end of the testicle.

Research was conducted at Colorado State University some years ago, in which some proud-cut geldings were surgically examined. It was found to make little difference in their behavior whether the epididymis had been removed or not. It has been theorized that these animals have male hormone production in their bodies from some site other than the testicles—perhaps from one of the other glands in the endocrine system. Many of the geldings who "act like stallions" after castration are those who were sexually aggressive as stallions, and had considerable sexual experience. They may still exhibit learned breeding behavior after being gelded. This may be a constant problem, or it may only be seen around mares or premises where they had previously exhibited sexual behavior. There is little or no cure for the gelding who remains "studdy" after he has been castrated. There isn't anything else to remove, except maybe his head!

However, if you have a gelding who REALLY acts like a stallion, and you don't know for sure how he was castrated, it is worth having him examined to see that he does not still have a testicle retained in his abdomen. Occasionally, someone will take a cryrptorchid stallion, remove the visible testicle, and then sell the animal as a gelding. Your veterinarian can usually tell you if the animal appears to have a testicle in his abdomen yet. In some cases, exploratory surgery may be necessary to determine whether or not this is the case. Which brings us to:

CRYPTORCHID STALLIONS

Cryptorchid refers to the situation where a horse has one or both testicles which have failed to descend into the scrotum. An old name for one of these animals is risling or ridgeling. They vary from animals who have one or both testicles under the skin in the flank area or in the inguinal canal to animals who have both testicles in the abdomen near the kidneys. If the testicle is in the inguinal canal, the animal is called a "high flanker." In the normal male horse, the testicles should be through the inguinal ring (in the flank area) by birth, and should be completely in the scrotum at birth or shortly afterward.

If the testicle or testicles are in the flank or in the inguinal canal, the surgery to retrieve and remove them may not be much different than a normal castration. If, however, they are retained in the abdomen, major abdominal surgery is necessary to remove them. Ideally, this operation should be performed in an adequate surgical facility under sterile conditions because it does open the abdomen and because the horse is more susceptible to infection than many other animals.

The difficulty of the operation varies with the animal. Some are relatively easy, while others are quite difficult and challenge the surgeon's abilities. The retained testicle is often quite small and misshapen, which can make it very hard to find. The animal will be completely anesthetized (asleep) during the surgery. Your veterinarian may go into the animal's abdomen through the inguinal area (near the scrotum), through the flank, or at the midline, depending on his facilities and experience.

Why remove this testicle or testicles at all? If they are not removed, they are a source of male hormones and the animal will continue to act like a stallion. Indeed, it seems that some of these animals act MORE like a stallion than a normal stallion. This makes them both unpleasant and dangerous to handle. They may be nervous and irritable. The second reason is that the problem is hereditary. A cryptorchid stallion with one normal testicle will be fertile and will produce stud colts who have the same problem, resulting in added expense and increased risk when their owners go to castrate them. This can severely decrease the saleability of the animal's colts, as well as perpetuating a hereditary defect. If both testicles are retained in the abdomen, the animal is often sterile and unable to reproduce, but will dispositionally still be a stallion.

The third reason is that retained testicles are much more prone to tumors than are normal testicles. These may eventually result in severe hormonal disturbances, as well as death of the horse. All in all, it's a defect we could do without in our horse population.

SPAYING MARES

Spaying a mare is the female equivalent of castrating a stud colt. It results in an animal free of hormonal influences. Her behavior is the same every day, much like a gelding. Spayed mares can be run with geldings without upsetting them. This surgery is often done with grade mares who are not needed for reproduction, and is especially popular with owners of dude and pack strings in some areas of the western United States.

Spaying may also be done with mares who have hormonal upsets so that they are in heat all the time. While it often brings relief in these cases, it is by no means 100% effective. It is speculated that female hormones may be produced in areas other than the ovaries (much like those in a "proud-cut" gelding). If this is the case, surgery may bring little or no relief to the animal's behavioral problem.

Because this is major abdominal surgery, it needs to be done by a veterinarian, under sterile conditions (much like a cryptorchid). The animal is usually fully anesthetized. The operation may be done through the midline with the animal either tied and rolled on her back, or with her hind legs tied to both ends of a singletree and elevated with a winch. It could also be done through some area of the flank. The technique used depends on the veterinarian's facility and on his training and preference. No one method is necessarily better than any other—they are merely different. The veterinarian removes both the animal's ovaries; the uterus is left intact. After surgery, the mare should be fed lightly for a few days, and kept confined with no exercise. The animal may be returned to riding or use after she is completely healed, usually two to four weeks.

Chapter 20

TOXINS AND POISONOUS PLANTS

Toxins
  Mycotoxins
Snakebite
Poisonous Plants
  Prevention of Plant Poisonings
  Oleander Poisoning
  Bracken Fern
  Horsetail
  Castor Bean
  Yew Poisoning
  Red Maple Leaf Poisoning
  Yellow Star Thistle, Russian Knapweed
  Lupine
  Locoweed Poisoning
  Timber Milk Vetch Poisoning
  Selenium Poisoning
  Nicotine Poisoning
  Cirrhosis of the Liver
  Ground Ivy
  Poison Hemlock
  Western Water Hemlock
  Forage Poisoning
  Larkspur
  Marijuana
  Sorghum and Sudan Grass Toxicity
  Bermuda Grass Tremors
  Chokecherry Poisoning
  Miscellaneous Poisonous Plants
  Plants Causing Mechanical Injury

This section is not designed, nor is it intended, to make you an expert in the diagnosis of toxic problems. That's one of the things well worth paying your veterinarian to do for you. Its purpose is to give an overview of some toxins which may affect horses and to make you aware of some of the ways in which horses may be poisoned.

Horse poisonings, fortunately, are uncommon. When seen, many of them can be confused with diseases, such as colitis-X, which come on with explosive rapidity. If your horse becomes suddenly, violently ill, call your veterinarian IMMEDIATELY.

While he is on the way, keep the horse as comfortable as possible. In hot weather, keep him in the shade. In cold weather, get him inside if at all possible and put a blanket on him if he is cold. If you don't have a barn or shed, a garage, shop, or other building is better than no shelter at all until the animal is treated and better accommodations can be found.

If the animal is in convulsions, put a halter and long lead rope on him so that you can pull his head away from fences or walls and yet stay safely out of the way of his flailing feet. Or tie jackets, towels, or packing quilts around the halter with pieces of string or baling twine to keep himself from hitting his head and injuring his eyes.

Look around to see what the horse might have eaten or drunk that could have caused his problem. If you know what the horse has gotten into, have the can or other container available for your veterinarian when he arrives. This may save precious minutes determining what the animal has ingested, and will allow the start of treatment without delay. The more specific the diagnosis, the more specific and correct the treatment can be, thus increasing the horse's chance of survival.

"Universal antidotes" or similar products should usually not be used unless absolutely no veterinary help is available. They may do little or no good, and thinking they will help can cause a delay in seeking expert assistance. The time wasted on this type of product may make the difference between life and death for a poisoned horse.

Do not rely on laboratory tests to diagnose the cause of a poisoning. The animal may be long dead before the results finally come back from the laboratory, even on a "rush" basis. Unfortunately, some toxicities are only diagnosed on necropsy. This is not a total loss, as it may save another horse on the premises from getting into the same toxin. A small percentage of poisonings are never diagnosed. There are so many toxicities which cause some of the same groups of symptoms that if it is not obvious what the horse ate, there may be no way to tell for sure what caused his illness or death.

TOXINS

Many illnesses which at first glance look like poisoning turn out to be explainable disease processes. Colitis-X is perhaps the best example of this. Remember that not all acute, sudden illnesses in the horse are poisonings, and that the great majority of poisonings are not malicious, but are accidental.

Many medications and chemicals can be poisonous to the horse. Some, like urea, must be present in fairly large quantities to cause poisoning, being well utilized in smaller amounts. Others cause toxicity when present in very small quantities. Some minerals, such as selenium, can cause toxicity when present in excess, yet in small amounts is an essential dietary component.

Monensin (Rumensin, Elanco Products Co., Indianapolis, IN 46285) is a substance which is commonly mixed with grain for feeder cattle and poultry. It is highly toxic to horses and may cause death in amounts as small as 1 to 2 mg per lb (½ to 1 mg per kg) of feed. No antidote is available for this toxicity, and monensin consumption is nearly always fatal. Horses who eat it show signs of severe colic. Giving activated charcoal or mineral oil (administered by a veterinarian via stomach tube) may lessen the effects of the intoxication.

Many petroleum products are toxic to horses. While they are not normally attractive to horses, they may be eaten by animals with a depraved appetite, or by confined animals having access to them. Poisoning may occur when kerosene or other petroleum products are used as "home remedies." Waste oil used to reduce dust may cause toxicity in some cases. Skin diseases, including hair loss and irritation, may occur when these items are applied to the animal's skin, or he rubs or lies on them. One "herbal" book recommends using waste oil for insect repellent. DON'T! The little money that might be saved is not worth the risk of problems—OR—the cost of treating them.

Excessive zinc intake may cause unthriftiness and abnormal bone growth in foals. Soil and forage contamination may cause these problems near zinc smelters. The animals may have generalized joint swellings and lameness due to the severe disturbance of their bone growth centers. Foals may show contracted flexor tendons. The animals may have an abnormal posture, with the head held low and the back arched and stiff. The animals move slowly and deliberately. The front legs are advanced a short step, and the hindlegs shuffled forward (almost in a hop), and placed well under the body, giving the impression that it is painful to flex the joints and place weight on the limbs. Foals are often emaciated. Lesions are found in the joint cartilage at necropsy. (86)

Lead poisoning can be encountered when horses lick old batteries or chew on paint cans. It can also be seen near lead smelters. It can come from consumption of or contact with petroleum products which contain lead. Pica (depraved appetite) in which horses eat odd substances may lead a horse to eat lead-based paint from a building or vehicle. Lead-based paints should not be used on fences, barns, or horse trailers. High lead concentrations may result from horses who graze near busy highways, although this problem may be reduced with the increasing use of unleaded gasoline.

Lead ingestion in horses results in peripheral nerve degeneration, causing paralysis in the larynx and pharynx. This symptom may cause it to be confused with rabies. Contact your veterinarian IMMEDIATELY if the horse seems to have a brain problem, or apparent difficult in swallowing. It may be rabies and not lead poisoning!

Removal of the source of lead is necessary to curing a case of lead poisoning. It does no good to treat the animal and get him back on his feet if he just goes back to eating whatever he was getting previously and comes down with the same problem again. (87)

Selenium poisoning (often called alkali disease) may be seen in horses who drink water containing too much selenium. It is also seen in horses who have eaten plants which pick up appreciable quantities of selenium from the soil. There is no good treatment for selenium poisoning—as with other toxicities, prevention is the best cure (see Poisonous Plants).

Fluorine toxicity can be seen when animals graze pastures contaminated by smelters or other industrial operations. Some mineral supplements, such as rock phosphates or water, may naturally contain excessively high levels of fluorine.

Fluorosis may cause damage to horses' teeth when intake of fluorine occurs during tooth formation. The enamel of the teeth becomes discolored and brittle. The weak, defective enamel may chip, exposing the underlying, softer material, which will wear excessively fast. Horses with fluorosis may eat less than normal, chew their food poorly, and slobber much of it out of their mouths. Because there may be some problems with bone involvement, the horse may appear stiff and lame. The bones may show enlarged areas. Horses, unlike humans, do not seem to need fluorine for normal tooth development.

Arsenic toxicity is occasionally seen as a malicious poisoning. The animal will show severe abdominal pain. He will be weak, staggering, and often in shock. There may be both salivation and diarrhea.

Mercury poisoning may be seen when horses eat large amounts of grain treated with mercurial antifungal products. The symptoms may resemble those of arsenic poisoning. The animal may tremble and show convulsions or coma.

Poisoning with insecticides such as organophosphates, carbamates, and chlorinated hydrocarbons usually results in central nervous system signs. The animal may appear hyperactive or nervous and twitchy. He may show excessive salivation and diarrhea. The muscular excitation may proceed into convulsions.

Most toxins meant to kill rodents (rats, mice, and gophers) are poisonous to horses. In addition, they are often in a grain base which makes them attractive for horses to eat. If large amounts are eaten, grain founder may complicate the problem. Warfarin (dicoumarin) is one of the common rodenticides used; others include strychnine, ANTU, thallium, arsenic, phosphorus, and zinc phosphide. Many of these products have NO antidote, and some may be toxic to horses in small quantities.

Strychnine poisoning may be seen when animals eat large amounts of rodent bait containing this poison. It is also (rarely) seen as a malicious poisoning. Horses with strychnine poisoning will be abnormally excitable, so that any small noise or motion will trigger a spasm or convulsions. They may twitch uncontrollably. With large amounts, the animal may fall down and go into convulsions before death occurs.

The best cure for rodenticide poisoning in the horse is to avoid it. Rodenticides should be placed where there is no possibility that a horse can get at them. Large quantities (as are often found on ranches or farms) should be stored in cans with securely latched lids (such as those that clamp onto the top of an oil drum) and placed inside a shed which is locked or barred for extra safety.

MYCOTOXINS

Mycotoxins (toxins produced by molds) may be present in moldy or spoiled feed. Aflatoxins (a type of mycotoxin produced by a mold called Aspergillus flavus) produce liver damage. Other types may produce colic or bloody diarrhea. They also may cause kidney problems, as well as defects in blood coagulation and in the body's immune system.

Toxins produced by a mold called Fusarium have been incriminated in horse deaths in Virginia. In those animals, the Fusarium toxins caused blindness, incoordination, problems with chewing, coma, and death. There is no effective treatment when the animal is showing signs of mold poisoning.

For this reason, uneaten feed should be removed from the feeder and carefully disposed of by placing it in a trash can with a tight lid or other safe means of disposal. Spoiled feed which one horse has not eaten may be quite attractive to another horse who gets out of his pen after you have dumped the feed on the ground. You may wish to put bad grain in a garbage bag and take it with you the next time you go to town. It will be much safer in a dumpster headed for the city landfill than it would be dumped on your own premises.

Feed which is obviously moldy should not be fed to horses, and may not be safe for other classes of livestock.

Feed need not show obvious signs of mold to be poisonous. Mycotoxins may remain in feeds long after the fungus which produced them has died. Milling and pelleting may kill the fungus, but not destroy its toxins. If you suspect toxic problems due to mycotoxins on feed, have a sample checked by a reliable laboratory.

SNAKEBITE

Snakebite is not a common problem in the United States, but when it does occur, it is usually due to a rattlesnake. Water moccasins and copperheads may cause bites to horses in the southern states. Coral snake bites are said to be uncommon in the horse. Most bites occur on warm days in the spring and summer when the snakes are active.

One of the most frequent sites for bite is the nose or elsewhere on the face. The horse hears the noise of the snake rattling and goes to investigate. Because of his poor close vision, he probably puts his head down to smell the snake, getting bit in the process. Bites on the leg also occur when the animal steps on or near a snake. Bites occur mostly on the front legs, but may be found on hind legs after the horse has stepped over the snake with his front legs and then gets hit. Bites on the legs are often hard to find because there is little soft muscle tissue there, and thus little swelling.

Bites on the head are rapidly followed by considerable swelling. In some cases, the nostrils may swell shut, causing breathing difficulty. If you catch the horse in time, cut pieces of garden hose or similar tubing about 5 inches long. Insert a piece into each nostril, and tape them into place. As the swelling gets larger, it will hold the chunks of hose firmly, allowing the horse to breathe. When the swelling recedes, the hose will tend to fall out of the nostril. In severe cases, it may be necessary for your veterinarian to perform a tracheotomy (cut a hole in the horse's windpipe) to allow him to breathe until the swelling goes down.

Swelling may extend far up the face, and the eyelids may be thickened and nearly swollen shut; the ears may be swollen. In short, a horse with a snakebit face is a miserable beast, and a peculiar-looking one, too. Some animals may show weakness and depression. While the majority of horses who are snakebitten do not die, they may have tissue damage which later develops into osteomyelitis (bone infection) or gangrene, leading to either death or the need for euthanasia. Animals who recover may take weeks or months to do so.

To minimize damage and have the best chance for successful treatment, therapy should be started as soon as possible. Older thinking had us making x-shaped cuts and applying suction to the bitten area. This is not a good idea for several reasons. It is easy to cut a major blood vessel and allow venom to flow directly into the animal's blood stream. As with humans, inexpert and often panicked hacking and slashing frequently does more harm than good. Instead, apply an ice pack to the area (but be careful of causing frostbite if you have to leave it in place for more than an hour or so).

Get the animal to a veterinarian for more extensive treatment as soon as you can. Trailer him instead of walking him if at all possible. Keep the animal as calm and quiet as you can and move him as little as possible. A tourniquet should NOT be used with equine snakebite.

POISONOUS PLANTS

When a horse dies suddenly and the cause cannot be determined, it is often lumped into the category of "poisoning," and a plant or chemical agent is suspected. Literally hundreds of poisonous plants have been indicted as causing illness or death in livestock, including horses.

Most diagnoses of poisoning are not based on laboratory experiments, but rather on field observation and experience. It is difficult to run clinical tests on poisonous plants, because not all plants are toxic at the same time. Nor are they equally poisonous when growing under different conditions, or when compared as fresh versus dried.

As with other toxicities, there are very few signs that are absolutely diagnostic for plant poisoning. And, few plants cause distinctive changes in a dead animal. In fact, many plants can kill animals without producing noticeable changes before the death occurs.

Weather conditions can influence toxicities. A storm prevented a group of horses from eating normally for several days. When the weather finally cleared, they were hungry and ate huge numbers of acorns. Several of the animals died. This may occur with other plants. When the animals finally eat again, they are so hungry that they may eat whatever is handy rather than what they would normally eat.

PREVENTION OF PLANT POISONINGS

As a general rule, poisonous plants are not palatable. A horse will usually avoid them if he has a choice of other, palatable feed—whether growing forage or adequate supplemental hay and grain. Horses may be forced to eat poisonous plants when pasture is overgrazed and no other feed is offered. Overgrazing not only reduces the supply of desirable feed species, but by its destruction of valuable range plants, may stimulate the spread of undesirable species.

Horses may consume poisonous plants in hay, where the animal cannot separate them out. This problem is less easily controlled. Horses may also be affected when poisonous plants are cut and left where the animals are accustomed to eating. The wilting of some plants can drastically increase their toxicity.

Horse owners should check hay as it is fed to make sure that it is not too weedy. Animals may be poisoned by plants, such as oleander, which have been baled with the hay. Buy hay from the same source all the time if possible, and know your supplier. Fortunately, most poisonous plants must be eaten in approximately 1 to 3% of the animal's body weight before toxicity occurs. A horse is unlikely to get this much in a feeding or two of hay. However, continued ingestion of small amounts of some poisonous plants in hay may cause toxicity.

If poisonous plants are noticed in the pasture, they can be removed by digging or using chemical weed killers. Be sure that the weed killer used is compatible with a grazing animal, or remove the horse from the pasture for the recommended length of time after treating the plants. With annual plants, mowing them before they go to seed can result in control of the offending plant within a couple of years. They should be raked up and removed from the pasture after mowing so the animals don't have access to them.

Ditches, fence rows, and spring or seep areas should be closely checked, as poisonous plants are often found there. Some plants are only poisonous at certain times of the year, and it may be necessary to take animals out of the pasture at this time. In California, for example, yellow star thistle grows mostly in the late summer and fall, when native pastures are dry. Care should be taken to provide the animals with supplemental feed, or they may eat the thistle. If the animals acquire a taste for the thistle, which they sometimes do, it may be necessary to completely remove them from the pasture.

Mineral deficiencies sometimes stimulate horses to eat certain plants. For example, plants high in nitrates may have a salty taste, and are thus palatable. If the pasture is short, it is desirable to provide mineral supplements.

Do not turn hungry horses out into strange pastures. At this point, they will eat anything, especially since they don't know what is there. If the first plants a horse finds are poisonous, he may eat them anyway. Fill the animals with hay and then turn them out, after the edge is off their appetite. Young horses are more curious than older ones, and will often eat dangerous plants.

OLEANDER POISONING (Nerium oleander)

Oleander is a shrub grown as an ornamental throughout California and the southern states. It is frequently planted by roadsides in California and Arizona. It is a very beautiful shrub, with white, pink, or red flowers. It is extremely poisonous; poisonings have occurred when humans have used twigs for food skewers. A single leaf is considered potentially lethal to a human being.

Horses will not normally eat leaves from the plant. Horse poisonings usually occur when trimmings are placed where the animal is used to eating hay. They also occur when the animal is fed lawn clippings containing oleander leaves, or when the leaves are baled with hay. About 40 to 60 green or dried leaves are enough to kill a horse. Horses should NEVER be tied to or near oleander bushes, as even a casual nibble of a few leaves may result in the animal's death. If you should have need to burn oleander stems and leaves, be careful. Even the smoke can be hazardous.

A profuse diarrhea begins several hours after the animal has eaten oleander; it may be bloody. The heartbeat becomes fast and irregular—the sounds are indistinct and beats may be frequently skipped. The heart is alternately strong and weak. The membranes of the eyes and mouth may be slightly cyanotic (bluish). The extremities are unusually cold; this is characteristic of oleander poisoning. The animal may sweat and show colic; later he may go down and thrash. Death often occurs within 8 to 24 hours after the animal eats the plant material.

There is no specific treatment for oleander poisoning. Call your veterinarian immediately if you suspect it, and he will treat the symptoms which he sees. He will administer one or more laxative substances to help move any remaining material out of the digestive tract. Good nursing and good luck may bring the animal through if he hasn't eaten too much.

BRACKEN FERN POISONING (Pteridium aquilinum)

Also called brake fern, bracken fern is found in woodland areas in much of the United States. Cases of poisoning are especially common in Oregon, Washington, and British Columbia. Bracken fern is a coarse perennial fern with fronds 3 to 6 feet in height. It thrives in either shade or sun, usually in sandy or gravelly soils. It is often one of the first plants to appear in burned-over or clear-cut forest areas. The poisoning is usually seen in the fall when the animal eats the fern because it is the only material which is still green.

All portions of the plant, whether green or dry, are poisonous to livestock. Animals accustomed to grazing fern-filled pastures rarely eat it. However, animals who are new to these pastures, or those driven to eat it because the grass is sparse may browse it freely. Feeding a horse hay containing 20% or more bracken fern will usually cause symptoms within a month. Horses bedded in poor hay containing the fern may eat enough of it to become poisoned.

The animal must eat the fern over a long period of time—as long as 30 to 60 days—before symptoms are seen. This is because it takes time for the plant to cause the thiamine deficiency and central nervous system disturbances which will cause clinical signs. For this reason, signs may be seen 2 to 6 weeks after the animal is removed from the pasture containing the fern. Because the poison is cumulative, animals who are getting even small

amounts in hay day after day may accumulate enough to cause illness or death. After eating the fern for some time, a horse may acquire a taste for it and continue to eat it even in the presence of adequate feed.

SIGNS

Horses usually develop bracken fern poisoning signs slowly, and the disease becomes chronic. Loss of weight and condition is often the first symptom noted. The animal then becomes unsteady when walking. He may be disinclined to move at all; when forced to walk, he shows incoordination. This progresses to swaying and staggering, leading to one of the names for the disease, the "fern staggers." He may stand with his legs apart as though bracing himself. In some cases, the horse may adopt a crouching stance with his back arched and legs apart. This is often accompanied by twitching muscles, which later become muscular tremors so severe that the animal is unable to remain standing. While the animal is down, he often makes violent attempts to get up, injuring himself in the process. Convulsions or spasms may be seen.

The animal may show rapid or difficult breathing. There may be marked depression. He may have general body weakness and a weak, fast pulse. The horse may push his head against stationary objects. Both temperature and appetite may remain normal until the disease is far advanced. Then, the temperature may be above or below normal. The animal may be anemic. If the disease is severe and untreated, death will occur several days to several weeks after symptoms are first seen.

TREATMENT

Recovery from bracken fern poisoning is often dramatic when horses are treated in all but the terminal stages. They respond to intramuscular or intravenous injections of thiamine hydrochloride at doses of 200 to 1000 mg. Marked improvement is seen within a day or two. Recovery is often complete within two to four days. Prevention depends on removing the horse from further access to the bracken fern.

NOTE: Several other species of fern are toxic to a greater or lesser extent, including some found in abundance in the eastern states. Not enough animals are poisoned to warrant taking the space to describe the symptoms, but you should be aware that bracken is not the only fern toxic to horses.

HORSETAIL (Equisetum species)

Also called mare's tail or scouring rush, horsetail causes symptoms similar to bracken fern. It is a common plant in bog areas and near streams. It grows throughout most of North America. All species of horsetail are poisonous. They can be recognized by their ridged, jointed stems. Horsetail may cause poisoning when meadow hay containing large amounts of it is cut and fed to horses. Animals poisoned by horsetail become quiet and comatose before death. Otherwise, signs and treatment are similar to those of bracken fern.

CASTOR BEAN POISONING (Ricinus communis)

The castor bean is the source of castor oil. The plant is also called castor oil plant and palma christi. It is grown as an ornamental plant throughout California and the southern tier of states. The toxin, called ricin, is a water soluble substance which causes severe irritation to the intestinal tract. Castor oil is not toxic because the toxin is not soluble in oil.

The seed is poisonous; the rest of the plant is relatively nontoxic. It should not be used as an ornamental plant around barns and corrals where animals will have access to it. Poisoning is usually not a problem except when new animals are brought into the area, or curious young animals nibble the beans.

All animals, including humans, are susceptible to poisoning by castor beans. Horses are the most susceptible. As little as 1/5 ounce (7 grams) of seeds have been reported to kill a horse. More commonly, it takes about 1-1/2 ounces (50 grams—about 150 beans) to kill a 1000 lb. horse. Poisoning may occur when feed grains become contaminated with castor-bean seeds.

Extreme irritation of the intestinal tract is seen with castor bean toxicity. Signs may not appear for several hours to as long as 2 to 3 days after the horse has eaten the beans. During this period, the animal appears completely normal. When signs do appear, they are acute and rapidly become worse. The animal is dopey and then becomes incoordinated. He will finally sweat profusely, and may show signs of shock.

There may be spasms in the neck and shoulder muscles. The heart beat may be so strong as to shake the whole body. The pulse is weak and rapid. The temperature may be elevated at first; occasional cases may go as high as 107 degrees F (41.5 C). The most characteristic sign is a profuse, watery diarrhea, usually without blood. Colicky pain may accompany the diarrhea, as evidenced by the animal grinding his teeth, humping his back, and kicking at his belly. The animal may progress into convulsions and finally die.

A high level of immunity to castor bean toxin can be built up in horses by an immunization process. Serum from such treated animals is an effective treatment for poisoned animals if given immediately or within a few hours after it has eaten a lethal dose of the seeds. Prompt veterinary treatment for the shock and allergic reaction may save some horses.

YEW POISONING (Taxus brevifolia)

The Western Yew is a small evergreen tree found in the Cascade Mountains and westward to the coast, as well as in other parts of the Pacific Northwest. Other Taxus species have also been found to be toxic.

Horses have been poisoned by consuming large amounts of twigs and fruits within a short time. As little as one mouthful can be toxic to a horse. Poisoning often occurs when horses have access to trimmings from these plants; it is very often seen in the spring and summer. Drying does not lessen the toxicity of the plant material. (88)

Death is very sudden, often occurring within five minutes after the horse has ingested the yew. The horse may be found dead without prior symptoms being noticed. The animal is often close to the yew, and may still have twigs or leaves in his mouth. Death in these cases is due to circulatory failure.

Animals who are less severely poisoned may show nervous signs before they die. These include difficulty in breathing, trembling, and collapse. Symptoms occur suddenly and the course is short. There is usually no time for treatment and no known antidote.

RED MAPLE LEAF POISONING

A severe, rapid hemolytic anemia may be seen in horses after they have eaten red maple leaves. Signs were seen in horses in Georgia 3 to 4 days after they had eaten wilted leaves from cut red maple (Acer rubrum) branches. The animals were weak and had rapid breathing and a rapid heart rate. The mucous membranes were yellow (icteric) or bluish (cyanotic). They were depressed. Both the blood and urine may show a brownish discoloration. The problem is often fatal. Toxicity may also be seen in horses who eat red maple bark. (89)

YELLOW STAR THISTLE POISONING AND RUSSIAN KNAPWEED POISONING

Commonly called "chewing disease," its technical name is nigropallidal encephalomalacia. This term refers to the softening of a particular part of the brain caused by the yellow star thistle, Centaurea solstitialis. This plant is a weed in California and other western states, usually in waste places and roadsides. It is a member of the sunflower family. It is an annual that grows 1 to 2½ feet high and has rigid, spreading stems which are branched from the base. The stems and leaves are whitened with a loose, cottony wool. Leaves around the base are 2 to 3 inches long and look somewhat like dandelion leaves. The flowers are bright yellow. Russian knapweed is a closely related species, causing the same problem, which may extend as far east as Colorado and Wyoming.

SIGNS

Horses must eat yellow star thistle over a 30 to 60 day period before signs will appear. Once signs have begun, most affected animals die. If the animal is only slightly affected, he may live with good nursing.

The disease appears suddenly. The first sign seen by the owner is usually difficulty in swallowing or chewing. The animal may spit food out. It may push its head into water, but be unable to drink. At this point, you should IMMEDIATELY call your veterinarian. With any brain/chewing problem, the possibility of rabies must be considered. Under no circumstances should you "reach into the animal's mouth to see what's stuck in his throat."

The tongue is not completely paralyzed, and the animal may move it in and out of his mouth. He will make characteristic chewing movements with no feed in the mouth. Or, he may chew with feed in the front part of his mouth and be unable to push it into the back. Twitching of the lips may be seen. The lips may be pulled back in a peculiar expression, and the mouth held halfway open. Spines from the plant may produce sores around the mouth; these may become infected, thus hindering eating and drinking.

The animal may be depressed, yawn frequently, and assume abnormal positions. Some horses may stand with their heads down in a vain attempt to get food. Often the disease will not progress any further than this stage, but the animal will become thin because he can neither eat nor drink. He will die of starvation or dehydration if not carefully nursed. Some animals may be depressed or dopey, but can be easily aroused. The gait is usually not affected, although some animals may appear slightly stiff or may wander aimlessly.

Animals with brain involvement will push against objects and show incoordination. They may fall down and show convulsive seizures. This is not common. Most cases show the paralysis in the throat and starvation. Because this disease softens the part of the brain involved in eating, there is no chance that the animal will recover; the damage is permanent and irreversible. Experimental animals have been fed via stomach tube and observed for long periods of time to see if they would recover the ability to swallow. Recovery does not occur. Euthanasia is the best course once the diagnosis is confirmed.

LUPINE POISONING

Lupines are a large genus of plants which usually have blue, purple, pinkish, or white flowers. All have pea-like flowers in bunches toward the top of a straight, upright stalk. They often grow along roadsides and in waste places. They range from sea beaches and prairie grassland to high mountain pastures, and from desert areas to moist meadows. Many species of lupine are nontoxic. Horses have an equally difficult time telling them apart. It is difficult for even a trained botanist to distinguish between harmful and harmless species.

Harmful lupines are poisonous throughout the year. Young plants and plants in the seed stage are most toxic. In the summer, these may be the only green plants available in a pasture. Poisonings which occur in the fall and winter are due to mature pods. Lupines may cause illness and death when the dried plants occur in hay. Dangerous concentrations of lupine seed may occur when infested grain fields are harvested. Lupine poison is not cumulative. Animals eating small amounts of it day after day will not be harmed. A lethal dose must be eaten within a short period of time to cause death.

The animal will have gastrointestinal irritation with diarrhea. The hair coat may be rough and dry. He may have a peculiar gait, lifting his feet higher than normal. He may be reluctant to move about and show twitching leg muscles and nervousness. The animal may be depressed and weak. This may progress to loss of all muscular control, prostration, convulsions, and coma. Chronic lupine poisoning produces a toxic hepatitis (liver problem). No treatment is known to be of value in lupine poisoning.

LOCOWEED POISONING

Found mostly in the western states, "locoweeds" belong to the genera Astraglus and Oxytropis. The name "locoweeds" comes from the Spanish word for crazy, and is used because of the peculiar actions of animals affected by them. Not all plants which are called locoweeds are poisonous. There are over 300 species of plants in these two genera, and only about 20 are poisonous. As with the lupines, it is often difficult to tell the good guys from the bad guys, even for an expert botanist.

Locoweeds range from low-growing plants two or three inches high to beautiful clumps of flowers two feet tall. These vary in color from cream or yellow to blue and purple. They are commonly found on foothills and plains and semiarid desert regions. They range from Canada to Mexico, from the Rocky Mountain states westward. The plants are poisonous at all stages of growth and throughout the year, even when matured and dried. All parts are toxic.

SIGNS

Horses must graze locoweed for a period of time before symptoms will be seen. Death in horses is said to occur after a horse has ingested about 30 percent of his weight over a period of six weeks. The most severe signs may not be seen until after the horse has stopped eating the plant.

Animals affected by locoweeds have an abnormal gait, and may wander in circles or straight lines. They may go into convulsions and throw themselves to the ground.

Mental attitudes range from dull or depressed to excited and frantic. Loco'ed horses may stay apart from others, and may carry the head in a peculiar attitude. The attitude of the head may be due to visual disturbances. Some horses' perception is apparently so altered that they run into objects or over cliffs.

The horse may be listless and not notice ordinary activities, and then become nervous, upset, and wild when stimulated by a sudden event. The animal may refuse to eat or drink and may be constipated. He may show an irregular gait or loss of muscle control, and may circle, stagger, or make exaggerated and abnormal leg movements. The incoordination usually increases with time. The animal may attempt to rear and fall to a sitting position instead. Horses in the early stages of loco poisoning are hazardous to ride or drive. The hair coat is often dull and dry. Loco'ed horses may bump into objects or press the head against objects for varying periods of time.

In chronic cases, the animal may become gradually more paralyzed until he has trouble eating. If the animal is excited, he may die from convulsions. Under pasture conditions, the animal may lose condition slowly, until he literally starves to death.

The toxic principle of locoweed is an alkaloid. It appears to be cumulative, with each day's grazing adding more until typical symptoms appear and the animal finally dies. Signs of poisoning appear after two to three weeks of continuous grazing. There is no effective treatment.

Animals who do not die usually have enough brain damage that they are never completely normal. They may have weird mental quirks, such as crashing over backwards from time to time, which make them dangerous and unpredictable to ride and handle.

By the time signs of locoweed poisoning appear, these animals are usually addicted to the plant. Allowed to graze on their own, they will seek out locoweeds and continue to eat them, often to the exclusion of good feedstuffs. Sometimes the appetite is transferred from one species of loco to another. The addicted horses may become thin and poor because of their insatiable urge to search out and eat these particular plants. This urge may be strong enough that if they can find a large enough number of plants, they will eventually die.

If the animal is confined and fed hay or moved to a range free of locoweeds, he may have a slow but uneventful recovery, if his symptoms have not progressed too far. In general, most loco'ed animals are at best only good for breeding. Incidentally, bees have been poisoned after "working" the flowers of one particular species of locoweed in Nevada.

TIMBER MILK VETCH POISONING

Timber milk vetch is a plant (or group of plants) which also belongs to the genus Astraglus (as do the locoweeds, above). It causes a disease in horses which is different from either locoweed poisoning or selenium poisoning, which can also be caused by some plants of the genus Astraglus.

Symptoms occur much more quickly than either locoweed poisoning or selenium poisoning—in 2 to 7 days rather than several weeks or months. When excited, an apparently normal animal quickly develops a roaring sound when he breathes out. He shows staggering and salivation. Sudden death from asphyxiation may occur.

SELENIUM POISONING

Various Astraglus species ("locoweeds") as well as other species of plants are involved in another type of poisoning, selenium toxicity. Some plants, called "selenium indicator plants," require large amounts of selenium for their metabolism. They pick it up from certain soils where it occurs in large quantities and concentrate it in their tissues. In addition to Astraglus species, other plants have been incriminated in selenium poisoning. One is "prince's plume" (Stanleya species); another is woody aster (Xylorrhiza species); "golden weeds" (Oonopsis species) also cause selenium toxicity.

When these plants are seen, they indicate that there is a large quantity of selenium in the soil. Selenium may constitute as much as 2% of the soil in some western states. It is soluble only under alkaline conditions. Selenium concentrations in plants have been reported approaching 15,000 ppm. (parts per million). As little as 5 ppm. may be toxic when consumed by the animal.

The horse is perhaps more affected by selenium poisoning than are other animals. If the animal then eats these plants, he is likely to come down with a case of selenium poisoning.

ACUTE SELENIUM POISONING

Consumption of large amounts of these plants over a short period of time will cause signs of acute poisoning. Animals will not eat these massive quantities at one time unless driven to it. Symptoms appear within one to two days.

The animal will be depressed and stop eating. The pulse is rapid and weak, and may sometimes be undetectable. He may pass more urine than normal. The brain is affected. There may be a dark diarrhea, and the animal may have an elevated temperature. Coma and death due to heart failure follow. The animals die within a few hours to a few days from the onset of symptoms.

CHRONIC SELENIUM TOXICITY (ALKALI DISEASE)

Some other species of plants are called secondary selenium absorbers. They do not require selenium in order to grow, but if they grow on soil containing this mineral, they will accumulate it in their tissues. Many common forage plants and grains are in this category, including oats, barley, corn, grass, and wheat. These plants can be eaten over a week to a month or more before symptoms appear. This problem is often seen in poor, wasteland pastures which have large quantities of alkali in the soil, thus the name, "alkali disease."

Alkali disease is characterized by the loss of hair and hooves. The mane and tail are often shed first. The animal will have a poor hair coat and may become emaciated. He may appear mentally dull, and may also be anemic. There may be lameness and a peculiar gait.

Hoof involvement usually indicates a greater consumption of the offending plants, or perhaps a greater sensitivity of the affected animal to excess selenium. Hooves which are affected often develop a crack around the top of the hoof wall, resulting in a separation between old and new hoof material. The process is very painful, and the old hoof tissue does not receive normal wear. Because of this, the hooves become severely deformed and bent forward with the lameness getting worse. The process may occur repeatedly. The animal may be in such severe pain that he grazes from a kneeling position; these horses often die of starvation or from lack of water. All four feet are usually equally affected. In severe cases, the hooves may completely fall off without adequate new hoof growth to cover the underlying tissues. It may be necessary to euthanize the animal (for humane reasons).

The only treatment is to remove the animal from access to selenium-bearing plants. The symptoms are treated as well as possible. In mild cases, good feed and nursing as well as giving the affected hooves whatever protection is possible, may lead to recovery. A high protein ration may help to lessen the effects of the disease.

NICOTINE POISONING

Many plants in the potato family (Solanaceae) are potentially poisonous; nicotine and its related compounds are toxic to horses. This alkaloid is found in various species of the wild tobaccos (genus Nicotiana). These plants grow throughout the western states and Hawaii, often in desert and waste areas. As with many other poisonous plants, horses will generally not eat them if desirable forage is available. Horses are reported to have been poisoned from eating leaves of harvested, domestic tobacco when stabled overnight in a tobacco barn.

Some of the earliest signs of nicotine poisoning are due to stimulation of the autonomic nervous system. The horse shakes, shivers, and may show muscle twitching, especially around the neck and shoulders. This is followed by staggering, weakness, and eventual prostration and paralysis. The heart may beat violently, but the pulse is weak and fast. Body temperature may be above normal, but the extremities are cold. Signs of colic, with or without diarrhea, may be seen. Breathing may be labored.

Large doses of nicotine produce rapid onset of symptoms often within 15 minutes. Smaller doses may not show signs for several hours. Death may occur a few minutes after the first signs are seen; in other cases, the animal may live for several days before dying. Most cases are seen in the paralytic stage if the owner even notices the illness before death occurs. There is no treatment for the poisoning.

CIRRHOSIS OF THE LIVER

Three unrelated groups of poisonous plants cause similar problems in the horse due to toxins which produce cirrhosis of the liver. The clinical signs of these problems are due to the liver damage. Most of these plants are unpalatable and are only eaten when other pasture plants are not available, or if they are included in baled hay or pellets. The plants grow in winter and early spring and are more common in first cutting hay.

Horses must eat the contaminated feed for a period of time before enough liver damage occurs to cause signs. For this reason, cases are often seen in late summer to early winter months. By the time damage is seen in the horse, none of the contaminated hay may be left to aid in diagnosis of the problem.

Amsinckia species, such as fiddleneck, tarweed, fireweed, yellow burr weed, and buckthorn, are involved in producing liver cirrhosis. These plants are common in the western United States, and are often found as a weed of wheat and other grain crops. They grow in semiarid lands of Washington, Idaho, Oregon, and California. The seeds are the most toxic part of the plant. Poisoning occurs when contaminated grain is threshed and fed to animals. In past years, cases were seen in early spring after horses were fed wheat straw or pastured on wheat stubble through the winter.

Senecio species are also involved in causing cirrhosis of the liver. This is one of the largest genera in the plant kingdom. Not all species of Senecio are poisonous, nor do all contain enough of the alkaloids to cause problems. One species which has been proven to be toxic is Senecio jacobaea; many others have been incriminated. Some of their common names include ragwort, groundsel, and "stinking willie." They are found over most of the midwest and western states. Senecio species are the cause of a problem called "Walking Disease" in Nebraska. Other common names are "Hard Liver Disease" and "Walla Walla Walking Disease" in the Pacific Northwest.

Crotalaria species are more common in the southeastern states. Two species known to be toxic to the liver are Crotalaria spectabilis and Crotalaria sagittalis. Common names include rattle weed, rattle box, and wild pea. They belong to the pea family. Crotalaria is used as a cover crop to improve soil in the southern states as far west as Texas. It may cause severe loss in horses. (90)

SIGNS

Liver cirrhosis causes hardening and inactivity of the liver. This results in disturbances of the central nervous system (because the liver is now unable to filter out toxic wastes). Symptoms may occur abruptly. Signs include aimless walking—about 80% of the horses which are affected will travel in a straight line for miles, often through fences and into obstructions. The animal will not walk around a building, and may press its head against a barn or other solid object, often becoming frenzied. In many instances, death occurs when the animal becomes tangled in a fence or walks over the edge of a ravine.

The horse may become reckless and charge, or appear delirious. They often walk in circles and may drag the rear legs or show a staggering gait or incoordination. This gives the disease one of its common names, the "sleepy staggers." The horse may hang its head and act sleepy or sluggish and depressed.

Some cases may have severe intestinal irritation, resulting in straining, diarrhea, and occasional rectal prolapse. There may be signs of colic. Small ulcers may develop on the mucous membranes of the mouth, often accompanied by an offensive odor.

The animal may show icterus (yellow membranes around the eyes and in the mouth). This may disappear in terminal stages of the disease when it is replaced by an anemia. The disease is usually chronic. The animal will look poor and thin and will have a rough coat. Once enough liver damage has occurred, the animal becomes weak and dies. The temperature is usually normal throughout the disease. As with any other disease involving brain problems, your veterinarian should be called IMMEDIATELY, because of the possibility that it might be rabies or a contagious encephalitis, such as VEE.

Treatment is of little value because cirrhosis of the liver is an irreversible type of damage. The only solution to the problem is to prevent it by eliminating access to Amsinckia screenings in grain or to Crotalaria or Senecio plants in hay or pasture.

GROUND IVY

Also called Creeping Charlie (Glechoma hederaceae), this is a low, creeping weed plant which exists throughout much of the world. If eaten in large quantity, it is poisonous to horses. Either fresh or cured in hay, it causes problems.

Animals poisoned by ground ivy froth at the mouth and show difficulty in breathing. There is extreme sweating. Severe cases may result in death.

POISON HEMLOCK (Cicuta species)

This range plant may kill horses who eat only a small amount of it. It is poisonous to sheep and cattle as are many of the other plants discussed here, and EXTREMELY toxic to humans. It grows 4 to 10 feet high, and may be confused with western water hemlock—a plant with a similar name that is even more deadly. Poison hemlock is also known as poison parsley, deadly hemlock, spotted hemlock, European hemlock, and Nebraska or California fern.

All parts of the plant are poisonous; the leaves are especially poisonous in the spring up to the time the plant flowers. Four or five pounds of fresh leaves have killed horses. (91)

Poison hemlock is found at roadsides, in creekbeds and irrigation ditches, on the edges of cultivated fields, and in waste areas. Poisoning may occur when humans confuse hemlock root with wild parsnips, or hemlock seed with anise. Whistles made from hollow stems of poison hemlock have caused death in children. Drying seems to neutralize the toxin; the plant is not a problem in hay.

Signs of poison hemlock toxicity occur within a few hours after the horse has eaten the plant. Some horses may collapse without any signs of the approaching problem; they will appear unaware of their surroundings. Animals poisoned by hemlock may show nervous trembling, salivation, lack of coordination (especially in the hindlimbs), and dilation of the pupils. The pulse is slow and weak and the membranes of the mouth may be bluish in color.

The animal may live several hours to a few days before death occurs, but he will probably be comatose much of the time. Severely affected animals usually die within 5 to 10 hours after onset of signs. Death follows respiratory paralysis and coma.

Stimulants and large amounts of mineral oil given via stomach tube may save animals which have not eaten an excessive amount of hemlock. Now the good news: animals who do recover rarely show any ill effects.

WESTERN WATER HEMLOCK

This is considered to be one of the most poisonous plants growing in the United States. It has many local common names, among which are poison parsnip, snakeroot, false parsley, and a dozen or so others. It may be confused with poison hemlock because of the similarity in names and the general appearance of the plants although western water hemlock only reaches a height of 2 to 3 feet, as compared to 4 to 10 feet for poison hemlock. Western water hemlock is a wetland plant and is commonly found in wet meadows and pastures and along banks of streams.

Only a small amount of the toxic alcohol contained in the water hemlock is needed to poison livestock or humans. Animals seldom eat western water hemlock if good forage is available. Most losses occur in early spring or after plants have been sprayed with 2,4-D, which increases their palatability. Underground portions of the plant, especially the tuberous roots, are very dangerous. Leaves and stems lose most of their toxicity with maturity.

Horses usually show signs of poisoning 15 minutes to 6 hours after eating the plant, and may die within an hour or so after symptoms appear. Excessive salivation is usually the first sign, with frothing at the mouth. There may be muscle twitching, tremors, and convulsions. The convulsions may be extremely violent, with the head and neck thrown rigidly back, the legs flexed as though running, and with chewing motions and grinding of the teeth.

Abdominal pain is usually present. There will be a rapid pulse, rapid breathing, and dilation of the pupils. The temperature may be several degrees above normal. Coma and death follow. There is no known treatment for western water hemlock poisoning. The toxin acts so rapidly that the affected animal can rarely be saved. If the affected horse lives five or six hours after symptoms are first seen, chances are good that he will survive.

FORAGE POISONING

Also called cornstalk disease and moldy corn poisoning, forage poisoning was first noticed when a large number of horse deaths were reported in the central plains states in the winter of 1934–35. It was estimated that more than 5000 horses were lost in Illinois alone. Most of the horses had been fed damaged corn or cornstalks. It was associated with a dry summer followed by an unusually wet fall.

Symptoms look exactly like virus encephalitis. However, when samples are taken from the brain of an animal who has died of forage poisoning, it can be clearly distinguished from sleeping sickness. Prevent forage poisoning by not feeding molded corn, and by not grazing horses in stalk fields where weather conditions may have caused the feed to mold.

LARKSPUR (Delphinium Species)

In the western United States, larkspur is second only to the locoweeds as a cause of livestock losses. It accounts for the death of many cattle each year, and occasionally causes losses in sheep. Under natural conditions, horses will eat larkspur, but will stop before they have eaten enough to kill themselves. Garden delphiniums belong to the same genus and should be considered poisonous.

MARIJUANA (Cannabis)

Marijuana is bitter and unpalatable and is rarely consumed by animals. Kingsbury reports the loss of several horses and mules in Greece caused by eating illegally grown marijuana. Shortly after eating it, they showed excitation, difficulty in breathing, and muscular trembling. They sweated and salivated profusely, although their body temperatures were below normal. Death occurred in all

affected animals within 15 to 30 minutes of ingestion. Keep your horse out of the pot patch! Also, be aware that hemp (marijuana) grows wild, particularly in the midwest where it was cultivated up to the Second World War as a source of fiber for rope-making.

SORGHUM AND SUDAN GRASS TOXICITY

Both sorghum and sudan grass show two distinct types of poisoning. The first is prussic acid (cyanide) poisoning. This toxin may form in the new growth after a frost or rapid growth or trampling. Cyanide poisoning is very rapid. Often the first sign is a horse who is seen dead or dying. Abnormal breathing may be noticed, along with trembling, nervousness, and muscle spasms or convulsions. These signs are followed by respiratory failure and death. Animals in the pasture who are not affected may be saved by prompt removal from the offending forage. Some species of sorghum have been bred especially for low cyanide-producing potential.

The second syndrome which is associated with sorghum and sudan grass is a problem with the urinary bladder. The animal will dribble urine constantly. Bladder infections may occur, and the urine may be very thick and viscous. Urine which has run down the animal's hind legs may cause hair loss. Most horses will show a characteristic incoordination when trotted, backed, or turned. Mares may appear to be constantly in heat. Mares who are pregnant may abort or give birth to deformed foals.

Death is often caused by the infection traveling up the urinary tract into the kidneys. This problem is progressive until the animal either dies or is euthanized because of its lack of recovery. It is not seen with hay made from these plants. However, caution should be observed when using sorghum or sudan grass hybrids as horse pasture. Johnson grass is a related plant which has caused similar problems.

BERMUDA GRASS TREMORS

Ergot is a fungus which grows on certain grasses and grains when the weather conditions are right. It appears as small brownish or black nodules which replace a few seeds in the seed head. It is very often seen on rye, and may be found on Bermuda grass or Dallis grass. When eaten by an animal, it causes a problem known as Bermuda Grass Tremors or Dallis Grass Shakes. This problem is more common in late summer, fall, and winter.

The affected horse may first be seen to have muscle tremors, incoordination, and varying degrees of excitement. The animal may hang its head or show peculiar head movements, tremors, and tongue lolling. Paralysis may follow.

The symptoms may continue for days or weeks after the animal is removed from the affected hay or pasture. The recovery is usually more rapid than that of cattle.

Some horses may recover overnight without treatment, while others may be intermittently affected for several days. Abortion may occur in pregnant mares who eat feed with ergot on it.

CHOKECHERRY POISONING (Prunus species)

Chokecherry is a bush which may be six to twelve feet high. It grows throughout most of the United States, often in creek bottoms and along roadsides. The berries which ripen in late summer and early fall can be made into a delicious jelly. However, the plant's leaves contain cyanide-producing materials. They are more toxic under abnormal conditions, such as when they have been wilted, frozen, stunted, or affected by drought.

Death can occur within minutes to hours after the horse has eaten the leaves. The animal appears to have trouble breathing and will have flared nostrils. The tail may be lifted, and the horse may urinate or have bowel movements, seemingly without control. He may be incoordinated and trembling, with muscular contractions and signs of agitation. The animal eventually falls to the ground and kicks its legs for a few minutes before it dies. If treatment is undertaken rapidly, some animals may be saved; however, most die so rapidly that they are dead by the time help arrives.

MISCELLANEOUS POISONOUS PLANTS

It is impossible to list all plants which have ever killed horses in a book this size—suffice it to say that many plants are toxic to certain animals at certain stages in their growth, or under certain conditions. This includes many of the domesticated plants which we take for granted. Common garden flowers, such as the iris and foxglove, may be toxic.

Horses have been poisoned by eating the bark of black locust posts or trees to which they were tied; horses are very susceptible to the toxin which is involved. They become severely ill within a few hours, showing lack of appetite, depression, and weakness. Later, paralysis occurs. Mild colic may be seen. Animals may die if they have eaten enough locust material. Others may recover after several days to several weeks.

Horses have died from eating acorns or oak leaves. A bush called whitebrush in Texas, Arizona, and Mexico causes lack of stamina, emaciation, lameness, or incoordination. Affected animals may sweat profusely and later become paralyzed, prostrate, dying about a week after the first symptoms have appeared.

Wild jasmine grows in waste places in Florida and Texas. It causes an imbalance in the calcium and vitamin D ratio within the body, leading to weight loss, lameness, and a short, choppy gait. The animal may appear humped up. The disease may regress if the horse is moved to a clean pasture and given good care.

Hay made from overripe crimson clover may cause death from impaction in horses. The fibers around the flower and seed form dense balls in the intestine.

Alsike clover may cause a poisoning in horses called dew poisoning. These animals will have sores which cover the muzzle; they may extend into the mouth, causing shallow ulcers of the gums and tongue. The animal may become markedly depressed or excited, and some may show corneal opacities. The animal may refuse to eat and become emaciated. The combination of liver problems and brain involvement is called hepatoencephalopathy. No treatment is effective for this disease. (92)

Death camas is found in plains and foothills areas from the Mississippi to the Rocky Mountains. The plant is normally unpalatable to horses, but poisoning may occur in the early spring when it is one of the few green plants available. Small amounts may cause death. Signs begin within a few hours after the horse has eaten the plant, although death may not occur for several days. The horse will salivate profusely and show depression and staggering. Prompt veterinary treatment may save some affected animals.

Horses have been poisoned by eating large quantities of fallen apples when they are turned into an orchard in the fall. Large quantities of onions, chives, or wild onions may cause toxicity.

PLANTS CAUSING MECHANICAL INJURY

Nontoxic plants may cause mechanical injury to an animal, resulting in illness and possibly death. Long-bearded grasses and spiny-surfaced plants can injure the muzzle and lips, eyes, and nostrils. The sores which result may make it impossible for the animal to eat, causing loss of weight and even starvation. If the sores become infected, loss of sight or loss of life may result.

Grass awns or the beards from small grains, such as barley, may become imbedded in the animal's mouth, causing sores and considerable pain and discomfort. A weed grass often found in hay, called foxtail, is one of the worst offenders. This grass can also cause problems if animals are grazed on pasture containing a large amount of mature foxtail and not enough good forage. Whether in hay or on pasture, foxtail awns cause tremendous, painful damage to a horse's mouth.

Cheat grass (Bromus tectorum, also called downy chess, downy brome, or June grass) is common across many parts of the United States, growing in neglected fields and waste places. This plant may cause problems when it is either baled and fed in hay or is grazed after it has dried. While in the green state, both foxtail and cheat grass are good and nutritious feed. They're definitely not desirable after they have dried, but may be used up to that point as pasture.

Yellow Bristle Grass (Setaria glauca, S. lutescens) is another grass which causes ulcers in the horse's mouth. It has short, sharp awns which embed themselves in the gums, tongue, and lips, causing irritation and ulcer formation.

Often the first clue to this problem is that the horse is getting thin. He is then noticed to be reluctant to eat and may dribble feed from his mouth. Lift the animal's lips and examine his mouth carefully. You will see masses of awns imbedded in sores in the cheeks, gums, and under the base of the tongue. There may also be sores on the surface of the tongue.

Remove as much of the offending material as you can, using tweezers or small pliers. If the animal is not cooperative, you may have to have your veterinarian sedate him in order to clean out his mouth. Rinse him out with a mouth wash as follows: have your druggist make up a quart or two of a 1:4000 solution of potassium permanganate. After you have cleaned as much of the offending material out of the animals's mouth as possible, rinse it with the mouth wash, using a large syringe or dose syringe.

Often all that is necessary to effect healing of damage from grass awns is to remove the offending material; when this is done, the sores heal rapidly. If the sores are badly infected, it may be necessary to help healing along by giving penicillin/streptomycin for three days. Animals with severe ulcers are especially helped by the mouthwash described above.

Change the animal immediately to a good quality feed without awns or beards in it. This will allow the animal to heal without further insult. If the problem occurred on pasture, keep the animal in and feed a good grade hay. Or put him on another pasture with something to eat besides foxtail or other offending feedstuff. If the animal is put back on the feed which caused the problem, it will only occur again, and the animal will continue to get thinner and thinner. You also risk getting a serious infection started because of the open, raw wounds in the mouth.

Chapter 21

MISCELLANEOUS CONDITIONS

Equine Infectious Anemia (Swamp Fever)
Nervous System Diseases
   Eastern Equine Encephalomyelitis
   Western Equine Encephalomyelitis
   Venezuelan Equine Encephalomyelitis
   Rabies
Botulism
Kidney and Bladder Problems
Heart Problems
Anhidrosis
Heat Exhaustion
Other Heat Problems
Cold Problems
Exhaustion
Emergencies
   Fractures
   Certain Wire Cuts
   Eye Injuries
   Shock
   Foaling
   Uterine Problems
   Burns and Smoke Inhalation
   Severe Colic or Founder
   Deep Puncture Wounds to The Chest or Abdomen
Euthanasia
   Chemical Methods
   How to Shoot a Horse
   Other Methods of Emergency Euthanasia
Necropsy
Letter to a Girl on the Death of Her Horse

Several virus diseases are discussed in other parts of this book, in sections relating to the specific areas where they cause problems. For example, warts and vesicular stomatitis are covered under skin problems. Rabies and sleeping sickness (encephalitis) will be discussed in this section. Another major disease which is caused by a virus is equine infectious anemia.

EQUINE INFECTIOUS ANEMIA (SWAMP FEVER, EIA)

This disease was reported in Europe in 1843 and was recognized not long after that in the United States. It currently affects about ½ of 1% of the horses in this country. The virus which causes the disease affects only horses, mules, and donkeys. It is not contagious to humans. It may persist in the blood of an infected animal for years. It may then be spread from the infected animal by secretions, such as milk and semen. It is also spread mechanically by the bites of horse flies (most common), stable flies, certain mosquitoes, and biting lice. It may be spread by using the same needle to vaccinate or treat more than one horse, as well as by worming equipment, dental floats, bits, and any other mechanical means that can transfer blood from one horse to another. This can occur at a race track or breeding farm. It can occur when equipment is loaned to someone else; do not borrow or lend equipment which may be contaminated with another horse's blood or saliva.

Normally, the disease will spread slowly within a group. Occasionally, it spreads rapidly as with the use of a common needle as mentioned above. The virus can persist for up to 96 hours on twitches, bits, and other objects which have become contaminated with blood from an infected horse. (93) It may also spread rapidly when a carrier animal is attacked by large numbers of insects who then carry their virus burden to other horses and inject it into susceptible animals via their bites.

Horse flies are thought to be especially important in spreading swamp fever. An outbreak suspected to be due to them occurred near Yellowstone National Park some years ago. Several horses at one camp of a wilderness outfitter came down with swamp fever. Checking the rest of the animals at this camp revealed others to be infected with EIA. The incubation period is usually around 14 days, although it may vary from a few days to three months or longer.

SIGNS

Swamp fever may occur as an acute, rapidly fatal disease, showing a sudden onset. The temperature rises to 105 to 108 degrees F (40.5 to 42 degrees C). The animal may have either a high, continuous fever, or a series of frequent, intermittent attacks. These may rapidly terminate in death. More often, however, the attacks decrease in frequency and intensity leaving the animal with a chronic case of the disease. A chronic carrier who shows no signs may have an acute relapse with stress and then the clinical fever will become evident.

In addition to the fever, the animal may have little or no appetite. He will usually have a rapid pulse. He may be very depressed. The horse may be incoordinated, weak in the hindquarters, and may frequently shift weight from one leg to another. He will urinate more often than usual. The conjunctiva may be reddened and/or yellowish. There may be small hemorrhages on the gums, under the tongue, and visible inside the nostrils. Laboratory examination will show a decrease in the number of red blood cells. A Coggins test will often be negative because the animal has not yet had time to develop antibodies against EIA upon which the test is based. In some horses, staggering and incoordination may be the only signs noticed.

The initial attack (in the animal who lives through it) usually lasts three to five days. At this time, the animal returns to normal. His temperature and red blood cell count return to normal, and he looks normal except for weight loss. In some animals, the initial attack will persist until the animal dies.

Subacute and chronic cases do not have as high a fever, and the intervals between attacks are longer. The attacks may become less frequent, with the animal becoming a recovered carrier. Or, they may end in death in one of the later attacks. If the disease becomes chronic, the animal usually looks very poor. He tends to be depressed and may appear weak. He may become emaciated and may show edema (filling with fluid) in the legs, underbelly, and sheath.

As the disease progresses, signs of anemia develop. The red blood cell count will be extremely low and the blood will appear thin and watery. The gums will appear pale. The pulse may be slow and weak. A pulse may be noticed in the jugular vein (in the groove in the lower third of the horse's neck). The heartbeat may be irregular.

Animals who survive the initial attack may have another bout or two of fever and then become inapparent carriers. Their temperatures are normal, and their blood count is normal. There may be no sign of infection for years, but they remain sources of infectious virus which may be carried to other animals. Hard work, stress, or another disease may cause EIA to become active. Or, they may recover completely, but still react to the Coggins test.

TREATMENT

As with other virus diseases, no specific cure for EIA is known at the present time. Treatment is not attempted because it is likely to result in an infected carrier who will be a source of the disease for the rest of his life. Other horses in the group should be tested with the Coggins test, and reactor animals sent to slaughter. Attempts to develop a vaccine against EIA have been unsuccessful to date.

Foals who are born to clinically ill mares are frequently infected, either in utero or through the colostrum. These foals should be isolated from other horses for at least six months. This will allow them to lose any antibodies which have been passed to them in the mother's milk. At this time, they can be tested to determine whether they are infected or free of the disease. It is recommended that infected horses not be used for breeding because of the possibility that they will infect the foal and that the foal will then be bitten by insects who will spread the disease to other horses.

THE COGGINS TEST

The Coggins test is required to move horses into most states, to racetracks, shows, and sales. If you are showing a horse or horses, it is easiest to keep their tests current. This will mean having them tested every six months to a year, depending on where you are taking them. Specific shows or sales may require a more current test—say within the last 15 or 30 days. This testing must be done by a veterinarian. He will draw a sample of blood from each animal, labeling it separately. He also has some rather long Federal forms which must be filled out. He will then submit the blood samples to a government-approved laboratory for testing.

The test itself takes as long as three days to incubate, and transportation each way takes another couple of days to several weeks or more, depending on the mail service. Plan accordingly when you need to move horses across state lines. Occasionally, if you must move an animal under emergency situations (such as taking him across state lines to a veterinary facility for treatment), the state veterinarian of the admitting state will issue a permit for the animal to be moved and tested upon his arrival in the recipient state. This is not guaranteed, and the permit may be very difficult to obtain after normal business hours or on weekends or holidays.

How accurate is the Coggins test? Its negatives are reliable. If the test says that the horse does not have the disease, chances are very good that he does not. The problem comes with the positives. One has no way of knowing whether the animal is a recovered carrier who may be infectious to other equines, or an animal who has recovered completely and has an immunity against the disease. A small percentage of the positives are probably completely false—due to other antibodies present in the serum or other factors. About 90% of the horses who have a positive Coggins test do not show any signs of the disease, even when kept under prolonged quarantine.

Herein lies the difficulty; what do you do with a positive animal? The government programs were originally designed to eliminate dangerously ill horses who might spread the disease to other equines. Most states currently require either immediate slaughter or lifetime quarantine; the animal may have to be kept in a screened, insect-free barn, or kept a specified distance from other equines. Reactors are generally freeze branded on the left jaw or left side of the neck. The brand consists of two numbers denoting the state followed by the letter "A." For instance, "86A" is used on a reactor in Arizona. Cheap horses are sent directly to a packing house. Which is fine (and eminently sensible) if you have a horse of low value, such as the pack horses mentioned near Yellowstone. You will get nearly as much for them as canners as they are worth otherwise, and you can be sure that there will be no infection carried from these animals to other horses. This was a definite consideration in the above case; the owner was a horse supplier who had a herd of over 700 horses. He could not afford to have EIA established in his herd.

If you have one single, very expensive animal who is not showing and has not shown any clinical signs of EIA, then you have to make a decision as to whether the precautions to prevent possible spread are worth the bother or not. You also have to decide whether you wish to keep the animal in confinement in a screened, insect-free facility for the rest of his life, which is basically what is required. If your horse is separated from all other equines by 200 yards or more, it may not be necessary to keep the horse in a screened area. The horse owner who has a positive animal must take responsibility for possibly spreading the disease to other equines. This is an ethical responsibility in addition to the legal requirements of state and Federal government.

It is worth having any horse that you are considering purchasing checked for EIA. Because it is not a common problem, this author would not hesitate to buy a horse and take it home pending the results of a Coggins test, but with the understanding (or contractual agreement) that the animal can be returned for full refund if the test should prove positive.

Horses who have been in contact with a horse who is positive should be tested immediately. Any who are found to be positive should be removed from the herd. Those who are negative should be retested about 28 days later, and again in four to six months. This gives them time to build antibodies against EIA, or to begin to develop the disease if they are going to. At this time, those who again test negative can be considered to be free of the disease. (94) For additional information on EIA, see DVM Newsmagazine, Feb. 1980, p. 46–51, and Journal of Equine Medicine and Surgery, Nov. 1978. See also JAVMA Vol. 184, No. 3, 1 February 1984, p. 279–301.

NERVOUS SYSTEM DISEASES

Several diseases afflict the horse's nervous system. The most common of these are eastern and western encephalomyelitis. Venezuelan equine encephalomyelitis is a related disease which appeared in 1971 in Texas, but is currently not found in the United States. However, it could reappear from Mexico or Central America at any time. For that reason, it will be discussed, as well as for the reason that several states require vaccination against it. The other, fortunately uncommon, disease which affects the nervous system is rabies.

EASTERN EQUINE ENCEPHALOMYELITIS (EEE)

Eastern Equine Encephalomyelitis is also called sleeping sickness, blind staggers, eastern encephalitis, or eastern viral encephalitis. It was described as early as 1831 in Massachusetts. EEE most commonly occurs in pastured animals in the summer. The virus does not occur only in the eastern states, although it is more common there. It is also reported in Mexico, Canada, Central and South America, and in the southwestern U.S.

The spread of the disease is not well understood. It is thought to involve mosquitoes and birds. The virus is thought to stay alive in certain mosquitoes. In some years, it enters the bird population and is spread from the birds by other mosquitoes, which then carry the disease to horses and man. Both man and the horse are considered to be dead-end hosts. This means that when either species is infected by the disease, there is not enough virus produced in the body to be spread to other humans or horses, either in bodily secretions or by blood-sucking insects.

SIGNS

The most obvious early signs of EEE are severe depression and a high fever—up to 105 degrees F (40.5 degrees C). The horse will stop eating and will usually show little or no response when touched. The lower lip may droop and the eyeballs may roll from side to side without control. The animal will be very incoordinated, especially when turned. In later stages of the disease, animals may act quite peculiar, doing things like trying to walk through the side of a building, climbing to the top of a woodpile, or knocking down fences or walls. Once the animal is lying down and unable to rise, it may dig a hole in the ground because of the nonstop running movement of the front legs. The disease usually does not last more than two to three days before the animal dies.

Diagnosis is confirmed by laboratory testing. Your veterinarian will draw a blood sample and send it in for analysis. Two samples are needed, taken a few days to several weeks apart, if the animal lives that long.

PROGNOSIS

The prognosis with EEE is extremely poor, as over 90% of clinically recognized cases die. In those who survive, there is often permanent brain damage. The damage may include vision problems and behavioral or learning problems. The horse may be a "dummy" for the rest of his life. Occasional animals will make a complete recovery.

TREATMENT

As with other viral diseases, no specific treatment works. Nursing, combined with the animal's strength and bodily defenses, will help make the difference between the animal's living and dying. The best of care may not save the animal, but it is the only chance that he has. Your veterinarian may give sedatives to help reduce thrashing and random activity. If dehydration occurs, he may administer intravenous fluids. He may also give drugs to lower fever if one is present. If the horse is unable to eat, he may pass a stomach tube and give nutrients or a nourishing gruel. In some cases, he may suture a stomach tube into the animal so that you can feed the horse through it. A gruel can be made of complete feed pellets mixed with water; this is pushed through the stomach tube with a pump. It may be necessary to give water in the same manner to help prevent dehydration if the horse will not drink.

The horse should have a nutritious diet. It should be slightly laxative to help prevent impaction. Keep the animal comfortable by any means possible. If the animal is staggering or thrashing, deep bedding will help to prevent injury. Stall walls may be padded with old carpet or packing quilts if the animal is injuring himself on the walls.

Keep the animal on his feet if at all possible. It is a good idea to keep leg wraps on the horse throughout the course of the disease to help prevent injury. If the horse goes down, try to keep him upright rather than lying flat; he may be propped up with hay bales or sandbags. If he is lying completely flat, turn him over every 4 to 5 hours to prevent fluid accumulation and subsequent pneumonia. Placing the animal in a wooden stocks fitted with a canvas sling may increase the animal's chance of survival if he is trying to collapse and go down.

PREVENTION

See Western Equine Encephalomyelitis, below.

WESTERN EQUINE ENCEPHALOMYELITIS (WEE)

Also called western encephalitis or sleeping sickness, WEE is primarily found in the western and midwestern states. There is a considerable area of overlap with EEE, especially in Texas and Louisiana. Perhaps pro-portionately more animals are involved with WEE than with the eastern variety of the disease; the 1938 outbreak is said to have involved over 100,000 animals.

WEE is also a greater public health menace than EEE. Outbreaks occur more frequently in humans, and are more severe than the eastern type. As with EEE, both the human and the horse are dead-end hosts. The significance of diagnosing the disease in horses is a warning that the same biting insects may transmit the disease to humans from the bird reservoirs at the same time. Cases are usually seen in horses two to five weeks before they are seen in humans in the same area. (95) It is also significant to the owner if his horse becomes permanently damaged or dies from the disease.

The primary method of spread of WEE is by mosquitoes. It is thought that birds act as a reservoir for the virus in outbreaks as with EEE, but the virus has also been recovered from reptiles and wild mammals. One of the largest differences between the two diseases is that only about half the animals affected with WEE die, as compared to about 90% mortality with EEE. So, if your horse gets WEE, he has about a 50/50 chance of recovery. The incubation period is one to three weeks after the animal is bitten by an infective mosquito. (96)

DIAGNOSIS

Signs of WEE are much the same as EEE (see above). Often, the only way of differentiating between the two diseases is that the horse is much more likely to survive with WEE. If he lives, this is most likely the disease that he had. Or, seriologic tests may be run on a couple of samples of blood. One of these is taken early in the disease, and the other is drawn some time after the animal is recovered. By comparing these two, a laboratory can tell which of the diseases the horse had. At this point, knowing which disease he had is purely academic. He has either lived or died by the time you find out.

PROGNOSIS

As mentioned above, if your horse acquires WEE, he has a 50/50 chance of surviving. The worst symptoms of WEE usually only last two or three days, but it may take two to three weeks for an animal to totally recover. If the horse remains standing and there are no complications, recovery may be complete. If he gets down and is unable to rise, chances are very poor that he will live through the disease. As with EEE, some animals are left dummies or so mentally abnormal that they are unusable.

TREATMENT

See EEE, above.

PREVENTION

Vaccines are available to prevent both eastern and western equine encephalomyelitis; they are generally combined in a single vaccine. The animal should receive two injections initially, two to four weeks apart, depending on the vaccine used. Then, he will need a booster every year, as the immunity does not reliably last in the horse from one season to another. The booster may be one or two injections, depending, again, on the vaccine used. In the northern states, the booster injections should be given approximately a month before mosquito season begins. In climates where the insects are present on a year-round basis, establish a convenient (usually twice-yearly) schedule for boosters and stick to it—religiously. (97)

These diseases are definitely more prevalent in some years than in others, probably depending on how plentiful the mosquitoes are. Do not count on protecting your horse by vaccinating when cases begin to occur in your area. If mosquitoes are carrying the disease, your horse may already have been bitten by one of them before you decide to vaccinate. Or, he may be infected with the disease during the time that it takes his body to develop an immunity after being vaccinated. However, vaccinating at the time of an outbreak is better than doing nothing, as protective levels of antibodies have been demonstrated as few as three days after vaccination in VEE (Venezuelan Equine Encephalomyelitis) studies. (98) If you vaccinate in August or September (when we usually start seeing cases in the Rocky Mountain States), you are way behind the proverbial 8-ball. Vaccinate in the spring and give your horse a chance. It is not known how durable an immunity horses get from having had sleeping sickness. For this reason, horses who have had it and recovered should still be vaccinated on a regular schedule. (98)

Foals who have maternal antibodies against equine encephalomyelitis (all three kinds) may not develop a good immunity against the disease when vaccinated. On the other hand, to wait until 7 months or older, when almost all response has gone, will leave some foals dangerously unprotected for a long period of time. The best way to deal with this problem is to give a series of immunizations against encephalitis, beginning at two to four months of age. This series should include two or three vaccinations each a month apart. This schedule will allow foals who have lost their colostral immunity to be stimulated to develop their own protection. Foals who are deprived of colostrum should be vaccinated around two months of age, and their exposure to mosquitoes should be kept to a minimum.

Mosquito control is worthwhile in terms of reducing the possibility of these diseases. It is also worthwhile because large numbers of mosquitoes drain considerable blood from the horse as well as making him miserable (see Mosquitoes).

VENEZUELAN EQUINE ENCEPHALOMY-ELITIS

VEE is caused by a virus similar to EEE and WEE. The disease itself differs from the other two in that the animal may die from systemic effects of the virus before signs of nervous system problems are seen. Another difference is that enough virus IS produced in the horse to infect humans or other horses either through secretions from his body or via insects.

You can see that if VEE became established in our horses, the implications to human health would be enormous. For this reason, considerable effort is being made to keep VEE out of the United States. Florida, Texas, and North Carolina currently require vaccination of equines for VEE. This is another reason why your veterinarian should be called any time you suspect a nervous system disease. If the disease turned out to be VEE, the family you save may be your own. Also, the fact that you may live in Montana or Vermont has nothing to do with being sure that you do not have this disease. Modern transportation can enable a horse to travel from Florida to Maine in a matter of days, bringing VEE with him.

VEE may occur as an encephalitis-type problem, looking much like EEE or WEE. Or, it may be a slow disease affecting the blood vessels. The disease starts with marked depression and fever. Diarrhea may be seen. The temperature usually drops below normal before death.

Like the other encephalitic problems, this disease is diagnosed by a blood samples taken by your veterinarian and forwarded to a laboratory.

Treatment is as described above in EEE (see above). The prognosis is poor, especially if the animal goes down and cannot stand.

Vaccine is available against this disease and should be used if required by your state. It is not necessary at the present time to vaccinate for VEE all over the United States. If an outbreak should occur in the future, immediate vaccination is recommended.

RABIES

In old times, this disease was called hydrophobia because it was believed that animals or humans who had rabies were afraid of water. What really happens is that the throat muscles become paralyzed and the human or animal is unable to drink, no matter how thirsty he may be. A rabid horse does not usually show the aggressive, biting activity which may be seen in dogs, skunks, and other animals. Thus, he is unlikely to spread it over a wide area. The danger lies with handling him; the virus may enter through a cut or scratch on your hand which comes into contact with his saliva. As with the encephalitis types previously discussed, rabies is caused by a virus.

The incubation period in horses ranges from 3 weeks to 3 months. The horse usually acquires the disease from the bite of a rabid skunk, fox, dog, or other animal. In South America, rabies spread by bats, especially vampire bats, is a significant cause of horse (and cattle) loss. Rabid bats have been reported from every state except Hawaii. While it is not practical to attempt to completely control the bat population, any bats nesting in or around horse housing should be eliminated, if at all possible. Seal any entry routes with screen or other material to help keep them out.

Any horse which is bitten by a bat or a wild carnivorous mammal, such as a fox, should be considered to have been exposed to rabies. If the biting animal is available for examination, it should be taken to your veterinarian immediately so that he can send its brain to a laboratory for examination. If you need to kill the animal, be careful not to shoot it in the head; this destroys the brain which is critical to rabies diagnosis. Do not get bitten in your attempts to capture the animal.

SIGNS

Rabies should be considered with any horse who has a peculiar mental attitude until he has been examined by a veterinarian and determined not to have rabies. Early in the disease, the horse may be excitable and vicious. If the bite which infected the animal has not already healed, the site may be inflamed. The horse may bite or tear his flesh at the site. As the disease progresses, the animal may show periods of aggressive behavior. One case of rabies was reported in which the horse suddenly went crazy and knocked down a woman and child and started biting them. (99) The animal may act normally between these episodes of aggression. Trembling and muscular spasms may be observed. The horse may be incoordinated. In the final stages, the horse may show paralysis in the hindlimbs. He will quit eating. Convulsions and death follow. The pulse and respiration rates are elevated from the time signs are seen until the animal's death. This usually occurs within five days of the time the first signs are noticed.

One of the greatest dangers to humans from rabies in a horse is that an animal who is out on pasture may go through the excitement, viciousness, and aggression without being noticed. By the time he is found, he is not eating and may act as if he is having trouble swallowing, which he probably is. The owner's first instinct is to open the animal's mouth and examine it for problems. His second thought, when he doesn't find anything in the mouth, is often to reach down the horse's throat to see if there is anything caught there. The owner may be exposed to the virus through any cut or scrape that he already has on his hands—or through a fresh abrasion made by the sharp edge of a tooth as he checks the animal's mouth. Another veterinarian, who helped me prepare this book, told me that the most horrible thing he could imagine would be reaching into a horse's mouth to remove a stick or other object—and find nothing! In recent years, there have been a number of people exposed to rabies in this manner, even veterinarians who know better. The situation is made worse by the fact that we are not quick to suspect rabies in the horse. Both owners and veterinarians in areas where rabies is common, such as Arizona and Texas, are conditioned to suspect it in dogs and cats, but less so in horses and cattle.

TREATMENT

Animals affected by rabies invariably die. Also, the danger is great that they will infect other animals with the disease if they are kept alive. An animal with a diagnosed case of rabies should be euthanized as soon as possible. He should NOT be shot in the head! He should be shot in the heart or central vital area. Do NOT handle the animal before killing it AND use gloves to handle it after it is dead. Your veterinarian will remove the horse's brain and send it to a laboratory for confirmation of the presence of rabies.

Horses who have been bitten by animals who are known to be rabid are NOT treated because of the danger they may develop the disease several months in the future, and may thus infect humans. Rabies vaccine should NEVER be given to a horse (or other animal) who is bitten by a rabid animal. No vaccines have been proved either safe or effective for use in animals in this situation. Using them may delay onset of the signs of rabies, or alter them so that the disease is not recognized, thus resulting in danger to humans who handle the horse.

Animals who are bitten by animals who might be rabid, but are not proven to be so, should be strictly quarantined and carefully observed for at least six months. If signs of rabies develop, the animal should be euthanized and the brain submitted for confirmation.

PREVENTION

Only one rabies vaccine is currently available in the United States for use in horses. This is Imrab (Pitman-Moore, Washington Crossing, NJ 08560). It gives immunity for one year and boosters must be administered annually. Other vaccines which are used for dogs and cats may NOT be used on horses. Do NOT use ANY rabies vaccine on horses unless current labeling indicates that it is to be used on horses. Use of the wrong vaccine may cause the disease that we are trying to prevent. Horses are not commonly vaccinated against rabies, especially in areas where it occurs only occasionally. However, this may be a worthwhile investment in areas where rabies is common in the wildlife, especially if you have a valuable horse who is out on pasture and may have occasion to contact a rabid wild animal. Keeping your dogs and cats current on their rabies vaccinations will help to reduce the chances of their transmitting rabies to your horses. Vaccination of horses and cattle is routine in areas of South America where bat-carried rabies is common.

A high percentage of veterinarians have availed themselves of prophylactic rabies immunizations since the disease is an occupational hazard for them. If you live in an area of high rabies activity and you or your horses could have frequent contact with wildlife, you may want to ask your physician about prophylactic rabies immunization for yourself.

BOTULISM

Botulism is caused in horses, as it is in humans, by ingesting food containing bacterial toxins produced by the bacterium, Clostridium botulinum. It is not an infectious disease, but is an intoxication. The toxins are present in the food before it is eaten. Botulism is not a common disease. It occurs in so-called "forage poisoning," and has been found in silage and hay. Hay containing decomposed bodies of rodents or other animals is often a source of botulism.

Botulism produces signs which relate mainly to the nervous system and brain. The animal may be reluctant to move or appear paralyzed. He may be weak. He usually has difficulty in picking up food, chewing, and swallowing. As the disease progresses, the animal will become totally unable to eat or drink. Death usually is due to respiratory paralysis.

If you think your horse may have botulism, call your veterinarian immediately to collect samples for laboratory confirmation of the intoxication and for prompt treatment of the animal. The best prevention is to keep the horse from getting any spoiled feed which may contain the toxin. Immunizing toxoids may be given if botulism is a problem in your area; consult your veterinarian for their current availability. Botulism is not contagious from one animal to another, but more than one animal may be affected if they are eating from the same contaminated food source.

KIDNEY AND BLADDER PROBLEMS

Many horsemen feel that their horses have kidney problems, and "won't urinate." These are among the commonest of horsemen complaints—and among the rarest of actual problems. The kidneys are deep under the back area, protected by heavy muscles and the lateral processes of the backbone. In the horse, a blow strong enough to cause damage to the kidney through all this protection would be more likely to break the animal's back! If that happens, you don't have to worry about kidney problems!

Much of the pain felt by horsemen to be "kidney trouble" is due to soreness of the back. A horse who has been ridden hard, especially by a heavy rider who sits far back or moves from side to side in the saddle, may have extremely sore back muscles. For this reason, he may appear uncomfortable when he stretches to urinate. His back will be extremely sore when it is touched. But that's not kidney problems—it's sore muscles. One of my clients had a racehorse sent back from the track for "kidney problems." Examination showed the horse to have an extremely sore back from the way she had been ridden—and no kidney problems at all.

Problems in the hock joint occasionally show a similar uneasiness and discomfort, which again is often interpreted to be kidney trouble. Stifle problems show a similar uneasiness and discomfort. The horse may be reluctant to stretch and urinate with either of these conditions.

So, when do we REALLY have kidney problems in the horse? The answer is: very rarely. When kidney problems do occur, they are often secondary to another disease. Treatment of a complicating kidney problem may be an important part of treating the underlying disease. Kidney problems may occur with toxicities due to lead, arsenic, and mercury poisoning, as well as with some other chemicals. Kidney problems are an important part of blister beetle poisoning. Bladder paralysis may be seen with sudan grass poisoning. In some cases, the paralysis may be permanent, necessitating euthanasia of the horse. Diabetes may be seen in the horse, but is extremely rare. Kidney failure may occasionally be seen in horses with severe exhaustion or dehydration. In these cases, the kidneys shut down because there is not enough fluid volume or blood pressure available to keep them working.

Recently, chronic renal (kidney) failure has been incriminated as a cause of weight loss in the horse. Again, it is uncommon, but worth checking in an animal who loses weight for no apparent reason. The animal may be noticed to continually shift its hind feet and to urinate small amounts frequently. Edema may appear along the lower abdomen.

Kidney and bladder stones may occasionally cause problems in the urinary tract. Animals with stones often show blood in the urine. This will appear fresh and red, rather than brownish or wine-colored as is seen with tying-up and similar muscular problems.

When do you correctly suspect urinary tract problems? One of the most common signs is when the horse seems to be drinking more water and urinating more than usual. It is important to know what is normal for your horse because some horses normally drink a lot of water and urinate a lot—especially some stallions and most mares who are nursing foals. Other signs of possible problems include blood or pus in the urine, an animal who urinates small amounts constantly, has edema along the lower abdomen, or a sudden unexplained weight loss. A horse's urine normally contains a fair amount of mucus, making it appear stringy, cloudy, or ropey. This is not pus. Excessive buildups of tartar on the teeth have been seen in some horses with kidney trouble. Consult your veterinarian if you suspect kidney problems. He can arrange a urinalysis and further examination of the animal, if necessary.

If the urinalysis indicates kidney abnormalities, your veterinarian may wish to take a biopsy of kidney tissue for further examination, to positively confirm or deny the presence of kidney disease. This is done with a long needle-like instrument through the body wall just below the back muscles. The tissue which is removed is then prepared for microscopic examination and checked. In some cases, this may be the only way to confirm that an animal does or does not have a kidney problem.

Occasional horses will refuse to urinate under certain circumstances. It is said that one of the top cutting horses some years ago could not be hauled early in his career because he fought the trailer badly. He would be fine the first day, and then each day he got worse and worse until he would nearly kick it to pieces, when he finally loaded after a considerable battle. A trainer realized that the horse was uncomfortable because he wasn't urinating—he didn't like the feeling of the urine splashing on his legs. Hauling the horse in a roomy trailer, bedded extra deep in sawdust, allowed him to urinate while being hauled. He learned to haul without fighting and in much more comfort. The animal went on to become a winning cutting horse.

HEART PROBLEMS

Heart problems are uncommon in the horse. When present, they are often diagnosed only by a veterinarian very skilled and experienced with his stethoscope, or by an electrocardiogram. For that reason, this section will only briefly mention a few signs that may signal cardiac disease, and leave it to you to consult your veterinarian if you think that your horse has a problem along this line. This is not to slight the importance of the heart, but to be realistic about the difficulty (even for the veterinarian) of diagnosing heart problems.

As mentioned in the section on pulse, it is not uncommon for a horse to have a slightly irregular heartbeat with occasional skipped beats. If the heartbeat becomes regular when the animal is exercised, no abnormality is present. Conversely, if the animal's heartbeat becomes irregular after he is worked, he should be examined for possible problems.

Signs of heart disease include stumbling or fading when worked, and fainting. The mucous membranes may appear bluish in color because they are not getting adequate oxygen due to inefficient heart action. One common sign of heart disease is edema in which all the animal's legs fill with fluid; this may include a fluid line along the animal's abdomen and occasionally fluid in the jaw area. Persistent edema is almost always a sign of more serious problems, such as heart disease or purpura hemorrhagica, and your veterinarian should be consulted.

ANHIDROSIS

Anhidrosis is the inability to sweat. It was first reported in Thoroughbred racehorses who were taken from temperate to tropical climates for polo or racing. Within five to eight weeks after arriving in their new homes, they lost the ability to perspire (sweat). This cripples the animal's ability to regulate his temperature in extreme heat because his normal method of heat removal is through sweating.

Today, anhidrosis is a serious problem on the Gulf Coast and in Florida, as well as in low altitude areas of tropical countries. It affects horses of all breeds, both those native to the area, and those who have been imported from other areas. It is most commonly seen in animals who are worked hard. It is thought that their high concentrate diet and heavy work schedule contribute to the problem.

As many as 20% of horses in the Miami area may be affected by the problem in the summer months. A decrease in the animal's athletic performance usually results. Many native animals lose the ability to sweat even without the stress of hard work. Some of the affected horses will sweat normally during the winter, but lose the ability to do so in the summer. A similar problem is seen in human soldiers who are sent to desert and tropical areas.

When asked to work or exercise, these horses may have rapid, labored breathing. One of the most common signs is hard blowing as the animal attempts to cool himself in hot weather. The body temperature is elevated above normal with exercise. It may be as high as 104 to 106 degrees F (40–41 degrees C) or higher. The heart rate is also elevated. The mucous membranes may be severely congested.

The animal may collapse with heatstroke if work is continued. His coat will be excessively dry and it may be dull. There may be hair loss in some cases, especially on the face. Some animals will show decreased appetite and become thin. The problem may come on either gradually or suddenly. Some animals will produce small amounts of sweat in some areas, such as under the mane and tail and on the chest.

Anhidrosis may be confirmed when your veterinarian administers drugs to make the animal sweat, and gets no response. (100) There is no known cure for this syndrome—only management to use the animal within his limitations. Make sure that the horse has adequate shelter from the sun. Exercise him only on cool days. Keep an eye on his temperature, pulse, and respiration during workouts because you will not be able to tell how warm he is by the amount of sweat as you can often do on a normal horse.

Some people feel that giving several tablespoons of corn oil daily in the horse's feed may be helpful. Also give Vitamin E at 2000 IU per day. Oral electrolyte therapy has been tried, but does not consistently give good results. Give the animal more alfalfa hay and less concentrate in his ration. Make sure that he has (and is drinking) adequate water. Free-choice salt should be available.

Other management changes are aimed at keeping the horse more comfortable by providing shade or fans, or even, in some cases, air conditioning the stable area. The horse can be clipped to help him stay cooler and he can be sponged or sprayed with water to help cool him. Some of these animals can continue in use if they are worked only during the cooler hours of the day.

In some cases, the only solution has been to stable and train the animals in higher, cooler areas of a country, and take them to the lower, hotter, areas only for matches or races. Or, the animal may be permanently moved to a more moderate climate. Acclimation does not have any role in the development or prevention of the disease, but heat stress does. (101) (102)

HEAT EXHAUSTION

Also called hyperthermia, heat exhaustion may be seen in poorly conditioned horses who are worked on a hot day. It may also be seen when animals are worked hard on exceptionally hot days. The heat which is generated by muscular activity may be greater than the animal can remove by sweating, especially if the day is humid. This will raise the body temperature. Horses who are dehydrated will not have fluid available to produce sweat even if the day is conducive to cooling in this manner.

Horses will show increased heart and respiratory rates with hyperthermia. In early stages, the animal may sweat profusely. As his temperature rises, he will become dehydrated and stop sweating. The dehydration may cause shock because of the drop in the animal's blood volume. He may be restless, dull, and incoordinated. Severely affected animals may collapse, go into convulsions, and die. If the horse's temperature remains above 107 to 109 degrees F (41.5 to 43 C) for more than a short period of time, death usually results.

Treat the animal by cooling him, but beware of shock which may occasionally follow extremely rapid cooling (as by icing the animal). Stand him in a cool stream if one is available, and pour water over him with a bucket. Or, run water over him with a hose. Use cool, not extremely cold, water. If he will not drink enough fluids to take care of the dehydration, it may be necessary to call a veterinarian to give him fluids intravenously or via stomach tube. Prompt treatment is also necessary if the animal goes into shock.

OTHER HEAT PROBLEMS

Care and consideration when hauling horses in hot weather is important to their usability when you arrive at the end of the trip, and indeed, to their survival in some cases. Lack of consideration may lead to heat stroke, exhaustion, or founder. Temperatures in the 90 to 100 degree range may cause problems. When it is necessary to move horses across extreme desert climates, such as the southern California or Arizona deserts, in midsummer, it is best to travel at night. Even if you have an air-conditioned horse van, what will happen to the animals if you break down in 120 degree F (49 C) heat when you are traveling during the day?

Trailers should be well ventilated. In extremely hot weather, carrying a couple of five-gallon containers of water will provide for the animal's comfort and add to the margin of safety. Horses should be exercised at night or in the early morning hours when the temperatures are coolest. The horse should be cooled out slowly and carefully.

A horse who is showing rapid breathing, fast pulse, elevated body temperature, heavy sweating, and signs of weakness or trembling may be in serious trouble. Those who stop sweating before being cooled out may be close to death. In hot weather, horses should be offered water more often than normally, and salt should be available. In some cases, it may be necessary to sponge the animal with water to help lower his body temperature.

COLD PROBLEMS

Horses live in many cold climates, and survive them. How well they survive may depend on the care they receive. Shelter is desirable if you have access to it. Even a shed or windbreak will help the animal to stay out of the cold winds and snow which drain so much of his body heat. Trees or heavy brush in the horse pasture will often provide some shelter. Horses who are left to winter in severe climates without adequate care may lose several hundred pounds by spring and may show problems, such as frostbitten ears. With some extra care, horses can live through extreme winters without any shelter at all. What is needed to make up for the lack of shelter?

Horses should be in good condition going into the winter, maybe even a little on the fat side. This gives them energy reserves to draw on. They should have their teeth floated so that they will be eating efficiently and should be wormed so that they are not supporting a parasite load. Even if the pasture seems to be adequate, it is often necessary to feed extra hay when the snow is very deep and the horses cannot paw down to get enough feed each day. Feeding hay also makes the digestive system work harder, providing extra heat to help keep the horse warm. Many horse owners feed grain all winter. If you cannot do that, at least feed grain when the temperature is very low. One of my clients had board horses who were given a gallon of grain apiece in the evening on nights when the temperature was going to be less than 20 degrees F below zero (−7 C). You can give grain to horses who are not on it all the time in this kind of weather without getting into problems IF you provide heated water so that the animals have enough to drink.

Tank heaters will keep water warmed to a few degrees above freezing. This allows the animals to drink water rather than taking in snow and having to use precious feed calories to melt it. The animals will drink more water and have less colic, impactions, and other problems if they have access to warmed water. If you have to choose one thing which makes the largest difference in the way horses will winter in an extremely cold climate, that choice would be to have heated water for them.

EXHAUSTION

Exhaustion is seen in horses on endurance and competitive trail rides who are ridden beyond their level of conditioning and physical ability. It may be seen with animals who are used on ranches or hunting trips when they are not properly conditioned for the work that is asked of them. It may occur with animals who are accustomed to a certain level of work (say, a given number of miles on the level) who are then asked to do the same or more miles up and down mountains, or who are accustomed to slow work and are asked to work excessively fast without proper conditioning. Factors such as heat and humidity may contribute to the problem; indeed, heat exhaustion may be a significant part of the animal's total exhaustion.

The exhausted horse may show any combination of the following signs, but will rarely show all of them: he will be depressed and have little interest in his surroundings. He will have no appetite and may not drink even when he is dehydrated. The eyes may be dull, sunken, and glazed, and the ears may hang limply. Some animals may have tense facial muscles and an anxious expression, especially if the problem is accompanied by colic or muscle problems. The mouth may be dry.

The horse will not cool out, and his temperature may rise to 106 degrees F (41 degrees C). When the thermometer is inserted, it will be noticed that the muscles of the anus are loose, and air may enter the rectum. If the anus is pinched, it may not respond by puckering closed. This is one of the best indications of severe exhaustion. Any feces which are passed may be hard and dry. Urine output is decreased due to kidney shutdown.

The heart and respiration rates are often well above normal and often do not return to normal when the animal is rested, as they would in a normal horse. In some cases, the respiration rate may remain faster than the heart rate. Breathing may occur in a pattern called "thumps" (synchronous diaphragmatic flutter), where the diaphragm contacts with the heartbeat, shaking the entire animal and giving him a rapid, inefficient breathing pattern. The horse may be severely dehydrated. Tying-up may occur along with the other symptoms, but most cases of tying-up are unrelated to exhaustion.

Get veterinary attention for the exhausted horse, if at all possible. If the horse will not drink, intravenous fluids may be necessary to help counteract the dehydration. Treatment for shock may be necessary in some cases. Oral electrolytes should be given if the horse will drink.

The horse will need rest and careful nursing, often for several days. If he is hot, sponge him with lukewarm or cool (NOT COLD) water. If he is cold or shivering or if he is still wet and the weather is damp, cold, or windy, blanket him. Get the horse into a stall with good, deep bedding if at all possible so that he may lie down and rest.

Horses who are used on endurance rides, as well as for other hard work, should be conditioned carefully so that they are able to handle what is demanded of them. They should be encouraged to drink as often as possible, and free-choice, loose salt should be available during the event. Excessive electrolyte supplementation should not be given before endurance rides, as the horse's body may become accustomed to allowing the unneeded minerals to pass through; this may make it difficult for him to absorb electrolytes when he desperately needs them. (103)

EMERGENCIES

What is an emergency? We all become upset when our horse is injured; it's a natural reaction. Go ahead—take thirty seconds and panic! Then, slow down, take a deep breath, and then gather all the information you can about the problem so that you and your veterinarian can make an intelligent decision about its severity.

Here's a list some problems which should be considered emergencies:

FRACTURES

Broken bones are often repairable with modern techniques, especially if the fracture is not compounded. A fracture must be promptly stabilized to prevent further damage to the bone or the surrounding tissues. The animal's chances of survival are greatly reduced if the bone is protruding through broken skin (compounded).

The most important first aid for a fracture in the horse is to stabilize the bone so that it cannot move, and to prevent its being compounded if it is not already. Do this first, and then worry about the next step.

Do not automatically shoot the horse unless you are in the middle of the mountains in a place where you cannot get help, or unless the animal is of little value to you. One horseman camped with his horse for five to six weeks in the mountains until the animal had healed enough to walk out!

You can stabilize a broken leg in several ways. If you don't have anything else, a couple of bed pillows or blankets and either adhesive tape or bandaging material—or strips of bedsheet or rags will steady the leg enough that the animal may be transported or can more comfortably wait for a veterinarian to arrive. Wrap the limb, including the joint ABOVE the break with padding until there are two to three inches of material around all sides of the leg. If using pillows, place them in the same manner to give a thick layer of protection. Then, wrap the whole padded area FIRMLY with several layers of tape. Duct tape or electrical tape can be used in an emergency. Pull it snugly around the soft padding. You are making the whole area into one big, soft, stiff splint. Pieces of plastic pipe, split lengthwise, can be used to stiffen the splint. Or, you can tape lightweight pieces of wood or metal to the outside of the bandage as splints.

Whether you transport the animal to a veterinary clinic or have a veterinarian come to you depends on several factors. If you are close to a veterinary hospital or university clinic, load the animal into a trailer (AFTER the leg is carefully stabilized) and take him to the facility. There, they can x-ray the break to determine the extent of the damage, and give you a good idea of whether the problem is repairable and what it will cost to do the repair. If you choose to fix it, the animal is right there where the surgery or fixation can be done.

If you have one available, use a trailer with a sling in it to help take the animal's weight off the leg. Inadequate stabilization before hauling can make a simple, easily repairable fracture into a compound fracture—a contaminated mess which may not be repairable. Extra time spent to get the leg carefully supported before moving the animal will mean more to his survival than driving 90 mph to get him to a hospital. Taking the time to do it right really can pay off.

If you live a long way from a veterinary clinic or the animal is in rough country, try to get the veterinarian to come to you. If there is no hospital in your area catering to horses, your horse will probably be better off at home with your nursing and with regular visits from a traveling veterinarian.

CERTAIN WIRE CUTS

Wire cuts should be considered dire emergencies if the horse is suffering severe, unstoppable bleeding, which leaves large clots of blood on the ground. Remember that a horse can take a small amount of blood (especially if spurting from a small artery) and spread it over a large area, making it look as if he were bleeding to death, when he really isn't.

Use direct pressure over the site of the bleeding as you would in treating a human with the same problem. Use sterile gauze compresses or sponges, if you have them available. If not, use a clean cloth, towel, or paper towels. Disposable diapers and sanitary napkins make good, absorbent materials with which to pack large wounds if sterile sponges or pads are not available. These may be moistened in sterile saline solution or in tamed iodine diluted in water to the color of weak tea. Do NOT use loose cotton, as the fibers become caught in the wound surface and cannot be removed when the wound is cleaned for suturing. It may break open later because of this.

Get a veterinarian within six hours of the time the wound has occurred, if at all possible (see Wound Treatment). An adult horse can easily lose a gallon of blood without harm. Do NOT use a tourniquet because it may cut off the blood supply to the leg, resulting in gangrene and loss of the horse. Don't put anything on or in the wound except a clean bandage. Especially do not use the blood-clotting powders which are made for use when dehorning cattle, since these will make it impossible to suture the wound.

When you call your veterinarian for a cut, be sure before you get too upset that it is indeed a fresh cut. One client called me away from the middle of treating another animal for a horse who had "just gotten cut clear across the neck, right over the jugular veins." On arrival, I found a horse who did indeed have a wire cut all the way across the bottom of his neck. Just missing both jugular veins, the cut continued up each side past them. The only problem was that the cut was at least three or four days old. The cut had pus oozing everywhere and was severely infected. It was not a dire emergency! The owner felt guilty about not finding the problem earlier, and so said that it had just happened. This is definitely NOT the way to win friends and influence your veterinarian!

EYE INJURIES

Cuts and scrapes on the surface of the cornea as well as severe bruising of the eyeball are definite emergencies. So are eyeball punctures. Keep the animal in a quiet, darkened stall and obtain veterinary help as soon as possible.

SHOCK

Severe shock can kill a horse because of blood pooling in his intestines and lowering his blood pressure. Shock may occur because of pain, injury, or foaling problems; it may be due to colitis-X (salmonellosis) or because of an anaphylactic reaction to a vaccine or medication.

Immediate treatment is necessary to save the horse's life.

Epinephrine should be a part of your first aid kit if you are vaccinating your own horses. If the shock is due to vaccination or drug administration, administer epinephrine immediately (see Anaphylactic Shock).

In any case of shock, fluid therapy and treatment with special corticosteroids may be necessary to save the animal. Get veterinary help as soon as possible.

FOALING

The mare's abdominal muscles are extremely strong and powerful. Once the mare starts into hard labor, she rarely strains for more than an hour without producing a foal. If she goes more than an hour, she is in trouble (treat as discussed under Foaling). While you are doing what you can for the mare, have someone call a veterinarian to help you. It is preferable to have the veterinarian arrive as you pull the foal out, rather than to work on the mare for several hours until she is badly in shock and exhaustion, and then call for help.

UTERINE PROLAPSE

Uterine prolapse is associated with foaling. As the foal emerges, or shortly afterward, the uterus turns inside out like a sock peeled off a foot. The mare usually goes into severe shock within a very short time. An injection of anesthetic into the space around the spinal cord is usually needed to keep her from straining to allow replacement of the uterus. Call for veterinary help immediately.

Meanwhile, keep the uterus clean. Wrap it in a sheet or towel moistened with a solution of 1 teaspoon of salt per quart of water. If the mare lies down, protect the uterus so that it does not become dirty or torn and so that she does not lie on it. Keep the mare calm, and keep her from thrashing, if possible.

It is sometimes useful to summon a neighbor or friend for extra help. It is often easier to replace the uterus if the mare is standing, and extra persons may be needed to help stabilize her and keep her on her feet.

BURNS AND SMOKE INHALATION

These problems can be very severe and life-threatening. If the animal is treated promptly, the chance of survival is much better. Cover large burned areas with bedsheets or other clean cloths moistened in cool water with a teaspoon of salt added per quart. Call for veterinary assistance.

SEVERE COLIC OR FOUNDER

A mild colic, while requiring veterinary assistance, is usually not an immediate emergency. It becomes an ex-

treme emergency when the animal is thrashing violently and you cannot keep him on his feet, or if he is battering himself by hitting his head on the ground or similar action. A severely foundered horse should be treated as soon as possible to relieve his pain and minimize damage to the feet.

DEEP PUNCTURE WOUNDS TO THE CHEST OR ABDOMEN

Wounds which penetrate the chest may result in a punctured or collapsed lung and/or a life-threatening infection. If the animal has a hole where you can hear air coming out and going in, plug it with something clean to stop the air from moving back and forth. Lung damage may also occur with injuries which cause broken ribs as well as from being gored by horned livestock.

Abdominal punctures have the same deadly potential. If there is something like a stick lodged in the wound, do NOT remove it. You may pull the intestines out the same hole. If they are hanging out, wrap the horse with a clean bedsheet or hold them in place with a clean towel. It is helpful to moisten the cloths with lukewarm water. Do whatever you can to keep more intestines from emerging until the veterinarian arrives.

THE EMERGENCY: YOU AND YOUR VETERINARIAN

When you call your veterinarian in an emergency situation, find out from his office how long it will be before he can get there. Describe your problem in as much detail as possible. This will give the veterinarian a chance to evaluate the call and see if he should respond or refer you to someone else if he cannot get away from other work in time to do your animal any good. If you call more than one veterinarian, be prepared to pay call charges to both. And, be aware that this might cause you a considerable amount of ill will from them. In dire emergencies, go ahead and do it anyway. Generally, they will understand that you wanted help in an emergency any way you could get it.

Another note: put in calls to one or two veterinarians and then stay off your phone! Don't call every friend and neighbor to tell them about your problem. There is nothing more frustrating to the veterinarian than to have a note about an emergency sitting on his desk or forwarded to him by an answering service, and then not be able to return the call! You will get service a lot faster if you stay off the phone and give us a chance to call you back.

EUTHANASIA

This term means an easy or painless death. Other terms often used include "putting the animal down," "putting him away," "putting him to sleep," etc.

IMPORTANT NOTE: Some veterinarians and horse-men also talk of "putting a horse down" or "putting him to sleep," when they are referring to anesthetizing the animal for a surgical procedure. Make sure when using these terms that you and the veterinarian are talking about the same thing. The terms "euthanasia" and "anesthesia" mean completely different things, are precise, and should be used.

Euthanasia means humanely killing the horse to end his suffering when it is apparent that he cannot be saved, or will not be able to function after he has recovered from his injury. This is never an easy decision to make, but it is far more fair to put the animal out of his misery than to torture him by keeping him alive.

Several factors should be considered when deciding to euthanize an animal. Let's go over some of them:

1) How much chance does the animal have of recovery? Are you willing to take a chance with a 50% possibility of recovery? Is it fair to subject him to pain and suffering when he has only the very slightest chance of making it? Is the problem progressive and irreversible? Will it continue to get worse until the animal eventually dies, and leave him alive in pain in the interim?

A good example of a difficult decision concerns a 5-year old stallion who was a wobbler. He had been born with the condition, and it had become progressively worse. The animal walked across his pen from the food to the water and back. There were weeds growing in other parts of the pen, which told me that he did not walk in these areas, and that he did not reach down to graze the weeds. When this author first examined the animal as a four-year-old, he could scarcely walk. It was shocking to see him again as a five-year old. There had been no improvement in his gait and travel, and the animal had grown thin to the point of emaciation. The owners elected to euthanize him. This was not easy, as he belonged to a fifteen-year old girl who had owned him from the time that he was quite small. But, there was no hope of his getting better, and he was, at this point, getting noticeably, progressively worse. It was not fair to keep the animal alive with no hope of recovery.

2) If the animal is repairable, how much will it cost to fix him? This is an economic decision based on your pocketbook. Can you afford to have him repaired? Bear in mind that the costs are not only economic: there may be a great deal of time and effort that you have to invest in addition to the money. Perhaps the best example of this is saving an orphan foal. Are you willing to get up several times during the night and do all the nursing chores that are associated with saving the foal? An injured leg may require constant cleaning and frequent bandage changes. Severed flexor tendons may require as much as five or six months of care before you will even know if the animal will heal or not.

3) What are you going to have if you save the animal? Will he be usable or a cripple? Will he be usable for breeding or totally useless? A gelding was brought in to the Colorado State University Veterinary Hospital who had shattered the second phalanx in a barrel race. The owners were told that he could be repaired by fusing the joints above and below the bone. There was a very good chance of healing, but what would they have? He would not be rideable, and obviously was not a breeding animal. The owners discussed the situation, and came back to tell us that they would have him repaired and turn him out to pasture because he had been a good horse. That's great if you have the money to spend to have him repaired and then to support an unusable animal. A mare or stallion in a similar situation will not be rideable, but can usually be used as a breeding animal. It is often worth salvaging an animal with good bloodlines for this purpose.

4) What kind of patient is the animal? A high-strung or nervous animal is often a terrible patient to handle and care for after surgery or repairs are completed. And conversely, animals who seem not to care and are very complacent and sedate often give up. The best patient is often a middle-of-the-road beast—one with enough try not to give up, yet calm and workable enough not to hurt himself.

5) Do you have or can you get or build the equipment that will be necessary in caring for the animal? For instance, an animal may need to be supported in a sling. Can you buy, borrow, or make one? Or, the horse may need shelter and you don't have a barn. Can you borrow one from a neighbor who doesn't have a horse? Or put him in an unused garage? Be creative to find a solution to the question. If you truly wish to save the animal, don't let the fact that you have no barn stand in your way. Think creatively and solve your problem. A large stock trailer may make a perfect barn for a foal or yearling if you can borrow it for a few weeks. Bed it deeply in shavings or other bedding just as you would a regular stall.

When a horse is involved in a severe accident, the first problem is to determine whether the extent of the injury warrants euthanasia. If a veterinarian is available, he should be consulted; many broken legs that meant death for an animal 20 years ago can now be repaired. Among the injuries that are generally too severe to be repaired are difficult fractures such as two breaks in one leg, or more than one broken leg in an adult horse. Compound fractures are often impossible to salvage because of the ease with which horses develop infections from this type of wound.

The difficulty of getting the horse out to "civilization" must also be considered. If the break is splinted or cast, do you still have to walk the horse many miles to get him to a trailer? Often, the value of the horse is an important consideration. A broken leg, even if repairable, can be expensive. The healing process can take months and there is always the possibility of complications. Since healing of the fracture often leaves the animal useless for riding, this must also be taken into consideration. A mare or stallion of good bloodlines might be worth salvaging for use as a breeding animal.

Ownership of the animal should be taken into account. An animal hit by a car cannot usually be legally put down without permission from the owner. If the horse is insured, permission must usually be obtained from the insurance company before destroying the animal—or the company might refuse to pay the claim. Most insurance companies have 24-hour phone numbers for this purpose—be sure to give it to anyone who is training or hauling a horse for you, while the animal is not in your possession.

CHEMICAL METHODS

Now that you have taken all factors into consideration, and have decided to euthanize the animal, how should it be done? There are several methods. One is to have a veterinarian use drugs to kill the animal. These drugs are basically an overdose of an anesthetic, with other drugs added to stop the heart. They must be placed in the jugular vein so that they will take effect quickly. Often a large quantity is required—say, 75 to 100 cc. or more.

Your veterinarian gives the drug into the vein as rapidly as he can, but may only be able to get part of the dose into the animal before it goes down. When he goes down, be sure to stand out of the way as the horse may collapse to the side, fall over backwards, or pitch forward; there is not much predictability as to the direction they fall. This is because the dose is given more rapidly than it would be if the vet were going to anesthetize the animal for surgery. It is also usually given without the preparatory sedatives and tranquilizers that are given before anesthesia, and so takes effect more rapidly and drastically.

By the time the animal is on the ground, he is usually unconscious or nearly so. At this point, the veterinarian locates the jugular vein again and gives the rest of the dosage. He will check several reflexes and listen to the heart with a stethoscope to be sure that the animal is dead before he leaves. It may take as long as five minutes or more for the animal to die after he goes down.

Rest assured that although he may be breathing and his heart is beating, he does not know where he is or what is happening. He is in deep anesthesia. Even if he groans or makes other noises or movements, this does not mean that he is conscious. This type of movement also occurs with normal anesthesia. I mention this because some horse owners are upset because the animal is not dead immediately and instantly. Knowing what to expect will make it easier for you if you are unfortunate enough to have to make the decision to euthanize your horse.

HOW TO SHOOT A HORSE

Putting down an injured horse in any circumstances is a difficult and unpleasant task. However, any horseman who is more than ten miles from the nearest veterinarian should know how to humanely kill a severely injured horse. Horsemen or law officers are often concerned with disposing of a horse after an automobile or trailer accident. As a veterinarian, this author has been asked more than once to ride 30 or 40 miles into the back country to a hunting camp to put an injured horse out of his misery.

When the decision has been made to euthanize the animal and you must use a gun, a primary consideration is selection of the weapon. A handgun is best, but a rifle can be used if a sidearm is not handy. Use the largest caliber available—.38, .44, .45, or a .357 magnum. A .22 caliber weapon will work, but obviously the placement of the bullet must be precise to insure a clean, humane death with one shot.

To locate the proper spot for the bullet, draw imaginary lines from the base of each ear to the eye on the opposite side of the face. The spot where the lines intersect in the middle of the forehead is the place to hold the muzzle of the weapon. The animal can be down or still on his feet. Regardless, the principle is the same. Be sure that everyone is out of the field of fire. Assistants should be standing behind the person doing the shooting.

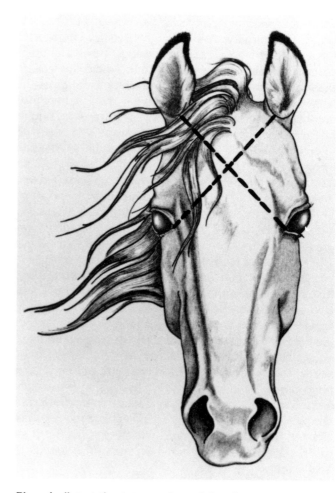

Place bullet at the intersection of the dotted lines.

Do not stand back eight or ten feet to attempt the shot. The emotions of the situation can make the best marksmen miss. Hold the muzzle of the gun ¼ to ½ inch (½ to 1 cm.) away from the horse's skull. It is possible that holding the gun directly against the skull may result in the same effect as if the barrel were plugged, and could possibly lead to the weapon exploding in your hands. Carefully squeeze the trigger and immediately step back to the end of the lead rope. While most horses instantly drop, some will flip over backwards so a step or two out of the way will prevent possible injury to you.

Even though dead, the animal might continue to twitch for several minutes. This is normal after a sudden death. If it becomes evident in a minute or two that the first shot was not fatal, a second bullet can be discharged into the same area. Again, make certain that people and other animals are out of the way.

Incidentally, the above method for determining the spot for placement of the bullet works on any large animal—a cow, sheep, pig, or game animal that is not quite dead.

And as a final suggestion, it is a good idea for organized groups traveling the back country to have a handgun available should the need arise to euthanize an injured animal. Of course, this is no problem with hunting parties. While it is true that firearms are generally unnecessary on a pleasure ride, someone in a group of organized riders should have a weapon. Years ago, one of the top trail-riding groups in the Rocky Mountains had an unfortunate incident when it was necessary to put down a horse and no weapon was available. Now that organization insures that a handgun is available during each year's ride. Only the ride management knows who has the weapon, but should the need arise to euthanize a horse, the means are there. But be sure to check local regulations before packing a firearm on the trail.

OTHER METHODS OF EMERGENCY EU-THANASIA

If you absolutely must put a horse out of his misery and there is no firearm available, what do you do? We shall assume that the animal is down and helpless or nearly so. One method is to cut the jugular vein with a VERY sharp knife. Stand behind the horse's neck when doing so, as there is danger of being struck by flailing front feet if you do not. Try to cut the vein cleanly in one stroke. It's not beautiful, but is better than letting an injured animal linger on in misery.

Another old method of killing a horse when it was not desirable to have blood running all over the place was to cut the animal's aorta, the main blood vessel just under the backbone, inside the horse. The person doing the procedure would hold a small, sharp knife or scalpel inside his hand, and reach inside the horse's rectum. Once inside to the length of his arm, he would make a deep, sweeping cut under the horse's backbone, severing the aorta. This way, the blood is all contained inside the horse's body. It is said that this method was used at racetracks and other places where the sight of blood would have been undesirable. Now, at tracks and shows, there is generally a trailer or skid available to move the animal out of sight to an area where an intelligent decision about his fate can be made.

NECROPSY

This word means the same as "autopsy" in humans; it refers to an examination of the deceased. "Postmortem" is another term with the same meaning. This is done by your veterinarian to determine why the animal died. A necropsy is usually necessary when an animal is insured. Upon the death of an insured animal, contact your insurance company immediately; they will usually request a necropsy. Necropsies are also a good idea when a horse dies suddenly and unexpectedly. This can help to tell if you have an infectious or contagious disease or a management problem on your premises that may affect other animals. While knowing what caused the horse to die will not bring him back, it may enable you to correct whatever caused his death to avoid losing other animals in the same manner.

In a certain number of animals, it is impossible to determine the cause of death. So, if your veterinarian can't tell you what has caused the animal's death, this is not necessarily his fault—it just happens in some cases.

To perform a necropsy, it is usually necessary to open the animal's chest and abdomen completely. If rabies is suspected, it will be necessary to open the skull to remove the brain. Performing a necropsy on a horse is brute labor, and most of us use tools which are brute tools: axes, large knives, and occasionally, chain saws. None of this procedure is pretty. Expect it to be ugly and messy and if there are children, you may want to send them away before the procedure begins. If you have a weak stomach or are quite attached to the animal involved, it may be a good idea to put the veterinarian to work and then go in the house and pour yourself a cold, stiff drink. Ask the vet to come up to the house and let you know when the job is finished. Reminisce about your friend, the horse.

LETTER TO A GIRL ON THE DEATH OF HER HORSE

Dear Kelly,

I know that when you asked me yesterday how I thought your horse was doing, you were looking for a last bright ray of hope. It really hurt not to be able to give you some encouragement that his problem could be healed. When we took him to where they were digging the grave, he hauled like the perfect gentleman that he was. When I gave him the injection, he laid down quickly and was unconscious in seconds. Although it took a few minutes for the drugs to take their final effect, he was in a total coma and feeling no pain until the end.

Saying that we've all got to go sometime does nothing to ease the pain of your loss. But if I had to choose a day to die, I would surely choose one like yesterday: a summer afternoon in June, not too warm nor too cool, in one of the wettest springs that I can remember. The fresh green grass stretched across the rolling hills as far as the eye could see. A crystal blue sky hung overhead with just a few marshmallow clouds on the horizon for contrast. A soft breeze kissed the brow of the hill, overlooking the river bottom in all its velvet green finery, stretching to the distant mountains. Dozens of different kinds of wild flowers splashed accents of red, yellow, and blue.

As I knelt to see if his heart had stopped, I noticed all around a wildflower that has been a favorite of mine since childhood. Lithe spiderworts were pregnant with buds and should be in bloom by the time you receive this letter. If you kneel and sniff several of these bright blue flowers, you will find one of the sweetest scents in the world—a fragrance to bring to memory happy times.

That's something else I'd like to mention—happy times. Kelly, please remember your friend not as he was with his problems, but as he would have been without them, and as I am sure that he is, even now. Remember him doing the horse things that he never could: galloping off across the hills with his proud Arabian head held high, and the wind whipping his tail behind him. Remember that the love you gave was never wasted, and that he also loved you. Even though he is gone, that love remains.

Sincerely,

Ruth B James DVM

Ruth B. James, D.V.M.

REFERENCES AND NOTES

1. Diseases of the Horse, U.S. Department of Agriculture, 1923, p. 13.
2. A Standard Guide to Horse and Pony Breeds, Elwyn Hartley Edwards, General Editor, McGraw-Hill Book Co., N.Y., N.Y., 1980, p. 193. This is both a valuable reference book and just plain interesting reading. It contains information on horse and pony breeds throughout the world, and has an informative section on conformation as related to performance and usage.
3. Cunha, Tony J., Horse Feeding and Nutrition, Academic Press, Inc (Harcourt Brace Jovanovich), N.Y., N.Y., 1980, p. 120.
4. The Intermountain Quarter Horse, Oct. 1981, p. 19.
5. Diseases of the Horse, 1923, p. 54.
6. Ibid, p. 57.
7. Journal of the American Veterinary Medical Association (JAVMA), Vol. 182, No. 3, 1 February 1983, p. 285–6.
8. Oklahoma State University Extension Facts Sheet #2072.
9. Current Therapy in Equine Medicine (Curr Ther Eq Med), N. Edward Robinson, Editor, W.B. Saunders Company, Philadelphia, 1983, p. 66.
10. Taylor, Louis, Harper's Encyclopedia of the Horse, Harper & Row Publishers, New York, 1973, p. 298.
11. Cunha, p. 192.
12. For additional information, see Dr. R. M. Miller, "The Corn Oil Trick," The Western Horseman, June 1979.
13. Taylor, p. 71.
14. Cunha, p. 117–119.
15. JAVMA, Vol. 182, No. 12, 15 January 1983, p. 1358–1369.
16. Proceedings of the American Association of Equine Practitioners (AAEP Proc), 1980, p. 66–7.
17. Ibid.
18. Curr Ther Eq Med, p. 78.
19. Curr Ther Eq Med, p. 608.
20. Modern Veterinary Practice (MVP), May 1980, p. 415–6.
21. Curr Ther Eq Med, p. 399.
22. Canadian Veterinary Journal (Can Vet J.), Vol. 22, March 1981, p. 72–76.
23. Can Vet J., Vol. 20, August 1979, p. 201–6.
24. Curr Ther Eq Med, p. 456.
25. Can Vet J., Vol. 20, No. 5, May 1979, p. xii.
26. Can Vet J., Vol. 17, No. 12, Dec. 1976, p. 301–307.
27. AAEP Proc., 1981, p. 209.
28. Curr Ther Eq Med., p. 417.
29. Rossdale, P. D., and S. W. Ricketts, Equine Stud Farm Medicine, Second Edition, Lea and Febiger, Philadelphia, 1980, p. 295.
30. Veterinary Annual, 22nd Edition, p. 157.
31. MVP, April 1979, p. 516–517.
32. Curr Ther Eq Med., p. 428–429.
33. MVP, February 1979, p. 140–142.
34. MVP, Movember 1982, p. 857–860.
35. Cunha, p. 258.
36. A Standard Guide to Horse and Pony Breeds, p. 311 & 315.
37. Cunha, p. 88.
38. Cunha, p. 120 & 217.
39. AAEP Proc., 1979, p. 377.
40. Adams, O. R., Lameness in Horses, 3rd Edition, Lea and Febiger, Philadelphia, 1974, p. 3.
41. Equine Medicine and Surgery (Eq Med & Surg), First Edition, American Veterinary Publications, Santa Barbara, California, 1963, p. 501.
42. AAEP Proc., 1981, p. 459–462.
43. Veterinary Clinics of North America, Large Animal Practice, (W.B. Saunders Co., Philadelphia), Vol. 2, No. 1, May, 1980, p. 19–24.
44. MVP, May 1978, p. 391–392.
45. AAEP Proc., 1979, p. 476.
46. JAVMA, Vol. 180, No. 3., 1 February 1982, p. 251–253.
47. Adams, 2nd Ed., p. 260.

48. Wintzer, in Michael Perron, Personal Communication, 1981.
49. Emery and others, in Michael Perron, Personal Communication, 1981.
50. Rossdale, p. 387.
51. Can Vet J., Vol. 22, May 1981, p. 130–133.
52. Can Vet J., Vol. 180, No. 3, Feb. 1982.
53. JAVMA, Vol. 181, No. 3, 1 August 1982, p. 255–258.
54. AAEP Proc., 1982, p. 107–111.
55. Veterinary Medicine/Small Animal Clinician (VM/SAC), July 1981, p. 1019–1020.
56. MVP, August 1978, p. 633–634.
57. For additional information, see JAVMA Vol. 183, No. 5, 1 September 1983, p. 519–524.
58. R. J. Rose in Newsletter of the AAEP, July 1983, as abstracted in JAVMA Vol. 183, No. 9, 1 Nov. 1983, p. 962.
59. AAEP Proc., 1979, p. 494.
60. Australian Veterinary Journal (Austr Vet J.), Vol. 56, March 1980, p. 119–122.
61. American Journal of Veterinary Research (Am J Vet Res) Vol. 43 (November 1982), p. 2019, abstracted in JAVMA Vol. 183, No. 5, 1 September 1983, p. 561.
62. Austr Vet J., Vol. 57, Feb. 1981, p. 57–60.
63. Emergency War Surgery, S.E.A. Publications, 2515 W. Orangethorpe, Fullerton, California, 92633, p. 9–17.
64. AAEP Proc., 1982, p. 73–83.
65. AAEP Proc., 1982, p. 97–105.
66. Can Vet J., Vol. 17, No. 10, Oct. 1976, p. 272.
67. AAEP Proc, 1979, p. 378.
68. Curr Ther Eq Med., p. 497.
69. Can Vet J., Vol. 21, Sept. 1980, p. 250–251.
70. Am J Vet Res., Vol. 42, 1981, p. 703–707.
71. JAVMA Vol. 18, No. 10, 15 November 1982, p. 1151.
72. Curr Ther Eq Med., p. 177.
73. MVP, July 1981, p. 547–548.
74. Can Vet J., Vol. 22, Oct. 1981, p. 300–301.
75. Curr Ther Eq Med., p. 24.
76. Can Vet J., Vol. 20, May 1979, p. 127–130.
77. Curr Ther Eq Med., p. 338, 393.
78. Rossdale, p. 455.
79. Curr Ther Eq Med., p. 271.
80. Eq Med & Surg, p. 390.
81. Eq Med & Surg, p. 232.
82. Curr Ther Eq Med., p. 266.
83. JAVMA, Vol. 180, No. 7, 1 April 1982, p. 752–753.
84. Vet. Annual, 22nd Ed., p. 152.
85. Curr Ther Eq Med., p. 268.
86. JAVMA Vol. 180, No. 3, 1 February 1982, p. 295–299.
87. Ibid.
88. Curr Ther Eq Med., p. 605.
89. JAVMA, Vol. 180, No. 3, 1 February 1982, p. 300–302.
90. Kingsbury, John M., Poisonous Plants of the United States and Canada, Prentice-Hall, Inc., Englewood Cliffs, New Jersey, 1964, p. 295.
91. Curr Ther Eq Med., p. 602.
92. MVP, April 1982, p. 307–309.
93. MVP, May, 1980, p. 419.
94. For further information, see DVM Newsmagazine, Feb. 1980, p. 46–51, and Journal of Equine Medicine and Surgery, Nov. 1978. See also JAVMA Vol. 184 No. 3, 1 Feb. 1984, p. 279–301.
95. Curr Ther Eq Med., p. 355.
96. Curr Ther Eq Med., p. 352.
97. Curr Ther Eq Med., p. 97.
98. Curr Ther Eq Med., p. 351.
99. VM/SAC, Sept. 1982, p. 1409–1410.
100. Curr Ther Eq Med., p. 170–171.
101. JAVMA Vol. 149, 15 December 1966, p. 1556–1560.
102. VM/SAC, 8 May 1981, p. 730–732.
103. For additional information, see Proc. AAEP, 1979, p. 459–482 on endurance horses and their response to exercise.

RECOMMENDED READING

Adams, O. R., Lameness In Horses, 3rd. Edition, Lea & Febiger, Philadelphia, Pa., 1974. 566 pp. $22.50.

This is a classic text on foot and leg problems in the horse, as well as other conditions affecting the animal's "using" soundness. It covers examination and diagnosis of lameness, and has extensive sections on each individual lameness. It also has good coverage of trimming and shoeing for special problems. It is written for veterinarians, but is valuable for the knowledgeable horse owner, and is often found in the libraries of the best horseshoers and racehorse trainers. Recommended for persons needing in-depth coverage of locomotor problems in the horse.

Cunha, Tony J., Horse Feeding and Nutrition, Academic Press, Inc. (Harcourt, Brace, Jovanovich), N.Y., 1980. $31.50.

This book should be on the shelf of every horseman who wishes to learn more about the nutrient requirements of the horse, and what feedstuffs do what. The book is extremely well-researched and complete. It is technical enough to provide good information, but still very readable and useful. Buy this one if you're interested in horse feeding. It may not be the last word on it, but is the best available at the present time.

Frandson, R. D., Anatomy and Physiology of Farm Animals, 3rd Edition, Lea and Febiger, Philadelphia, Pa., 19106. 1981. 533 pp. $24.50.

This is an excellent text for those who would like to learn more about the structure of their animals. It bridges the gap between simple, superficial treatments of animal anatomy and the intricate, extremely technical texts used by veterinarians and veterinary students. For instance, it discusses bone structure, how bones grow, and how they heal after fractures, as well as how the skeleton is constructed. It will give the horse owner a good idea of how the different systems of his animal are put together and how they function.

Kingsbury, John M., Poisonous Plants of the United States and Canada, 3rd Edition, Prentice-Hall, Inc., Englewood Cliffs, New Jersey, 07632. 1964. $34.95.

If you are using pastures which have (or might have) any poisonous plants, this book is excellent. It gives good descriptions of the medical problems which occur with each poisonous plant. The reader must be a little bit botanist, however, as the descriptions of the plants are put in purely botanical terms, and most of the illustrations are line drawings. If you need good technical information in this area, this is the book. If you require colored pictures to visualize the plants, check with your county agent or write to your state agricultural extension service to see if there are any illustrated publications available for your area. Many states publish excellent information of this kind.

The Merck Veterinary Manual, 5th Edition, Merck & Co., Inc., Rahway, New Jersey, 07065. 1979, $18.95.

This is a compact text which covers most diseases of domestic animals and poultry. The information is concise and comprehensive, but sometimes short on specifics for horses. A good reference book, with an excellent section on medications, drug dosages, and ingredients of some old prescriptions.

Rossdale, P. D., and S. W. Ricketts, Equine Stud Farm Medicine, Second Edition, Lea and Febiger, Philadelphia, Pa., 19106. 1980. 564 p. $58.50.

This superb and highly technical text covers all aspects of breeding management of horses, from the hormones which make it all happen to the nuts and bolts of handling animals during breeding. Expensive, but worth it if you are breeding horses seriously.

Rooney, James R., Biomechanics of Lameness in the Horse, Robert E. Krieger Publishing Co., 645 New York Avenue, Huntington, New York, 11743. 1969. 272 p. $19.50.

This book is a discussion of Dr. Rooney's thinking, formed over a lifetime of studying causes of lameness in horses. It is highly detailed and technical, and explains many of the problems by way of calculus. If you are ready for "isocurtal, loxodromic curves," and "non-Newtonian, thixotropic properties," this is your book!

Rooney, James R., The Lame Horse: Causes, Symptoms, and Treatment. Melvin Powers, The Wilshire Book Company, 12015 Sherman Road, North Hollywood, California, 91605. C. 1974 by A.S. Barnes and Co. Paperback. $5.00.

This gives a good, understandable, concise description of lameness problems and their treatment, in laymen's terms. Well worth the price.

INDEX

A

Abdomen, Normal, 8
  Puncture Wounds, 338
Abortions, 73
  Due to Respiratory Infections,
    243
Abrasions, 219
Abscesses, Sole, 125
Acupuncture, 184
Ageing Horses, 91, 254
Alfalfa, 29
Alkali Disease, 321
Allergies, 276
Amputation, 236
Anabolic Steroids, 201
Anaphylactic Shock, 187
Anemia, 13
  Equine Infectious, 327
Anesthetics, 209
Anhidrosis, 334
Antibiotics, 202
Antidiarrheals, 208
Anti-inflammatory Agents, 199
Antiseptics, 204
Appetite, 6
Arthritis, 237
Artificial Insemination, 71
Artificial Lighting, 60
Ascarids, 300
Avascular Necrosis, 237
Azoturia, 133

B

Back, 159
  Conformation, 159
  Examination, 160
Back Back Teeth, 99

Bandages, 211
  Emergency, 214
  Foot, 213
  Leg, 214
  Robert Jones, 215
Bandaging, 211
  Materials, 211
  Techniques, 213
Barker Foals, 81
Base Narrow, 93
  Hindlegs, 98
  Toe In, 96
  Toe Out, 96
Base Wide, 93
  Hindlegs, 98
  Toe Out, 96
  Toe In, 96
Bedding, 20
Behavior, 4
Bermuda Grass Tremors, 324
Biopsy, Endometrial, 65
Biting, 106
Bladder Problems, 333
Blindfold, 177
Blindness, 99
Blind Spavin, 156
Blister Beetle Poisoning, 33
Blistering, 184
Blocks, Nerve, 118
Blood, 14
  Normal Values, 15
Blood Spavin, 156
Blowflies, 288
Bog Spavin, 102, 156
Boluses, 186
Bones, 234
Bone Spavin, 102, 154
Bots, 300
Botulism, 333

Bowed Tendons, 146
Bow Legs, 96
Brain, 9
Bran, 38
Bracken Fern, 318
Breeding, 68
  Exam, Mares, 62
  Hobbles, 176
  Pasture, 66
  Stallions, Feeding, 50
  Timetable, 65
Bridles, War, 176
Broodmares, 56
  Choosing, 56
  Feeding, 49, 50
  Preparation for Breeding, 59
Bruising, Sole, 125
Bucked Knees, 96
Bucked Shins, 150
Bucking, 106
Burns, 279
  as Emergency, 338
  Chemical, 280
  Rope, 280

C

Caesarean Section, 81
Calf Knees, 96
Camped
  Behind, 98
  In Front, 97
Cancer, Skin, 292
Capped
  Elbows, 101
  Hocks, 101
Caps, Retained, on Teeth, 257
Carpal Bones, Fractures, 152
Carpitis, 151

Carpus, Hygroma of, 151
Caslick's Operation, 62
Cast Horses, 158
Casting Harness, 176
Castor Bean, 319
Castration, 310
  Complications, 312
Cataracts, 100, 274
Cattle Grubs, 292
Central Nervous System, 9
Cervical Cultures, 64
Chains, Lip, 176
Chapped
  Hocks, 283
  Knees, 283
Charging, 106
Chemical Burns, 280
Chest, Puncture Wounds, 338
Chestnuts, 119
Chewing, Wood, 41, 107
Chloramphenicol, 203
Choke, 260
Chokecherry, 325
Chronic Colic, 266
Cinch Sores, 281
Circular Work, 22
Cirrhosis of the Liver, 322
Cleft Palate, 257
Closed Wounds, 233
Coat, 7
Coggins Test, 328
Coffin Bone, Fracture of, 138
Cold (for Treatment), 182
Cold Problems, 335
Colic, 266
  Chronic, 100, 266
  Mixtures, 208
  Sand, 266
  Severe, as Emergency, 338
Colostrum, 85
Concentrates, 35
Conformation, Defects, 93, 97
Conjunctivitis, 273
Contagious Equine Metritis, 70
Contracted
  Feet, 102, 121
  Tendons, 145
Corn, 35
Corneal Injuries, 272
Corns, 102, 125
Corticosteroids, 199
Cough Mixtures, 208
Counterirritants, 185
Counterirritation, 184
Cow Hocks, 97
Cow Kicking, 106

Cracks, Sand, 123
Cribbing, 99, 106
Crooked
  Neck, 100
  Legs, 152
Crossties, 167
Cryptorchidism, 100
Cryptorchid Stallions, 313
Cultures, Cervical, 64
Curb, 103, 156
Cuts, 223
Cycles, Heat, 61

D

Deer Flies, 288
Diarrhea, 267, 269
Diaphragmatic Hernias, 310
Digestive System, 6, 41, 251
Disinfectants, 204
Displaced Patella, 102
Distemper, 241
DMSO, 198
Drenching, 185
Drug Resistance, 302
Dummy Foals, 81

E

Earing, 169
Ear Problems, 294
Ear Ticks, 290
Eastern Equine Encephalomyelitis,
  329
EEE, 329
EIA, 327
Elbows, 101
Electrical Stimulation, 184
Embryo Transfers, 70
Emergencies, 336
Emphysema, 100, 248
Encephalomyelitis,
  Eastern Equine, 329
  Venezuelan, 331
  Western Equine, 330
Endometrial Biopsy, 65
Enemas, 187
Environment, Clean, 20
Epinephrine, 204
Epiphysitis, 141
Epistaxis, 240
Equine Infectious Anemia, 327
Equipment, for Restraint, 164
Ergots, 119
Euthanasia, 338
  Chemical Methods, 340

Emergency Methods, 341
  Shooting, 340
Ewe Neck, 100
Exercise, 22, 184
  After Meals, 43
  For Mature Horses, 24
Exhaustion, 336
  Heat, 335
External Parasites, 287
Eye Injuries, as Emergency, 337
Eyelids
  Lacerations, 273
  Spasm, 275
Eyes, 271
  Examination, 271
  Medicating, 273
  Removal, 275
  Sunburned, 279
  Tumors, 274
Eyeworms, 274

F

Face Flies, 289
Feces, 8
Feeding, 26
  Breeding Stallions, 50
  Fat Horses, 53
  Growing Horses, 49
  How Much, 46
  How To, 44
  Idle Horses, 48
  Lactating Mares, 50
  Pregnant Mares, 49
  Schedules, 43
  Sick Horses, 55
  Techniques for Foal, 87
  Thin Horses, 51
  Tired Horses, 43
Feeds
  Complete, 32
  Measuring, 48
Feed Supplements, 37
Feed, Wolfing, 45, 109
Fences, 17
Feet, 119
  Contracted, 102, 121
  Functions of, 120
  Malformed, 121
Fever, Swamp, 327
Fighting, 107
Firing, 184, 185
First Phalanx, Fractured, 151
Fistula of Withers, 294
Flexion Tests, 114
Flies, 287

Foaling, 75
    Complications, 81
    as Emergency, 338
Foals
    Barkers and Dummies, 81
    Early Care, 80
    Feeding and Care, 84
    Immature, 80
    Older Foals, 85
    Premature, 80
    Septicemia, 83
    Weaning, 88
Foot Care, 21
Forage Poisoning, 324
Formulas, 87
Founder, 102, 128
    as Emergency, 338
Fractures
    Carpal Bones, 152
    Coffin Bone, 138
    First Aid, 235, 336
    First Phalanx, 151
    Jaw, 259
    Navicular Bone, 138
    Second Phalanx, 151
    Sesamoid, 144
    Splint, 149
Frostbite, 281

G

Gait Problems, 103
Geldings, Proud-Cut, 312
Goat's Milk, 87
Grain, 35
    Mixtures, 36
Gravel, 123
Greenhead Flies, 288
Grooming, 20
Ground Ivy, 323
Growing Horses, Feeding, 49
Grubs, Cattle, 292
Gut Sounds, 14

H

Habronemiasis, 292
Halter Pulling, 108
Harness, Casting, 176
Hay
    Alfalfa, 29
    Alfalfa/Grass, 30
    Grain, 30
    Grass, 29
    Miscellaneous, 30

Selection, 33
    Straw, 30
Hay Cubes, 31
Heart
    Problems, 334
    Rate, 13
Heat (for Treatment), 183
Heat Cycles, 61
Heat Exhaustion, 335
Heaves, 100, 248
Heels
    Low, 127
    Sheared, 127
Hemlock
    Poison, 323
    Western Water, 323
Hemorrhage, Pulmonary, 240
Herbal Remedies, 210
Hernias, 104, 308
    Diaphragmatic, 310
Hip, Knocked Down, 101
History, Breeding, 61
Hives, 277
Hobbles, 175
    Breeding, 176
    Four-Leg, 176
Hocks
    Capped, 101
    Chapped, 283
    Cow, 97
    Sickle, 98
Holding the Horse, 166
Home Cures, 210
Hoof
    Care, 21
    Punctures, 126
    Testers, 114
Hormones, 72
Horse Flies, 288
Horsetail, 318
How to Shoot A Horse, 340
Hygroma of Carpus, 151

I

Immature Foals, 80
Incisors, Retained, 258
Induction of Labor, 82
Inguinal Hernia, 308
Inhalation, Smoke, 338
Injections, 187
    Intra-articular, 197
    Intradermal, 197
    Intramuscular, 189
    Intravenous, 196
    Legal Complications, 188

Reactions, Local, 188
    Routes, 189
    Subcutaneous, 196
Injuries, 217
    Corneal, 272
    Eye, 272, 337
Insect Repellents, 205
Insemination, Artificial, 71
Intra-articular Injections, 197
Intradermal Injections, 197
Intravenous Injections, 196
Intramuscular Injections, 189
Internal Parasites, 297
Isoerythrolysis, Neonatal, 81

J

Jaw, Undershot, 99
Joint Ill, 83

K

Keratoma, 122
Kicking, 108
Kidney Problems, 333
Knapweed, Russian, 319
Knees
    Chapped, 283
    Popped, 101, 151
Knocked Down Hip, 101
Knock Knees, 96

L

Labor, Induction of, 82
Lacerations, Eyelid, 273
Lactating Mares, Feeding, 50
Lameness, 110
    Chronic, 100
    Examination, 112
    History, 111
Laminitis, 102, 128
Lampas, 260
Laparoscopic Examination, 65
Larkspur, 324
Leading the Horse, 165
Leg Restraints, 173
Lice, 289
Lighting, Artificial, 60
Lightning Strike, 281
Liniments, 185, 206
Lip Chains, 176
Lips, Sunburned, 279
Liver, Cirrhosis of, 322
Locoweed, 320
Longeing, 23

Lotions, 206
Low Heels, 127
Lupine, 320

M

Malformed Feet, 121
Mange, 291
Marijuana, 324
Mares' Milk, 84
Mares, Spaying, 313
Massage, 184
Mastitis, 85
Masturbation, 108
Medications, 198
    Oral, 185
    Wound, 206
Membranes, at Foaling, 79
Metritis, Contagious Equine, 70
Milk
    Cow's, 87
    Goat, 87
    as Human Food, 85
    Mare's, 84
Milk Replacer, 87
Minerals, 39
Molasses, 37
    Chopped Hay with, 31
Monday Morning Sickness, 133
Mosquitoes, 288
Mouth
    Injuries, 259
    Smooth, 259
    Wave, 259
Movement, 5
Mucous Membranes, 7
Mycotic Diarrhea, 268
Mycotoxins, 316

N

Navel Ill, 83
Navicular Disease, 103, 135
Navicular Fractures, 138
Neck, 91
    Ewe, 100
Neck Cradle, 177
Necropsy, 341
Necrosis, Avascular, 237
Nerve Blocks, 118
Nerved, 103
Nervous System Diseases, 329
Neonatal Isoerythrolysis, 81
Neurectomy, 103
Nicotine Poisoning, 322

Nonsteroidal Anti-Inflammatory
    Agents, 199
Nose, Sunburned, 279
Nosebleed, 240
Nursing, 180

O

Oats, 35
Obstructive Pulmonary Disease,
    250
Occlusion of Tear Duct, 274
Occult Spavin, 156
Oleander Poisoning, 317
Onchocerciasis, 292
Opening, Mares, 64
Ophthalmia, Periodic, 100, 274
Oral Medications, 185
Orphan Foals, Feeding, 85
Osteomyelitis, 236
Overfeeding, 48
Overweight, 23
Oxytocin, 203

P

Palpation
    for Lameness, 116
    Rectal, 72
Parasites
    External, 287
    Internal, 297
Parrot Mouth, 98, 257
Pasterns
    Long, Sloping, 97
    Upright, 97
Pastes, 186
Pasture, 28
    Finding, 46
Patella, Displaced
    (Upward Fixation of), 102, 153
Pawing, 108
Penicillin, 202
    with Streptomycin, 202
Periodic Ophthalmia, 100, 274
Photosensitization, 278
Pigeon Toes, 93
Pinworms, 301
Plants, Poisonous, 314
Pleurisy, 247
Pleuritis, 247
Pneumonia, 246
Poison Hemlock, 323
Poisonous Plants, 314, 317
Poll Evil, 294
Post-Legged, 98

Post, Solid, 167
Posture, 5
Poultices, 216
Pregnancy
    Care of Mares, 73
    Diagnosis, 72
Pregnant Mares, Feeding, 49
Premature Foals, 80
Premolars, Retained, 258
Prolapse of Uterus, 82
    as Emergency, 338
Prostaglandins, 71
Protozoal Diarrhea, 268
Proud-Cut Geldings, 312
Proud Flesh, 232
Punctures, Hoof, 126
Puncture Wounds, 220
    Abdomen, 338
    Chest, 338
Pulling, Halter, 108
Pulmonary Hemorrhage, 240
Pulse, 11
Pyometra, 70
Pyoderma, 283

Q

Quittor, 103, 143

R

Rabies, 331
Rachitic Ringbone, 141
Rearing, 108
Rectal Palpation, 72
Red Maple, 319
Remedies, Herbal, 210
Replacer, Milk, 87
Respiration Rate, 13
Respiratory Tract Infections, 243
Rest, 184
Restraint, 163
    Equipment, 164
    Foal, 177
    Facilities, 167
Restraints
    Front Leg, 174
    Hand, 169
    Hind Leg, 175
    Leg, 173
Retained Caps, 257
Ringbone, 103, 140, 141
Ringworm, 284
Roaring, 100, 239
Roll, Shoulder, 169
Root Cellars, 19

Rope Burns, 280
Roughages, 28
    Miscellaneous, 32
Routes of Injection, 189
Rubbing, Tail, 294
Running Away, 108
Ruptured Flexor Tendons, 146
Rupture of Uterine Blood Vessels, 82
Russian Knapweed, 319

S

Saddle Marks, 282
Saddle Sores, 281
Safety, 163
Salt, 40
Sand Cracks, 123
Sand Colic, 266
Sarcoids, 293
Schedules, Feeding, 26
Scours, 267
Scratches, 220, 283
Screwworms, 288
Scrotal Hernias, 308
Second Phalanx, Fracture, 151
Seedy Toe, 127
Selenium Poisoning, 321
Septicemia, Foal, 83
Septic Tanks, 19
Sesamoid Fractures, 144
Sesamoiditis, 143
Sheath, Washing, 294
Shelter, 19
Shins, Bucked, 150
Shivering, 103
Shock, 337
Shock, Anaphylactic, 187
Shoulder, Roll, 169
Shoulder, Stick In, 170
Shying, 108
Sick Horses, Feeding, 55
Sidebone, 103, 142
Sidelining, 175
Side Stick, 177
Silage, 32
Skin Cancer, 292
Skin Grafts, 229
Skin
    Normal, 7
    Problems, 276
    Virus Diseases, 285
Slings, 178
Small Strongyles, 299
Smoke Inhalation, 338
Smooth Mouth, 259

Snakebite, 316
Soaking Solution, 183
Sole
    Abscesses, 125
    Bruising, 125
Sorghum, 324
Sores
    Cinch, 281
    Saddle, 281
Soundness, 90
Spavin
    Blind, 156
    Blood, 156
    Bog, 102, 156
    Bone, 102, 154
    Occult, 156
Splay-Footed, 93
Splint Fractures, 149
Splints, 101, 147
Spots, White 282
Stall Walking, 108
Standing Under In Front, 97
Steroids, Anabolic, 201
Stethoscope, 12
Stick in the Shoulder, 170
Stimulation, Electrical, 184
Stocks, 168
Stomach Tube, 186
Stomatitis, Vesicular, 286
Strangles, 241
Straw, 30
Streptothricosis, 291
Striking, 108
Stringhalt, 101
Strongyles, 298
    Control Programs, 303
    Drug Resistance, 302
    Small, 299
Strongyloides, 300
Stumbling, 109
Subcutaneous Injections, 196
Sudan Grass, 324
Sulfa Drugs, 201
Summer Pasture-Associated Pulmonary Disease, 250
Sunburned
    Eyes, Noses, Lips, 279
    Udders, 279
Supplements, Feed, 37
Swamp Fever, 327
Swellings, 233

T

Tablets, 186
Tail Rubbing, 109, 294

Tail Wringing, 109
Tapeworms, 301
Tear Duct, Occlusion, 274
Tears in Uterus, 82
Teasing, Mares, 67
Teeth, 91
    Bad Back, 99
    Examination, 253
    Normal, 251
    Retained, 257
Temperature, 9
Tendons
    Bowed, 146
    Contracted, 145
    Ruptured Flexor, 146
Testers, Hoof, 114
Tests
    Flexion, 114
    Wedge, 116
Tetanus, 218
Tetracyclines, 203
Thin Horses, Feeding, 51
Thistle, Yellow Star, 319
Thrush, 124
Thumps, 247
Ticks, 209
    Ear, 290
Timber Milk Vetch, 321
Tired Horses, Feeding, 43
Toe In, 93
Toe Out, 93
Torsion, Uterine, 81
Toxins, 314, 315
Tranquilizers, 209
Transfers, Embryo, 70
Treatment Methods, 180
Tube, Stomach, 186
Tumors, 292
    Eye Area, 274
Twitching, 170
Tying the Horse, 166
Tying-Up, 133
Tying Up a Hindleg, 175

U

Udder, Sunburned, 279
Ultrasound, for Pregnancy Diagnosis, 73
Umbilical Hernias, 309
Undershot Jaw, 99, 257
Unsoundness, 98, 104
    Breeding, 104
Upward Fixation of Patells, 102, 153
Urea, 39

Urine, 8
Uterine Prolapse, 82
    as Emergency, 338
Uterine Torsion, 81
Uterus
    Rupture of Blood Vessels, 82
    Tears In, 82

V

Vaccines, 210
Vaginal Discharge, 8
Venezuelan Equine Encephalomy-
    elitis, 331
Ventral Hernias, 310
Vesicular Stomatitis, 286
Vices, 106
Viciousness, 109
Virus Diarrhea, 268
Vitamins, 39
Voice, 6
Vomiting, 261

W

War Bridles, 176
Warts, 285
Washing the Sheath, 294
Water, 40
Watering, 45
Wave Mouth, 259
Way of Going, 103
Weaning, Foals, 88
Weaving, 109
Western Equine Encephalomyelitis,
    330
Western Water Hemlock, 323
White Spots, 282
Windpuffs, 139
Withers, Fistula of, 294
Wire Cuts, 337
Wobblers, 104, 157
Wolfing Feed, 45, 109
Wood Chewing, 41, 107
Working Horses, Feeding, 51

Wormers, 301
Worming Methods, 305
Worm Problems, Prevention, 304
Wound Medications, 206
Wounds
    Bullet, 221
    Closed, 233
    Complications in Open, 230
    Complications in Sutured, 229
    Deep Puncture, as Emergencies,
        338
    Open, 230
    Puncture, 220
Wry Neck, 100

X

X-Rays, 119, 158

Y

Yellow Star Thistle, 319

A Do-It-Yourself Veterinary Guide for
DOG OWNERS

NEW!

**100%
Money-Back
Guarantee for
One Full Year!**

If, for ANY reason,
you are not
satisfied with this
book, return it
within 1 year from
date of purchase
for a full,
courteous refund.

FREE
**postage
and
handling!**

**Also available at
better feed
stores, tack
shops, and
bookstores.**

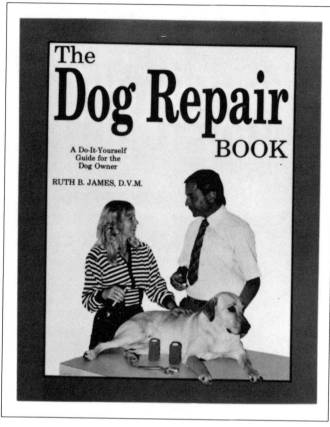

with Dr. Ruth B. James

TOPICS
INCLUDE:

Choosing a Dog
Housebreaking
Common
  Behavioral
  Problems
Worms and
  Worming
External Parasites
The Canine
  Gourmet
Skin Diseases
Emergency Care
Eye and Ear
  Problems
Care of the
  Elderly Dog
Reproduction
  and Puppy Care
Lameness and
  Back Problems

Dr. James, a respected veterinary practitioner, has written this book in the same easy-to-read style as her many articles in the Vet's Corner of *WESTERN HORSEMAN*. This book's 252 pages cover the latest breakthroughs and newest treatments, as well as tried-and-true remedies that really work! You'll know how to give your own injections, saving time and money. Most importantly, you'll know when you should call your vet, and when you can take care of a problem yourself. This book contains 23 chapters, with numerous photos, diagrams and drawings. A quality, stitched binding and tough plastic-coated cover make this a durable addition to your tack room or library.

Dealer Inquiries Invited.

A Wealth of Money-Saving Information for only $16.95. SEND TODAY!

We Hope. . .
    You've enjoyed reading this book as much as we've enjoyed writing and publishing it.

Please. . .
    Help us to help others keep their horses healthy and save money on horse care.
    Give this page to a neighbor or friend, or use it to order a copy for a gift.
    Remember, the postage is FREE on all shipments!

Please complete and include the following if this book is a gift or institutional purchase:

Person sending gift:

Shall we enclose a gift card?   ☐Yes.

Name _____

Occasion_____

Address _____

(Christmas, Birthday, Graduation, Mothers' or
Father's Day, Valentines, etc.)

City _____

Schools or Libraries:
    Purchase Order Number _____

State_____ Zip_____

Each book is shipped promptly in a custom mailing package:

Please send, postage paid:

____How to Be Your Own Veterinarian
    (Sometimes) at $19.95   _____
____The Dog Repair Book at $16.95   _____
(Canadian and foreign orders payable in
    U.S. funds)
Wyoming residents only add 3% sales tax   _____

                    Total Enclosed _____

☐Check Enclosed   ☐MasterCard   ☐VISA

Card No._____ Expiration Date_____

Card Holder's Signature _____

Our Guarantee

We are convinced that this book will help you to care for your horse(s), and that the information contained in it will help you avoid problems and save money.

If, for any reason, during ONE YEAR following the date of purchase, you are not satisfied with this book, you may return it for a full, courteous refund. Send it, with the receipt with purchase price circled, to:

Alpine Press
P.O. Box 1930
Mills, Wyoming, 82644

Sincerely,

Lynn Wilson

Lynn Wilson
Production Assistant